Get Ready for a Whole New Mastering Health Experience

New! **Ready-to-Go Teaching Modules** help instructors find the best assets to use before, during, and after class to teach the toughest topics in Personal Health. These curated sets of teaching tools save you time by highlighting the most effective and engaging videos, quizzing, coaching, self-assessment, and behavior change activities to assign within **Mastering™ Health**.

Donatelle, *My Health*, 3rd edition
Donatelle, *Health: The Basics*, 13th edition

Ready-To-Go Teaching Modules

My Health

Health

Ready-To-Go Teaching Modules make use of teaching tools for before, during, and after class, including new ideas for in-class activities.

The modules incorporate the best that the text, Mastering Health,™ and Learning Catalytics have to offer and guide instructors through using these resources in the most effective way.

Psychological Health	Stress
Reproductive Choices	Addiction and Drug Abuse
Alcohol and Tobacco	Nutrition
Fitness	CVD and Cancer
Infectious Conditions	Violence and Unintentional Injuries

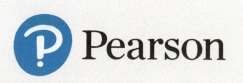
Pearson

A Focused Approach to Engage
Students in Health Content

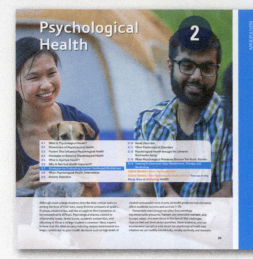

NEW! **A Mindfulness Theme** throughout the book relates mindfulness research and practices to topics ranging from relationships to mindful eating to stress management and more. Mindfulness modules are highlighted on the chapter opener page and signaled with a blue banner at the start of the module. In addition, there is increased coverage of diversity and access to health care and of sleep and health.

NEW! **Think About It** questions added to the end of each end-of-chapter Study Plan provide students the opportunity to strengthen their critical thinking skills.

Continuous Learning
Before, During, and After Class

BEFORE CLASS

Mobile Media and Reading Assignments Ensure That Students Come to Class Prepared.

NEW! Interactive Pearson eText gives students access to the text anytime, anywhere. Pearson eText features include:

- Offline access on smartphones/tablets
- Seamlessly integrated videos and other rich media.
- Interactive Self-Assessment Worksheets
- Accessible (screen-reader ready)
- Configurable reading settings, including resizable type and night reading mode
- Instructor and student note-taking, highlighting, bookmarking, and search

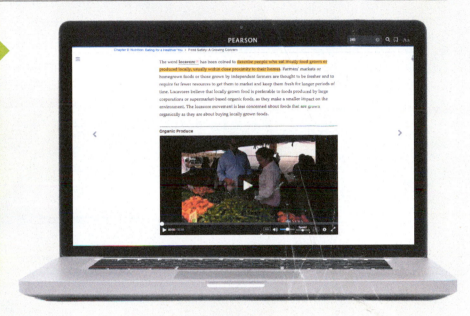

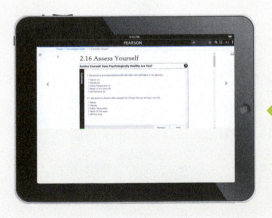

UPDATED! All Self-assessment worksheets formerly in the book are now offered online only and assignable in Mastering Health.

Pre-Lecture Reading Quizzes are easy to customize and assign

Reading Questions ensure that students complete the assigned reading before class. Reading Questions are 100% mobile ready and can be completed by students on mobile devices.

and Empower Them with Behavior Change Strategies

Hallmark Feature! The modular organization ensures that students spend their study time efficiently and remain engaged. Student learning outcomes provide concrete learning goals, and Check Yourself questions provide the opportunity for students to immediately test their own understanding.

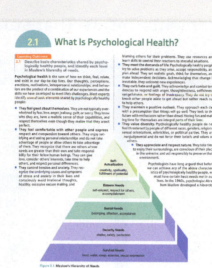

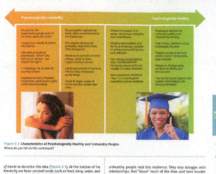

Skills for Behavior Change

Challenge the Thoughts That Sabotage Change

Are thought patterns and beliefs holding you back? Try these strategies:

- **"I don't have enough time!"** Chart your activities for 1 day. What are your highest priorities? What can you eliminate or reduce? Plan to make some time for a healthy change next week.
- **"I'm too stressed!"** Assess your major stressors right now. List those you can control and those you can change or avoid. Then identify two things you enjoy that can help you reduce stress now.
- **"I'm worried what others may think."** How much do other people influence your decisions about drinking, sex, eating habits, and the like? What is most important to you? What actions can you take to act in line with your values?
- **"I don't think I can."** Just because you haven't done something before doesn't mean you can't do it now. To develop confidence, take baby steps and break tasks into small chunks of time.
- **"I can't break this habit!"** Habits are difficult to break, but not impossible. What triggers your behavior? List ways you can avoid triggers. Ask for support from friends and family.

Hallmark Feature! Skills for Behavior Change strategies give students the tools they need to make immediate changes for healthier lifestyles. Strategies such as "How to Challenge Thoughts that Sabotage Change" or "Responding to an Offer of Drugs" empower students with the tools to create healthy change in their lives.

with Mastering Health

DURING CLASS

Engage Students with Learning Catalytics.

What has teachers and students excited? Learning Catalytics, a "bring your own device" student engagement, assessment, and classroom intelligence system, allows students to use their smartphone, tablet, or laptop to respond to questions in class. With Learning Catalytics, you can:

- Assess students in real time using open-ended question formats to uncover student misconceptions and adjust lectures accordingly.
- Automatically create groups for peer instruction based on student response patterns, to optimize discussion productivity.

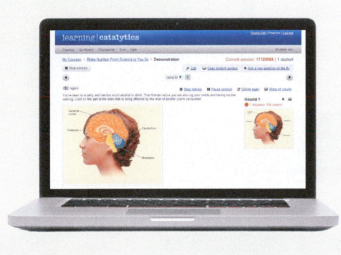
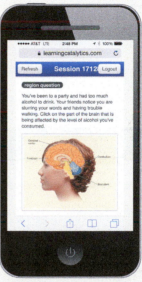

AFTER CLASS

Mastering Health Delivers Automatically Graded Health and Fitness Activities

NEW! Interactive Behavior Change Activities—Which Path Would You Take? Have students explore various health choices through an engaging, interactive, low-stakes, and anonymous experience. These activities show students the possible consequences of various choices they make today on their future health and are made assignable in Mastering Health with follow-up questions.

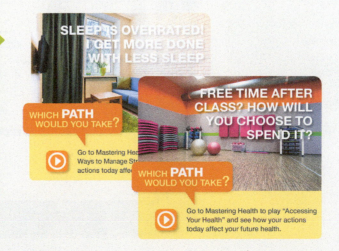

Continuous Learning
Before, During, and After Class

AFTER CLASS

Easy to Assign, Customize, Media-Rich, and Automatically-Graded Assignments

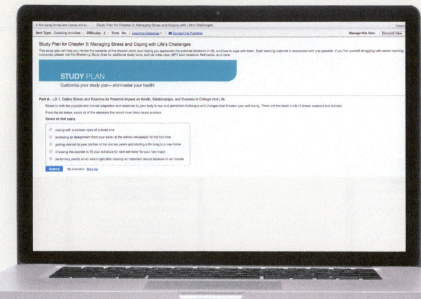

UPDATED! Study Plans Plans tie all end-of-chapter material (including chapter review, pop quiz, and Think About It questions) to specific numbered Learning Outcomes and Mastering assets. Assignable study plan items contain at least one multiple choice question per Learning Outcome and wrong-answer feedback.

HALLMARK! Video Tutors highlight a book figure or discussion point in an engaging video, covering key concepts such as how drugs act on the brain, reading food labels, and the benefits of regular exercise. All Video Tutors include assessment activities and are assignable in Mastering Health.

with Mastering Health

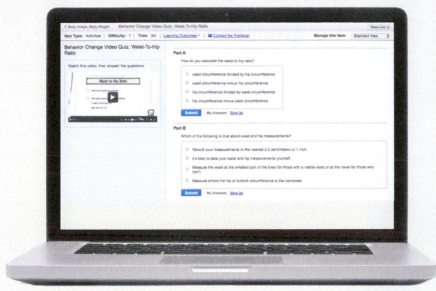

HALLMARK! **Behavior Change Videos** are concise whiteboard-style videos that help students with the steps of behavior change, covering topics such as setting SMART goals, identifying and overcoming barriers to change, planning realistic timelines, and more. Additional videos review key fitness concepts such as determining target heart rate range for exercise. All videos include assessment activities and are assignable in **Mastering Health.**

HALLMARK! *ABC News* **Videos** bring health to life and spark discussion with hot topics. Activities tied to the videos include multiple-choice questions that provide wrong-answer feedback to redirect students to the correct answer.

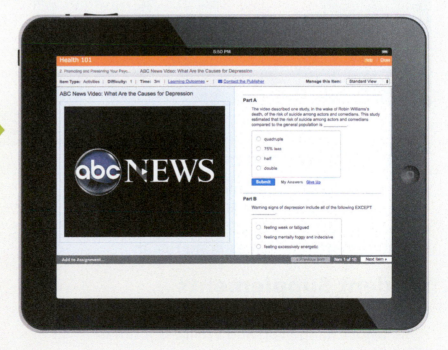

Resources for YOU, the Instructor

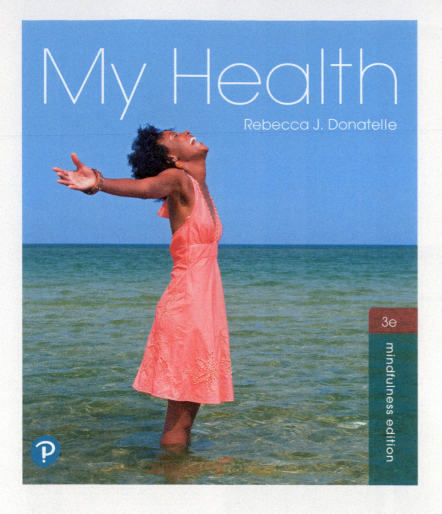

My Health

Rebecca J. Donatelle

3e
mindfulness edition

Mastering Health provides you with everything you need to prep for your course and deliver a dynamic lecture, in one convenient place. Resources include:

Media Assets For Each Chapter

- *ABC News* Lecture Launcher videos
- PowerPoint Lecture Outlines
- PowerPoint clicker questions and Jeopardy-style quiz show questions
- Files for all illustrations and tables and selected photos from the text

Test Bank

- Test Bank in Microsoft Word, PDF, and RTF formats
- Computerized Test Bank, which includes all the questions from the printed test bank in a format that allows you to easily and intuitively build exams and quizzes

Teaching Resources

- **New!** Ready-to-Go Teaching Modules
- Instructor Resource and Support Manual in Microsoft Word and PDF formats
- Learning Catalytics: Getting Started
- Getting Started with Mastering Health

Student Supplements

- Take Charge of Your Health Worksheets
- Behavior Change Log and Wellness Journal
- Eat Right!
- Live Right!
- Food Composition Table
- Study Area in Mastering Health, including flashcards, practice quizzes, MP3 Tutor Sessions, and more.

Measuring Student Learning Outcomes?
All of the Mastering Health assignable content is tagged to book content and to Bloom's Taxonomy. You also have the ability to add your own learning outcomes, helping you track student performance against your learning outcomes. You can view class performance against the specified learning outcomes and share those results quickly and easily by exporting to a spreadsheet.

My Health

Rebecca J. Donatelle

3e

mindfulness edition

Courseware Portfolio Manager: Michelle Yglecias
Content Producer: Lizette Faraji
Managing Producer: Nancy Tabor
Courseware Director, Content Development: Barbara Yien
Courseware Senior Analysts: Alice Fugate, Erin Strathmann
Courseware Editorial Assistants: Nicole Constantine, Crystal Trigueros
Rich Media Content Producer: Timothy Hainley, Keri Rand
Full-Service Vendor: Heather Winter, SPi Global
Copy Editor: Barbara Willette
Art Coordinator: Morgan Ewald, Lachina Publishing Services

Design Manager: Mark Ong
Interior and Cover Designer: Tamara Newnam
Rights & Permissions Project Manager: Donna Kalal, Cenveo Publishing Services
Rights & Permissions Management: Ben Ferrini
Photo Researcher: Cenveo Publisher Services
Manufacturing Buyer: Stacey Weinberger, LSC Communications
Marketing Manager: Alysun Burns
Senior Field Marketing Manager: Mary Salzman

Cover Photo Credit: UpperCut Images/Alamy Stock Photo

Library of Congress Cataloging-in-Publication Data

Names: Donatelle, Rebecca J., 1950- author.
Title: My health / Rebecca J. Donatelle, Oregon State University.
Description: The mastering health edition/3e. | New York : Pearson,
    [2019] | Includes bibliographical references and index.
Identifiers: LCCN 2017052164| ISBN 9780134729275 | ISBN 0134729277
Subjects: LCSH: Health. | Health behavior. | Medicine, Preventive.
Classification: LCC RA776 .D6635 2019 | DDC 613—dc23 LC record
available at https://lccn.loc.gov/2017052164

ISBN 10: 0-134-72927-7; ISBN 13: 978-0-134-72927-5 (Student edition)
ISBN 10: 0-134-80122-9; ISBN 13: 978-0-134-80122-3 (Instructor's Review Copy)

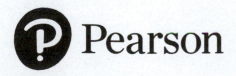

www.pearson.com

About the Author

Rebecca J. Donatelle, Ph.D.

Oregon State University

Rebecca Donatelle has served as a faculty member in the Department of Public Health, College of Health and Human Sciences, at Oregon State University for the last two decades. In that role, she has chaired the department and been program coordinator for the Health Promotion and Health Behavior Program (bachelor's degree, master of public health, and Ph.D. degree programs), and she has served on more than 50 national, state, regional, and university committees focused on improving student academic success and improving the public's health. Most important to her, she has taught and mentored thousands of undergraduate and graduate students. She is proud of the many outstanding accomplishments of her students! Many of these students gained community-based intervention and research skills while working on Dr. Donatelle's funded projects, and those experiences have led to exciting career paths nationally and internationally. Other students have gone on to receive advanced degrees in public health and have assumed leadership roles in a wide range of academic, community, and health care system positions. "I believe that my successes are measured in large part by the successes of the students I have worked with and the fact that, even when times are challenging, they continue to work for positive changes and improved health status for all," says Dr. Donatelle.

Dr. Donatelle has a Ph.D. in community health/health promotion and health education with specializations in health behaviors, aging, and chronic disease prevention from the University of Oregon; a master of science degree in health education from the University of Wisconsin, La Crosse; and a bachelor of science degree from the University of Wisconsin, La Crosse, with majors in health/physical education and English. In recent years, Dr. Donatelle has received several professional awards for leadership, teaching, and service within the university and for her work on developing nationally ranked undergraduate and graduate programs in the health promotion/health behavior areas.

Her primary research and scholarship areas have focused on finding scientifically appropriate means of motivating behavior change among resistant populations. Specifically, her work uses incentives, social and community supports, and risk communication strategies in motivating diverse populations to change their risk behaviors. She has worked with pregnant women who smoke in an effort to motivate them to quit smoking, obese women of all ages who are at risk for cardiovascular disease and diabetes, prediabetic women who are at risk for progression to type 2 diabetes, and individuals with a wide range of other health issues and problems. Her earlier research projects focused on decision making and factors influencing the use of alternative and traditional health care providers for treatment of low back pain, illness and sick role behaviors, occupational stress and stress claims, and worksite health promotion.

More recently, through her writing, she has been working to provide scientifically defensible, engaging ways to help students understand today's complex health and health care challenges, to ask the tough questions, and to understand that there are often no simple solutions to the myriad of health issues we face both in the United States and internationally. With this text in particular, she has worked to motivate students to approach their challenges in a mindful, thoughtful way; to take time to notice and to look within and outside themselves to really see, hear, and feel the life experience; and to act compassionately toward self and toward other people who are struggling with personal challenges. In particular, she challenges students to ask, *"How can I make the world a better place, for me, for others, and for future generations?* How can I live more healthfully and with more enthusiasm?" Whether it be working to improve personal health behaviors, working to help others who are struggling, or working to improve the social, political, and macro health environment, her goal is to motivate students to become more engaged and be the health change agents of the future.

In addition to her writing, Dr. Donatelle enjoys playing acoustic guitar, gardening, camping and socializing with friends and family, and walks with her three rambunctious Westies!

Brief Contents

Contents

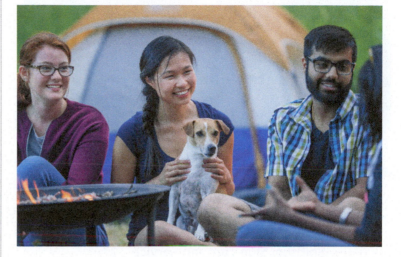

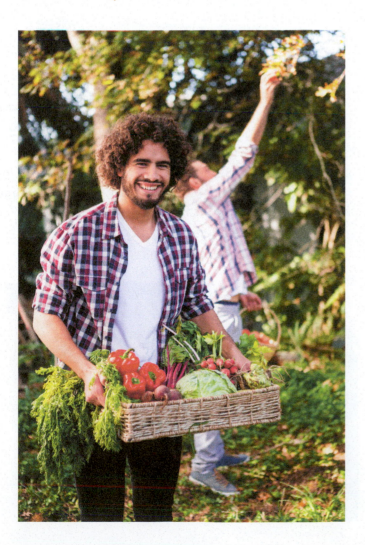

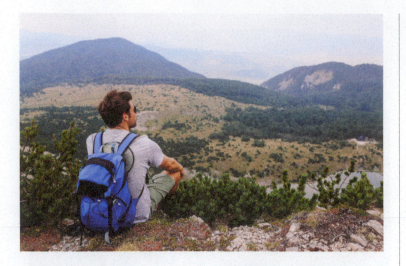

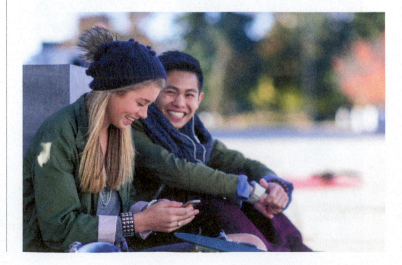

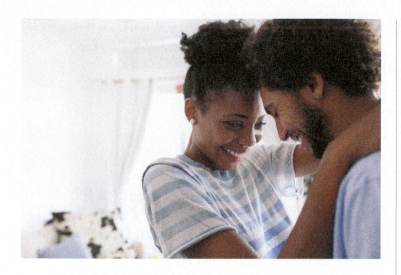

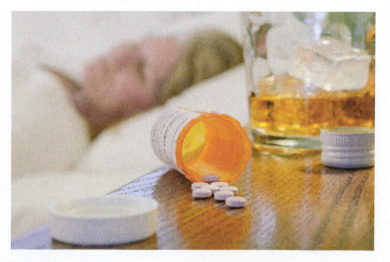

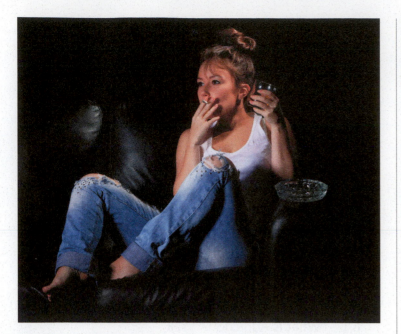

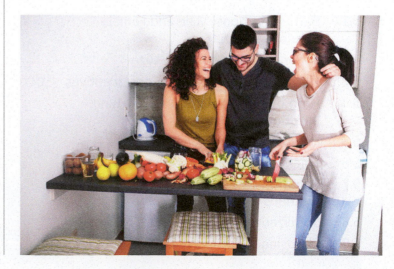

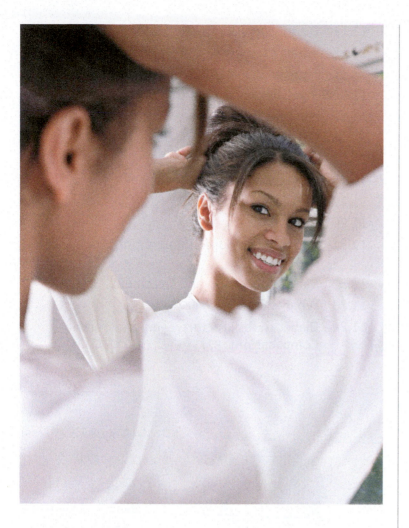

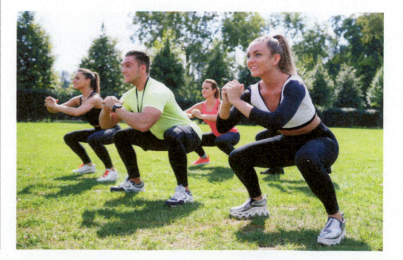

11   Cardiovascular Disease, Cancer, and Diabetes   249

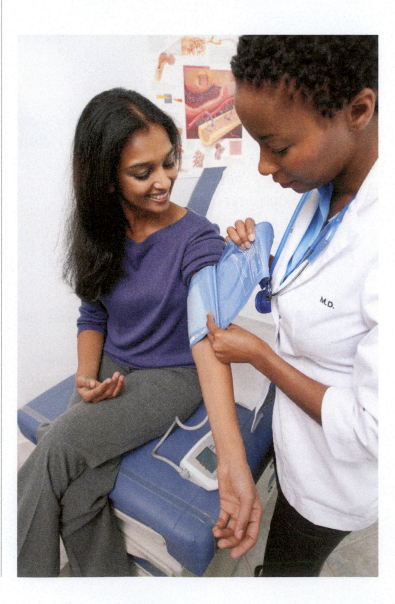

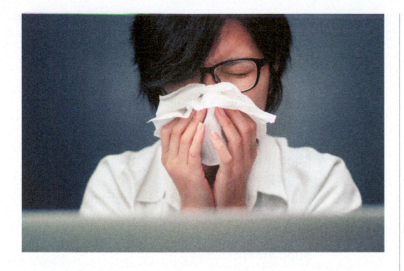

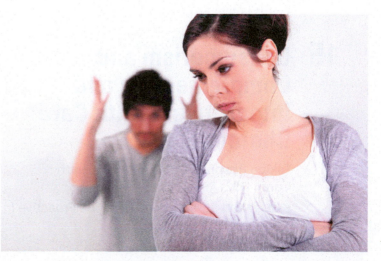

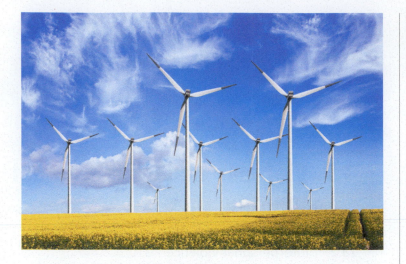

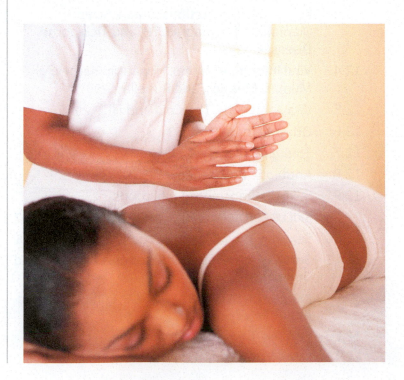

Preface

Today, health is headline news—the kind of news that all too often can result in depression, fear, anxiety, anger, and frustration among viewers. If you are like most people, you might want to ask, "Isn't there any good news out there?" From the latest cases of strange new pathogens carried into our homes by ticks, mosquitoes, or birds or passed on by a careless sexual relationship to the violence in the streets and threats of terrorism or nuclear bombs from other nations to the real-time catastrophic floods, fires, hurricanes, and other natural disasters brought on by climate change to the epidemic rates of diabetes, obesity, and soaring rates of mental health problems among youth and adults—the issues can seem overwhelming. However, although many things that influence our health are beyond our control, we are lucky that we do have control over many of the health risks we face. Health is multifaceted, and achieving it is a personal and societal responsibility. We can shape many of the things that influence us. It takes time, effort, patience, and a mindful approach.

As I have taught personal health courses over the past two decades, I have seen changes in students, especially regarding their health, their health concerns, and the way they assimilate information and make decisions about their health and the health of those around them. A new mode of instruction and a new approach to learning are required for instructors and textbook authors to present and relay scientifically valid information, create learning environments that meet diverse needs, and motivate students to engage in their own learning experiences. Students today want their information to be organized and concise. They want to know what they should be learning, see the relevance in knowing the information so that they can apply it to real world situations, and be able to test themselves to confirm that they understand the material and why it is important. What's more, students and their instructors want to be able to demonstrate that they know more about their health, see things with a more critical eye, and have options for making changes to improve their health and the health of others as a result of a particular course or course sequence. When they want to delve more deeply into a given topic, they will have the skills and resources to get more information. While there will always be new and formidable challenges in achieving personal health and health equity for all, individuals who are armed with information, who listen and hear others' points of view, and who take a reasoned approach to problem solving have the best chance of creating environments where people thrive. Creating a classroom and extended learning culture in which young minds ask themselves regularly, "What can I do to make the world a better place—a place where people can increase their years of healthy life?" has been a lifelong goal. For these reasons and more, I decided that the time had come to bring to fruition a new textbook that would change the health text marketplace. I decided to tap the creative minds of my colleagues and students and work with a great publishing company in writing the Mindfulness Edition of *My Health*.

Key Features of This Text

My Health: The Mindfulness Edition, Third Edition, maintains many features that this text is known for and includes exciting new features, including the following:

- **The modular organization,** which presents information in one- and two-page spreads, helping students to pace their learning and highlighting the most essential, up-to-date information about each topic in a synthesized, easy-to-understand format.
- **NEW! The mindfulness theme** throughout the text provides students with research and tools to incorporate mindfulness practices in all aspects of their health, helping them to be more focused in their academic and personal lives. Mindfulness coverage is contained within new modules and signaled by a blue banner.
- **NEW! Modules** on high interest topics such as Sleep, Diversity, and Health Equity.
- **Student learning outcomes,** which give instructors and students a measurable goal for each module and are matched specifically to the content in each module in the text. These take the guesswork out of the question that students inevitably ask: "What do I need to know for this exam or this performance outcome?"
- **Check Yourself questions** to help students confirm that they have mastered the content of each module.
- **Skills for Behavior Change boxes,** which are featured in many modules and are designed to help students develop the skills necessary to use what they have learned in making practical and important improvements in their health behaviors.
- **Striking figures and photos** on every page to engage students and encourage learning.
- **A streamlined approach,** helps students focus on the core health content, allowing them to follow the narrative without interruptions and feature boxes, and apply what they have learned at the end of each module.
- **New! Think About It critical thinking questions** are included in the end-of-chapter Study Plan material.

Student learning outcomes are a critical part of this book. Learning outcomes are a powerful tool to set clear expectations for students and to assess their level of mastery of a subject area. Outcomes for this text were developed on the basis of foundational personal health content appropriate for college-level learners. These outcomes were then revised and edited on the basis of careful review and input from health instructors and other experts from representative colleges and universities throughout the country (their names are listed later in the Acknowledgments section). Each module has a specific outcome that students must try to achieve to be successful. This mastery approach helps students home in on the relevant information and focus attention on achieving this learning outcome.

At the end of each module, students are challenged by Check Yourself questions. If students can successfully answer these questions, they are ready to move on to the next module. If they have difficulty answering the questions, they are able to go back through the material and focus on key points until they have mastered the module content.

We know that students are often pressed for time and may be able to read through only a few pages of this book in one sitting. With the learning outcomes and the Check Yourself questions, students can learn the material in one or two modules, test themselves, and know that they have accomplished a measurable portion of their reading goal, even if they can complete only part of a reading assignment.

In addition to the modular organization, learning outcomes, and Check Yourself questions, you will notice Skills for Behavior Change boxes throughout the chapters. Using the skills learned from these boxes, students can engage in behaviors that will contribute to improved health. You will also see that these are the only feature boxes in the text. To keep the book streamlined and focused on essential points, the type of information that has traditionally been relegated to a feature box has been included in the text, if it is important for student understanding, or has been omitted. I hope that you will agree that this provides students with a clear, concise presentation of the most important health information.

Chapter-by-Chapter Revisions

My Health: The Mindfulness Edition, Third Edition, has been thoroughly updated to reflect the most cutting-edge, scientifically valid, and relevant information available and includes additional references that will allow students to glean additional information from key sources in the area. Portions of modules have been reorganized to improve the flow of topics, while figures, tables, and photos have all been added, improved on, and updated. The following is a chapter-by-chapter listing of some of the most noteworthy changes, updates, and additions.

Chapter 1: Healthy Change
- New mindfulness module on how mindfulness influences health
- New module on diversity
- Reorganized section on *Healthy People 2020*, including adding description of leading health indicators
- New coverage of the Affordable Care Act (ACA) and issues with health care in the United States today
- New Think About It end-of-chapter questions

Chapter 2: Psychological Health
- New mindfulness module on meditation
- New mindfulness module on mindfulness therapies
- New Skills for Behavior Change box on relationships
- New module on the importance of spiritual health
- New Assess Yourself on spiritual health
- Added coverage of Seligman's happiness theory (PERMA)
- New Think About It end-of-chapter questions

Chapter 3: Stress
- New mindfulness module on relaxation and stress reduction
- Increased coverage on sleep
- New section on happiness and flourishing
- New section titled "Men and Women Respond to Stress Differently"
- New section on shift and persist
- New Think About It end-of-chapter questions

Chapter 4: Relationships and Sexuality
- New mindfulness module on mindful listening and nonverbal skills
- New module on relationships and social media
- New module on using technology responsibly
- New Think About It end-of-chapter questions

Chapter 5: Reproductive Choices
- New section on abortions in the developing world
- New section on contingency planning for parents
- Expanded coverage of nutrition and exercise in prenatal care
- New Think About It end-of-chapter questions

Chapter 6: Addiction and Drug Abuse
- New mindfulness module on treatment, recovery, and relapse prevention
- New figure on college students who use drugs and employment rates
- New information about medicinal and legal marijuana
- New content on harm reduction strategies
- New Think About It end-of-chapter questions

Chapter 7: Alcohol and Tobacco
- New mindfulness module on smoking cessation
- New content on e-cigarettes
- New content on different ethnicities and alcoholism
- New Think About It end-of-chapter questions

Chapter 8: Nutrition
- New mindfulness section on mindful eating
- New module on the health benefits of functional foods
- New content on the Dietary Reference Intakes (DRIs)
- New Think About It end-of-chapter questions

Chapter 9: Weight Management and Body Image
- New mindfulness module on mindless versus mindful eating
- New Skills for Behavior Change box on portion distortion
- New figure showing an overview of methods to measure body composition
- Expanded coverage of treatment of anorexia and bulimia
- New table on popular diet programs and their effectiveness
- New Think About It end-of-chapter questions

Chapter 10: Fitness
- New mindfulness module on fitness plans and staying motivated
- Expanded coverage of SMART fitness goals and objectives

- New coverage of physical inactivity
- New coverage of alcohol and exercise
- New Think About It end-of-chapter questions

Chapter 11: CVD, Cancer, and Diabetes
- New mindfulness module on mindfulness-based interventions for cancer patients
- New table on the signs of a heart attack in men and women
- New Skills for Behavior Change box on recognizing the signs of a stroke
- Increased coverage on diabetes prevalence rates and risks
- New Skills for Behavior Change box on reducing your risk for diabetes
- New module on diabetes diagnosis and treatment
- New Think About It end-of-chapter questions

Chapter 12: Infectious Conditions
- New mindfulness module on infection risk factors
- New cold and flu module
- New sections on mumps, measles, and rubella
- Expanded discussion of other pathogens and new pathogens such as Powassan
- New Think About It end-of-chapter questions

Chapter 13: Violence and Unintentional Injuries
- New section on rape on U.S. campuses and government policies on violence
- New section on coping in the event of campus violence
- Added new statistics and information related to distracted driving, texting and driving, and other preventable issues, including the statistics on injuries and deaths among college-age adults
- New Think About It end-of-chapter questions

Chapter 14: Environmental Health
- New mindfulness module on environmental mindfulness
- Updated scientific evidence that climate change is real and why you should be concerned
- New section on fracking and potential threats to the environment
- New information on sustainable ways to use consumer electronics
- Expanded coverage related to green cities and campuses
- New Think About It end-of-chapter questions

Chapter 15: Consumerism and Complementary and Integrative Health Care Choices
- New mindfulness module on meditation and mind and body practices
- New table on common nonherbal supplements
- New figure on where our health care dollars are spent
- New Think About It end-of-chapter questions

Supplementary Materials

Available with *My Health: The Mindfulness Edition*, Third Edition, is a comprehensive set of ancillary materials designed to enhance learning and to facilitate teaching.

Instructor Supplements

- **Mastering™ Health.** Mastering Health coaches students through the toughest health topics. Instructors can assign engaging tools to help students visualize, practice, and understand crucial content from the basics of health to the fundamentals of behavior change. **Coaching Activities** guide students through key health concepts with interactive mini-lessons, complete with hints and wrong-answer feedback. **Reading Quizzes** (20 questions per chapter) ensure that students have completed the assigned reading before class. *ABC News* Videos stimulate classroom discussions and include multiple-choice questions with feedback for students. **NutriTools Coaching Activities** in the nutrition chapter allow students to combine and experiment with different food options and learn firsthand how to build healthier meals. **MP3s** relate to chapter content and come with multiple-choice questions that provide wrong-answer feedback.
- **NEW! Ready-to-Go Teaching Modules** in the Instructor Resources section help instructors efficiently make use of the available teaching tools for the toughest topics. Before-class assignments, in-class activities, and after-class assignments are provided for ease of use in efficient course setup. Instructors can incorporate active learning into their courses with the suggested activity ideas, clicker questions, or Learning Catalytics questions.
- **UPDATED Learning Catalytics™** is a student response tool that generates classroom discussion, guides your lecture, and promotes peer-to-peer learning with real-time analytics. Students use their smartphones, tablets, or laptops to engage them in more interactive tasks and thinking. Instructors, you can:
  - **NEW!** Upload a full PowerPoint® deck for easy creation of slide questions.
  - **NEW!** Name teams the way you want to—team names are no longer case sensitive.
  - Help your students develop critical-thinking skills.
  - Monitor responses to find out where your students are struggling.
  - Rely on real-time data to adjust your teaching strategy.
  - Automatically group students for discussion, teamwork, and peer-to- peer learning.
- **Digital Instructional Resources (Download Only).** The Digital Instructional Resources include everything instructors need to prepare for their course and deliver a dynamic lecture in one convenient place. Resources include *ABC News* videos, Video Tutor videos, clicker questions, Quiz Show questions, PowerPoint lecture outlines, all figures and tables from the text, PDF and Microsoft Word files of the *Instructor Resource and Support Manual* and the Test Bank, the Computerized Test Bank, the User's Quick Guide, *Teaching with Student Learning Outcomes, Teaching with Web 2.0, Behavior Change Log Book and Wellness Journal, Eat Right!, Live Right!*, and *Take Charge of Your Health* worksheets.
- *ABC News* **Videos** and **Video Tutors.** Fifty-one new *ABC News* videos, each 5 to 10 minutes long, and 22 brand-new brief videos assignable in Mastering Health help instructors

stimulate critical discussion in the classroom. Videos are provided already linked within PowerPoint lectures and are also available separately in large-screen format with optional closed captioning on the Teaching Toolkit DVD and through Mastering Health.

- *Instructor Resource and Support Manual (Download Only).* This teaching tool provides chapter summaries and outlines of each chapter. It includes information on available PowerPoint lectures, integrated *ABC News* video discussion questions, tips and strategies for managing large classrooms, ideas for in-class activities, and suggestions for integrating Mastering Health and MyDietAnalysis into your classroom activities and homework assignments.

- **Test Bank.** The Test Bank incorporates Bloom's Taxonomy of Educational Objectives to help instructors create exams that encourage students to think analytically and critically rather than simply to regurgitate information. Test Bank questions are tagged to global and book-specific student learning outcomes.

- **User's Quick Guide.** Newly redesigned to be even more useful, this valuable supplement acts as your road map to the Digital Instructional Resources.

- *Teaching with Student Learning Outcomes.* This publication contains essays from 11 instructors who are teaching using student learning outcomes. They share their goals in using outcomes and the processes that they follow to develop and refine them, and they provide many useful suggestions and examples for successfully incorporating outcomes into a personal health course.

- *Teaching with Web 2.0.* From Facebook to Twitter to blogs, students are using and interacting with Web 2.0 technologies. This handbook provides an introduction to these popular online tools and offers ideas for incorporating them into your personal health course. Written by personal health and health education instructors, each chapter examines the basics about each technology and ways to make it work for you and your students.

- *Behavior Change Log Book and Wellness Journal.* This assessment tool helps students track daily exercise and nutritional intake and create a long-term nutritional and fitness prescription plan. It also includes a Behavior Change Contract and topics for journal-based activities.

Student Supplements

- **The Study Area of Mastering Health** is organized by chapter, with study resources organized by learning areas: *Read It* houses the new Pearson eText 2.0, with which users can create notes, highlight text in different colors, create bookmarks, zoom, click hyperlinked words for definitions, and change page view. *See It* includes 51 *ABC News* videos on important health topics and the key concepts of each chapter. *Hear It* contains MP3 Study Tutor files and audio case studies. *Do It* contains critical-thinking questions and Web links. *Review It* contains study quizzes for each chapter. *Live It* helps jump start students' behavior-change projects with assessments and resources to plan change; students can fill out a Behavior

Change Contract, journal and log behaviors, and prepare a reflection piece.

- **NEW! Pearson eText:**
  - Now available on smartphones and tablets. Offline access is available through the Pearson App.
  - Seamlessly integrated videos, interactive self-assessments worksheets, and other rich media.
  - Accessible (screen-reader ready).
  - Configurable reading settings, including resizable type and night reading mode.
  - Instructor and student note-taking, highlighting, book-marking, and search.

- *Behavior Change Log Book and Wellness Journal.* This assessment tool helps students track daily exercise and nutritional intake and create a long-term nutrition and fitness prescription plan. It includes Behavior Change Contracts and topics for journal-based activities.

- *Eat Right! Healthy Eating in College and Beyond.* This booklet provides students with practical nutrition guidelines, shopper's guides, and recipes.

- *Live Right! Beating Stress in College and Beyond.* This booklet gives students useful tips for coping with stressful life challenges during college and for the rest of their lives.

- **Digital 5-Step Pedometer** Take strides to better health with this pedometer, which measures steps, distance (miles), activity time, and calories and provides a time clock.

- **MyDietAnalysis** (www.mydietanalysis.com). Powered by ESHA Research, Inc., MyDietAnalysis features a database of nearly 20,000 foods and multiple reports. It allows students to track their diet and activity using up to three profiles and to generate and submit reports electronically.

Flexible Options

My Health: The Mindfulness Edition, Third Edition, is also available in alternate print and electronic versions:

- **Mastering with eText**: students can purchase access to Mastering Health with eText in lieu of purchase a print text and have access to all of the assignments and study tools within Mastering Health, as well as their entire textbook in a mobile and accessible electronic format.

- **Books a la Carte** offers the exact same content as *My Health: The Mindfulness Edition* in a convenient, three-hole-punched, loose-leaf version. Books a la Carte offers a great value for your students—this format costs 35% less than a new textbook!

- **Vitalsource eTextbooks** are an alternative to purchasing the print textbook. Students can subscribe to the same content online and save 40% off the suggested list price of the print text. Access the Vitalsource eText at www.vitalsource.com.

- Creating a customized version of the book from the **Pearson Custom Library**, with only the chapters that you select, is also possible. Contact your Pearson sales representative for more details.

A Note on the Text

From my earliest years of college instruction, I have believed that in order to be motivated to focus on their health, students need to understand the complex health world that people live in, to appreciate how the macroenvironment and culture influence health decision making, and to recognize that there is no "best" recipe for health. Helping students access the best information available and motivating them to ask the right questions and be thoughtful in their analysis of issues, as well as *mindful in their approach to healthy change*, have been part of my overall approach to teaching, learning, and writing.

Today's students have been raised on a steady dose of health information, some of which sounds good but may be highly questionable in terms of accuracy. Helping them sift through the changing sands of health information, examine their own risks, and make positive changes that affect them, their loved ones, and others in the community is key to improving health. Writing a text such as this one has helped keep me current in my teaching and tuned in to the needs of twenty-first-century students and the instructors who teach classes such as this one. This text, focused on a more technology-based, interactive, and challenging approach to learning, cuts to the chase in delivering essential information and thought-provoking questions. Consistent with an ever-evolving and "information at your fingertips" approach, this format is designed to help students navigate the seemingly endless world of health and bring it to life in a colorful and fresh format. In keeping with the times, this text is a "work in continual progress," and it will benefit greatly from your feedback and suggestions. As an author, I'd love to hear from you!

Acknowledgments

The process of writing and developing a textbook is truly a team effort. Each step along the way in planning, developing, and translating critical health information to students and instructors requires a tremendous amount of work from many dedicated professionals, including contributors who are at the top of their games in their knowledge of health science and behaviors and publishing professionals who personify all that is the absolute "best" in terms of qualities an author looks for in bringing a text to fruition. I cannot help but think how fortunate I have been to work with the gifted contributors to this text and the extraordinary publishing professionals at Pearson. Through time constraints, exhaustive searches for cutting-edge background research, and the writing process, these contributors were outstanding.

From painstaking efforts in development, design, editing, and editorial decision making to highly skilled marketing and dedicated sales efforts, the Pearson group handled every detail, every obstacle with patience, professionalism, and painstaking attention to detail. From this author's perspective, these personnel personify key aspects of what it takes to be successful in the publishing world: (1) drive and motivation; (2) commitment to excellence; (3) fantastic job and performance skills; (4) a vibrant, youthful, forward-thinking and enthusiastic approach; and (5) personalities that motivate an author to continually strive to produce market-leading texts. I have been amazed at the way that this team continually works to be well ahead of the curve in terms of cutting-edge information. Asking "What do students need to know?" and "What will help instructors and students thrive in today's high-pressure academic settings?" was at the heart of our efforts. I am deeply indebted to everyone who has played a role in making this book come alive for students and getting it into the hands of instructors.

In particular, credit goes to my development editor for this edition, Alice Fugate, who painstakingly merged and synthesized content and provided additional insight and expertise in making this new edition accessible to students. Alice did an extraordinary job of streamlining and revising material to fit within the constraints of the modular outline while retaining accuracy and readability. Without her, this book would not exist—thank you!

Further praise and thanks go to the highly skilled and hardworking executive editor Sandra Lindelof, who was responsible for the conceptualization of this text and helped to spearhead its initial development in the marketplace, doing the necessary work to procure the cutting-edge technology and skilled professionals that were key to its success. Her successor, Michelle Yglecias, quickly took charge of the list after Sandy's departure and worked to ensure that this text provided the necessary framework to meet the needs of an increasingly demanding group of instructors and students.

Although these women were key contributors to the finished work, there were many other people who worked on *My Health: The Mindfulness Edition*. Thanks go to Lizette Faraji, Michelle Gardner, and Heather Winter at SPi Global, who reliably kept us on track with flexibility and dedication. Design director Mark Ong and designer Tamara Newnam refreshed the visually impactful design while keeping students and instructors in mind. We could not have created this book without their creativity and dedication. Dinesh Deivendiran gets major kudos for overseeing the supplements package. Senior Rich Media Content Producer Timothy Hainley and Rich Media Content Producer Keri Rand put together an innovative and comprehensive set of assets for *My Health: The Mindfulness Edition*. Additional thanks go to the rest of the team at Pearson, especially Editorial Assistants Nicole Constantine and Crystal Trigueros, Managing Producer Nancy Tabor, and Director of Development Barbara Yien.

The editorial and production teams are critical to a book's success, but I would be remiss without thanking another key group who ultimately help determine a book's success: the textbook sales group and Senior Field Marketing Manager Mary Salzman and Product Marketing Manager Alysun Burns. With the support of Mary and Alysun, the Pearson sales representatives traverse the country, promoting the book, making sure that instructors know how it compares to the competition, and providing support to customers. From directing an outstanding marketing campaign to the everyday tasks of being responsive to instructor needs, Mary and Alysun do a superb job of making sure that *My Health* gets into instructors' hands and that adopters receive the service they deserve. In keeping with my overall experiences with Pearson, the marketing and sales staff is among the best of the best. I am very lucky to have them working with me on this project and want to extend a special thanks to all of them!

This book was developed in part from material from my other textbooks, *Access to Health* and *Health: The Basics*. I would like to thank the contributors to those books, particularly Dr. Patricia Ketcham of Western Oregon University and past president of the American College Health Association; Dr. Susan Dobie, associate professor in the School of Health, Physical Education, and Leisure Services at the University of Northern Iowa; Dr. Kathy Munoz, professor in the Department of Kinesiology and Recreation Administration at Humboldt State University; Dr. Erica Jackson, associate professor in the Department of Public and Allied Health Sciences at Delaware State University; and Laura Bonazzoli, who has worked on my texts for years and has done an outstanding job in providing updates and original work for many chapters. She is amazing! A special thanks to Niloofar Bavarian of Oregon State University, who drafted the original student learning outcomes on which the book is based.

Thanks also to the talented people who contributed to the supplements package: Lisa Tunks who updated the *Instructor Resource and Support Manual*; Laura Bonazzoli, who updated the Test Bank; and Michelle Lomonaco, who updated the PowerPoint lecture slides and PowerPoint quiz show slides.

Reviewers

This book is the result of not only my efforts, but also the invaluable contributions of the many reviewers. From the initial idea to the fine-tuning of each and every learning outcome, the thoughtful comments from reviewers shaped this book in many ways. I am extremely grateful for your feedback.

I am forever grateful to all of those who contributed in large and small ways to the success of this text and all of my texts. It really does take a village to make things happen, and this village was extraordinary!

Rebecca J. Donatelle, PhD

Reviewers for the Third Edition

Michelle Alexander
Thomas Nelson Community College

Daniel Armstrong
Queensborough Community College

Lisa Beck
Ball State University

LaNita Harris
University of Central Oklahoma

Ryan Donovan
Colorado State University Ft. Collins

Trudy Moore-Harrison
UNC Charlotte

Kathy Hutcheson
Colorado State University Ft. Collins

Dena Pistor
Rollins College

Grace Pokorny
Long Beach City College

Dominique Rose
Southern Illinois University

Giovanna Sabatini
Western Michigan University

Anthoney Stock
Mesa Community College

Deborah Dailey Stone
Louisiana State University

Erika Vargas
James Madison University

Reviewers for the Second Edition

Debbie Allison
Guilford Technical Community College

Nicole Clark
Indiana University of Pennsylvania

Henry Counts
University of South Carolina

Teresa Dolan
Lincoln University

Kathy Finley
Indiana University Bloomington

Ari Fisher
Louisiana State University

Chris Isenbarth
Weber State University

Ellen Larson
Northern Arizona University

Cynthia Smith
Central Piedmont Community College

Mastering Health Faculty Advisor Board Reviewers

Daniel Armstrong
Queensborough Community College

Anthoney Stock
Mesa Community College

Kris Jankovitz
California Polytechnic State University

Stasi Kasianchuk
Oregon State University

Lynn Long
University of North Carolina at Wilmington

Ayanna Lyles
California University of Pennsylvania

Steven Namanny
Utah Valley University

1

Healthy Change

Got health? That may sound like a simple question, but it isn't; health is a process, not something we just "get." People who are healthy in their forties, fifties, sixties, and beyond aren't just lucky or the beneficiaries of hardy genes. In most cases, those who are healthy and thriving in their later years have set the stage for good health by making it a priority in their early years. You've probably heard others say that your college years are some of the best years of your life. Whether your story is filled with good health, happiness, great relationships, and fulfillment of your life goals is largely dependent on the health choices you make—beginning right now.

We aspire to be fit; we want to be more environmentally conscious; we search for relationships that are meaningful, loving, and lasting; and we want to live to a healthy, happy old age. How does what you do today influence you and those around you?

1.1 Discuss definitions of health used throughout history, and distinguish among the dimensions of health and wellness.

Over the centuries, several models have been put forth attempting to define what it means to be "healthy." Earlier models focused primarily on hygiene and the absence of disease. Today's models view health in a broader context that includes individuals and their macro environment. The choices we make affect our own health, but they can also affect others. For example, you might be a great specimen of physical health, but are a chronic "worrier" and suffer from debilitating stress that affects your academic performance and can result in problems in your interactions with others (Figure 1.1).

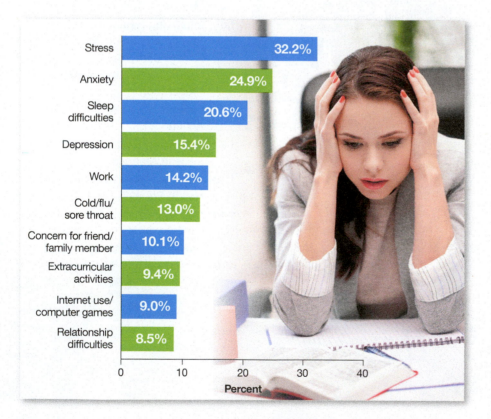

Figure 1.1 Top 10 Reported Impediments to Academic Performance—Past 12 Months

In a recent survey by the National College Health Association, students indicated that stress, poor sleep, recurrent minor illnesses, and anxiety, among other things, had prevented them from performing at their academic best.

Source: Data are from American College Health Association, *American College Health Association—National College Health Assessment II (ACHA-NCHA II) Reference Group Data Report, Fall 2016* Hanover, MD: American College Health Association, 2017. Available at www.acha-ncha.org.

Models of Health

Before the twentieth century, if you made it to your fiftieth birthday, you were regarded as lucky. Survivors were believed to be of healthy stock—having what we might refer to today as "good genes." During this time, perceptions of health were dominated by the **medical model**, in which health status focused primarily on the individual and his or her tissues and organs. The surest way to improve health was to cure the individual's disease, either with medication to treat the disease-causing agent or through surgery to remove the diseased body part. Government resources focused on initiatives that led to disease treatment rather than prevention.

In the early 1900s, researchers begin to recognize that entire populations of poor people, particularly those living in certain locations, were victims of environmental factors—such as polluted water, air, and food—over which they often had little control. Experts then began to realize that disease and health are related to more than just physical factors. A field of study examining interactions between the social and physical environment evolved, leading to a more comprehensive **ecological** or **public health model**.

Recognition of the public health model enabled health officials to control contaminants in water, for example, by building adequate sewers and to control burning and other forms of air pollution. Over time, public health officials began to recognize and address other forces affecting human health, including hazardous work conditions, negative influences in the home and social environment, stress, unsafe behavior, diet, and sedentary lifestyle.

By the 1940s, progressive thinkers began calling for policies, programs, and services to improve individual health and that of the population as a whole. Their focus shifted from treatment of individual illness to **disease prevention**, reducing or eliminating the factors that cause illness and injury. For example, childhood vaccination programs reduced the incidence and severity of infectious disease, and laws governing occupational safety reduced worker injuries and deaths. In 1947, at an international conference focusing on global health issues, the World Health Organization (WHO) proposed a new definition of health that rejected the old medical model: "Health is the state of complete physical, mental, and social well-being, not just the absence of disease or infirmity."[1]

Alongside prevention, the public health model emphasized **health promotion**—policies and programs promoting behaviors known to support health. Such programs identify people engaging in **risk behaviors** (behaviors increasing susceptibility to negative health outcomes) and motivate them to change their actions by improving their knowledge, attitudes, and skills.

Wellness and the Dimensions of Health

In 1968, René Dubos proposed an even broader definition of health. In his book *So Human an Animal,* Dubos defined *health* as "a quality of life, involving social, emotional, mental, spiritual, and biological fitness on the part of the individual, which results from adaptations to the environment."[2] This concept of adaptability became a key element in our overall understanding of health.

Eventually, the word **wellness** entered the popular vocabulary, further enlarging Dubos's definition of health by recognizing levels—or gradations—of health within each category. Today, the words *health* and *wellness* are often used interchangeably to mean the dynamic, ever-changing process of trying to achieve one's potential in each of the following six interrelated dimensions (**Figure 1.2**):

- **Physical health.** Physical health includes characteristics such as body size and shape, sensory acuity and responsiveness, susceptibility to disease and disorders, body functioning, physical fitness, and recuperative abilities. Newer definitions of physical health include our ability to perform normal *activities of daily living (ADLs),* or those tasks necessary to normal existence in society, such as getting up from a chair, bending to tie your shoes, or writing a check.
- **Social health.** The ability to have satisfying interpersonal relationships with friends, family members, and partners is a key part of overall wellness. This implies being able to give and receive love, to be nurturing and supportive in social interactions, and to interact and communicate with others.
- **Intellectual health.** The ability to think clearly, reason objectively, analyze critically, and use brainpower effectively to meet life's challenges are all part of this dimension. This includes learning from successes and mistakes; making sound, responsible decisions that consider all aspects of a situation; and having a healthy curiosity about life and an interest in learning new things.
- **Emotional health.** This is the feeling component—being able to express emotions when appropriate, and to control them when not. Self-esteem, self-confidence, self-efficacy, trust, and love are all part of emotional health.
- **Spiritual health.** This dimension involves having a sense of meaning and purpose in your life. This may include believing in a supreme being or following a particular religion's rules and customs. It may also include the ability to understand and express one's purpose in life; to feel part of a greater spectrum of existence; to experience peace, contentment, and wonder over life's experiences; and to care about and respect all living things.
- **Environmental health.** This dimension entails understanding how the health of the environments in which you live, work, and play can affect you; protecting yourself from hazards in your own environment; and working to protect and improve environmental conditions for everyone.

Achieving wellness means attaining the optimal level of well-being for your unique limitations and strengths. For example, a physically disabled person may function at his or her optimal level of performance; enjoy satisfying interpersonal relationships; work to maintain emotional, spiritual, and intellectual health; and have a strong interest in environmental concerns. In contrast, someone who spends hours lifting weights to perfect each muscle but pays little attention to social or emotional health may look healthy but may not maintain a balance in all dimensions. The perspective on wellness we need is *holistic,* emphasizing balanced integration of mind, body, and spirit.

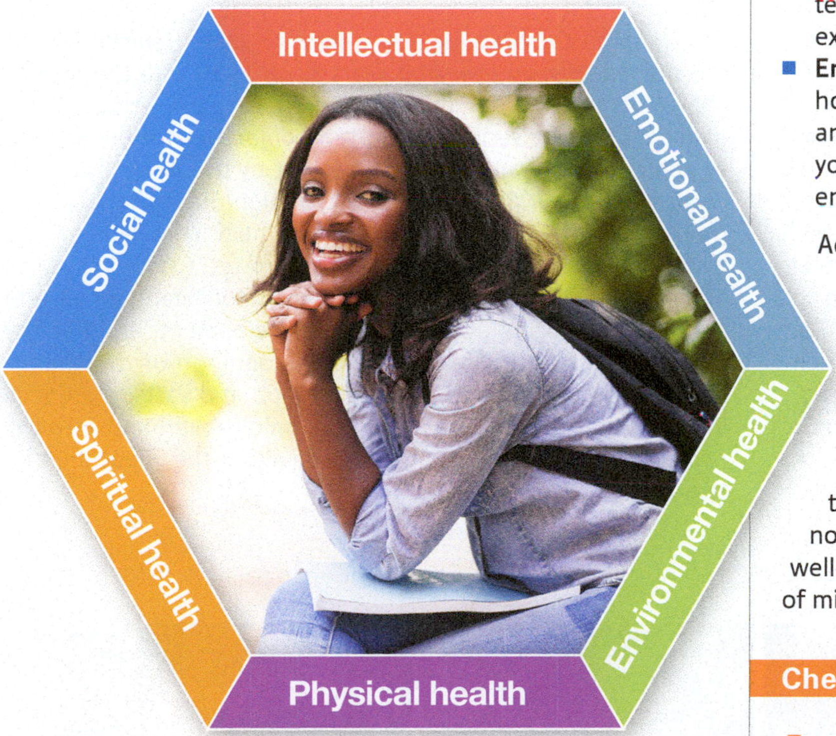

Figure 1.2 The Dimensions of Health
When all dimensions of health are in balance and well developed, they can support your active and thriving lifestyle.

▶ **Mastering Health & Nutrition** Dimensions of Health

Check Yourself

- How have definitions of health changed over time?
- What are the dimensions of health? Explain the differences among them?
- When you think of someone as being "healthy," what comes to mind? Are your criteria consistent with modern definitions?

3

1.2 Health in the United States

1.2 Specify major present-day health issues affecting the United States population, and explain the overall goals of *Healthy People 2020*.

Our health choices are not only personal; they affect the lives of others in many ways. For example, overeating and inadequate physical activity contribute to individual obesity, but obesity also burdens the U.S. health care system and economy. Obesity also costs the public indirectly, for example, by increased disability payments and health insurance rates. Similarly, smoking, excessive consumption of alcohol, and use of illegal drugs place an economic burden on our communities and our society as a whole—not to mention social and emotional burdens on families and caregivers.

How Healthy Are We?

According to current **mortality** statistics—which reflect the proportion of deaths within a population—average **life expectancy** at birth in the United States is projected to be 78.8 years for a child born in 2015.[3] In other words, American infants born today will live to an average age of over 78 years, much longer than the 47-year life expectancy for people born in the early 1900s.

In the last century, with the development of vaccines, antibiotics, and other public health successes, as well as advances in medications, diagnostic technologies, surgery, and cancer treatments, life expectancy increased dramatically. The leading cause of death shifted to **chronic diseases**, such as heart disease, cerebrovascular disease (which leads to strokes), cancer, and diabetes.

Unfortunately, life expectancy in the United States is several years below that of many other nations. Factors contributing to premature mortality and thus limiting U.S. life expectancy include obesity, tobacco and alcohol abuse, and drug overdose, which is now the leading cause of accidental death.[4] Our highly fragmented system of health care, lower quality of care for chronic disease, social inequality, and poverty are also part of the complex, multifactorial influences on our lower life expectancy.[5]

Lifestyle factors are strongly linked to four leading causes of death in the United States: heart disease, cancer, chronic respiratory disease, and stroke (Table 1.1).[6] In fact, the four leading causes of these chronic diseases are all under our individual control (Figure 1.3).

Clearly, healthful choices increase life expectancy. But they also increase **healthy life expectancy**—the years of full health a person enjoys without disability, chronic pain, or significant illness. For example, if we could delay the onset of diabetes until age 60 rather than 30, there would be a 30-year increase in that individual's healthy life expectancy. The prevalence of health issues affecting the U.S. population highlights the need to focus on healthy life expectancy as a cornerstone of public health.

Healthy People 2020: Setting Health Objectives

The Surgeon General's health promotion plan, *Healthy People,* has been published every 10 years since 1990 with the goal of improving quality of life and years of life for all Americans. Each plan consists of a series of long-term objectives for the decade to come. The overarching goals set out by the newest version, *Healthy People 2020,* are to (1) attain high-quality, longer lives free of preventable diseases; (2) achieve health equity, eliminate disparities, and improve health of all groups; (3) create social and physical environments that promote good health for all; and (4) promote quality of life, healthy development, and healthy behaviors across all life stages.[7] In recognition of the changing demographics of the U.S. population and vast differences in health status based on racial or ethnic background, *Healthy People 2020* included strong language about the importance of reducing disparities.

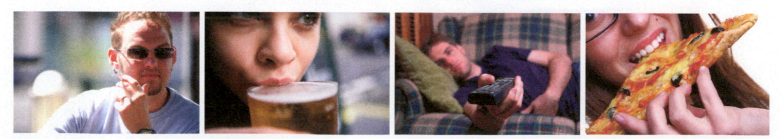

Figure 1.3 Four Leading Causes of Chronic Disease in the United States.
Tobacco use, excessive alcohol consumption, lack of physical activity, and poor nutrition—all modifiable health determinants—are the four most significant factors leading to chronic disease among Americans today.

1.1 Leading Causes of Death in the United States, 2014, Overall and by Age Group (15 and older)

All Ages	Number of Deaths
Diseases of the heart	614,348
Malignant neoplasms (cancer)	591,700
Chronic lower respiratory diseases	147,101
Accidents (unintentional injuries)	135,928
Cerebrovascular diseases (stroke)	133,103
Aged 15–24	
Accidents (unintentional injuries)	11,797
Suicide	5,090
Assault (homicide)	4,171
Malignant neoplasms (cancer)	1,569
Diseases of the heart	953
Aged 25–44	
Accidents (unintentional injuries)	33,366
Malignant neoplasms (cancer)	14,891
Diseases of the heart	13,709
Suicide	13,289
Assault (homicide)	6,769

Source: Data from M. Heron, "Deaths: Leading Causes for 2014, Table 1," *National Vital Statistics Reports* 65, no. 5 (June 2016), www.cdc.gov/nchs/data/nvsr/nvsr65/nvsr65_05.pdf.

At the root of *Healthy People 2020* are "foundation health measures" designed to indicate progress toward reaching these four goals:

- Measures of *general health status,* including life expectancy, healthy life expectancy, and chronic disease prevalence
- Measures of *health-related quality of life and well-being,* including physical, mental, and social factors and participation in common activities
- *Determinants of health,* which are the personal, social, economic, and environmental factors that influence health status
- Measures of *disparities* and inequity, including differences in health status based on race/ethnicity, gender, physical and mental ability, and geography

Healthy People 2020's comprehensive. comprehensive approach includes 42 topic areas, each representing a public health priority, such as diabetes, physical activity, or substance abuse.[8] Under each area is an overview describing health issues within its scope, objectives for the nation to achieve during the decade to come, and resources for communities and individuals. For instance, objectives for the nutrition topic include "Increase the proportion of schools that offer nutritious foods and beverages outside of school meals" and "Increase the proportion of physician office visits that include counseling or education related to

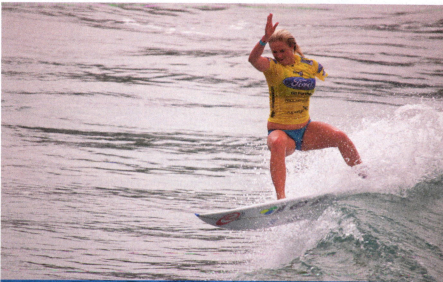

How are *health* and *quality of life* related?

Just because a person has a disability doesn't mean his or her quality of life is necessarily low. Surfer Bethany Hamilton lost her arm in a shark attack while surfing at age 13, but she returned to surfing just 1 month after the attack and has since traveled around the world competing professionally.

nutrition or weight." For each objective, the report lists baseline statistics and a target goal for the year 2020.

Within the 42 topic areas, a smaller set of topics, called *leading health indicators,* indicate high-priority health issues and actions. Topics include access to health services and reproductive and sexual health, among others.[9]

Perhaps the most revealing aspects of the report are the 13 topic areas newly added for this decade, which reflect concern over health disparities, the relationship of lifestyle and wellness, and issues affecting the young and the very old.[10] These include adolescent health; global health; lesbian, gay, bisexual, and transgender health; older adults' health; sleep health; and health-related quality of life and well-being. Health is a comprehensive system encompassing the individual and the society, with influences both intensely personal and broadly global in scope.

Healthy People 2030 goals are currently being developed. To check out how decisions are made about what goes into the document and how they are finalized, go to: https://www.healthy-people.gov.

Check Yourself

- What are four key health issues in the United States?
- How are national health objectives used to improve health among Americans?

1.3 Describe the major factors affecting an individual's ability to attain optimal health, and explain the connection between lifestyle and health outcomes.

If you're lucky, aspects of your world promote health: Your family is active and fit; there are fresh apples on sale at the neighborhood farmers market; and a new walking trail opens along the river. If you're not so lucky, aspects of your world discourage health: Your family eats a high-fat diet; cigarettes, alcohol, and junk food dominate the corner market; and you wouldn't dare walk along the river for fear of being mugged. This variety of influences explains why seemingly personal choices aren't totally within an individual's control.

Public health experts refer to the factors that influence health as **determinants of health,** a term the U.S. Surgeon General defines as "the range of personal, social, economic, and environmental factors that influence health status" (**Figure 1.4**).[11]

Biology and Genetics

In the domain of health determinants, *biology* refers to an individual's genetics, ethnicity, age, and gender. Biological determinants—what health experts refer to as *nonmodifiable determinants*—are things you can't change or modify. Your sex is a key biological determinant: Compared to men, women have an increased risk for low bone density and autoimmune diseases (in which the body attacks its own cells), whereas men have an increased risk for heart disease compared to women. Biology also includes family history; for example, if your parents developed diabetes in their forties, that's a biological determinant for you. Your history of illness and injury factors in, too; a serious injury might influence your ability to participate in physical activity, which in turn may predispose you to weight gain.

Individual Behavior

In contrast to biological factors, *behaviors* are responses to internal and external conditions. By definition, behaviors are changeable; health experts refer to them as *modifiable determinants*. They significantly influence your risk for chronic disease, which is responsible for 7 out of 10 deaths in the United States.[12] Just four modifiable determinants are responsible for most illness and early death related to chronic diseases:[13]

- **Lack of physical activity.** Low levels of physical activity contribute to over 200,000 deaths in the United States annually.[14]

- **Poor nutrition.** Diets low in fruits and vegetables have been linked in multiple studies with an increased risk of death by any cause.[15]
- **Excessive alcohol consumption.** Alcohol causes 88,000 deaths in adults annually, through cardiovascular disease, liver disease, cancer, and other conditions, as well as traffic accidents and violence.[16]
- **Tobacco use.** Tobacco smoking and the cancer, high blood pressure, and respiratory disease it causes are responsible for about 1 in 5 deaths in American adults.[17]

Another major contributor to disease and mortality among Americans is our rising abuse of prescription and illegal drugs, especially opioid pain relievers and heroin. Between 1999 and 2015, the number of overdose deaths involving these drugs quadrupled. Every day, 91 Americans die from an opioid overdose.[18]

Social Factors

Social determinants of health refer to the social factors and physical conditions in the environment in which people are born or live. Your social environment includes your exposure to crime, mass media, technology, and poverty, as well as availability of healthful foods, transportation, living wages, social support, and educational or job opportunities.

Among the most powerful determinants of health in the social environment are economic factors; even in affluent nations such as the United States, people in lower socioeconomic brackets have substantially shorter life expectancies and more illnesses than do people who are wealthy.[19] Economic disadvantages exert their effects on health in areas such as access to high-quality education, safe housing, nourishing food, warm clothes, medication, and transportation.

The effects of family on health can be both biological and environmental. Genetics determine some of your health status, but the actions and values of your family also have a strong influence on health.

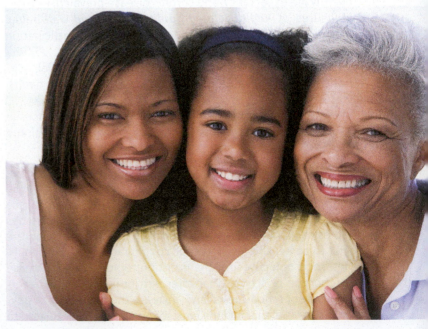

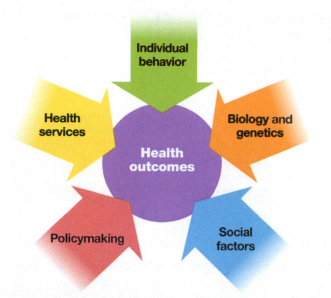

Figure 1.4 *Healthy People 2020* **Determinants of Health**
The determinants of health often overlap one another. Collectively, they impact the health of individuals and communities.

The physical environment is anything—from skyscrapers to snowfall—that you can perceive with your senses. It also includes less tangible things such as radiation and air pollution. Individuals and communities exposed to toxins, radiation, irritants, and infectious agents can suffer significant harm. And the effects go beyond the local; the pollutants one region produces, or the diseases it harbors, can affect people worldwide. Examples include the burning of the South American rainforest, which is contributing to global warming, and the swift transmission of strains of severe influenza across populations.

The built environment includes anything created or modified by human beings, from buildings to transportation to electrical lines. Changes to the built environment can improve the health of community members.[20] These include increased construction of parks, sidewalks, pedestrian-only areas, bike paths, public transit systems to which commuters typically walk or bike, and improved safety strategies, with better lighting and increased security. Some communities are enticing supermarkets to open in underserved neighborhoods to increase residents' access to fresh fruits and vegetables.

Health Services

The health of individuals and communities is also determined by access to quality health care, not only provider services but also accurate information and products such as eyeglasses, medical supplies, and medications.

Policymaking

Public policies and interventions can have a powerful effect on the health of individuals and communities. Examples include campaigns to prevent smoking, laws mandating seatbelt use, vaccination programs, and public funding for mental health services.

Policymaking also includes health insurance legislation. Although the Affordable Care Act had reduced the numbers of uninsured Americans by 20 million people by the end of 2016, millions remained without insurance, and the current status of health insurance coverage in the United States is uncertain.[21]

Health Disparities

Among the factors that can influence an individual's ability to attain optimal health are **health disparities**. Health disparities can arise from a variety of factors, including the following:

- **Race and ethnicity.** Research indicates dramatic health disparities across racial and ethnic backgrounds. Socioeconomic differences, stigma based on "minority status," poor access to care, cultural barriers and beliefs, discrimination, and limited education and employment opportunities can all affect health.
- **Inadequate health insurance.** A large and growing number of the *uninsured* or *underinsured* face unaffordable payments or co-payments, high deductibles, or limited care in their area.
- **Sex and gender.** At all stages of life, men and women experience differences in rates of disease and disability. For instance, men smoke more than do women, but women who smoke have higher rates of lung disease. In contrast, men have much higher rates of drug-induced deaths and deaths from suicide and homicide. Overall, men have a lower healthy life expectancy than females.
- **Economics and education.** Poverty may make it difficult to afford healthy food, preventive medical visits, or medication. Economics also influences access to safe, affordable exercise. Moreover, poor Americans with a low level of education experience increased rates of illness, premature death, and risk-taking behaviors such as smoking and binge drinking.
- **Geographic location.** Whether you live in an urban or a rural area and have access to public transportation or your own vehicle can have a huge impact on what you eat, your physical activity, and your ability to visit the doctor or dentist.
- **Sexual orientation.** Gay, lesbian, bisexual, or transgender individuals may lack social support, are often denied health benefits because of their unrecognized marital status, and face unusually high stress levels and stigmatization by other groups.
- **Disability.** Disproportionate numbers of disabled individuals lack access to health care services, social support, and community resources.

Check Yourself

- **What are the determinants that affect health identified in this section?**
- **Give three examples of the connection between lifestyle and health outcomes.**

1.4 How Does Mindfulness Influence Health?

Recently, many media outlets have been promoting a shift to *mindful* behavior as a path to optimum health. If you've seen these claims, you may be wondering if they're backed by evidence, and if so, how to practice mindfulness in your own life. In this section, we introduce the concept of mindfulness, the research that supports it effectiveness, and some simple strategies for living more mindfully. In later chapters of this text, we'll provide further research, resources, and tips for you to include mindfulness as part of a comprehensive plan for living your best, most healthful life!

Definitions of Mindfulness

Definitions of **mindfulness** include being present "in the moment" through greater awareness of yourself—including your sensations, thoughts, and feelings—and your environment. Some people have called mindfulness an extended "stop and smell the roses" moment that becomes a total approach to your daily life. Other people describe it as a way of looking at yourself and the world without judging or trying to "fix," but instead with gentleness and compassion. One of the keys to mindfulness is focusing—bringing your complete attention to the present rather than re-hashing the past or dwelling on future fears. In fact, one of the clearest definitions found in the popular media is: "Keeping your feet in the now!"

Mindfulness is believed to have originated around 1500 BCE or earlier as an element of the Hindu practices of yoga and meditation. Buddhism, which evolved from Hinduism around 600 BCE, incorporated mindfulness as one of its core practices. Today, mindfulness is no longer solely affiliated with Eastern religions, and those who practice it may follow other religions or no religion at all.

Health Benefits of Mindfulness

A growing body of research evidence links mindfulness to improved health. Studies associate it with pain relief, as well as stress reduction, lower levels of anxiety and depression, improved sleep, improved memory and attention, weight loss, reduced risks for CVD, and improvements in relationships. Although research in these areas is in its early stages, examples of some of the areas where positive results have been shown include:

Stress Level and Psychological/Mental Health Improvements: Theories of mindfulness and a growing amount of research support the idea that in the presences of negative emotions or threat, mindfulness activities can help with self-regulation and control

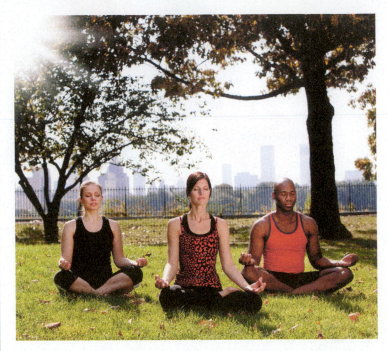

Yoga comes in many variations, but all yoga practices incorporate a focus on the here and now through breathing, attention, and gratitude.

of negative reactions and can help you stay centered and more focused. According to recent research, the more frequently you practice mindfulness meditation and overall mindfulness strategies, the greater the likelihood of a stress control and anxiety reduction, to name two of the most promising areas of benefit.[22]

Benefits of Specific Activities Such as Yoga: A recent "study of studies" (meta-analysis) focused on the benefits of yoga indicates that yoga and overall mindfulness meditation can improve mental and physical health.[23]

Possible Help with Addictions: Results of a small Oregon pilot study indicated promising results with individuals in a methadone treatment program who engaged in a mindfulness-based relapse prevention program (MBPP). Those in the MBPP program showed statistically significant improvements in depression levels, cravings, and trauma symptoms at the end of treatment compared to those in a methadone treatment program only.[24]

Relief of Low Back Pain: A recent study by RAND Corporation, Kaiser Permanente, Washington Health Research Institute, and the University of Washington randomly assigned 342 adults with chronic back pain to an 8-week, 2-hour weekly session of either mindfulness-based stress reduction (MBSR), cognitive-behavioral therapy (CBT), or usual therapy or care. Published in the journal

Spine, results indicated that MBSR, in particular, may offer significant pain relief and cost benefits over usual care.[25]

Aids in Sleep Quality: A large meta-analysis of studies examining the role of cognitive-behavioral sleep interventions—including mindfulness—appear to show that sleep quality, daytime sleepiness, depression, and anxiety improve and are maintained with these strategies. More large scale randomized controlled trials are recommended to examine this association.[26]

How to Practice Mindfulness

Although there are many ways to incorporate mindfulness into your daily life, here are a few steps you can take to tune in to life around you and gain a greater appreciation for yourself and your place in the world. This is just a brief introduction. Other chapters of this book will provide specific skills for helping you develop mindfulness.

You can practice mindfulness at any time, in any place. According to mindfulness guru Jon Kabat-Zinn, it requires only a willingness to examine who you are, your view of the world, and your place in it, and to appreciate each moment.[27] The path to mindfulness differs for each of us, however. It might include formal actions, such as carving out times to meditate or practice yoga. Alternatively, it might comprise informal actions, such as increasing your attention to your relationships, food choices, or the environment. It might also include working to build your compassion for others or pausing to acknowledge the things in your life that you're thankful for. The following are some basic mindfulness skills.

Cultivate Compassion The word *compassion,* derived from the Latin phrase "to suffer together," is a recognition of another's pain and a sincere desire to help. You cultivate compassion for others by supporting loved ones going through difficult times, or by volunteering to help others who are less fortunate. You cultivate compassion for yourself by learning to recognize critical thoughts that say you're not good enough and setting them aside. You may then remind yourself of your positive qualities, achievements, and loving relationships. Practicing yoga can help you drop your internal critic and develop self-confidence. You might also take a vow to avoid engaging in negative thinking about yourself and others for a single day.

Some simple ways to practice compassion include meeting others' eyes as you pass, acknowledging that you're aware of their presence. Smile. When friends criticize others, try to listen fully to what's behind the words, and respond with gentleness and honesty.

Start Each Day with Intention How do your values guide your actions? What might you wish to do differently today? What will success look like? Each morning, jot down some intentions—perhaps to listen more, to stop procrastinating, or to think before you act. During the day, try to stay mindful of how your actions align with these intentions. Then, before bed each night, take a moment to consider—without judgment—how well you lived your intentions that day.

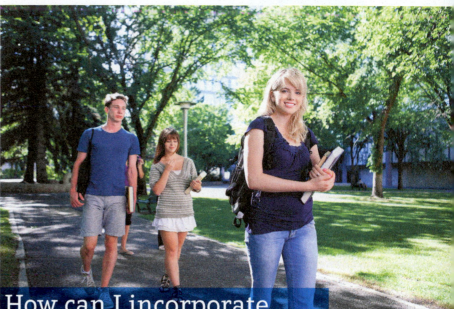

How can I incorporate mindfulness into my hectic life?

You can practice mindfulness at almost any time of the day. Try focusing on the present by paying attention to the sights, smells, and sounds you encounter during your daily walk through campus or your community.

Examine the Way You Deal with Life's Challenges Perhaps you became angry with a friend or got stressed out by homework. One method for confronting challenges with mindfulness is to acknowledge what you felt, then try to determine why. Was the event really as negative as you felt it to be at the time? Could you have responded differently? In future, would you prefer to let go of your attachment to particular outcomes, say "It is what it is," and move on? One way to do this is to acknowledge that nothing in life—and no one—is perfect, including you. For yourself and for others, seek goodness rather than perfection.

Check Yourself

- What is mindfulness? Summarize health benefits that are associated with it.

- How might mindfulness, with its emphasis on the present, help overcome feelings of anxiety about the future or depression about the past?

- Describe several ways in which you could add mindfulness into your daily life.

Models of Behavior Change

1.5 Describe models of behavior change.

A wide variety of factors influence your health status. But the factors over which you have by far the most control fall into one category: individual behaviors (otherwise known as *modifiable determinants*).

Clearly, change is not always easy. But your chances of successfully changing negative habits improve when you first identify a behavior that you want to change, then develop a plan for gradual transformation—one that allows you time to unlearn negative patterns and substitute positive ones. Many experts advocate breaking any health behavior you want to change into small parts, then working on them one at a time in "baby steps."

In other words, to successfully change a behavior, you need to see change not as a singular *event* but instead as a *process*—one that requires preparation, consists of several stages, and takes time to succeed.

Over the years, social scientists and public health researchers have developed a variety of models to reflect the multifaceted process of behavior change. We explore three such models in this section.

The Health Belief Model

Many people see changing health behaviors as a straightforward process: When rational people realize that their behaviors put them at risk, they will change those behaviors and reduce that risk. But for many (even most) of us, it's more complicated than that. Consider the number of health professionals who smoke, eat junk food, and act in other unhealthy ways. They surely know better, but "knowing" is disconnected from "doing." One classic model of behavior change proposes that our beliefs may help to explain why this occurs.

A **belief** is an appraisal of the relationship between some object, action, or idea (e.g., smoking) and some attribute of that object, action, or idea (e.g., "smoking is expensive, dirty, and causes cancer"—or "smoking is sociable and relaxing"). Psychologists studying the relationship between beliefs and health behaviors have determined that although beliefs may subtly influence behavior, they may or may not cause people to actually behave differently. In 1966, psychologist I. Rosenstock developed a classic theory, the **health belief model (HBM),** to show when beliefs about health affect behavior change.[28] The HBM holds that, before change is likely to happen, our beliefs must reflect the following:

- **Perceived seriousness of the health problem.** The more serious the perceived effects, the more likely that action will be taken.
- **Perceived susceptibility to the health problem.** People who perceive themselves at high risk are more likely to take preventive action.
- **Perceived benefits.** People are more likely to take action if they believe that this action will benefit them.
- **Perceived barriers.** People who believe an action is too expensive, difficult, or inconvenient must overcome or acknowledge these barriers as less important than the perceived benefits.
- **Cues to action.** People who are reminded or alerted about a potential health problem are more likely to take action.

People follow the health belief model many times every day. Take, for example, smokers. Older people who smoke are likely to know other smokers who have developed serious heart or lung problems. They are thus more likely to perceive tobacco as a threat to their health than are teenagers who have just begun smoking. The greater the perceived threat of health problems caused by smoking, the greater the chance a person will quit.

But many chronic smokers know the risks yet continue to smoke. Why do they miss these cues to action? According to Rosenstock, some people do not believe that they, personally, are susceptible to a severe problem, and so they act as though they are immune to it. Such people are unlikely to change their behavior.

The Social Cognitive Model

The **social cognitive model (SCM)** developed from the work of several researchers and their models over the years, though it is

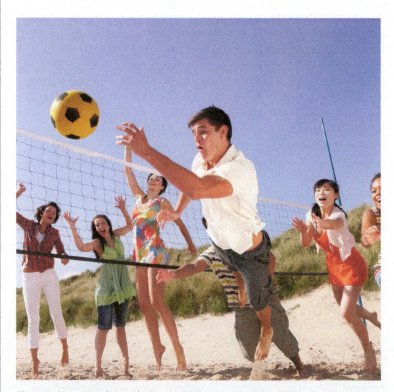

The top New Year's resolution in 2016 was to enjoy life, according to a survey of over 5,000 Americans by GoBankingRates.

most closely associated with the work of psychologist Albert Bandura. Fundamentally, SCM proposes that three factors interact in a reciprocal fashion to promote and motivate change. These are the social environment in which we live, our thoughts or cognition (including our values, perceptions, beliefs, expectations, and sense of self-efficacy), and our behaviors. We change our behavior, in part, by observing models in our environment—from childhood to the present moment—reflecting on our observations, and regulating ourselves accordingly.

The social cognitive model is often used to design health promotion programs. For example, one public health initiative in the southeast United States used the SCM to develop an after-school program for preteens that focused on nutrition and physical activity. The program supported participants in mastering certain physical activities and self-regulation of eating habits. Participants improved not only their eating and activity patterns, but also their body weight, cardiovascular endurance, mood, and ability and their confidence in regulating their behaviors.[29]

The Transtheoretical Model

Why do so many New Year's resolutions fail before Valentine's Day? According to Drs. James Prochaska and Carlos DiClemente, it's because most of us aren't really prepared to take action. Their research indicates that behavior changes usually do not succeed if they start with the change itself. Instead, we must go through a series of stages to adequately prepare ourselves for an eventual change.[30]

According to Prochaska and DiClemente's **transtheoretical model** of behavior change (also called the *stages of change model*), our chances of keeping those New Year's resolutions will be greatly enhanced if we have proper reinforcement and help during each of the following stages:

1. **Precontemplation.** People in the precontemplation stage have no current intention of changing. They may have tried to change a behavior before and given up, or they may be in denial and unaware of any problem.
2. **Contemplation.** In this phase, people recognize that they have a problem and begin to contemplate the need to change. Despite this acknowledgment, people can languish in this stage for years, realizing a problem but lacking the time or energy to make the change.
3. **Preparation.** Most people at this point are close to taking action. They've thought about what they might do and may even have come up with a specific plan.
4. **Action.** In this stage, people begin to follow their action plans. Those who have prepared for change appropriately and made a plan of action are more ready for action than those who have given it little thought.
5. **Maintenance.** During the maintenance stage, a person continues the actions begun in the action stage and works toward making them a permanent part of his or her life. In this stage, it is important to be aware of the potential for relapses and to develop strategies for dealing with such challenges.

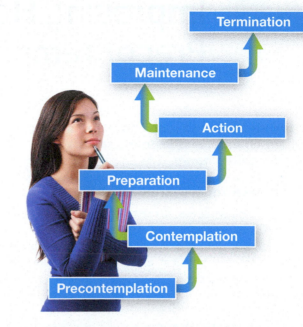

Figure 1.5 Transtheoretical Model
People don't move through the transtheoretical model stages in sequence. We may make progress in more than one stage at one time, or we may shuttle back and forth from one to another—say, contemplation to preparation, then back to contemplation—before we succeed in making a change.

6. **Termination.** By this point, the change in behavior is so ingrained that constant vigilance may be unnecessary. The new behavior has become an essential part of daily living.

See It! Videos

How can you change your habits and stick with it? Watch **New Year's Resolutions** in the Study Area of Mastering Health.

We don't necessarily go through these stages sequentially. They may overlap, or we may shuttle back and forth from one to another—say, contemplation to preparation, then back to contemplation—for a while before we become truly committed to making the change (Figure 1.5). Still, it's useful to recognize where we are with a change, so we can consider the appropriate strategies to move us forward.

Check Yourself

- Compare and contrast models of behavior change.

- Which model of behavior change reflects your experiences most accurately? Why?

- Why do people typically not go through the stages of behavior change sequentially?

1.6 Improving Health Behaviors: Precontemplation and Contemplation

1.6 Identify strategies to use before and during behavior change, and examine factors that affect behavior change.

Step One: Increase Your Awareness

Before you can decide what you want to change, you'll need to learn about both the behaviors that affect your health and the health determinants in your life. What aspects of your biology, behavior, and social and physical environment support your health, and which are obstacles to overcome?

Step Two: Contemplate Change

Examine Your Health Habits and Patterns Do you routinely stop at Dunkin' Donuts for breakfast? Smoke when you're stressed? Party too much? Get to bed way past 2 a.m.? When considering habits, ask yourself the following:

- How long has this been going on?
- How often does it happen?
- How serious are its consequences?
- What are your reasons for the behavior?
- What situations trigger it?
- Are others involved? If so, how?

Health behaviors involve personal choice but are also influenced by determinants that make them more or less likely. Some are *predisposing factors*—for instance, if your parents smoke, you're more likely to start smoking than is a child of nonsmokers. Some are *enabling factors*—for example, peers who smoke enable one another's smoking.

Reinforcing factors can also contribute to habits. If you decide to stop smoking but your friends all smoke, you may lose your resolve. In such cases, it can be helpful to employ the social cognitive model and deliberately change your environment—spending more time with nonsmoking friends who model behavior you want to emulate.

Identify a Target Behavior Ask yourself these questions:

- **What do I want?** Is your ultimate goal to lose weight? Exercise more? Reduce stress? Have a lasting relationship? Get a clear picture of your outcome.
- **Which change is my priority now?** Suppose you're gaining unwanted weight. Rather than saying, "I need to eat less and start exercising," identify one specific behavior that contributes to your problem, and tackle that first.
- **Why is this important to me?** Do you want to change for your health? To improve academic performance? To look better? To win someone's approval? It's best to target a behavior because it's right for you rather than because you think it will please others.

Learn about the Target Behavior Get solid information from reliable sources (see the **Do Your Research** section on the following page). Look at the behavior, its effects, and aspects of your world that could hinder your success. Let's say you want to meditate daily. You need to learn what meditation is, how it's practiced, and its benefits. Consider what else might pose an obstacle: Do you think of yourself as hyper? Do you live in a noisy dorm? Are you afraid your friends might find meditating weird? To prepare for change, learn everything you can about your target behavior now.

Assess Your Motivation and Readiness To change, you need not just desire but also **motivation**—a social and cognitive force that directs your behavior. To understand motivation, think about the health belief model (HBM) and the social cognitive model (SCM).

According to the HBM, beliefs affect ability to change. Smokers may think, "I'll stop tomorrow" or "They'll have a cure for lung cancer before I get it." These beliefs

Find reliable health information at your fingertips!

allow them to continue smoking—they dampen motivation. Ask yourself the following:

- Do you believe your current pattern could lead to a serious problem? For example, over 70 countries have laws requiring cigarette packages to display graphic warning labels with images of the physical effects of smoking, from diseased organs to chests sawed open for autopsy. Research shows that these graphic labels have reduced smoking among adolescents and young adults and increased smoking cessation among established smokers. Countries have reported that 25, 50, and even 60 percent of current smokers have attempted to quit as a result of these labels.[31]

- Do you see yourself as personally likely to experience the consequences of your behavior? Losing a loved one to lung cancer could motivate you to stop smoking.

If you're struggling to perceive a behavior as serious or its consequences as personal, use the SCM. You could interview people struggling with the consequences of the behavior and ask if when they were engaging in the behavior they believed it would harm them. And don't ignore the motivating potential of positive role models. Do you know people who have successfully lost weight, stopped drinking, or quit smoking? Hang out with them!

Mindfulness can help. A recent study of physical activity among adults found that mindfulness practices increased study participants' exercise motivation and participation.[32] *Readiness* precedes behavior change. People who are ready to change possess the knowledge, skills, and external and internal resources that make change possible.

Develop Self-Efficacy **Self-efficacy**—a belief that one is capable of achieving certain goals or of influencing events in life—is one of the greatest influences on health. People who exhibit high self-efficacy are confident that they can succeed and approach challenges positively. They may therefore be more likely to succeed. Conversely, someone with low self-efficacy may give up easily or never try to change.

Cultivate an Internal Locus of Control People with a strong *internal* **locus of control** believe that they have power over their own actions. In contrast, individuals with an *external* locus of control feel that they have limited control over their lives; they may easily succumb to feelings of anxiety and disempowerment and give up.[33] For example, a recent study among cancer patients found that, compared to those with a high internal locus of control, people with an external locus of control were more likely to respond with depression to their diagnosis.[34]

Do Your Research The Internet is a wonderful resource for finding answers to your questions, but it can also be a source of *misinformation*. To ensure that the sites you visit are trustworthy, follow these tips:

- Look for websites sponsored by government agencies (identified by *.gov* extensions—e.g., the National Institute of Mental Health at www.nimh.nih.gov); universities or colleges (*.edu* extensions—e.g., Johns Hopkins University at www.jhu.edu); or hospitals/medical centers (often *.org*—e.g., the Mayo Clinic at www.mayoclinic.org). Major philanthropic foundations (such as the Robert Wood Johnson Foundation and the Kellogg Foundation) and

national nonprofit organizations (such as the American Heart Association and the American Cancer Society) are good, authoritative sources. Most foundation and nonprofit sites have *.org* extensions.

- Search for peer-reviewed journals such as the *New England Journal of Medicine* (content.nejm.org) and *Journal of the American Medical Association* (JAMA; jama.ama-assn.org). Although some of these sites require an access fee, many colleges give students free access to them.

- Other reliable sites include the Centers for Disease Control and Prevention (www.cdc.gov), the World Health Organization (www.who.int/en), FamilyDoctor.org (familydoctor.org), MedlinePlus (www.nlm.nih.gov/medlineplus), Go Ask Alice! (www.goaskalice.columbia.edu), and WebMD (my.webmd.com).

- Don't believe everything you read. Cross-check information against reliable sources. Be wary of websites selling you something. When in doubt, check with your health care provider or health professor.

Skills for Behavior Change

Maintain Your Motivation

- **Pick one specific behavior you want to change.** Trying to change many things at once can be overwhelming and can cause you to lose motivation.

- **Assess the behavior you wish to change.** Why is it important to change? If you can't find a compelling reason to motivate yourself, you probably shouldn't address this behavior right now.

- **Set achievable and incremental goals.** Developing short- and long-term goals and taking small steps to meet them improves your chances of staying motivated.

- **Reward yourself.** Create a list of things you find rewarding; link each to a specific goal. Having something to look forward to can help you stay focused and motivated.

- **Avoid or anticipate barriers and temptations.** Control or eliminate the environmental cues that provoke the behavior you want to change.

- **Remind yourself why you're trying to change.** List the benefits you'll get from this change, both now and down the road, as well as the risks of doing nothing.

- **Enlist the support of others.** They can serve as role models, a cheering squad, or partners in change. Let the people you care about know your plans, and ask for help.

- **Don't be discouraged.** Everyone, no matter how committed, experiences setbacks. A brief lapse doesn't mean the cause is lost. Look for new strategies, set new short-term goals, and then get back on track.

Check Yourself

- What should I do before undertaking a behavior change?

- What are some common behavior change strategies?

- Name important factors that influence behavior and behavior change decisions.

Improving Health Behaviors: Preparation

1.7 Set a behavior change goal, and identify obstacles to behavior change.

Prepare for Change

You've contemplated change for long enough—now it's time to set a realistic goal, anticipate barriers, reach out to other people, and commit.

Set a SMART Goal Unsuccessful goals are vague and open-ended—for instance, "Get into shape by exercising more." In contrast, successful goals are SMART:

- **S**pecific. "Attend the Tuesday/Thursday aerobics class at the YMCA."
- **M**easurable. "Reduce my alcohol intake on Saturday nights from three drinks to two."
- **A**ction-oriented. "Volunteer at the animal shelter on Friday afternoons."
- **R**ealistic. "Increase my daily walk from 15 to 20 minutes."
- **T**ime-oriented. "Stay in my strength-training class for the full 10-week session, then reassess."

A SMART goal is one that you truly can achieve—not someday, when things in your life change, but within the circumstances of your life right now. Knowing that your goal is attainable increases your motivation. This, in turn, leads to a better chance of success and to a greater sense of self-efficacy—which can in turn motivate you to succeed even more.

Use Shaping **Shaping** is a process of making a series of small changes. Suppose you want to start jogging 3 miles every other day, but right now you get tired and winded after half a mile. Shaping would dictate a process of slow, progressive steps, perhaps beginning with walking 1 hour every other day at a slow, relaxed pace for the first week; walking for an hour every other day but at a faster pace that covers more distance the second week; and speeding up to a slow run the third week.

Regardless of the change you plan, remember that your current habits didn't develop overnight and they won't change overnight, either.

Prepare your goals and your plan of action with these shaping points in mind:

- Start slowly to avoid hurting yourself or causing undue stress.
- Keep the steps of your program small and achievable.
- Be flexible and ready to change your original plan if it proves uncomfortable.
- Master one step before moving on to the next.

Anticipate Barriers to Change Anticipating *barriers to change*, or possible stumbling blocks, will help you prepare fully and adequately for change. For example, if you want to lose weight, you may face several barriers to change, including social determinants (your family members and friends are overweight), aspects of the built environment (the only food vendors on or near your campus are convenience stores and fast-food outlets), or lack of adequate health care (you have an inexpensive health insurance policy that doesn't cover treatment for weight loss). In addition to negative determinants, the following are a few general barriers to change that you may need to overcome:

- **Overambitious goals.** Remember the advice to set realistic goals? Even with the strongest motivation, overambitious goals can derail change. Most people cannot lose weight, stop smoking, and begin running 3 miles a day all at the same time. Wanting to achieve dramatic change within unrealistically short time frames—for example, aiming to lose 20 pounds in 1 month—tends to be equally unsuccessful. Habits are best changed one small step at a time.
- **Self-defeating beliefs and attitudes.** As the health belief model explains, believing you're too young or fit or lucky to have to worry about the consequences of your behavior can keep you from making a solid commitment to change. Likewise, seeing yourself as helpless to change your eating, smoking, or other habits can undermine your efforts. Greater self-efficacy and more positive expectations may help.
- **Failing to accurately assess your current state of wellness.** You might assume that you will be able to walk the 2 miles to campus each morning, for example, only to find yourself aching and winded after only a mile. Failing to make sure that the planned change is realistic for *you* can leave you with weakened motivation and commitment.

To reach your behavior change goals, you need to take things one step at a time.

- **Lack of support and guidance.** If you want to cut down on your drinking, peers who drink heavily may be powerful barriers to that change. To succeed, you will need to recognize the people in your life who can't support, or might even actively oppose, your decision to change, then limit your interactions with them.
- **Emotions that sabotage your efforts and sap your will.** Sometimes the best laid plans go awry because you're having a bad day or are fighting with someone you care about. While emotional reactions to life's challenges aren't inherently bad, they can sabotage your efforts to change by distracting you and draining your reserves. Seek help for more severe psychological problems, and recognize that you may need to focus on those before you can effect significant change in other aspects of your health.

Enlist Others as Change Agents The social cognitive model recognizes the importance of our social contacts in successful change. Most of us are highly influenced by the approval or disapproval (real or imagined) of close friends, family members, and the social and cultural groups to which we belong. In addition, watching others successfully change their behavior can give you ideas and encouragement for your own change. This **modeling**, or learning from role models, is a key component of the social cognitive model of change. Observing a friend who is a good conversationalist, for example, can help you improve your communication skills. Or find someone to share your plan for change! For instance, get your roommate to commit to taking a daily walk or run with you or sign a contract with a friend stipulating that you will never let each other drink and drive.

Family Members From the time of your birth, your parents and other family members have given you strong cues about which actions are and are not socially acceptable. Your family has also influenced your food choices, your activity patterns, your political beliefs, and many of your other values and actions. Strong and positive family units provide care, trust, and protection; are dedicated to the healthful development of all family members; and work together to reduce problems.

When a loving family unit does not exist or when it does not provide for basic human needs, a child can find it difficult to learn positive health behaviors. Healthy families provide the foundation for a clear and necessary understanding of what is right and wrong, what is positive and negative. Without this fundamental grounding, many young people have great difficulties.

Friends Just as your family influences your actions during your childhood, your friends and significant others influence your behaviors as you grow older. Most of us desire to fit the "norm." If you deviate from the actions expected in your hometown or among your friends, you may suffer ostracism, strange looks, and other negative social consequences. But if your friends offer encouragement, or even express interest in joining you in a behavior change, you are more likely to remain motivated. Cultivating and maintaining close friends who share your personal values can greatly affect your behaviors and improve your chances of success.

FREE TIME AFTER CLASS? HOW WILL YOU CHOOSE TO SPEND IT?

WHICH PATH WOULD YOU TAKE?

 Go to Mastering Health to play "Accessing Your Health" and see how your actions today affect your future health.

Professionals Sometimes the change you seek requires more than the help of well-meaning family members and friends. Depending on the type and severity of the problem, you may want to enlist support from professionals such as your health instructor, PE instructor, coach, health care provider, academic adviser, or religious adviser. As appropriate, consider counseling services offered on campus, as well as community services such as smoking cessation programs, Alcoholics Anonymous support groups, and your local YMCA.

Sign a Contract It's time to get it in writing! A formal *behavior change contract* serves many powerful purposes. It functions as a promise to yourself, a public declaration of intent, an organized plan that lays out start and end dates and daily actions, a list of barriers you may encounter, a place to brainstorm strategies to overcome barriers, a list of sources of support, and a reminder of the benefits of sticking with the program.

Writing a behavior change contract will help you clarify your goals and make a commitment to change. In the next module, you will see an example of a completed behavior change contract, and later in the chapter, a blank behavior change contract. Fill out the blank contract in Module 1.11 to put your behavior change plan in writing.

Check Yourself

- What is your behavior change goal? Does it fit the SMART system?
- What are some obstacles to change that you expect to face? What strategies will you employ to overcome them?
- Why is it so important to enlist other people in your plan for behavior change?

1.8 Improving Health Behaviors: Action

1.8 Employ behavior change strategies to make a behavior change.

Take Action to Change

It's time to put your plan into action! Behavior change strategies include visualization, countering, controlling the situation, changing your self-talk, rewarding yourself, and journaling. The options don't stop here, but these are a good place to start.

Visualize New Behavior Mental practice can transform unhealthy behaviors into healthy ones. Using an **imagined rehearsal** to visualize an action ahead of time can help you reach your goals. Careful mental and verbal rehearsal of how you intend to act will help you anticipate problems and greatly improve the likelihood of success.

Learn to "Counter" Substituting a desired behavior for an undesirable one is called **countering**. If you want to stop eating junk food on your break, for example, toss a banana in your backpack to eat instead.

Control the Situation Sometimes, the right setting or the right group of people will positively influence your behaviors. Any behavior has both antecedents and consequences. *Antecedents* are aspects of a situation that come beforehand, cueing or stimulating a person to act in certain ways. *Consequences*—the results of behavior—affect whether a person repeats an action. Both antecedents and consequences can be events, thoughts, emotions, or the actions of others.

Keeping a journal noting your undesirable behaviors and the settings in which they occur can be useful in helping you determine the antecedents and consequences. Once you have recognized the antecedents of a given behavior, use **situational inducement** to modify those that are working against you—consider which settings help and which hurt your effort to change. Identifying substitute antecedents that support a more positive result helps you control the situation further.

Change Your Self-Talk There is a close connection between what people say to themselves, known as **self-talk,** and how they feel. When we feel we have little

control, it's tempting to engage in negative self-talk, which can sabotage our best intentions. According to psychologist Albert Ellis, most emotional problems and related behaviors stem from irrational statements that people make to themselves when events in their lives are different from what they would like them to be.[35]

For example, suppose you say to yourself, "I can't believe I flunked that exam. I'm so stupid." Changing such irrational, negative self-talk into rational, positive statements about what is really going on can increase the likelihood of positive change: "I didn't study enough for that exam. I'm not stupid; I just need to prepare better for the next test." Positive self-talk can help you recover from disappointment and take steps to correct problems.

Another technique for changing self-talk is to practice blocking and stopping negative thoughts. For example, suppose you're

---

Behavior Change Contract

My behavior change will be:
To snack less on junk food and more on healthy foods.

My long-term goal for this behavior change is:
Eat junk food snacks no more than once a week

These are three obstacles to change (things that I am currently doing or situations that contribute to this behavior or make it harder to change):
1. The grocery store is closed by the time I come home from school.
2. I get hungry between classes, and the vending machines only carry candy bars.
3. It's easier to order pizza or other snacks than to make a snack at home.

The strategies I will use to overcome these obstacles are:
1. I'll leave early for school once a week so I can stock up on healthy snacks in the morning.
2. I'll bring a piece of fruit or other healthy snack to eat between classes.
3. I'll learn some easy recipes for snacks to make at home.

Resources I will use to help me change this behavior include:
a friend/partner/relative: my roommates: I'll ask them to buy healthier snacks instead of chips when they do the shopping.
a school-based resource: The dining hall: I'll ask the manager to provide healthy foods we can take to eat between classes.
a community-based resource: The library: I'll check out some cookbooks to find easy snack ideas
a book or reputable website: The USDA nutrient database at www.nal.usda.gov/fnic I'll use this site to make sure the foods I select are healthy choices.

In order to make my goal more attainable, I have devised these short-term goals:
short-term goal Eat a healthy snack 3 times per week   target date September 15   reward new CD
short-term goal Learn to make a healthy snack   target date October 15   reward concert tickets
short-term goal Eat a healthy snack 5 times per week   target date November 15   reward new shoes

When I make the long-term behavior change described above, my reward will be:
ski lift tickets for winter break   target date: December 15

I intend to make the behavior change described above. I will use the strategies and rewards to achieve the goals that will contribute to a healthy behavior change.

Signed: Elizabeth King   Witness: Susan Bauer

Figure 1.6 Example of a Completed Behavior Change Contract

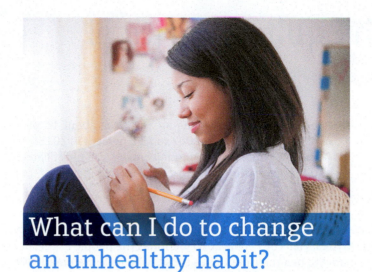

What can I do to change an unhealthy habit?

One of the best tools for helping you change your habits is journaling. Keeping track of your goals, behaviors, feelings, accomplishments, and setbacks can reinforce the healthy changes you are trying to make and provide motivation to continue. Other useful tools include shaping, enlisting supports, visualization, countering, controlling the situation, changing your self-talk, and rewarding yourself.

preoccupied with your ex-partner, who left you for someone else. By refusing to dwell on negative images and by forcing yourself to focus elsewhere, you can avoid wasting energy, time, and emotional resources and move on to positive change.

Reward Yourself Promote positive behavior change with **positive reinforcement**. Each of us is motivated by different positive reinforcers. Most of these fall into one of the following categories:

- *Consumable reinforcers* are edible items, such as a favorite fruit or snack mix.
- *Activity reinforcers* are opportunities to do something enjoyable, such as going on a hike or taking a trip.
- *Manipulative reinforcers* are incentives, such as reduced rent in exchange for mowing the lawn or the promise of a better grade for doing an extra-credit project.
- *Possessional reinforcers* are tangible rewards, such as a new gadget or car.
- *Social reinforcers* are signs of appreciation, approval, or love, such as hugs or praise.

Successful positive reinforcement often lies in choosing choosing an incentive that motivates you to change. Your reinforcers may initially come from others (*extrinsic* rewards), but as you see positive changes in yourself you will begin to reward and reinforce yourself (*intrinsic* rewards).

Reinforcers should immediately follow a behavior, but beware of overkill; if you reward yourself with a movie every time you go jogging, the reinforcer will soon lose its power. It would be better

to give yourself such a reward after, say, a full week of adherence to your jogging program.

Journal Writing down personal experiences, interpretations, and results in a journal is an important skill for behavior change. You can log your daily activities, monitor your progress, record your feelings, and note ideas for improvement.

Let's Get Started

Once you have the skills to support successful behavior change, you can apply them to your target behavior. In Module 1.11, you can create a behavior change contract incorporating the goals and skills discussed here. Place it where you'll see it every day as a reminder that change doesn't "just happen." (See Figure 1.6 for an example.) Reviewing your contract helps you stay alert to potential problems, be aware of your alternatives, maintain a firm sense of your values, and stick to your goals under pressure.

Skills for Behavior Change

Challenge the Thoughts That Sabotage Change

Are thought patterns and beliefs holding you back? Try these strategies:

- **"I don't have enough time!"** Chart your activities for 1 day. What are your highest priorities? What can you eliminate or reduce? Plan to make some time for a healthy change next week.
- **"I'm too stressed!"** Assess your major stressors right now. List those you can control and those you can change or avoid. Then identify two things you enjoy that can help you reduce stress now.
- **"I'm worried what others may think."** How much do other people influence your decisions about drinking, sex, eating habits, and the like? What is most important to you? What actions can you take to act in line with your values?
- **"I don't think I can."** Just because you haven't done something before doesn't mean you can't do it now. To develop confidence, take baby steps and break tasks into small chunks of time.
- **"I can't break this habit!"** Habits are difficult to break, but not impossible. What triggers your behavior? List ways you can avoid triggers. Ask for support from friends and family.

Check Yourself

- Describe the behavior change strategies that you have used. What were the benefits and disadvantages of each strategy?

- What types of reinforcers do you think would be most helpful to you?

1.9 Achieving Health Equity: A Critical Issue in America

Learning Outcome

1.9 Explain why health equity is a critical issue in 21st century America.

The founders of the United States proclaimed in a *Declaration of Independence* that we are all created equal. Ironically, despite this national proclamation of equality, the U.S. has consistently ranked lowest in *health equity* among the world's eleven wealthiest industrialized nations.[36]

What Is Health Equity?

The World Health Organization (WHO) defines *equity* as "the absence of avoidable or remediable differences among groups of people."[37] Thus, a society characterized by **health equity** has worked to prevent or reverse conditions such as persistent poverty and discrimination that undermine health. A society lacking health equity has a high level of health disparities. Health disparities are fundamentally unjust, reflecting an unfair distribution of health risks and health resources.[38]

America: A Nation of Increasing Diversity America is a country of increasing racial and ethnic **diversity** (**Figure 1.7**). Immigration is expected to continue to diversify the U.S. population throughout the 21st century.[39]

Other ways in which the U.S. is becoming more diverse include:

- **Age composition.** The population of Americans under age 18, is expected to increase only slightly between 2014 and 2060, from 74 million to 82 million. In contrast, the population of Americans age 65 or older will more than double, from 46 million to 98 million.[40]
- **Self-identity.** The percentage of Americans identifying as LGBT (lesbian, gay, bisexual, or transgender) more than doubled between 2000 and 2017, from 2 percent to 4.1 percent, and among millennials (born between 1980 and 1998) the percentage is now 7.3 percent.[41,42]
- **Religion.** The percentage of Americans who identify as Christian has been declining for decades, whereas the non-Christian religious have increased. The percentage who are religiously unaffiliated has been rising as well, from about 15 percent of all Americans in 2007 to 22.8 percent in 2015.[43,44] About 36 percent of young millennials are unaffiliated, and this generational trend is expected to increase.[45]

Certain Population Groups Are More Vulnerable to Health Disparities *Healthy People 2020* identifies the people especially vulnerable to health disparities as those "who have systematically experienced greater obstacles to health based on their racial or ethnic group; religion; socioeconomic status; gender; age; mental health; cognitive, sensory, or physical disability; sexual orientation or gender identity; geographic location; or other characteristics historically linked to discrimination or exclusion."

In addition to their emotional and physical burdens, health disparities exert significant financial costs. Every year racial and ethnic health disparities cost the U.S. economy an estimated $35 billion in direct medical expenditures, $10 billion in lost productivity, and nearly $200 billion in premature deaths.[46]

Health disparities are associated with financial costs because when people do not have adequate access to preventative care, they often do not seek help when it is needed, or when they do seek help, it is in the emergency room, where the cost of care

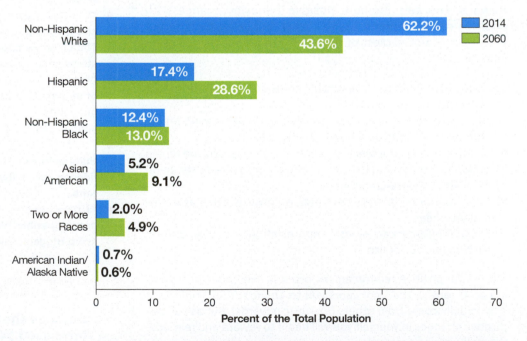

Figure 1.7 The racial and ethnic diversity of the United States population is expected to increase between 2014 and 2060. Source: S.L. Colby and J. M. Ortman, "Projections of the Size and Composition of the U.S. Population: 2014-2060, U.S. Census Bureau, March, 2015. Available at www.census .gov/content/dam/Census/library/publications/2015/demo/p25-1143.pdf

is very high. By the time someone seeks care, it may be too late to reverse or treat the illness.

Social Determinants of Health

Recall from module 1.3 that social determinants of health influence health disparities both directly and indirectly. Health disparities are avoidable. If as a society we are to reduce them, we need to understand the social, economic, and environmental disadvantages to which they are closely linked.[47]

Important social determinants of health include:

- **Economic stability.** Since 1980, the gap between rich and poor Americans has widened dramatically.[48] Today, 43.1 million Americans live in poverty.[49] Decades of research support a close association between poverty and poor health.[50] Males in the lowest 10 percent of income have an average life expectancy 14 years below that of males with income in the top 10 percent; for females, the gap is 13 years.[51]

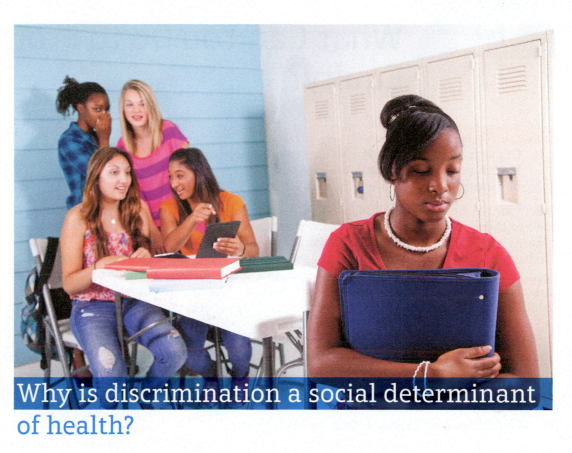

Why is discrimination a social determinant of health?

Even the anticipation of discrimination may trigger the stress response.

- **Educational attainment.** Low educational attainment increases with increasing poverty. Education enhances health in multiple ways: It directly increases access to information about nutrition, physical activity, alcohol use, and other lifestyle choices influencing health. It also leads to better job opportunities and, in turn, better working conditions. Better jobs often include such health promoting benefits as sick leave, paid vacation, health insurance coverage, and other benefits. People with higher incomes have better access to high-quality housing, nutritious food, and other essentials.[52]
- **Discrimination.** Discrimination is a key contributor to stress and poor health.[53] A recent report from the American Psychological Association (APA) identified an increased risk for discrimination among members of the following five groups: *the poor, the disabled, racial/ethnic minorities, LGBT Americans, and older Americans.*[54] Americans who report experiencing extreme levels of stress are twice as likely to also report fair or poor health, compared to those with low stress levels.[55] In other words, discrimination alone can lead to health inequities.
- **Health literacy.** Health literacy Is the ability to obtain, process, and understand health information and services needed to make appropriate health decisions.[56] People with low health literacy may have problems communicating with health providers, obtaining recommended tests, and taking medications correctly. They may suffer complications from poor disease management, and they have a higher mortality rate.[57]

- **Environment.** Neighborhood characteristics, such as walkability, presence of healthy food stores, density of recreational facilities, safety, appropriate lighting and infrastructure, higher quality schools, adequate low income housing, adequacy and availability of appropriate community, public health and mental health services influence health.[58] Pollution in air, water, and soil contributes to health disparities.[59, 60] Exposure to neighborhood violence is another powerful social determinant, contributing directly to traumatic injuries and deaths, and indirectly to disparities in mental and physical health as well as increased risks for several chronic diseases.[61, 62, 63, 64, 65]

Check Yourself

- **In what ways is the U.S. population becoming more diverse?**
- **Relate the social determinants of health discussed in this module to America's health issues.**
- **In your community, what are the biggest sources of health inequity?**

What Can You Do to Promote Health Equity?

Learning Outcome

1.10 Discuss specific actions you can take to promote health equity in yourself, on campus, in your community, and in the U.S. as a whole.

"Health for all" means living in communities that offer opportunities to thrive—physically, mentally, economically, and socially. It means access to healthy nutrition, physical activity, safe and affordable housing, education from early childhood through adulthood, jobs paying living wages, career opportunities, social support, community resources, freedom from discrimination, quality health care, and other social resources. This is where, as a society, we want to go. The question is, how do we get there?

The factors contributing to health disparities are complex and interconnected, and solutions can seem overwhelming. However, you can start by addressing health disparities on a smaller scale, in your own mind and in your neighborhood.

Use Mindfulness to Examine Your Assumptions

Be aware that your age, gender identity, race/ethnicity, abilities and disabilities, life experiences, and countless other factors have contributed to who you are, including how you perceive others and how they perceive you. As discussed in Module 1.4, mindfulness is a highly effective strategy for challenging the beliefs and attitudes that limit us.

Participants in a recent mindfulness training program enhanced their ability to pay attention to their own unconscious biases;

increased their insights into and understanding of the unconscious aspects of others' behavior; and adopted a more "us" versus "them" approach to interactions with others.[66] Another study offering a single session of mindfulness training to college students found that those who received the training demonstrated reduced racial and age biases and fewer negative behaviors that commonly result from such biases.[67] The researchers attributed this reduction in bias to dampening the brain's activation of automatic negative associations. In other words, when we pay close attention to what is actually occurring within our mind and our surroundings, we disable previously established, habitual neurological pathways by which we perceive, interpret our perceptions, and respond.[68]

Enjoy the Benefits of Diversity

Diversity is a great teacher. Interacting every day with others who are different from you challenges your assumptions, exposes you to new ideas, and expands your world. The skills you develop in working across differences are likely to improve your career prospects, even preparing you for international job opportunities. This deeper self-awareness can support you in making decisions about your coursework, social life, and future plans.[69] Building relationships with those who are different can expose you to new ideas, as well as new foods, new sports, new music, new authors . . . and a lot of fun!

Increase Access to Health Care

To achieve a more equitable distribution of health care in the United States, public health experts propose the following initiatives:

- **Increase minority providers.** Minorities are more likely to seek care from health care providers of their own race/ethnicity.[70] Educational programs and policies should encourage minority Americans (racial/ethnic minorities, LGBT Americans, and disabled Americans) to pursue careers in the health professions.[71]
- **Increase diversity training.** All health care providers should be required to obtain diversity training to increase their ability to communicate health information in the language and at the literacy level of the client they are serving.[72]
- **Increase preventive services.** Municipalities, employers, school districts, and health care organizations should partner to offer preventive services such as mental health services, dental exams and cleanings, vision care, vaccinations, blood pressure screenings, and other services for underserved populations.

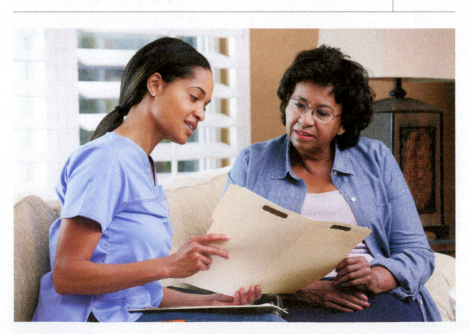

Minorities are more likely to seek care from health providers of their own race or ethnicity.

- **Expand access to health insurance.** The national initiative that has had perhaps the greatest effect on increasing access to health care for all population groups is the Affordable Care Act (ACA). Under the ACA, the percentage of poor and near-poor Americans who are uninsured dropped from 27 and 29 percent respectively in 2013 to 17 and 18 percent in 2015.[73] While reaching a goal of 100 percent insurance for all Americans is a goal, these decreases in uninsured percentages are a significant achievement. Currently, provisions of the Affordable Care Act are being questioned, with some members of Congress saying it goes too far and others saying it doesn't go far enough. Stay tuned!

Reduce the Social Determinants That Contribute to Health Disparities

In addition to increasing access to quality care, we must reduce the social determinants that contribute to health disparities. As these determinants are intertwined, they must be counteracted by systemic measures.[74] Specific strategies to reduce social determinants affecting the physical environment include:[75]

- Constructing high-quality, safe, and affordable housing
- Identifying and working to remediate sources of pollution
- Increasing neighborhood walkability
- Building parks and playgrounds
- Establishing after-school programs for tutoring, physical activity, and social support
- Offering incentives to chain grocers to open healthy food stores
- Building community gardens
- Supporting meetings between law enforcement officers and community members to foster collaboration and establish neighborhood watch programs
- Using libraries and community centers to increase health literacy

Initiatives on Campus College can provide unique opportunities for students from underserved communities to develop more healthful habits, via access to the student health center, healthy meal options in the student union and in the dorms, fitness facilities, and security services. Some college and university campuses have food service providers committed to offering healthy foods. Others sponsor community gardens or offer a food pantry for student use. Conduct some research on campus-based programs to advance health equity, and recommend model programs for your own campus that will help reduce disparities in health.

Advocate for Yourself and Others

And finally, be an advocate for yourself and others. For strategies, see the Skills for Behavior Change.

Skills for **Behavior Change**

Becoming Your Own Advocate

If you've experienced stereotyping or discrimination, you might be tempted simply to accept the situation and move on. But a more healthy way to respond is to become your own advocate. Here are some suggestions:

- Actively reject the negative messages you've received. Remind yourself of your goodness, your core values, and your life purpose.
- Don't dwell on the negative. Focus on what you can do to improve the narrative in your own head.
- If you experience a particularly troubling situation, talk with someone such as family members, friends, members of student diversity groups, and leaders at campus diversity centers, or with a mental health professional. Focus on how it made you feel, and talk about how you could have changed the dynamics and felt better about the situation.
- If you are likely to engage in the future with the individual who treated you unfairly, decide in advance how you would like your interactions to change. Make mental or written notes about the message you want to communicate and how to do it calmly, clearly, and effectively.
- Remember that you have a right to speak up for your interests. Someone else disagreeing with you or becoming defensive does not negate the importance of your needs or your right to make them known.
- If you believe you have been harrassed or discriminated against, file a complaint. For example, for job discrimination, contact the U.S. Equal Opportunity Employment Commission at www.eeoc.gov.
- Remember that you are helping others by speaking out.

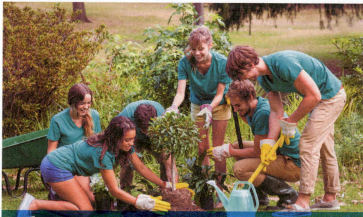

What can I do to create health equity in my neighborhood?

Community gardens can help reduce health disparities by increasing everyone's access to nourishing food.

Check Yourself

- Describe several initiatives that you think would reduce health disparities.
- What do you think are indicators of health disparities on your campus? In your community?
- How might you use mindfulness to reduce health disparities in your community?

1.11 **Complete a behavior change contract.**

Complete the Assess Yourself questionnaire. After reviewing your results and considering the various factors that influence your decisions, choose a health behavior that you would like to change, starting this quarter or semester. Sign the contract at the bottom to affirm your commitment to making a healthy change, and ask a friend to witness it.

My behavior change will be:

_____

My long-term goal for this behavior change is:

_____

These are three obstacles to change (things that I am currently doing or situations that contribute to this behavior or make it harder to change):

1. _____
2. _____
3. _____

The strategies I will use to overcome these obstacles are:

1. _____
2. _____
3. _____

Resources I will use to help me change this behavior include:

a friend/partner/relative: _____

a school-based resource: _____

a community-based resource: _____

a book or reputable website: _____

To make my goal more attainable, I have devised these short-term goals:

short-term goal	target date	reward
short-term goal	target date	reward
short-term goal	target date	reward

When I make the long-term behavior change described above, my reward will be:

_____ target date: _____

I intend to make the behavior change described above. I will use the strategies and rewards to achieve the goals that will contribute to a healthy behavior change.

Signed: _____ Witness: _____

■ **Do you think that completing this contract will make it more likely that you will succeed in your behavior change? Why or why not?**

Summary

LO 1.1 Health is the process of fulfilling one's potential in physical, social, emotional, spiritual, intellectual, and environmental dimensions of life. Wellness means achieving the best health possible in several dimensions.

LO 1.2 The goals of *Healthy People 2020* are to increase life span and the quality of life and to reduce and eliminate health disparities.

LO 1.3 Health is influenced by *determinants,* which the Surgeon General's health promotion plan, *Healthy People 2020*, classifies as individual biology and behavior, the social environment, the physical environment, access to quality health care, and policies and interventions.

LO 1.4 Mindfulness—nonjudgmental attention to the present moment—enhances health in all dimensions.

LO 1.5 Models of behavior change include health belief, social cognitive, and transtheoretical (stages of change) models. You can increase the chance of changing a behavior by viewing change as a process.

LO 1.6 When contemplating change, examine current habits, learn about a target behavior, and assess readiness.

LO 1.7 When preparing to change, set incremental goals, anticipate barriers to change, enlist support, and sign a behavior change contract.

LO 1.8 When taking action, visualize new behavior, practice countering, control the situation, change self-talk, reward yourself, and keep a log or journal.

LO 1.9 Health disparities and increasing diversity of the U.S. population, combined with social determinants that affect health, are challenges we face in achieving health equity.

LO 1.10 We can take action to become more mindful of our attitudes, address social determinants that undermine health, and improve living standards and health care for all members of the population.

Pop Quiz

Visit Mastering Health to personalize your study plan with Chapter Review Quizzes and Dynamic Study Modules.

LO 1.1 1. Janice displays both high self-esteem and high self-efficacy. The dimension of health this relates to is the
   a. social dimension.
   b. emotional dimension.
   c. spiritual dimension.
   d. intellectual dimension.

LO 1.2 2. *Healthy People 2020 is*
   a. a blueprint for actions designed to improve U.S. health.
   b. a projection for life expectancy rates in the United States in the year 2020.
   c. an international plan for achieving global health priorities for the environment by the year 2020.
   d. a set of specific goals that states must achieve in order to receive federal funding for health.

LO 1.3 3. Which of the following is a *non-modifiable* determinant for health?
   a. Physical activity
   b. Genetics
   c. Nutrition
   d. Tobacco use

LO 1.5 4. Cody has decided that he needs to improve his diet. He observes his roommates' healthy meal choices and decides to adopt some of their eating habits. This is an example of which model of behavior change?
   a. Social cognitive
   b. Health belief
   c. Transtheoretical
   d. Stages of change

LO 1.6 5. Jake is exhibiting *self-efficacy* when he
   a. claims he will never be able to bench-press 125 pounds.
   b. doubts he'll ever bench-press the weight he hopes for.
   c. believes that he can and will be able to bench-press 125 pounds in his specified time frame.
   d. does not believe he possesses personal control over this situation.

LO 1.6 6. Because Craig's parents smoked, he is 90 percent more likely to start smoking than someone whose parents didn't. This is an example of what factor influencing behavior change?
   a. Circumstantial factor
   b. Enabling factor
   c. Reinforcing factor
   d. Predisposing factor

LO 1.7 7. Suppose you want to lose 20 pounds. To reach your goal, you start by counting calories. After 2 weeks, you begin an exercise program and gradually build up to your desired fitness level. What behavior change strategy are you using?
   a. Shaping
   b. Visualization
   c. Modeling
   d. Reinforcement

LO 1.7 8. What strategy is advised for an individual in the preparation stage of change?
   a. Seeking recommended readings
   b. Finding ways to maintain positive behaviors
   c. Setting realistic goals
   d. Publicly stating the desire for change

LO 1.7 9. After Kirk and Tammy pay their bills, they reward themselves by watching TV together. This type of positive reinforcement is a(n)
   a. activity reinforcer.
   b. consumable reinforcer.
   c. manipulative reinforcer.
   d. possessional reinforcer.

LO 1.7 10. Aspects of a situation that cue or stimulate a person to act in certain ways are called
   a. reinforcers.
   b. antecedents.
   c. consequences.
   d. cues to action.

LO 1.9 11. Which of the following social determinants of health contributes significantly to chronic stress?
   a. Poverty
   b. Discrimination
   c. Exposure to neighborhood violence
   d. All of the above

Answers to these questions can be found on page A-1. If you answered a question incorrectly, review the module identified by the Learning Outcome. For even more study tools, visit Mastering Health.

Think About It!

LO 1.1 **1.** How are the words *health* and *wellness* similar? What, if any, are important distinctions between these terms? What is health promotion? Disease prevention?

LO 1.2 **2.** How healthy is the U.S. population today? What factors influence today's disparities in health?

LO 1.3 **3.** Describe several factors that can affect a person's health. How do these factors affect you?

LO 1.4 **4.** Could mindfulness help you improve your academic performance this semester? If not, why not? If so, how?

LO 1.5 **5.** What is the health belief model? How may this model be working when a young woman decides to smoke her first cigarette? Her last cigarette?

LO 1.7 **6.** Using our plan for behavior change, discuss how you might act as a change agent to help a friend stop smoking. Why is it important that your friend be ready to change before trying to change?

LO 1.9–1.10 **7.** What initiatives do you think would help promote health equity in your community? On your campus?

Psychological Health

Although most college students describe their college years as among the best of their lives, many find the pressures of grades, finances, relationships, and the struggle to find themselves to be extraordinarily difficult. Psychological distress caused by relationship issues, family issues, academic competition, and adjusting to life as a college student is common. Many experts believe that the often anxiety-inducing campus environment is a major contributor to poor health decisions such as high levels of alcohol consumption and, in turn, to health problems that ultimately affect academic success and success in life.

Fortunately, even though we often face seemingly insurmountable pressures, humans are remarkably **resilient**; able to cope, adapt, and even thrive in the face of life's challenges. How we feel and think about ourselves, those around us, and our environment can tell us a lot about our psychological health and whether we are healthy emotionally, socially, spiritually, and mentally.

2.1 What Is Psychological Health?

2.1 Describe basic characteristics shared by psychologically healthy people, and identify each level in Maslow's hierarchy of needs.

Psychological health is the sum of how we think, feel, relate, and exist in our day-to-day lives. Our thoughts, perceptions, emotions, motivations, interpersonal relationships, and behaviors are the product of a combination of our experiences and the skills we have developed to meet life's challenges. Most experts identify several basic elements shared by psychologically healthy people:

- **They feel good about themselves.** They are not typically overwhelmed by fear, love, anger, jealousy, guilt, or worry. They know who they are, have a realistic sense of their capabilities, and respect themselves even though they realize that they aren't perfect.
- **They feel comfortable with other people and express respect and compassion toward others.** They enjoy satisfying and lasting personal relationships and do not take advantage of people or allow others to take advantage of them. They recognize that there are others whose needs are greater than their own and take responsibility for their fellow human beings. They can give love, consider others' interests, take time to help others, and respect personal differences.
- **They control tension and anxiety.** They recognize the underlying causes and symptoms of stress and anxiety in their lives and consciously avoid irrational thoughts, hostility, excessive excuse making, and blaming others for their problems. They use resources and learn skills to control their reactions to stressful situations.
- **They meet the demands of life.** Psychologically healthy people try to solve problems as they arise, accept responsibility, and plan ahead. They set realistic goals, think for themselves, and make independent decisions. Acknowledging that change is inevitable, they welcome new experiences.
- **They curb hate and guilt.** They acknowledge and combat tendencies to respond with anger, thoughtlessness, selfishness, vengefulness, or feelings of inadequacy. They do not try to knock other people aside to get ahead but rather reach out to help others.
- **They maintain a positive outlook.** They approach each day with a presumption that things will go well. They look to the future with enthusiasm rather than dread. Having fun and making time for themselves are integral parts of their lives.
- **They value diversity.** Psychologically healthy people do not feel threatened by people of different races, genders, religions, sexual orientations, ethnicities, or political parties. They are nonjudgmental and do not force their beliefs and values on others.
- **They appreciate and respect nature.** They take time to enjoy their surroundings, are conscious of their place in the universe, and act responsibly to preserve their environment.

Psychologists have long argued that before we can achieve any of the above characteristics of psychologically healthy people, we must have certain basic needs met in our lives. In the 1960s, psychologist Abraham Maslow developed a *hierarchy*

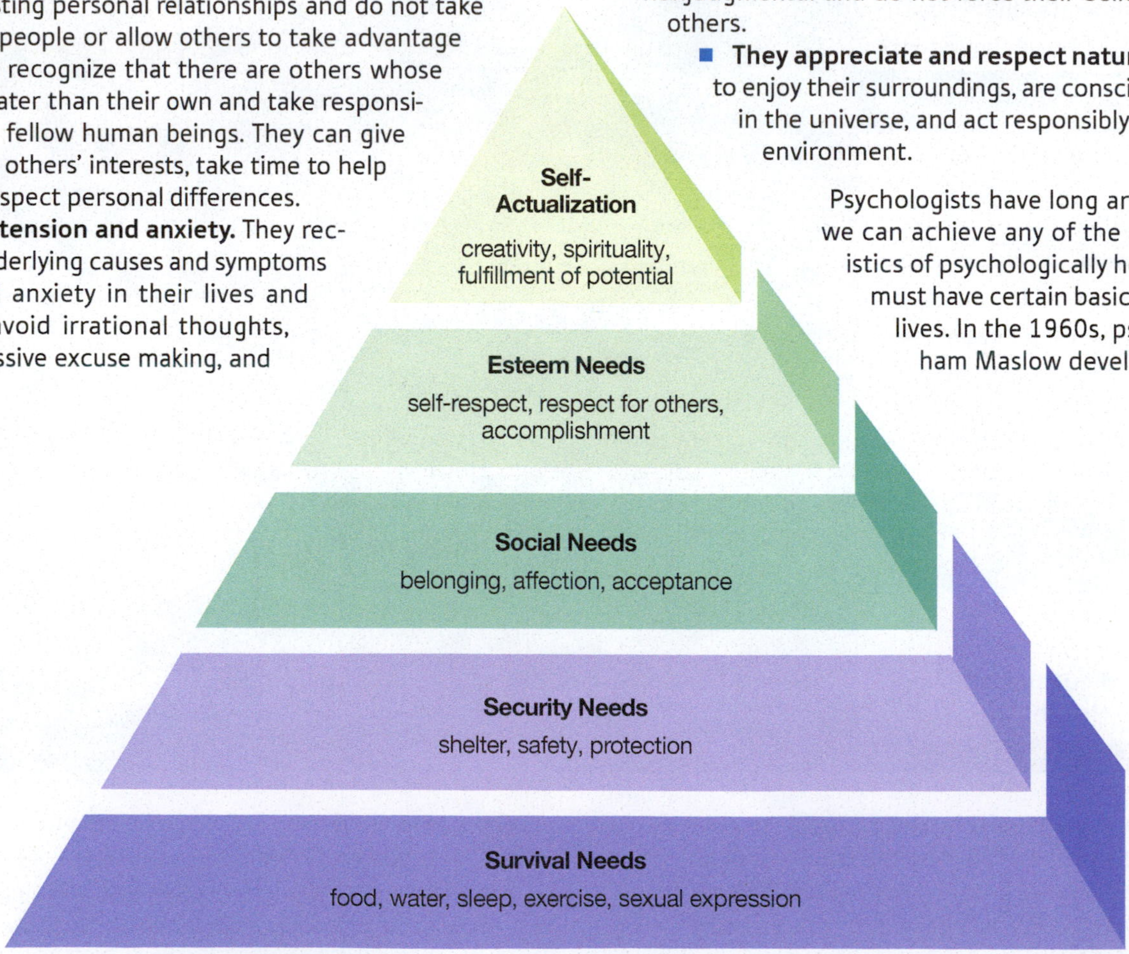

Self-Actualization
creativity, spirituality, fulfillment of potential

Esteem Needs
self-respect, respect for others, accomplishment

Social Needs
belonging, affection, acceptance

Security Needs
shelter, safety, protection

Survival Needs
food, water, sleep, exercise, sexual expression

Figure 2.1 Maslow's Hierarchy of Needs

▶ **Mastering** Health & Nutrition Maslow's Hierarchy of Needs

No zest for life; pessimistic/cynical most of the time; spiritually down

Laughs, but usually at others, has little fun

Has serious bouts of depression, "down" and tired much of time; has suicidal thoughts

A "challenge" to be around, socially isolated

Experiences many illnesses, headaches, aches/pains, gets colds/infections easily

Shows poorer coping than most, often overwhelmed by circumstances

Has regular relationship problems, finds that others often disappoint

Tends to be cynical/critical of others; tends to have negative/critical friends

Lacks focus much of the time, hard to keep intellectual acuity sharp

Quick to anger, sense of humor and fun evident less often

Works to improve in all areas, recognizes strengths and weaknesses

Healthy relationships with family and friends, capable of giving and receiving love and affection

Has strong social support, may need to work on improving social skills but usually no major problems

Has occasional emotional "dips" but overall good mental/emotional adaptors

Possesses zest for life; spiritually healthy and intellectually thriving

High energy, resilient, enjoys challenges, focused

Realistic sense of self and others, sound coping skills, open minded

Adapts to change easily, sensitive to others and environment

Has strong social support and healthy relationships with family and friends

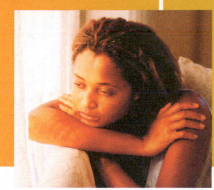

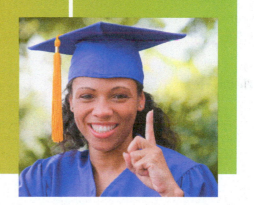

Figure 2.2 Characteristics of Psychologically Healthy and Unhealthy People
Where do you fall on this continuum?

of needs to describe this idea (**Figure 2.1**). At the bottom of his hierarchy are basic *survival needs*, such as food, sleep, water, and sexual expression. At the next level are *security needs*. Security needs include shelter, safety, and protection. *Social needs* make up the third level and include a sense of belong and affection. At the fourth level are *esteem needs*, self-respect, respect for others, and accomplishment. Finally, at the top are needs for *self-actualization* and self-transcendence.

According to Maslow's theory, a person's needs must be met at each of these levels before that person can ever truly be healthy. Failure to meet any of the lower levels of needs will interfere with a person's ability to address upper-level needs. For example, someone who is homeless or worried about threats of violence will be unable to focus on fulfilling social, esteem, or actualization needs.[1]

In sum, psychologically healthy people are emotionally, mentally, socially, and spiritually resilient. They most often respond to challenges and frustrations in appropriate ways, despite occasional slips (see **Figure 2.2**). When they do slip, they recognize that fact and take action to rectify the situation. Psychologically

unhealthy people lack this resilience. They may struggle with relationships, feel "down" much of the time, and have trouble focusing.

Attaining psychological well-being involves many complex processes. This chapter will help you understand not only what it means to be psychologically well, but also why we may run into problems in our psychological health. Learning how to assess your own health and take action to help yourself are important aspects of psychological health.

Check Yourself

- What are the basic characteristics shared by psychologically healthy people?

- What are basic characteristics of psychologically unhealthy people?

- At which level of Maslow's hierarchy of needs do you face the most challenges?

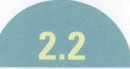

2.2 Dimensions of Psychological Health

Psychological health includes mental, emotional, social, physical, and spiritual dimensions (see **Figure 2.3**).

Mental Health

The term **mental health** is used to describe the "thinking" or "rational" dimension of our health. A mentally healthy person perceives life in realistic ways, can adapt to change, can develop rational strategies to solve problems, and can carry out personal and professional responsibilities. In addition, a mentally healthy person has the intellectual ability to learn and use information effectively and strive for continued growth. This is often referred to as *intellectual health*, a subset of mental health.[2]

Emotional Health

The term **emotional health** refers to the feeling, or subjective, side of psychological health. **Emotions** are intensified feelings or complex patterns of feelings that we experience on a regular basis, including love, hate, frustration, anxiety, and joy. Typically, emotions are described as the interplay of four components: physiological arousal, feelings, cognitive (thought) processes, and behavioral reactions. As rational beings, we are responsible for evaluating our individual emotional responses, their causes, and the appropriateness of our actions.

Emotionally healthy people usually respond appropriately to upsetting events. Rather than reacting in an extreme fashion or behaving inconsistently or offensively, they can express their feelings, communicate with others, and show emotions in appropriate ways. Emotionally unhealthy people are much more likely to let their feelings overpower them. They may be highly volatile and prone to unpredictable emotional responses, which may be followed by inappropriate communication or actions.

Emotional intelligence is the ability to identify, use, understand, and manage one's emotions in positive and constructive ways. Emotional intelligence consists of four core abilities: *self-awareness*, *self-management*, *relationship management*, and *social awareness*. Developing your emotional intelligence can help you build strong relationships, succeed at work, and achieve your goals.[3]

Emotional health also affects physical, social, and intellectual health. People who feel hostile, withdrawn, or moody may become socially isolated. Because they are not much fun to be around, friends may avoid them at the very time they are most in need of emotional support. A concern for students is the impact of emotional trauma on academic performance. Have you ever tried to study for an exam after a fight with a close friend or family member or after a sleepless night? Emotional turmoil can seriously affect your ability to think and act rationally.

Social Health

Social health includes a person's interactions with other people individually and in groups, the ability to use social resources and support in times of need, and the ability to adapt to a variety of social situations. Socially healthy individuals enjoy a wide range of interactions with family, friends, and acquaintances and are able to have healthy interactions with an intimate partner. Typically, socially healthy individuals can listen, express themselves, form healthy attachments, act in socially acceptable and responsible ways, and find the best fit for themselves in society. Studies have documented the importance of positive relationships in overall well-being and longevity.[4]

Social bonds, which reflect the level of closeness and attachment that we develop with other individuals, are the

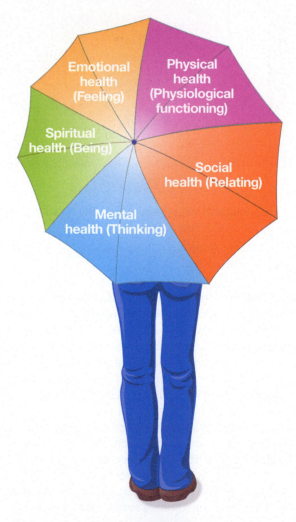

Figure 2.3 Psychological Health
Psychological health is a complex interaction of the mental, emotional, social, physical, and spiritual dimensions of health. Possessing strength and resiliency in these dimensions can maintain your overall well-being and help you weather the storms of life.

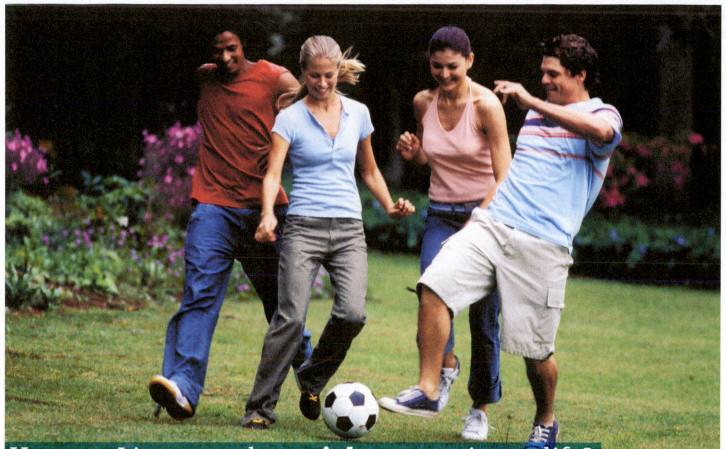

How can I increase the **social support** in my life?

Fostering a solid social support group can be as simple as spending time playing a game with friends. Physical health affects mental health, so doing something active with others is doubly beneficial.

very foundation of human life. They provide intimacy, feelings of belonging, opportunities for giving and receiving nurturance, reassurance of one's worth, assistance and guidance, and advice. Social bonds take multiple forms, the most common of which are social support and community engagements.

The concept of **social support** refers to the people and services with whom we interact and share social connections. These ties can provide *tangible support*, such as babysitting services or money to help pay the bills, or *intangible support*, such as encouraging you to share your concerns. Research shows that college students with adequate social support have higher GPAs, higher perceived ability in math and science courses, less stress and depression, less peer pressure for binge drinking, lower rates of suicide, and higher overall life satisfaction.[5]

The communities we live in can provide social support, as can religious institutions, schools—including your own campus community—clinics, public health programs and services, social services, and local businesses that work to provide support for people in need.

Spiritual Health

It is possible to be mentally, emotionally, and socially healthy and still not achieve optimal psychological well-being. What is missing?

For many people, the difficult-to-describe element that gives purpose to life is the spiritual dimension.

Spirituality is broader in meaning than religion; it goes beyond material values and can be defined as an individual's sense of purpose and meaning in life and sense of peace and connection to others and the social and physical environment.[6]

Spirituality may be practiced in many ways, including through religion; however, religion does not have to be part of a person's spiritual life. **Spiritual health** refers to the sense of belonging to something greater than the purely physical or personal dimensions of existence. For some, this unifying force is nature; for others, it is a feeling of connection to other people; for still others, the unifying force is a god or other higher power.

Check Yourself

- When you think of someone as being mentally healthy, what characteristics come to mind?

- Name the dimensions of psychological health.

- Assess your psychological health in each of the dimensions discussed here.

2.3 Factors That Influence Psychological Health

Learning Outcome

2.3 Identify factors that affect your psychological health, and describe the interaction between psychological well-being and health.

The Family

Families have a significant influence on psychological development. Healthy families model and help develop the cognitive and social skills necessary to solve problems, express emotions in socially acceptable ways, manage stress, and develop a sense of self-worth and purpose. In adulthood, family support is one of the best predictors of health and happiness.[7] Children who are brought up in **dysfunctional families**—in which there is violence, distrust, anger, dietary deprivation, drug abuse, significant parental discord, or abuse—may run an increased risk of psychological problems.[8] However, not everyone who is raised in a dysfunctional family becomes psychologically unhealthy, and not everyone from a healthy environment becomes well adjusted.

Support System

Initial social support may be provided by family, but as we develop, the support of peers becomes more and more important. We rely on friends to help us figure out who we are and what we want to do with our lives. We often bounce ideas off friends to find out whether they think we are being logical, smart, or fair. Having people in our lives who provide positive support and whom we can rely on is important to our psychological health.

Community

Our communities can affect our psychological health through collective actions. For example, neighbors may come together to pick up trash, participate in a neighborhood watch, or initiate a community picnic. You are part of a campus community, which can support psychological health by creating a safe environment in which to develop your mental, emotional, social, and spiritual dimensions.

Self-Efficacy and Self-Esteem

During our formative years, successes and failures in school, athletics, friendships, relationships, jobs, and every other aspect of life subtly shape our beliefs about our personal worth and abilities. These beliefs in turn become influences on our psychosocial health.

Self-efficacy describes a person's belief about whether he or she can successfully engage in and execute a specific behavior. Self-efficacy is a result of life experiences and our successes and failures. **Self-esteem** refers to one's sense of self-respect or self-worth. People with high levels of self-efficacy and self-esteem tend to express a positive outlook on life. However, excessive self-esteem taken to extremes might result in a narcissistic and "me first" philosophy of life that can be detrimental.

Self-esteem results from the relationships we have with our parents and family growing up; with our friends as we grow older; with our significant others as we form intimate relationships; and with our teachers, coworkers, and others throughout our lives.

Psychologist Martin Seligman proposed that people who continually experience failure may develop a pattern of responding known as **learned helplessness**, in which they give up and fail to take action to help themselves. Seligman ascribes this response in part to society's tendency toward *victimology*—blaming one's problems on other people and circumstances.[9] Although viewing ourselves as victims may make us feel better temporarily, it does not address the underlying causes of a problem. Ultimately, it can erode self-efficacy.

Your outlook on life is determined in part by your social and cultural surroundings, and your general sense of well-being can be strongly affected by the positive or negative nature of your social bonds. In particular, family members shape your psychological health. As you were growing up, they modeled behaviors and skills that helped you develop cognitively and socially. Their love and support can give you a sense of self-worth and encourage you to treat other people with compassion and care.

How do other people influence my psychological well-being?

Many self-help programs use elements of Seligman's principle of **learned optimism**—the idea that by changing our self-talk, examining our reactions, and blocking negative thoughts, we can "unlearn" negative thought processes that have become habitual.

Personality

Your personality is the unique mix of characteristics that distinguishes you from others, as influenced by heredity, environment, culture, and experience. Personality determines how we react to the challenges of life, interpret our feelings, and resolve conflicts.

Recent psychological theories promote the idea that we have the power to understand and change our behavior, thus molding our own personalities.[10] A leading personality theory distills personality into five traits[11]:

- **Agreeableness.** People who score high are trusting, likable, and demonstrate friendly compliance and love; low scorers are critical and suspicious.
- **Openness.** People who score high demonstrate curiosity, independence, and imagination; low scorers are more conventional and down-to-earth.
- **Neuroticism.** People who score high are anxious and insecure; low scorers show the ability to maintain emotional control.
- **Conscientiousness.** People who score high are dependable and demonstrate self-control, discipline, and a need to achieve; low scorers are disorganized and impulsive.
- **Extroversion.** People who score high adapt well to social situations, demonstrate assertiveness, and draw enjoyment from the company of others; low scorers are more reserved and passive.

Lifespan and Maturity

Our temperaments change as we grow, and most of us learn to control our emotions as we age. The college years mark a transition period for young adults as they move away from families and become independent. This transition is easier for those who have accomplished earlier developmental tasks such as learning how to solve problems, to make and evaluate decisions, to define and adhere to personal values, and to establish both casual and intimate relationships. People who have not fulfilled these earlier tasks may find their lives interrupted by recurrent crises left over from earlier stages. For example, those who did not learn to trust others in childhood may have difficulty establishing intimate relationships as adults.

Happiness and the Mind–Body Connection

Your emotional states can affect your overall health, especially in conditions of stress. At the core of this mind–body connection is the study of **psychoneuroimmunology (PNI)**, or how the brain and behavior affect the body's immune system.

One area of study that appears to be particularly promising in enhancing health is **positive psychology**. According to psychologist Martin Seligman, positive psychology is the scientific study of human strengths and virtues.[12] People who are described as mentally healthy have certain strengths and virtues in common:

- They have high self-esteem.
- They are realistic.

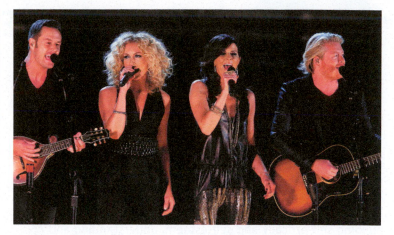

The hit song "Happy People" by country music group Little Big Town celebrates the positive elements of being happy, in sharp contrast to a world that seems to be increasingly dark.

- They value close relationships with others.
- They approach life with excitement and energy.
- They think things through and examine things from all sides.

Positive psychology interventions have proven effective in enhancing emotional, cognitive, and physical health, reducing depression, lessening disease and disability, and increasing longevity.[13]

Seligman suggests that we can develop well-being by practicing positive psychological actions. He describes five elements of well-being—**P**ositive emotion, **E**ngagement, **R**elationships, **M**eaning, and **A**ccomplishment (PERMA)—that help humans flourish.[14]

The study of **happiness**—a collective term for several positive states in which individuals actively embrace the world around them—is part of the study of positive psychology.[15] Happy people share four characteristics: *health* (knowing and partaking in healthy habits); *intimacy* (being able to enjoy the company of friends and family and to practice empathy); *resources* (possessing a certain agency over one's conditions in life); and *competence* (the knowledge of and ability to learn new skills).[16] People who experience more feelings of happiness have fewer mental health issues (depression, anxiety, and obsessive–compulsive disorders), behavioral health issues, and physical health issues (cardiovascular disease, obesity, cancer, etc.).[17] Some research, however, shows that happiness has no direct effect on mortality.[18]

Check Yourself

- What factors affect your psychological health?

- How does a person's psychological state affect his or her health?

- List three elements of happiness that help humans flourish. In thinking of your close friends and family, what characteristics about them indicate that they are happy?

2.4 Strategies to Enhance Psychological Health

2.4 Describe behavior change strategies to improve psychological health.

As we have seen, psychological health involves four dimensions. Attaining self-fulfillment is a lifelong, conscious process that involves enhancing each of these components. Strategies include building self-efficacy and self-esteem, understanding and controlling emotions, maintaining support networks, and learning to solve problems and make decisions. Try the following strategies to support and improve your own psychological health:

- **Develop a support system.** One of the best ways to promote self-esteem is through a support system of peers and others who share your values. Members of your support system can help you feel good about yourself and force you to take an honest look at your actions and choices.

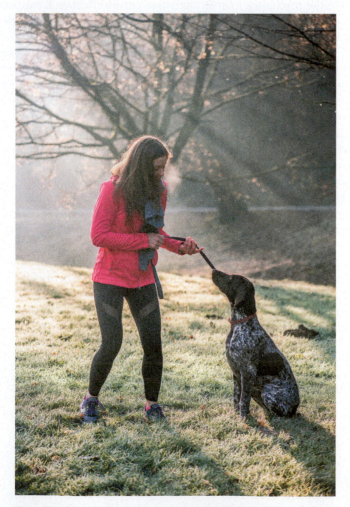

Spending time in the fresh air with your best friend is a simple thing you can do to facilitate better psychological health.

- **Complete required tasks to the best of your ability.** A good way to boost your sense of self-efficacy is to learn new skills and develop a history of success. Most college campuses provide study groups and learning centers that can help you manage time, develop study skills, and prepare for tests.
- **Form realistic expectations.** If you expect perfect grades, a steady stream of dates, and the perfect job, you may be setting yourself up for failure. Assess your current resources and the direction in which you are heading. Set small, incremental goals that you can actually meet.
- **Make time for you.** Taking time to enjoy your life is another way to boost your self-esteem and psychosocial health. View a new activity as something to look forward to and an opportunity to have fun.
- **Maintain physical health.** Regular exercise fosters a sense of well-being. More and more research supports the role of exercise in improved mental health.
- **Examine problems and seek help when necessary.** Knowing when to seek help from friends, support groups, family, or professionals is an important factor in boosting self-esteem. Sometimes you can handle life's problems alone; at other times you need assistance.
- **Get adequate sleep.** Getting enough sleep on a daily basis is a key factor in physical and psychological health. Not only do our bodies need to rest to conserve energy for our daily activities, but we also need to restore supplies of many of the neurotransmitters that we use up during our waking hours.

Skills for Behavior Change

Tips to Enhance Your Support Network and Maintain Positive Relationships

- **Keep in contact.** Call, e-mail, or visit the people you are close to. Old friends and important family members can provide a foundation of unconditional love that will help you through life transitions.
- **Lend a listening ear.** Pay attention to your friends' emotions, and be there for your friends when they're down. They'll be more likely to reciprocate for you when you're in a rough spot.
- **Make time for others.** Chatting with a classmate after class, sharing a story over coffee with a coworker, or inviting a new friend to hang out are all ways to foster lasting relationships.

Check Yourself

- Which of these strategies do you think would be most effective for you?
- List five things you think would improve the psychological health of college students today.

2.5 Define spirituality, and describe how religion and values affect spirituality.

According to UCLA's Higher Education Research Institute (HERI), many American college students share a desire to find a sense of purpose, meaning, and harmony in life.[19] Of the 1.5 million students at 1,574 colleges and universities who were surveyed as they entered college in the fall of 2015, more than 37 percent rated themselves as above average in spirituality (when asked to compare themselves to the average person their age).[20]

What Is Spirituality?

Spirituality tends to defy the boundaries that strict definitions impose. The word's root, *spirit*, in many cultures refers to *breath*, or the force that animates life. When you're "inspired," your energy flows. You're not held back by doubts about the purpose or meaning of your work and life. Indeed, many definitions of spirituality incorporate this sense of transcendence, focused on how our work and life mesh with our psychological and emotional well-being. **Spirituality** has been defined as an internal, or personal, search for meaning and answers about life, the sacred, or the transcendent,[21] whether that be a higher power or being, the essential goodness of life, or our relationship with nature or forces we cannot explain.

Spirituality and religion are not the same thing. Religion is a set of rituals, beliefs, symbols, and practices intended to enable a feeling of connection to the holy or divine, often represented by specific deities (such as God, Allah, or Buddha, among others). It is possible to be spiritual and not religious, to be religious and not spiritual, and to be both spiritual and religious. In fact, while one global survey revealed that 4 of 5 people worldwide are religiously affiliated, it also showed 16 percent (1.1 billion) are not affiliated, making them the third largest group surveyed.[22] Many people without religious affiliation still have certain religious or spiritual beliefs.[23] Research suggests that so-called Millennials, people born between roughly the years 1981 and 1996, are less likely than older Americans to say that religion is very important to them. In contrast, they were just as likely as older Americans to report the importance of spirituality.[24] One explanation for why Millennials may be less religious may be that their Baby Boomer parents taught them to think for themselves, follow their own moral compass and have a do-it-yourself-' attitude, perhaps making it less likely that they would be obedient and give power to others, including a higher being.[25] Spirituality is not bound by affiliation with a religious affiliation, ceremony, buildings, or doctrine; however individuals have the option to choose whatever path or paths allows them to find meaning and a sense of purpose in life.

Elements of Spirituality

Another definition of spirituality integrates three facets: relationships, values, and purpose in life (**Figure 2.4**).[26]

Have you ever wondered whether someone you were attracted to is right for you? Have you wished you had more friends, or that you were a better friend to yourself? Such questions about relationships are often triggers for spiritual growth. At the same time, healthy relationships are a sign of spiritual well-being. When we think well of ourselves, and consequently treat others with respect, honesty, integrity, and love, we are manifesting our spiritual health.

Our **values** are our principles—the set of fundamental rules by which we conduct our lives. When we attempt to clarify our values and to live according to them, we're engaging in spiritual work.

What career do you plan to pursue? Do you hope to marry? Do you plan to have or adopt children? What things make you feel "complete"? Contemplating such questions about one's purpose in life fosters spiritual growth. People who are spiritually healthy are able to articulate their purpose, and to make choices that manifest that purpose.

Our relationships, values, and *sense of purpose* together contribute to our overall **spiritual intelligence (SI)**. This term was introduced by physicist and philosopher Danah Zohar, who defined it as "an ability to access higher meanings, values, abiding purposes, and unconscious aspects of the self."[27] Zohar includes self-awareness, spontaneity, and compassion in her definition, explaining that SI helps us use meanings, values, and purposes to live richer and more creative lives.

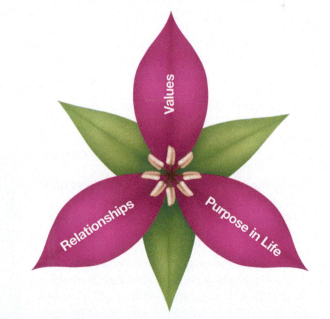

Figure 2.4 Three Facets of Spirituality
Most of us are prompted to explore our spirituality because of questions relating to our relationships, values, and purpose in life. At the same time, these three facets together constitute spiritual well-being.
Source: Data from B. L. Seaward, *Managing Stress: Principles and Strategies for Health and Well Being*, 7th ed. (Sudbury, MA: Jones and Bartlett, 2012).

▶ **Mastering** Health & Nutrition Facets of Spirituality

■ **What are some components of spirituality and spiritual intelligence?**

2.6 Why Is Spiritual Health Important?

Learning Outcome

2.6 Explain how spirituality contributes to physical and psychosocial health.

A broad range of large-scale surveys have documented the importance of the mind–body connection to human health and wellness.

Physical Benefits

The emerging science of mind–body medicine is a research focus of the National Center for Complementary and Integrative Health (NCCIH) and an important objective of the organization's *2016 Strategic Plan*. One area under study is the ways in which mind–body interventions affect well-being and general health, with specific attention to the impact on the brain and nervous system. The NCCIH is researching how these interventions (mindfulness, acupuncture, meditation, massage, etc.) can change our perceptions and control of pain, in addition to other health outcomes.[28] Increasing numbers of studies are examining the effect that certain spiritual practices, such as yoga, deep meditation, and prayer, have on the mind, the body, social and emotional health, and behavior and how these practices may improve health and promote healthy behaviors.[29]

The National Cancer Institute (NCI) contends that when we get sick, spiritual or religious well-being may help to restore health and improve our quality of life in the following ways[30]:

- Decreasing anxiety, depression, anger, discomfort, and feelings of isolation
- Decreasing alcohol and drug abuse
- Decreasing blood pressure and the risk of heart disease
- Increasing the ability to cope with the effects of illness and with medical treatments
- Increasing feelings of hope and optimism, freedom from regret, satisfaction with life, and inner peace.

Several studies show an association between spirituality and/or religion and a person's ability to cope with a variety of physical illnesses, including cancer.[31] However, other research has questioned the efficacy of many of these studies, citing small sample size and methodological issues.[32]

One recent study of over 33,000 adults found that indicators of "social capital" such as visiting friends or relatives, visiting neighbors, attending church, belonging to clubs, and attending club meetings were associated with improved biomarkers such as cholesterol and blood pressure.[33]

A review of literature found that measures of spirituality were related to biomarkers such as blood pressure, immune factors, cardiac reactivity, and the progression of disease.[34] In addition, spiritual well-being and spiritual growth have been shown to be associated with reports of overall good physical health.[35] Recent studies of college students found a relationship between personal spirituality and healthy behaviors such as physical activity, reduced alcohol use, and reduced non-suicidal self-harm behaviors.[36]

3 out of 5

entering first-year college students report that they are actively "searching for meaning and purpose in life."

Psychological Benefits

Current research also suggests that spiritual health contributes to psychological health. For instance, the NCI and independent studies have found that spirituality reduces levels of anxiety, stress, and depression.[37] In the case of student outcomes, practices that enhance spirituality may provide a protective factor against burnout. A review of meditation interventions in schools showed modest effects of meditation on student outcomes including well-being, social competence, and academic achievement.[38]

When people undergo psychological trauma, their understanding of the meaning of life can be severely challenged. Counselors

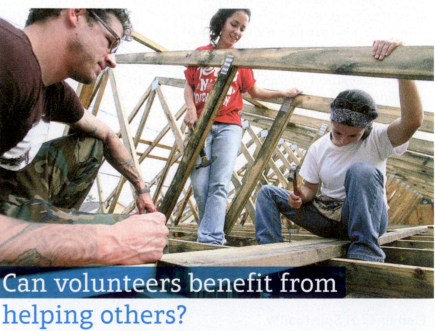

Can volunteers benefit from helping others?

Volunteering, and the associated "helper's high," can positively affect your overall health. Many students contribute their time and skills to volunteer organizations, as these students are doing by working to build homes for Habitat for Humanity.

work with trauma survivors to help them find meaning in their trauma, change their ways of thinking, and move them toward involvement in meaningful life experiences. Psychologists at the U.S. Department of Veterans Affairs have done extensive clinical work with veterans who are experiencing *posttraumatic stress disorder (PTSD)* as a result of their combat service. Research suggests that, after trauma, powerful emotions such as anger, rage, and wanting to get even are moderated, or softened, by psychological or emotional actions such as forgiveness, compassion, or the application of other spiritual beliefs and practices.[39]

People who have found a **spiritual community**—a group of people meeting together for the purpose of enriching and expanding their spirituality—also benefit from increased social support. For instance, participation in charitable organizations, religious groups, book clubs, meditation circles, social gatherings, fund-raising to help people in trouble, or spiritual learning experiences can help members think critically about their values and actions and to avoid isolation. A community may include retired members who offer childcare for working parents, support for people with addictions or mental health problems, shelter and food for the homeless, or transportation to medical appointments. Spiritually active members may volunteer or receive help from other volunteers, all of which may enhance feelings of self-worth, security, and belonging. This benefits the individual participants as well as the community as a whole.

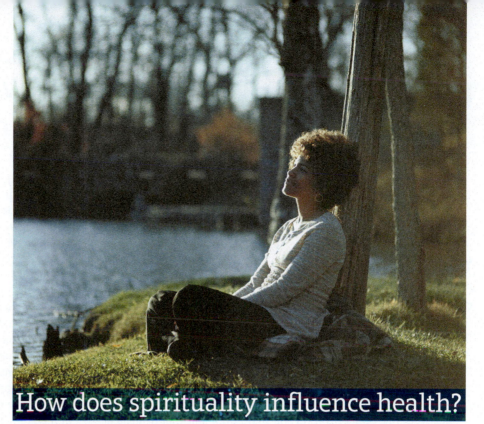

How does spirituality influence health?

Spirituality is widely acknowledged to have a positive impact on health and wellness. The benefits range from reductions in overall morbidity and mortality to improved abilities to cope with illness and stress.

Stress Reduction Benefits

The NCI also cites stress reduction as one probable mechanism among spiritually healthy people for improved health and longevity and for better coping with illness.[40] In addition, several small studies support the contention that positive religious practices aid in effective stress management.[41] Studies also suggest that increasing mindfulness through meditation reduces stress levels not only in people with physical and mental disorders, but also in healthy people.[42] For more on stress reduction, see Chapter 3.

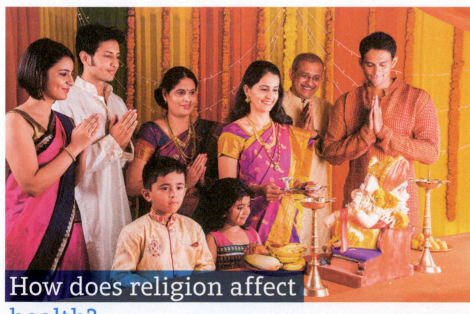

How does religion affect health?

Many people find that religious practices help them to focus on their spirituality. Spiritual well-being, including the use of prayer, can Improve the ability to cope and decrease stress.

Check Yourself

■ **List three benefits of spiritual health.**

2.7 Strategies for Cultivating Spiritual Health and Mindfulness

Tune in to Yourself and Your Surroundings

Focusing on your spiritual health can be likened to tuning in a station on a radio: Spirituality is perpetually available to us, but if we fail to tune our "receiver," we won't be able to focus through all the "static" of daily life. Four ancient practices used throughout the world can help you tune in: *contemplation*, *mindfulness*, *meditation*, and *prayer*.

Contemplation In the domain of spirituality, **contemplation** usually refers to concentrating the mind on a spiritual or ethical question or subject, a view of the natural world, or an icon or other image representative of divinity. Most religious and spiritual traditions advocate engaging in the contemplation of gratitude, forgiveness, and unconditional love. This engagement can take many forms, such as journaling or blogging.

Mindfulness A stated in chapter one, **mindfulness** is the ability to be fully present in the moment; to focus your thoughts and engage in nonjudgmental observation. Mindfulness involves "tuning in" rather than living your life worrying or on "autopilot" much of the time.[43] The range of opportunities to practice mindfulness is as infinite as the moments of our lives. Living mindfully means allowing ourselves to observe, to register what you are seeing and be wholly aware of what we are feeling in each moment (**Figure 2.5**).[44]

Meditation **Meditation** is a practice of cultivating a still or quiet mind. In many ways, meditation and mindfulness go hand in hand.

For thousands of years, humans of different cultures and traditions have found that achieving periods of meditative stillness each day enhances their spiritual health. Today, researchers are beginning to discover why.

Studies suggest that people who engage in mindfulness and compassion meditation show a significantly increased level of *empathy*—the ability to understand and share another person's experience—as well as increased levels of compassion toward others.[45] Studies also suggest that mindfulness meditation improves the brain's ability to process information; reduces stress, anxiety, and depression; reduces insomnia; improves concentration; and decreases blood pressure.[46]

New research has shown actual differences in the brain structures of experienced meditators compared to people with no history of meditation.[47] Other studies have shown mindfulness meditation to boost gray matter density in parts of the brain that are critical to learning and memory and improved psychological and emotional health, compassion, and introspection.[48] At the same time, mindfulness meditation may decrease gray matter areas of the brain that are known to play a key role in anxiety and stress.[49]

See It! Videos

Can meditation help reduce your stress and improve your grades? Watch **Meditation Becoming More Popular Among Teens** in the Study Area of Mastering Health.

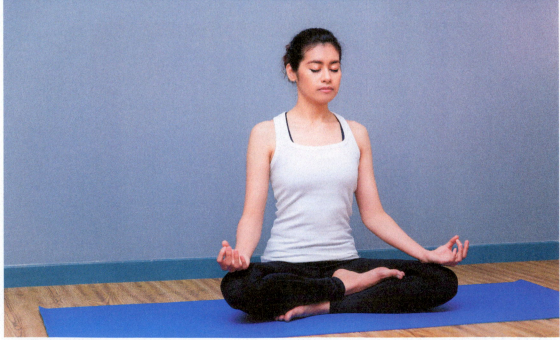

What type of meditation should I try?

Figure 2.5 Qualities of Mindfulness
Experts suggest trying different meditation techniques and picking the one that works best for you.
Source: M. Greenberg, "Nine Essential Qualities of Mindfulness," *Psychology Today*, February 22, 2012, www.psychology today.com.

Options for meditation include the following:

- **Mantra meditation.** Focus on a *mantra*, a single word such as *Om*, *Amen*, *Love*, or *God*, and repeat this word silently. When a distracting thought arises, simply set it aside. It may help to imagine the thought as a leaf, and visualize placing it on a gently flowing stream. Do not fault yourself for becoming distracted. Simply notice the thought, release it, and return to your mantra.
- **Breath meditation.** Count each breath. Pay attention to each inhalation, the brief pause that follows, and the exhalation. Together, these equal one breath. When you have counted ten breaths, return to one. As with mantra meditation, release distractions as they arise, and return to following the breath.
- **Color meditation.** When your eyes are closed, you may perceive a field of color, such as a deep, restful blue. Focus on this color. Treat distractions as in other forms of meditation.
- **Candle meditation.** With your eyes open, focus on the flame of a candle. Allow your focus to soften as you meditate on this object. Treat distractions as in the other forms of meditation.

Prayer In **prayer**, an individual focuses the mind in communication with a transcendent Presence. For many people, prayer offers a sense of comfort, a sense that we are not alone. It can be the means of expressing concern for others, for admission of transgressions, for seeking forgiveness, and for renewing hope and purpose. Focusing on the things we are grateful for can move people to look to the future with hope and give them the strength to get through the most challenging times. Research has shown that spiritual practices can improve the ability to cope and decrease stress among cancer patients.[50]

You can expand your awareness of different spiritual practices further by taking classes or involving yourself in spiritual or religious groups and/or services, joining meditation, yoga and other mindfulness practices, or studying sacred texts. In each case, evaluate the messages and ideas you encounter, and decide which practices or beliefs hold meaning for you and may be helpful to others.

Train Your Body

For thousands of years, in regions throughout the world, spiritual seekers have pursued transcendence through physical means. One of the foremost examples is the practice of **yoga**. Although many people in the West tend to picture yoga as having to do with a number of physical postures and some controlled breathing, more traditional forms also emphasize chanting, meditation, and other techniques that are believed to encourage unity with the *Atman*, or spiritual life principle of the universe.

The practices of *tai chi* or *qigong* can also increase physical activity and mental focus. With roots in Chinese medicine, both have been shown to have beneficial effects on bone health, stress, cardiopulmonary fitness, mood, balance, and quality of life.[51]

Training your body to improve your spiritual health doesn't necessarily require you to engage in a formal practice. Mindfulness *while* exercising or engaging in physical pursuits can enhance the physical benefits.

Reach Out to Others

Altruism, the giving of oneself out of genuine concern for others, is a key aspect of a spiritually healthy lifestyle. Volunteering time, donating money or other resources to a food bank or other program, and even spending an afternoon picking up litter in your neighborhood are all ways to serve others and simultaneously enhance your own spiritual and overall health. Researchers have referred to the benefits of volunteering as a "helper's high," a specific feeling connected with helping others.[52] Altruism in the form of volunteering can benefit the individual helper, the people who receive the help, and the community in which they live through increased satisfaction and interconnectedness of residents.[53]

Skills for **Behavior Change**
Finding Your Spiritual Side Through Service

Recognizing that we are all part of a greater system with responsibilities to and for others is a key part of spiritual growth. Volunteering your time and energy is a great way to connect with other people and help make the world a better place while improving your own health. Here are a few ideas:

- Offer to help elderly neighbors with lawn care or simple household repairs.
- Volunteer with Meals on Wheels, a local soup kitchen, a food bank, or another program that helps people obtain adequate food.
- Organize or participate in an after-school or summertime activity for neighborhood children.
- Participate in a highway, beach, or neighborhood cleanup; restoration of park trails and waterways; or other environmental preservation projects.
- Volunteer at the local humane society.
- Apply to become a Big Brother or Big Sister, and mentor a child who may face significant challenges or have poor role models.
- Join an organization working on a cause such as global warming or hunger, or start one yourself.
- Volunteer in a neighborhood challenged by poverty, low literacy levels, or a natural disaster. Volunteer with an organization such as Habitat for Humanity to build homes or provide other aid to developing communities.

Check Yourself

- How do physical, mental, and contemplative strategies affect spiritual health?
- What are some of the benefits of including spiritual health and mindfulness among the dimensions of health?

2.8 When Psychological Health Deteriorates

Learning Outcome

2.8 Define mental illness and discuss its prevalence.

Sometimes circumstances overwhelm us to such a degree that we need help to get back on track. Stress, anxiety, loneliness, financial upheavals, and other traumatic events can derail our coping resources, causing us to turn inward or act in ways outside the norm. Chemical imbalances, drug interactions, trauma, neurological disruptions, and other physical problems may also contribute.

Mental illnesses are disorders that disrupt thinking, feeling, moods, and behaviors, causing varying degrees of impaired functioning in daily living. They are believed to be caused by a variety of biochemical, genetic, and environmental factors.[54] Among the most common risk factors are a genetic or familial predisposition

and excessive, unresolved stress, particularly due to trauma or war or devastating natural or human-caused disaster. Changes in biochemistry due to illness, drug use, or other imbalances may trigger unusual mental disturbances. Car accidents or occupational injuries that cause physical brain trauma are among common threats to brain health. In addition, a mother's exposure to viruses or toxic chemicals while pregnant may play a part, as can having a history of child abuse or neglect.[55]

Mental illnesses can range from mild to severe and can exact a heavy toll on quality of life, both for people with the illnesses and for those who are in contact with them.

Mental disorders are common in the United States and worldwide. The basis for diagnosing mental disorders in the United States is the fifth edition of the *Diagnostic and Statistical Manual of Mental Disorders (DSM-5)*. An estimated 17.9 percent of Americans age 18 and older—just slightly under 1 in 5 adults—suffer from a diagnosable mental disorder in a given year, and nearly half of them have more than one mental illness at the same time.[56] About 5 percent, or approximately 1 in 20, suffer from a serious mental illness requiring close monitoring, residential care in many instances, and medication.[57]

Mental disorders are the leading cause of disability worldwide for people age 15–44, costing more than $464 billion annually in the United States alone.[58]

Among college students, mental health problems are growing in both number and severity.[59] The most recent National College Health Assessment survey found that approximately 38.2 percent of undergraduates reported "feeling so depressed it was difficult to function" at least once in the past year, and 10.4 percent of students reported "seriously considering attempting suicide" in the past year.[60]

In all, more than 1 in 4 college students are diagnosed or treated by a professional for a mental health issue each year.[61] Anxiety is the most common reported mental health issue (19.1 percent), with depression (15.2 percent) not far behind.[62] Although these numbers may appear alarming, it is important to note that increases in help-seeking behavior, in addition to actual increases in overall prevalence of disorders, may contribute to the available data. **Figure 2.6** shows the mental health concerns reported by American college students.

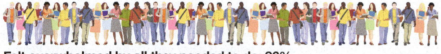

Felt overwhelmed by all they needed to do: 86%

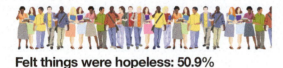

Felt things were hopeless: 50.9%

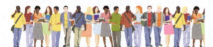

Felt so depressed that it was difficult to function: 38.2%

Seriously considered suicide: 10.4%

Intentionally injured themselves: 6.9%

Attempted suicide: 1.9%   **= 2%**

Figure 2.6 Mental Health Concerns of American College Students, Past 12 Months

Source: Data from American College Health Association, *American College Health Association, National College Health Assessment II (ACHA-NCHA II): Reference Group Data Report, Fall 2016* (Hanover, MD: American College Health Association, 2017).

Check Yourself

- **What is mental illness?**

- **Is mental illness more common or less common than you expected?**

2.9 Anxiety Disorders

Learning Outcome

2.9 **Describe common anxiety disorders and their causes.**

Anxiety disorders, are characterized by persistent feelings of threat and worry and are the largest mental health problem in the United States, affecting more than 40 million people each year. These disorders are most prevalent among 13- to 17-year-olds.[63] Approximately 19.1 percent of U.S. undergraduates report having been diagnosed with or treated for anxiety in the past year.[64]

To be diagnosed with **generalized anxiety disorder (GAD)**, the person must exhibit at least three of the following symptoms on most days during a 6-month period: restlessness or feeling keyed up or on edge, being easily fatigued, difficulty concentrating or mind going blank, irritability, muscle tension, and/or sleep disturbances.[65] GAD often runs in families and is readily treatable.

Panic disorder is characterized by **panic attacks**, acute anxiety bringing on an intense physical reaction. Approximately 9.6 percent of college students report having been diagnosed or treated for panic attacks in the last year.[66] Panic attacks and disorders are increasing in incidence, particularly among young women. Although highly treatable, panic attacks may become debilitating and socially isolating. Panic attacks typically begin abruptly, peak within 10 minutes, last about 30 minutes, and leave the person tired and drained. Symptoms include increased respiration, chills, hot flashes, shortness of breath, stomach cramps, chest pain, difficulty swallowing, and a sense of doom or impending death.[67]

Phobias, or phobic disorders, involve persistent and irrational fear of a specific object, activity, or situation, often out of proportion to circumstances. Between 5 and 12 percent of American adults suffer from specific phobias, such as fear of spiders, snakes, or riding in elevators.[68] Another 7.4 percent of American adults suffer from **social anxiety disorder**, also called *social phobia*,[69] a persistent fear and avoidance of social situations. A person with social anxiety disorder dreads these situations for fear of being humiliated, embarrassed, or perhaps even looked at. Some individuals experience difficulties only in specific situations, such as public speaking. In extreme cases, a person avoids all contact with others.

People who feel compelled to perform rituals over and over again; who are fearful of dirt or contamination; who have an unnatural concern about order, symmetry, and exactness; or who have persistent intrusive thoughts may be suffering from **obsessive-compulsive disorder (OCD)**. Approximately 1 percent of Americans age 18 and over have OCD.[70]

Unlike a perfectionist, a person with OCD often knows that the behaviors are irrational yet is powerless to stop them. Although the exact cause of OCD is unknown, genetics, biological abnormalities, learned behaviors, and environmental factors have all been considered. Symptoms of OCD usually first appear in childhood or the teen years; most people with OCD are diagnosed before age 20.[71]

People who have experienced or witnessed a natural disaster, violent assault, combat, or other traumatic event may develop **posttraumatic stress disorder (PTSD)**. Although PTSD has historically been listed as an anxiety disorder and shares many characteristics with anxiety disorders, changes in the *DSM-5* have moved PTSD to its own section of mental disorders, "Trauma and Stressor-Related Disorders." About 7 percent of Americans will experience PTSD in their lifetimes. Rates for women are twice as high as those for men.[72] Fourteen percent of U.S. combat veterans who fought in Iraq and Afghanistan have experienced PTSD.[73] However, the "worst stressful experiences" reported frequently by people with PTSD are not war-related but rather the unexpected death, illness, or injury of someone close, sexual assault, natural disasters, serious accidents, violent assault, and terrorism.[74] PTSD is not rooted in weakness or an inability to cope; traumatic events can actually cause chemical changes in the brain, leading to PTSD.[75]

Symptoms of PTSD include the following:

- Dissociation, or perceived detachment of the mind from the emotional state or even the body
- Intrusive recollections of the traumatic event—flashbacks, nightmares, or recurrent thoughts
- Acute anxiety or nervousness in which the person is hyper-aroused, may cry easily, or may experience mood swings
- Insomnia and difficulty concentrating
- Intense physiological reactions, such as shaking or nausea, when reminded of the traumatic event.

PTSD may be diagnosed if a person experiences symptoms for at least 1 month after a traumatic event. However, in some cases, symptoms don't appear until months or even years later.

Anxiety disorders vary in complexity and degree, and scientists have yet to find clear reasons why one person develops them and another doesn't. The following are cited as possible causes[76]:

- **Biology.** Positron-emission tomography (PET) scans can identify areas of the brain that react during anxiety-producing events. We may inherit tendencies toward anxiety disorders.
- **Environment.** Although genetic tendencies may exist, experiencing a repeated pattern of reaction to certain situations programs the brain to respond in a certain way. For example, if your sibling screamed whenever he saw a spider, you might react with anxiety to spiders later in life.
- **Social and cultural roles.** Because men and women are taught to assume different roles in society, women may find it more acceptable to express extreme anxiety. Men, in contrast, may learn to repress such anxieties rather than act on them.

See It! Videos

Learn about depression and ways to cope. Watch **What Are the Causes for Depression?** in the Study Area of Mastering Health.

Check Yourself

- **What are the most common anxiety disorders?**

2.10 Describe common mood disorders and their causes.

Chronic mood disorders are disorders that affect how you feel. In any given year, approximately 10 percent of Americans age 18 or older suffer from a mood disorder.[77]

Major Depression

Major depression or *clinical depression* is the most common mood disorder, affecting approximately 9 percent of the U.S. population in a given year.[78] Major depression is characterized by a combination of behavioral and emotional symptoms that may interfere with work, study, sleep, appetite, relationships, and enjoyment of life. Symptoms can last for weeks, months, or years and may vary in intensity.[79] Sadness and despair are the main symptoms of depression.[80] Examples of symptoms may include the following:

- Loss of motivation or interest in pleasurable activities
- Preoccupation with failures and inadequacies
- Difficulty concentrating, indecisiveness, memory lapses
- Loss of sex drive or interest in close interactions with others
- Fatigue and loss of energy, slow reactions
- Sleeping too much or too little, insomnia
- Feeling agitated, worthless, or hopeless
- Withdrawal from friends and family
- Diminished or increased appetite
- Significant weight loss or gain
- Recurring thoughts that life isn't worth living, thoughts of death or suicide.

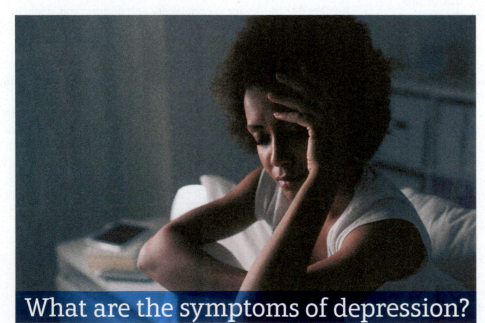

What are the symptoms of depression?

There is more to depression than simply feeling blue. A person who is clinically depressed finds it difficult to function, sometimes struggling just to get out of bed in the morning or to follow a conversation.

Depression in College Students Depression can be a major obstacle to healthy adjustment and success in college. In a recent survey by the American College Health Association, 15.4 percent of college students reported that depression had had a serious impact on their academic performance in the past 12 months.[81]

Being far from home can exacerbate problems and make coping difficult. International students are particularly vulnerable to depression and other mental health concerns. Most campuses have counseling centers, cultural centers, and other services available, though many students do not use them because of persistent stigma.

Other Mood Disorders

Persistent depressive disorder (PDD), formerly called *dysthymic disorder* or *dysthymia*, is a less severe form of chronic mild depression. Individuals with PDD may appear to function well but may lack energy or may fatigue easily; may be short-tempered, overly pessimistic, and ornery; or may not feel quite up to par without any significant overt symptoms. People with PDD may cycle into major depression over time. For a diagnosis, symptoms must persist for at least 2 years in adults or 1 year in children. This disorder affects approximately 1.5 percent of the adult population in the United States in a given year.[82]

People with **bipolar disorder**, also called *manic-depressive illness*, often have severe mood swings, ranging from extreme highs (mania) to extreme lows (depression). Swings can be dramatic and rapid or more gradual. When in the manic phase, people may be overactive, be talkative, and have tons of energy; in the depressed phase, they may experience symptoms of major depression.

Although the cause of bipolar disorder is unknown, biological, genetic, and environmental factors, such as drug abuse and stressful or psychologically traumatic events, seem to be triggers. Once diagnosed, people with bipolar disorder have several counseling and pharmaceutical options; most can live a healthy, functional life while being treated. In the United States, bipolar disorder affects approximately 2.6 percent of adults and 11.2 percent of 13- to 18-year-olds.[83]

Seasonal affective disorder (SAD) strikes during the winter and is associated with reduced exposure to sunlight. People with SAD suffer from irritability, apathy, carbohydrate craving and weight gain, increased sleep, and general sadness. Several factors are implicated in the development of SAD, including disruption in the body's natural circadian rhythms and changes in levels of the hormone melatonin and the brain chemical serotonin.[84] Over 500,000 people in the United States suffer from SAD. Nearly three-fourths of those with SAD are women in early adulthood, particularly those living at high latitudes with long winter nights.[85]

The most beneficial treatment for SAD is light therapy, using lamps that simulate sunlight. Other treatments include diet change, increased exercise, stress management, sleep restriction (limiting hours slept in a 24-hour period), psychotherapy, and prescription medications.

Causes of Mood Disorders

Mood disorders are caused by multiple factors, including biological differences, hormones, inherited traits, life events, and early childhood trauma.[86] The biology of mood disorders is related to levels of brain chemicals called *neurotransmitters*. Several types of depression, including bipolar disorder, appear to have a genetic component. Depression can also be triggered by serious loss, difficult relationships, financial problems, and pressure to succeed. Early trauma, such as loss of a parent, may cause permanent changes in the brain, making the person more prone to depression. Research has also shown that changes in physical health can be accompanied by mental changes, particularly depression. Stroke, heart attack, cancer, Parkinson's disease, chronic pain, diabetes, certain medications, alcohol, hormonal disorders, and a range of other afflictions can trigger depression.

Depression across Gender, Age, and Ethnicity

Although depression affects a wide range of people, it does not always manifest itself in the same way across populations. Women are almost twice as likely to experience depression as men are, partially as a result of hormonal changes. However, attributing depression to hormones alone would ignore the many other factors in women's lives that increase their risk for depression. Women often face stressors related to multiple responsibilities—work, childrearing, single parenthood, household work, and elder care—at rates higher than those of men. These responsibilities can lead to sleep deprivation, interference with social life and exercise, and questions about success in life. Unintended pregnancy and postpartum depression, violence and abuse in the home, and issues with career, control, and other issues can also lead to depression. Researchers have observed gender differences in coping strategies (responses to certain events or stimuli) and have proposed that some women's strategies make them more vulnerable to depression.[87]

Depression in men is often masked by alcohol or drug abuse or by the socially acceptable habit of working excessively. Typically, depressed men present as irritable, angry, and discouraged. Work problems, money problems, relationship problems, loss, and a host of other problems may lead to depression in men. Men who are depressed are four times more likely than men who are not depressed to commit suicide. Men are less likely to admit that they are depressed and view depression as a weakness to even talk about it. Therefore, doctors are less likely to suspect it. Depression is associated with increased risk of heart disease in both men and women but with a higher risk of death by heart disease in men.[88]

Depression affects nearly 3 percent of children in the United States. Boys have more depression up until age 10, and girls have higher rates after age 16. Between ages 12 and 17, rates of depression soar, and nearly 13 percent of adolescents are depressed. Other conditions such as bipolar disorder, attention-deficit disorder, and obsessive-compulsive behaviors may mask underlying depression for years. Depressed youth may have difficulties in school, sleep incessantly, and engage in self-mutilation and/or drug use and other behaviors. They may be antisocial and lonely. Depressed people have a suicide rate that is 12 times that of their nondepressed peers.

Before adolescence, boys experience more suicide before age 10, after which rates level off for a period. After age 16, girls experience more depression. As in their adult counterparts, causes of depression may be due to a wide range of social and environmental situations. Issues of self-esteem and fitting in, perceptions of success and approval, and increased risk of trauma from childhood sexual abuse, poverty, and drugs and violence in the home increase risk.[89]

Depression among older adults is a major problem, and only 10 percent of cases are diagnosed and treated. Uninsured people with low incomes are particularly vulnerable and have little access to resources. Symptoms of depression may be mistaken for dementia or other problems, and medications given to these individuals may exacerbate depression. Suicide rates among older adult men are higher than the rates in the general population.[90]

Rates of depression are higher among African Americans and Latinos than among Whites. However, true rates among minority populations are difficult to determine because members of these groups may have difficulty accessing mental health services because of economic barriers, social and cultural differences, language barriers, and lack of culturally competent providers. African American males, specifically, may avoid professional help because of the stigma attached to mental illness in the African American community as well as greater distrust of physicians and poor patient-physician communication. Data indicate that African Americans who do report depression symptoms to a health care provider are significantly less likely to receive a depression diagnosis than are non-Hispanic Whites, and those who are diagnosed are less likely to be treated for depression.[91]

Skills for **Behavior Change**

Dealing With and Defeating Depression

If you think you might have depression symptoms, make an appointment with a counselor. Depression is often a biological condition that you can't just "get over" on your own. You may need talk therapy, sometimes combined with antidepressant medication, to help you reach a place where you can play a greater role in getting well. Once you've started along a path of therapy and healing, these strategies may help you feel better faster:

- Be realistic and set appropriate personal goals.
- Break large tasks into small ones, set priorities, and do what you can as you can.
- Try to be with other people and to confide in someone.
- Mild exercise and religious or social activities may help.
- Try meditation, yoga, tai chi, or another mind–body practice. These disciplines can help you connect with your feelings, release tension, and clear your mind.
- Expect your mood to improve gradually, not immediately.
- Before deciding to make a significant transition, change jobs, or get married or divorced, discuss the situation with people who know you well.
- Let family and friends help you.
- Continue working with your counselor. If he or she isn't helpful, look for another.

Check Yourself

- What are the most common mood disorders?
- What are causes of mood disorders?

Other Psychological Disorders

2.11 Describe personality disorders, schizophrenia, learning disabilities, and neurodevelopmental disorders.

Personality Disorders

A **personality disorder** is an "enduring pattern of inner experience and behavior that deviates markedly from the expectation of the individual's culture and is pervasive and inflexible."[92] People dealing with individuals who suffer from personality disorders often find interactions with these individuals challenging and sometimes destructive.

Paranoid personality disorder involves pervasive, unfounded mistrust of others; irrational jealousy; and secretiveness, often with delusions of being persecuted. *Narcissistic personality disorders* involve an exaggerated sense of self-importance and self-absorption; sufferers are overly needy and demanding and feel "entitled" to nothing but the best. *Antisocial personality disorders* involve a long-term pattern of manipulation and taking advantage of others. Symptoms include disregard for others' safety, arrogance, anger, and lack of remorse. Men with antisocial personality disorder far outnumber women.[94]

Borderline personality disorder (BPD) is characterized by severe emotional instability, impulsiveness, mood swings, and poor

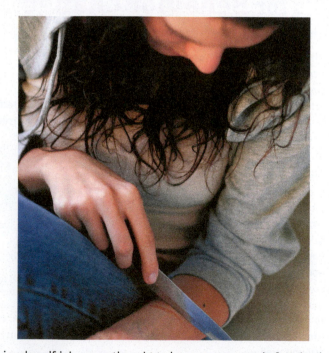

Previously, self-injury was thought to be more common in females, but recent research indicates that rates are generally the same for men and women, with 6.9 percent of college students engaged in self-injury in the last year.

Source: Data from American College Health Association, *American College Health Association, National College Health Assessment II (ACHA-NCHA II): Reference Group Data Report, Fall 2016* (Hanover, MD: American College Health Association, 2017).

self-image,[95] and erratic and risky behaviors, including gambling, unsafe sex, illicit drug use, and daredevil driving.[96] The symptoms of BPD usually appear during adolescence or early adulthood.[97] Many people with BPD engage in **self-injury**, or deliberately causing harm to one's own body, such as by cutting or burning, to cope with their emotions.[98] Many people who inflict self-harm suffer from other mental health conditions and have experienced abuse as children or adults. If you or someone you know is engaging in self-injury, seek professional help.[99]

Schizophrenia

Schizophrenia is a severe psychological disorder that affects about 1 percent of the U.S. population.[100] Schizophrenia is characterized by alterations of the senses (including auditory and visual hallucinations); the inability to sort out incoming stimuli and make appropriate responses; an altered sense of self; and radical changes in emotions, movements, and behaviors. Typical symptoms include fluctuating courses of delusional behavior, hallucinations, incoherent and rambling speech, inability to think logically, erratic movement, odd gesturing, and difficulty with activities of daily living.[101] Symptoms usually appear in men during the late teen years and twenties, while women generally present symptoms in their late twenties and early thirties.[102]

Schizophrenia is a biological disease, perhaps caused by brain damage that occurs as early as the second trimester of fetal development. At present, it is treatable but not curable. With medication, support, and therapy, many schizophrenics lead normal lives.

Learning Disabilities and Neurodevelopmental Disorders

Learning disabilities and neurodevelopmental disorders are brain-based disorders that are not mental illnesses.

Attention-deficit/hyperactivity disorder (ADHD) is a learning disability usually associated with school-age children, but symptoms may persist into adulthood. People with ADHD and attention-deficit disorder (ADD) are distracted much of the time and find concentrating and organizing things difficult.

Dyslexia, a language-based learning disorder, can pose problems in reading, writing, and spelling. Less known but equally challenging are *dyscalculia* (a learning disability involving mathematics) and *dysgraphia* (a learning disability involving writing).

Autism spectrum disorder (ASD) is a neurodevelopmental disorder (an impairment in brain development). People with ASD will continue to learn and grow intellectually throughout their lives but struggle to master communication and social behavior skills.

- What are causes of personality disorders, schizophrenia, learning disabilities, and neurodevelopmental disorders?

Psychological Health through the Lifespan: Successful Aging

2.12 Describe psychological conditions associated with aging, and explain the impact of loss on psychological health.

Most older adults lead healthy, fulfilling lives. However, some older people do suffer from mental and emotional disturbances.

Depression

Depression is the most common psychological problem among older adults, though the rate of major depression is lower in older adults than in younger adults. Regardless of age, people who have a poor perception of their health, have multiple chronic illnesses, take many medications, abuse alcohol and other drugs, lack social support, and do not exercise face more challenges that may require emotional strength.

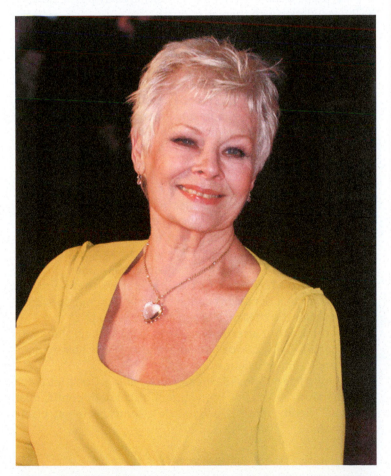

The people we often think of as aging gracefully—such as actress Dame Judi Dench—are those who continue to be active and productive; who are not frightened or ashamed of growing older; who adapt to the changing circumstances of their lives; and who strive to be healthy, vibrant, and alive at any age.

Dementia

Memory failure, errors in judgment, disorientation, and erratic behavior can occur at any age and for various reasons. The term *dementing diseases*, or **dementias**, are used to describe either reversible symptoms or progressive forms of brain malfunctioning.

One of the most common dementias is **Alzheimer's disease (AD)**. Affecting an estimated 1 in 10 Americans over the age of 65 (5.5 million),[103] this incurable disease kills its victims gradually, first through slow loss of personhood (memory loss, disorientation, personality changes, and eventual loss of independent functioning) and then through deterioration of body systems.

Patients with AD live for an average of 4 to 6 years after diagnosis, although they may continue to live for up to 20 years.[104] Although often associated with older adults, AD has been diagnosed in people in their forties. In AD, areas of the brain that affect memory, speech, and personality develop "tangles" that impair nerve cell communication, causing cell death. It progresses in stages marked by increasingly impaired memory and judgment. In later stages, many patients become depressed, combative, and aggressive. In the final stage, the person becomes dependent on others; loss of identity and speech problems are common. Eventually, control of bodily functions may be lost.

Researchers are investigating possible causes of Alzheimer's disease, including genetic predisposition, immune malfunction, a slow-acting virus, chromosomal or genetic defects, chronic inflammation, uncontrolled hypertension, and neurotransmitter imbalance. No treatment can stop AD, but medications can slow or relieve some symptoms.

Coping with Loss

Coping with the loss of a loved one is extremely difficult. Understanding feelings and behaviors related to death can help you comprehend the emotional processes associated with it.

Bereavement is the loss or deprivation a survivor experiences when a loved one dies. In the lives of the bereaved or of close survivors, the loss of loved ones leaves "holes" and inevitable changes. Loneliness and despair may envelop survivors. Understanding of these normal reactions, time, patience, and support from loved ones can help the bereaved person heal and move on.

Grief occurs in reaction to significant loss, including one's own impending death, the death of a loved one, or a loss (such as the end of a relationship or job) involving separation or change in identity. Grief may be a mental, physical, social, or emotional reaction, and it often includes changes in eating, sleeping, working, and even thinking. Symptoms vary in severity and duration. However, the bereaved person can benefit from emotional and social support.

- **What are three particular psychological issues associated with aging?**

2.13 When Psychological Problems Become Too Much: Suicide

Learning Outcome

2.13 **Identify warning signs associated with suicide, and discuss strategies for suicide prevention.**

Suicide is the second leading cause of death both for 15- to 19-year-olds and for 20- to 24-year-olds.[105] According to the 2016 *National College Health Assessment*, approximately 9 percent of students have seriously considered suicide at some point in their life, and 1 percent have attempted to kill themselves in the past year.[106] However, young adults who do not attend college are also at risk; in fact, suicide rates for young adults are higher in the general population than among college students.[107]

Risk factors include a family history of suicide, previous suicide attempts, excessive drug and alcohol use, prolonged depression, financial difficulties, serious illness in oneself or a loved one, and loss of a loved one. Lesbian, gay, bisexual, and transgender (LGBT) people are significantly more likely to have thought about or attempted suicide than their heterosexual counterparts, transgender individuals having the highest rates.[108]

Whether men are more likely to attempt suicide than women or are more often successful, nearly four times as many men die by suicide as women.[109] The most commonly used method of suicide among men is firearms; for women, the most common method is poisoning.[110]

Warning Signs

People who commit suicide usually indicate their intentions, although other people do not always recognize their warnings.[111]

If you notice warning signs of suicide in someone you know, it is imperative that you take action.

Anyone who expresses a desire to kill himself or herself or who has made an attempt is at risk. Common signs a person may be contemplating suicide include the following:[112]

- Recent loss and a seeming inability to let go of grief
- History of depression
- Change in personality—withdrawal, irritability, anxiety, tiredness, apathy
- Change in behavior—inability to concentrate, loss of interest in classes or work, unexplained demonstration of happiness following a period of depression
- Sexual dysfunction or diminished sexual interest
- Expressions of self-hatred and excessive risk-taking
- Change in sleep or eating habits or in appearance
- A direct statement such as "I might as well end it all"
- An indirect statement such as "You won't have to worry about me anymore"
- Final preparations: writing a will or giving away possessions
- Preoccupation with themes of death.

Preventing Suicide

Most people who attempt suicide want to live but see death as the only way out of an intolerable situation. Crisis counselors and suicide hotlines may help temporarily, but the best prevention is to get rid of conditions and substances that may precipitate attempts, including alcohol, drugs, isolation, and access to guns. If someone you know displays warning signs of doing so, do the following[113]:

- **Monitor signals.** Ensure that there is someone around the person as often as possible. Don't leave him or her alone.
- **Take threats seriously.** Don't brush threats off as "just talk."
- **Tell the person you can and want to help.**
- **Ask directly.** Ask the person, "Are you thinking of hurting or killing yourself?" Ask whether the person has a plan.
- **Don't belittle feelings.** Don't tell the person that he or she doesn't mean it or couldn't commit suicide. To some, such comments offer the challenge of proving you wrong.
- **Help think about alternatives.** Offer to go for help along with the person. Call a suicide hotline, and use all available community and campus resources.
- **Tell your friend's loved ones or counselor.** Don't let a suicidal friend talk you into keeping your discussions confidential. If your friend succeeds in a suicide attempt, you may blame yourself.

Check Yourself

- **What are five warning signs that someone may be contemplating suicide?**

2.14 Seeking Professional Help: Mindfulness, Therapy, and Medication

Learning Outcome

2.14 Recognize feelings and behaviors that may warrant seeking help from a mental health professional, and describe possible treatment options, including mindfulness therapies.

A physical ailment will readily send most people to the nearest health professional, but many people resist seeking help for psychological problems. Although about 20 percent of adults have some kind of mental disorder, only 13 percent of adults use mental health counseling services.[114] Consider seeking help in the following situations:

- You feel that you need help or feel out of control.
- You experience wild mood swings or inappropriate responses to normal stimuli.
- Your fears or feelings of guilt distract you.
- You have hallucinations.
- You feel worthless or feel that life is not worth living.
- Your life seems to be nothing but a series of crises.
- You are considering suicide.
- You turn to drugs or alcohol to escape.

Common misconceptions about people with mental illness are that they are dangerous, are irresponsible, or "need to get over it." The stigma of mental illness often leads to shame and isolation. Many people with mental illness report that the stigma was more disabling at times than the illness itself.[115]

If you're considering treatment for a psychological problem, first see a health professional for a checkup to rule out any physical causes for your symptoms.

Types of Mental Health Professionals

Mental health professionals include psychiatrists, psychologists, social workers, counselors, psychoanalysts, and licensed marriage and family therapists. When choosing a therapist, the most important criterion is whether you feel that you can work with this person. Here are questions to ask:

- Can you interview the therapist before starting treatment?
- Do you like the therapist? Can you talk to him or her comfortably?
- Does the therapist demonstrate professionalism? Be concerned if your therapist frequently breaks appointments, suggests outside social interaction, talks inappropriately about himself or herself, has questionable billing practices, or resists releasing you from therapy.
- Will the therapist help you set goals to work on between sessions?

Types of Therapy

Counseling options include individual or group therapy. *Psychodynamic therapy* focuses on the psychological roots of emotional suffering.[116] *Interpersonal therapy* focuses on social roles and relationships.[117] *Cognitive therapy* focuses on the impact of thoughts and ideas on feelings and behavior, and *behavioral therapy* focuses on what we do.[118]

Mindfulness Therapies

Mindfulness training, such as mindfulness-based stress reduction (MBSR) and mindfulness-based cognitive therapy (MBCT), show promising results for treating anxiety and depression. Mindfulness-based therapies emphasize acceptance of the present moment without ruminating over past events or catastrophizing over future events.

A recent study found mindfulness-based therapy just as effective as traditional therapy for treating anxiety and depression. Mindfulness-based therapy may be less expensive and easier to implement than more traditional therapies. It may also be helpful for individuals whose symptoms do not respond to medications.[119]

Pharmacological Treatment

Drug therapy can be important in the treatment of many psychological disorders. However, the medications aren't without side effects and contraindications. For example, the U.S. Food and Drug Administration requires warning labels on antidepressant medications about suicidal thinking and behavior in people age 18 to 24.[120]

Talk to your health care provider to understand the risks and benefits of any medication prescribed; tell your doctor of any adverse effects. With some therapies, such as antidepressants, you might not feel effects for several weeks. Finally, compliance with your doctor's recommendations for beginning or ending a course of any medication is very important.

See It! Videos

When should you consider professional psychological help? Watch **Psychological Disorders** in the Study Area of Mastering Health.

Check Yourself

- Give four examples of feelings and behaviors that may warrant seeking help from a mental health professional.

- What are some advantages and disadvantages of the various treatment options described?

Summary

LO 2.1 Psychological health is the sum of how we think, feel, relate, and exist in our daily lives.

LO 2.2 Mental, emotional, social, and spiritual dimensions are all components of psychological health.

LO 2.3 Many factors influence psychological health, including life experiences, family, the environment, other people, self-esteem, self-efficacy, and personality.

LO 2.3 The mind–body connection is an important link in overall health and well-being. Positive psychology emphasizes happiness as a key factor in determining overall reaction to life's challenges.

LO 2.4 Developing self-esteem and self-efficacy, making healthy connections, having a positive outlook, and maintaining physical health enhance psychological health.

LO 2.5-2.6 Spirituality is having a purpose and meaning in life that's guided by values. Spirituality is distinct from religion and has numerous physical and psychological benefits.

LO 2.7 Practicing mindfulness, meditation, yoga, prayer, and altruism can all contribute to spiritual health.

LO 2.8-2.9 Anxiety disorders include generalized anxiety disorder, panic disorder, phobic disorders, obsessive-compulsive disorder. Posttraumatic stress disorder shares many characteristics with anxiety disorders but is classified separately.

LO 2.8, 2.10 Mood disorders include major depression, persistent depressive disorder, bipolar disorder, and seasonal affective disorder. College is a high-risk time for developing depression or anxiety disorders because of high stress levels, pressures for grades, and financial problems, among others.

LO 2.11 Other psychological disorders include personality disorders, schizophrenia, and learning disabilities and neurodevelopmental disorders.

LO 2.12 Aging changes the mind in many ways. Potential mental problems include depression and Alzheimer's disease.

LO 2.12 Grief is the state of distress felt after a significant loss. People differ in their responses to grief.

LO 2.13 Suicide is a result of negative psychosocial reactions to life. People who intend to commit suicide often give signs of their intentions. Such people can often be helped.

LO 2.14 Mental health professionals include psychiatrists, psychoanalysts, psychologists, social workers, and counselors. Many therapy methods exist, including psychodynamic, interpersonal, cognitive, behavioral, and mindfulness therapies.

Pop Quiz

Visit Mastering Health to personalize your study plan with Chapter Review Quizzes and Dynamic Study Modules.

LO 2.2 **1.** The term that most accurately refers to the feeling or subjective side of psychological health is
a. social health.
b. mental health.
c. emotional health.
d. spiritual health.

LO 2.3 **2.** A person with high self-esteem
a. possesses feelings of self-respect and self-worth.
b. believes that he or she can successfully engage in a specific behavior.
c. believes that external influences shape psychosocial health.
d. has a high capacity for altruism.

LO 2.3 **3.** All the following traits have been identified as being related to psychological well-being *except*
a. conscientiousness.
b. introversion.
c. openness to experience.
d. agreeableness.

LO 2.3 **4.** In Seligman's theories of positive psychology, PERMA refers to
a. the five elements of well-being.
b. the permanent components of one's personality.
c. the permanent presence of positive emotions.
d. a psychological disorder.

LO 2.3 **5.** People who have experienced repeated failures at the same task may eventually quit trying altogether. This pattern of behavior is termed
a. posttraumatic stress disorder.
b. learned helplessness.
c. self-efficacy.
d. introversion.

LO 2.7 **6.** Kayla is a diver who enjoys the deep concentration needed to perform perfect spring dives. She is engaging in which aspect of spiritual health?
a. Altruism   c. Meditation
b. Mindfulness   d. Contemplation

LO 2.9 **7.** The disorder characterized by a need to perform rituals over and over is
a. personality disorder.
b. obsessive-compulsive disorder.
c. phobic disorder.
d. posttraumatic stress disorder.

LO 2.9 **8.** What is the number one mental health problem in the U.S.A.?
a. Depression
b. Anxiety disorders
c. Alcohol dependence
d. Schizophrenia

LO 2.10 **9.** Every winter, Jose suffers from irritability, apathy, weight gain, and sadness. He most likely has
a. panic disorder.
b. generalized anxiety disorder.
c. seasonal affective disorder.
d. chronic mood disorder.

LO 2.12 **10.** Which of the following statements is *correct*?
a. Depression is a significant mental health problem affecting people from youth through older age.
b. Although depression is a major problem for older adults, it is often misdiagnosed or underdiagnosed, and only about 10 percent of older adults are diagnosed and treated.
c. Mindfulness-based therapy has been shown to be as effective as traditional cognitive-based therapies for depression and anxiety.
d. All of the above are correct.

Answers to these questions can be found on page A-1. If you answered a question incorrectly, review the module identified by the Learning Outcome. For even more study tools, visit Mastering Health.

Think About It!

LO 2.1 **1.** What is psychological health? What indicates that a person is or is not psychologically healthy? Why might the college environment provide a challenge to psychological health?

LO 2.2 **2.** Which psychological dimensions do you need to work on? Which are most important to you, and why? What actions can you take today?

LO 2.3 **3.** Consider the factors that influence your overall level of psychological health. Which factors can you change? Which ones may be more difficult to change?

LO 2.8 2.11 **4.** What proportion of the student population suffers from some type of mental illness? What type of support networks exist on your campus?

LO 2.9 2.10 **5.** What are the symptoms of anxiety disorders? Panic attacks? Major depression? What are risk factors for each and how are they treated?

LO 2.13 **6.** What are the warning signs of suicide? Why are some people more vulnerable to suicide than others? What could you do if you heard a classmate say to no one in particular that he was going to "do the world a favor and end it all"?

LO 2.14 **7.** Describe the various types of mental health professionals and types of therapies. If you felt depressed about breaking off a long-term relationship, which professional and which therapy do you think would be most beneficial to you?

Stress

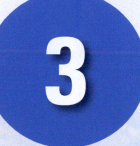

3

ASSESS YOURSELF: What's Your Stress Level? Find out in the Study Area at **Mastering** Health.

In today's fast-paced, 24/7-connected world, stress can cause us to feel overwhelmed and can zap our energy. It can also encourage us to push ourselves to improve performance, it can bring excitement, and it can help us thrive. Chronic stress is a growing public health crisis among people of all ages. According to recent American Psychological Association studies, the health care system is not giving Americans the support they need to cope with stress and build healthy lifestyles.[1] Here are some key findings:

- Americans consistently report high stress levels (20% report extreme stress), and teenagers are reporting stress levels on a par with those of adults.
- Lower-income populations, Blacks and Latinos, Millennials, Gen-Xers, and women are among those likely to report higher levels of stress.
- Only about half of all teens say they feel confident in their ability to handle personal problems.

Both men and women report above-average levels of stress, but women are more likely to report stress levels that are on the rise and more extreme.[2] Women are also more likely to report experiencing negative stress symptoms that affect their eating habits and prevent them from making lifestyle changes.[3] Additionally, although men may recognize and report stress, they are much less likely to take action to reduce it.[4]

3.1 What Is Stress?

Most current definitions state that **stress** is the mental and physical response and adaptation by our bodies to the real or perceived changes and challenges in our lives. A **stressor** is any real or perceived physical, social, environmental, or psychological event or stimulus that strains our abilities to cope.

Several factors influence one's response to stressors, including the *characteristics of the stressor* (Can you control it? Is it predictable? Does it occur often?); *biological factors* (e.g., your age or gender); and *past experiences or fears* (e.g., things that have happened to you, their consequences, and how you responded). Stressors may be *tangible*, such as a failing grade on a test, or *intangible*, such as the angst associated with meeting your significant other's parents for the first time.

Distress, or negative stress, is more likely to occur when you are tired, under the influence of alcohol or other drugs, or coping with an illness, financial trouble, or relationship problems. In contrast, **eustress**, or positive stress, presents the opportunity for personal growth and satisfaction and can actually improve health. It can energize you, motivate you, and raise you up when you are down. Getting married or winning a major competition can give rise to the pleasurable rush associated with eustress.

There are several types of stress. **Acute stress** is typically intense, flares quickly, and disappears quickly. Seeing your crush could cause your heart to race and your muscles to tense while you appear cool, calm, and collected. Or anticipating a class presentation could cause shaking hands, nausea, headache, cramping, or diarrhea, along with a galloping heartbeat, stammering, and forgetfulness.

Episodic acute stress is the state of *regularly* reacting with wild, acute stress to various situations. Individuals experiencing episodic acute stress may complain about all they have to do and focus on negative events that may or may not occur. These "awfulizers" are often reactive and anxious, but their thoughts and behaviors can be so habitual that to them they seem normal.

Although **chronic stress** may not feel as intense, it can linger indefinitely and wreak silent havoc on your body's systems. Caregivers are especially vulnerable to prolonged physiological stress as they watch a loved one struggle with a major disease or disability.

When a loved one dies, survivors may struggle to balance the need to process anger, grief, loneliness, and guilt with the need to stay caught up in classes, work, and everyday life.

11.4% of college students report experiencing "tremendous stress" over the past 12 months.

Another type of stress, **traumatic stress**, is often a result of witnessing or experiencing events like major accidents, war, shootings, assault, or natural disasters. Effects of traumatic stress may be felt for years after the event and cause significant disability, potentially leading to *post-traumatic stress disorder (PTSD)*.[5]

On any given day, we all experience both eustress and distress, each triggered by a wide range of both obvious and not-so-obvious sources. Several studies in recent years have examined sources of stress among various populations in the United States and globally.

One of the most comprehensive studies is conducted annually by the American Psychological Association. Recent stress surveys have consistently found that concerns over money, work, family responsibilities, personal and family health, and the economy were the biggest reported causes of stress for American adults. However, early in 2017, a new APA survey not only found that America's overall stress level had increased significantly for the first time in

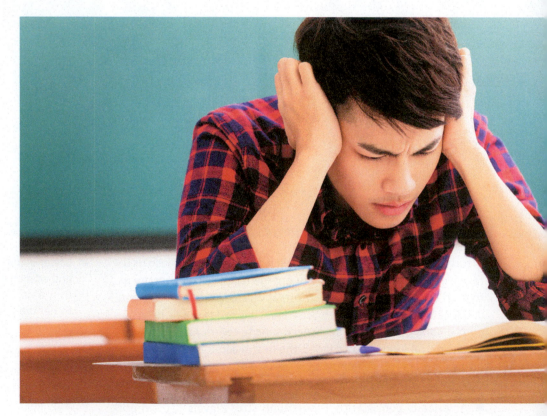

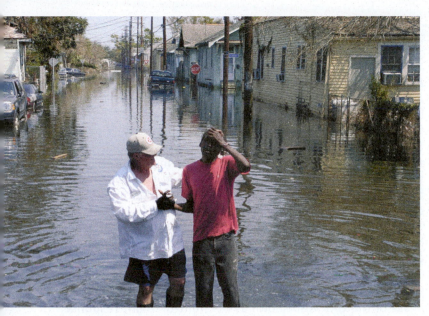

Natural disasters are among the most stressful events people can experience. The immediate event is traumatic and is followed by months of trying to get life back to "normal." Some people lack the resources and support needed to fully recover.

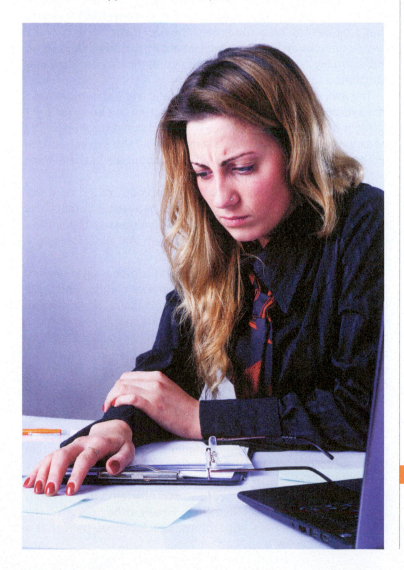

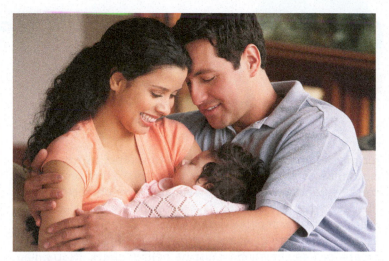

A moderate level of stress—especially eustress arising from new experiences—can actually help you live life to the fullest. Too much stress can affect your health for the worse, but so can too little stress; we need change and challenge to keep us fulfilled and growing.

10 years—with 2/3 of those surveyed concerned about America's future. Specific concerns were the political climate, terrorism, police violence against minorities, and personal safety—but that younger adults, women, and minorities experienced the highest levels of stress.[7]

College students, in particular, face stressors that come from internal sources, as well as external pressures to succeed in a competitive environment that is often geographically far removed from the support of family and hometown friends.

While key sources of stress are similar for men and women (money, work, and the economy), huge gender differences exist in how people experience, report, and cope with stress.

The good news is that increasing numbers of Americans recognize the physical and mental effects of stress on health and are seeking psychological help for problems as well as engaging in mindfulness-related activities to avoid, prevent, or control stressors.[8]

Awareness of the sources of the stress in your life can do much to help you develop a plan to avoid, prevent, and control the things that cause you stress.

Check Yourself

- How do distress and eustress differ?

- Do you have more trouble managing acute stress or chronic stress? Why?

Learning Outcome

3.2 Explain the purpose of the general adaptation syndrome, and the physiological changes that occur during each phase.

Our physiological responses evolved to protect us from harm. Thousands of years ago, if your ancestors didn't respond to stress by fighting or fleeing, they might have been eaten by a saber-toothed tiger or killed by a marauding enemy clan. Today when we face real or perceived threats, these same physiological responses kick into gear, but our instinctual reactions to fight, scream, or flee the enemy must be held in check. Restraining these responses rather than allowing them to run their course can make us physiologically charged for longer periods—sometimes chronically. Over time, a simmering stress response can wreak havoc on the body.

The General Adaptation Syndrome

When stress levels are low, the body is often in a state of **homeostasis**: All body systems are operating smoothly to maintain equilibrium. Stressors trigger a "crisis-mode" physiological response, after which the body attempts to return to homeostasis by means of an **adaptive response**. First characterized by Hans Selye in 1936, the internal fight to restore homeostasis in the face of a stressor is known as the **general adaptation syndrome (GAS)** (**Figure 3.1**). The GAS has three distinct phases: alarm, resistance, and exhaustion.[9] Regardless of whether you are experiencing distress or eustress, similar physiological changes occur.

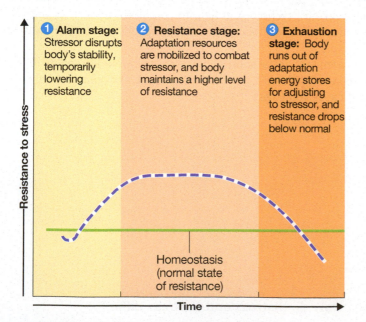

① **Alarm stage:** Stressor disrupts body's stability, temporarily lowering resistance

② **Resistance stage:** Adaptation resources are mobilized to combat stressor, and body maintains a higher level of resistance

③ **Exhaustion stage:** Body runs out of adaptation energy stores for adjusting to stressor, and resistance drops below normal

Homeostasis (normal state of resistance)

Resistance to stress

Time

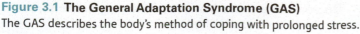

Figure 3.1 The General Adaptation Syndrome (GAS)
The GAS describes the body's method of coping with prolonged stress.

Alarm Phase Suppose you are walking to your residence hall on a dimly lit campus after a night class. You hear someone cough behind you, and you sense someone approaching rapidly. You walk faster, only to hear the quickened footsteps of the other person. Your senses become increasingly alert, your breathing quickens, your heart races, and you begin to perspire. In desperation, you stop, rip off your backpack, and prepare to fling it at your attacker to defend yourself. You turn around quickly and let out a blood-curdling yell.

To your surprise, the only person you see is a classmate. She has been trying to stay close to you out of her own anxiety about walking alone in the dark. She screams and backs off the sidewalk into the bushes, and you both start laughing with startled embarrassment. You and your classmate have just experienced the alarm phase of the GAS. Also known as the **fight-or-flight response**, this physiological reaction is one of our most basic, innate survival instincts.[10]

When the mind perceives a real or imaginary stressor, the cerebral cortex, the region of the brain that interprets the nature of an event, triggers an **autonomic nervous system (ANS)** response that prepares the body for action. The ANS is the portion of the central nervous system that regulates body functions that we do not normally consciously control, such as heart and glandular functions and breathing.

The ANS has two branches: sympathetic and parasympathetic. The **sympathetic nervous system** energizes the body for fight or flight by signaling the release of several stress hormones. The **parasympathetic nervous system** slows all the systems stimulated by the stress response; in effect, it counteracts the actions of the sympathetic branch.

The responses of the sympathetic nervous system to stress involve a series of biochemical exchanges between different parts of the body. The brain's **hypothalamus** functions as the control center of the sympathetic nervous system and determines the overall reaction to stressors.

When the hypothalamus perceives that extra energy is needed to fight a stressor, it stimulates the adrenal glands, which are located near the top of the kidneys, to release the hormone **epinephrine**, also called *adrenaline*. Epinephrine causes more blood to be pumped with each beat of the heart, dilates the airways in the lungs to increase oxygen intake, increases the breathing rate, stimulates the liver to release more glucose (which fuels muscular exertion), and dilates the pupils to improve visual sensitivity (see **Figure 3.2**).

In addition to the fight-or-flight response, the alarm phase can also trigger a longer-term reaction to stress. The hypothalamus uses chemical messages to trigger the pituitary gland within the brain to release a powerful hormone, *adrenocorticotropic hormone (ACTH)*. ACTH signals the adrenal glands to release **cortisol**, a hormone that makes stored nutrients more readily available to meet energy demands. Finally, other parts of the brain and body release endorphins, which relieve pain that a stressor may cause.

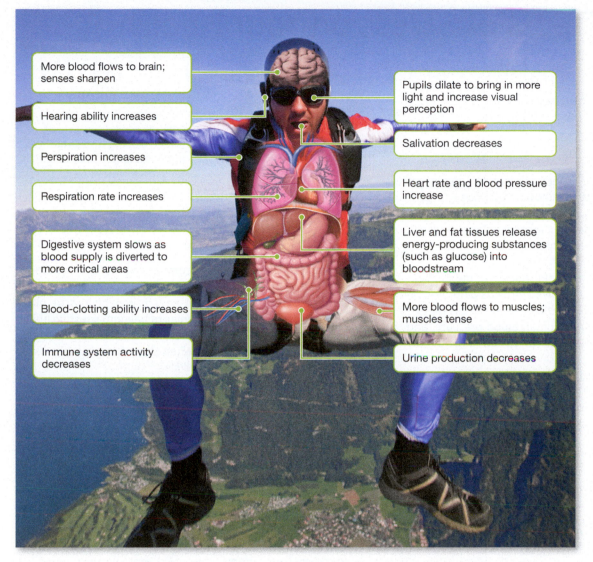

Figure 3.2 The Body's Acute Stress Response

More blood flows to brain; senses sharpen

Hearing ability increases

Perspiration increases

Respiration rate increases

Digestive system slows as blood supply is diverted to more critical areas

Blood-clotting ability increases

Immune system activity decreases

Pupils dilate to bring in more light and increase visual perception

Salivation decreases

Heart rate and blood pressure increase

Liver and fat tissues release energy-producing substances (such as glucose) into bloodstream

More blood flows to muscles; muscles tense

Urine production decreases

Figure 3.2 The Body's Acute Stress Response
Exposure to stress of any kind causes a complex series of involuntary physiological responses.

Mastering Health & Nutrition Body's Stress Response

immunocompetence, or the ability of the immune system to respond to attack. In turn, this increases the risk of diabetes, cardiovascular disease, and other chronic diseases.[11]

Men and Women Respond to Stress Differently

Ever since Walter Cannon's landmark studies in the 1930s, it's been thought that humans respond similarly to stressful events via the "fight-or-flight" response. However, several researchers now believe that men and women may respond differently to stressors.

While men may be prone to fighting or fleeing, women may be more likely to "tend and befriend" by either trying to befriend the enemy or obtaining social support from others to ease stress-related reactions.[12]

Many believe that the neurotransmitter *oxytocin* is key to this response. Essentially, women under stress appear to have higher oxytocin levels than men under similar circumstances and are more likely to form tight social alliances, be empathic, and seek out friends for support when stress levels are high. In contrast, men are more likely to withdraw when highly stressed.[13]

Resistance Phase In the resistance phase of the GAS, the body tries to return to homeostasis by resisting the alarm responses. However, because some perceived stressor still exists, the body does not achieve complete calm or rest. Instead, the body stays activated or aroused at a level that causes a higher metabolic rate in some organ tissues.

Exhaustion Phase In the exhaustion phase of the GAS, the hormones, chemicals, and systems that trigger and maintain the stress response are depleted, and the body returns to *allostasis*, or balance. You may feel tired or drained as your body returns to normal. In situations where stress is *chronic*, triggers may reverberate in the body, keeping body systems at a heightened arousal state. The prolonged effort to adapt to the stress response leads to **allostatic load**, or exhaustive wear and tear on the body.

As the body adjusts to chronic unresolved stress, the adrenal glands continue to release cortisol, which remains in the bloodstream for longer periods of time as a result of slower metabolic responsiveness. Over time, cortisol can reduce

Check Yourself

- How does the general adaptation syndrome help us understand our reaction to stressors?

- How does the body react during each phase of the general adaptation syndrome?

- What are the differences between the *fight-or-flight* and the *tend-and-befriend* stress responses?

Physical Effects of Stress

The higher the levels of stress you experience and the longer that stress continues, the greater the likelihood of damage to your physical health (see **Figure 3.3**).[14] Ailments related to chronic stress include heart disease, diabetes, cancer, headaches, ulcers, low back pain, depression, and the common cold.

Stress and Cardiovascular Disease Perhaps the most documented health consequence of unresolved stress is cardiovascular disease (CVD). Research indicates that chronic stress plays a significant role in heart rate problems, high blood pressure, and atherosclerosis, as well as increased risk for a wide range of cardiovascular diseases.[15]

In recent decades, research into the relationship between stress and CVD contributors has shown direct links between the incidence and progression of CVD and stressors such as job strain, caregiving, bereavement, and natural disasters.[16]

Stress and Weight Gain Higher stress levels may increase cortisol levels in the bloodstream, which contribute to increased hunger and seem to activate fat-storing enzymes. Animal and human studies support the theory that cortisol plays a role in increasing belly fat and encouraging eating behaviors.[17]

Stress and Headaches The most common type of headache is a *tension-type headache*.[18] Symptoms may include dull pain; tightness; and tender scalp, neck, and shoulder muscles.[19] Tension headaches are generally caused by muscle tension in the neck or head. **Migraines** are more severe headaches whose symptoms include moderate to severe throbbing pain that interferes with activity, nausea, and sensitivity to light and sound.[20] Prescription and over-the-counter medications often help migraine sufferers.

Stress and Hair Loss The most common type of stress-induced hair loss is *telogen effluvium*. Often seen in individuals who have lost a loved one or experienced severe weight loss or other trauma, this condition pushes colonies of hair into a resting phase. Over time, hair begins to fall out. A similar stress-related condition known as *alopecia areata* occurs when stress triggers white blood cells to attack and destroy hair follicles.[21]

Stress and Diabetes People under lots of stress often don't get enough sleep, are depressed, suffer from anxiety, don't eat well, and may drink alcohol or take other drugs to help them get through a stressful time. All of these behaviors can alter blood sugar levels and appear to increase the risks of type 2 diabetes.[22] Stress hormones, particularly cortisol, may affect blood glucose levels directly.[23]

Stress and Digestive Problems Although stress doesn't directly cause digestive problems, it is clearly related to them and may make symptoms worse.[24] For example, people who feel tense are more susceptible to dehydration, inflammation, and other digestive problems.[25]

Stress and Impaired Immunity A growing area of scientific investigation known as **psychoneuroimmunology (PNI)** analyzes the intricate relationship between the mind's response to stress and the immune system's ability to function effectively. Several recent research

"Why do I always get sick during finals week?"

Students are particularly vulnerable to stress-related infections like the flu or a cold during periods of high stress and short sleep (final exams!). Plan ahead to not leave everything to the last minute and make some "ME time" for relaxation and mindfulness during high stress periods.

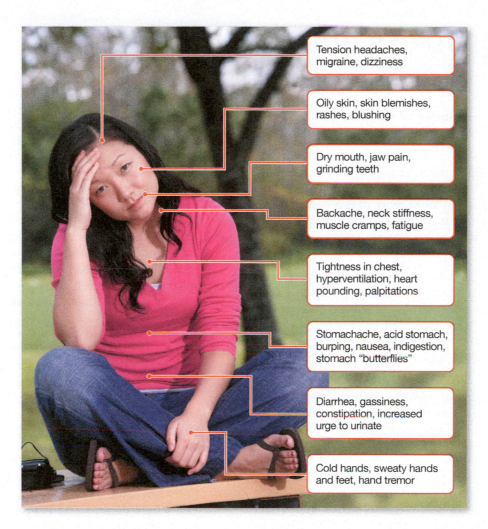

Tension headaches, migraine, dizziness

Oily skin, skin blemishes, rashes, blushing

Dry mouth, jaw pain, grinding teeth

Backache, neck stiffness, muscle cramps, fatigue

Tightness in chest, hyperventilation, heart pounding, palpitations

Stomachache, acid stomach, burping, nausea, indigestion, stomach "butterflies"

Diarrhea, gassiness, constipation, increased urge to urinate

Cold hands, sweaty hands and feet, hand tremor

Figure 3.3 Common Physical Symptoms of Stress
You may not even notice how stressed you are until your body starts sending you signals. Do you frequently experience any of these physical symptoms of stress?

reviews suggest that too much stress over a long period can negatively affect various aspects of the cellular immune response. This increases risks for upper respiratory infections and certain chronic conditions.[26] More prolonged stressors, such as the loss of a loved one or living with a disability, can impair the natural immune response over time.[27]

Intellectual and Psychological Effects of Stress

In a recent national survey of college students, nearly 51 percent of respondents said they felt overwhelmed by all that they had to do within the past 2 weeks (39 percent of men and 56 percent of women), and a similar number reported that they felt exhausted.[28] Stress can play a huge role in whether students stay in school, get good grades, and succeed on their career path.

Stress, Memory, and Concentration Animal studies suggest that *glucocorticoids*—stress hormones released from the adrenal cortex—may affect memory and concentration. In humans, memory is impaired when acute stress bombards the brain with hormones and neurotransmitters, affecting how we think, make decisions, and respond in stressful situations.[29] Prolonged

exposure to cortisol has been linked to shrinking of the hippocampus, the brain's major memory center.[30] Other research indicates that prolonged exposure to high levels of stress hormones may predispose women, in particular, to Alzheimer's disease.[31]

Psychological Effects of Stress Chronic stress may cause structural degeneration and impaired function of the brain, as well as an overactive *amygdala* (region of the brain associated with emotional responses) that may increase rates of violence.[32]

See It! Videos

Can a test identify your risk for stress-related illnesses? Watch **Stress Can Damage Women's Health** in the Study Area of Mastering Health.

Check Yourself

- What are four possible effects of stress on your physical and psychological health?

- Give an example of an instance in which psychological stress had a physical effect on you.

Stress and Sleep Problems

3.4 Describe the importance of sleep to good health, and list strategies for ensuring restful sleep.

In a recent survey by the American College Health Association, only 11.8 percent of students reported getting enough sleep to feel well rested in the morning six or more days a week.[33] Sixty-three percent of students said that they feel tired, dragged out, or sleepy during the day three to seven days each week.[34]

The Importance of Sleep

Sleep is much more important than people realize. Sleep conserves body energy and restores you physically and mentally. Many people do not get enough sleep. While most people need 7 or more hours of sleep, children need even more. Women need more hours of sleep than men do.

Sleep has beneficial effects on most body systems:

- **Sleep helps maintain your immune system.** The common cold, strep throat, flu, mononucleosis, cold sores, and a variety of other ailments are more common when your immune system is depressed. If you aren't getting enough sleep, your immune response is weakened.[35]
- **Sleep helps reduce your risk for cardiovascular disease.** Studies suggest a link between short sleep duration and increased risk of cardiovascular disease, stroke, high blood pressure, metabolic syndrome, obesity, and other cardiovascular risks.[36] New research points to a strong association between short-duration sleep and increased risk of developing and/or dying from cardiovascular disease.[37]

- **Sleep contributes to a healthy metabolism.** Chemical reactions in your body's cells break down food and synthesize compounds that the body needs. The sum of all these reactions is called *metabolism*. Several recent studies suggest that sleep contributes to healthy metabolism and possibly a healthy body weight.[38]
- **Short sleep increases risk of type 2 diabetes.** There is evidence that sleep deficiencies can increase the risk of *type 2 diabetes*, a disorder of glucose metabolism.[39]
- **Sleep may be a factor in reproductive health.** Young males who suffer from chronic sleep deficits have reduced semen concentration, reduced sperm quality and motility, and smaller testicular size than men with higher sleep levels. Women with chronic sleep deficits have increased issues with conception and overall fertility.[40]
- **Sleep contributes to mental function.** Restricting sleep can cause a wide range of mental problems, including lapses of attention, slowed or poor memory, reduced cognitive ability, difficulty concentrating, and a tendency for your thinking to get "stuck in a rut."[41] Studies of college students consistently show pulling an all-nighter to be a bad idea if you want to perform well on exams or be productive.[42]
- **Sleep improves motor tasks.** Sleep also has a restorative effect on motor function, that is, the ability to perform tasks such as shooting a basket or driving a car. Motor function is affected by sleep throughout the lifespan among otherwise healthy individuals.[43] Last year, over 35,000 people died in auto crashes. Between 7 and 20 percent of those deaths are thought to have involved a drowsy driver.[44]
- **Sleep plays a role in stress management and mental health.** The relationship between sleep and stress is complex: Stress

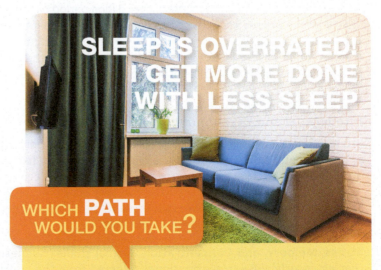

SLEEP IS OVERRATED! I GET MORE DONE WITH LESS SLEEP

WHICH **PATH** WOULD YOU TAKE**?**

 Go to Mastering Health to play "Finding Ways to Manage Stress" and see how your actions today affect your future health.

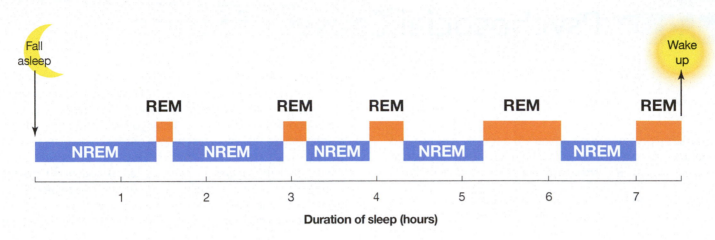

Figure 3.4 The Nightly Sleep Cycle
As the number of hours you sleep increases, your brain spends more and more time in REM sleep. Thus, sleeping for too few hours could mean that you're depriving yourself primarily of essential REM sleep.

can cause or contribute to sleep problems, and sleep problems can cause or increase your level of stress. The same is true of depression and anxiety disorders: Reduced or poor-quality sleep can trigger these disorders, but it's also a common symptom resulting from them. Individuals who suffer from chronic insomnia have over twice the risk of developing depression.[45]

Stages of Sleep

Researchers distinguish between two primary sleep stages: During **REM sleep**, rapid eye movement and dreams occur, and brain-wave activity appears similar to that when you are awake. **Non-REM (NREM) sleep**, in contrast, is the period of restful sleep with slowed brain activity that does *not* include rapid eye movement.

During the night, you alternate between periods of NREM and REM sleep, repeating one full cycle about once every 90 minutes (see **Figure 3.4**).[46] Overall, you spend about 75 percent of each night in NREM sleep and 25 percent in REM sleep. Research indicates that deep phases of NREM sleep consolidate and organize the day's information, while REM sleep stabilizes consolidated memory.[47] Without adequate sleep, your short-term memory may suffer.

Getting A Good Night's Sleep Researchers agree that adults should sleep 7 or more hours each night. Getting fewer than 7 hours of sleep per night on a regular basis increases the risks of adverse health outcomes.[48] Ways to ensure a good night's sleep include the following:

- **Let there be light.** Stay in sync with your circadian rhythm by spending time in the daylight.
- **Stay active.** Exercisers are much more likely to feel rested than those who are sedentary.
- **Sleep tight.** Comfortable pillows, bedding, and mattress can help you sleep more soundly.

- **Create a sleep "cave."** As bedtime approaches, keep your bedroom quiet, cool, dark, and free of technology.
- **Condition yourself into better sleep.** Go to bed and get up at the same times each day.
- **Avoid foods and drinks that keep you awake.** Large meals, nicotine, energy drinks, caffeine, and alcohol close to bedtime can affect your ability to fall asleep and stay asleep. Although alcohol may make you sleepy initially, it disturbs other stages of sleep, keeping you from the restorative, deeper levels of sleep you need.[49]
- **Don't drink large amounts of liquid before bed.** This prevents having to get up in the night to use the bathroom.
- **Don't toss and turn.** If you're not asleep after 20 minutes, read or listen to gentle music. Once you feel sleepy, go back to bed.
- **Don't nap in the late afternoon or evening.** Also, don't nap for longer than 30 minutes.
- **Don't read, study, watch TV, use your laptop, talk on the phone, eat, or smoke in bed.** Emotionally intense phone conversations can also make it hard to calm yourself enough to sleep.
- **Don't take sleeping pills.** Don't take sleep aids unless prescribed by your health care provider. Over-the-counter sleep aids can interfere with progression through the stages of sleep.

3.4

Stress

Check Yourself

- Why is it important for your health to sleep well?

- What are three common reasons for poor sleep, and how can you overcome them?

Psychosocial Causes of Stress

3.5   Discuss and classify psychosocial sources of stress.

Psychosocial stressors refer to the factors in our daily routines and in our social and physical environments that cause us to experience stress (Figure 3.5). Which of these are most common in your life?

Adjustment to Change   Any change, whether good or bad, occurring in your normal routine can result in stress. The more changes you experience and the more adjustments you must make, the greater the chances are that stress will have an impact on your health. The enormous changes associated with starting college, while exciting, can also be among the most stressful you will face in your life. Moving away from home, trying to fit in and make new friends from diverse backgrounds, adjusting to a new schedule, learning to live with strangers in housing that is often lacking in the comforts of home—all of these things can cause sleeplessness and anxiety and keep your body in a continual fight-or-flight mode.

Hassles   Some psychologists have proposed that little stressors, frustrations, and petty annoyances, known collectively as *hassles*, can be just as stressful as major life changes.[50] Listening to classmates who talk too much during lectures, being near people chatting on the phone and texting while you are trying to study, not finding parking on campus, and a host of other small but bothersome situations can trigger frustration, anger, and fight-or-flight responses.[51]

Technostress   Technostress is stress created by a dependence on technology and the constant state of connection, which can include a perceived obligation to always respond or be ever present. Research supports the concept that being "wired" 24/7 can lead to anxiety, obsessive compulsive disorder, narcissism, sleep disorders, frustration, time pressures, and guilt—some of the negative consequences known as iDisorders. According to a new study, college students who can't keep their hands off their mobile devices are reporting higher levels of anxiety, less satisfaction with life, and lower grades than peers who use their devices less often. The average student surveyed spent nearly 5 hours per day using his or her cell phone for everything from calling and texting to Facebook, e-mails, gaming, and more.[52]

To reduce technostress, set limits on your technology use, and make sure that you devote sufficient time to face-to-face interactions with people you care about, cultivating and nurturing your relationships. You don't always need to answer your phone or respond to a text or e-mail immediately. Leave your devices at home or turn them off when you are out with others or on vacation. Tune in to your surroundings, your loved ones and friends, your job, and your classes.

The Toll of Relationships   Relationships can trigger enormous fight-or-flight reactions—whether we're talking about the exhilaration of new love or the pain of a breakup, the result is often lack of focus, lack of sleep, and an inability to focus on anything but the love interest. And although we may think first of love relationships, even relationships with friends, family members, and coworkers can be the sources of overwhelming struggles, just as they can be sources of strength and support. These relationships can make us strive to be the best that we can be and give us hope for the future, or they can diminish our self-esteem and leave us reeling from a destructive interaction.

Academic and Financial Pressure   It isn't surprising that today's college and university students face mind-boggling amounts of pressure as they compete for grades, athletic positions,

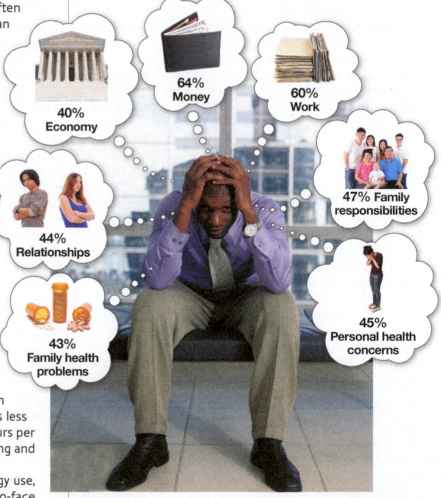

Figure 3.5 What Stresses Us?

A new survey indicates that in addition to the concerns shown in this figure, adults are also stressed about the political climate, terrorism, police violence toward minorities, and personal safety.

Source: Data from American Psychological Association, "Stress in America: Paying with our Health," 2015, http://www.apa.org/news/press/releases/stress/2014/stress-report.pdf..

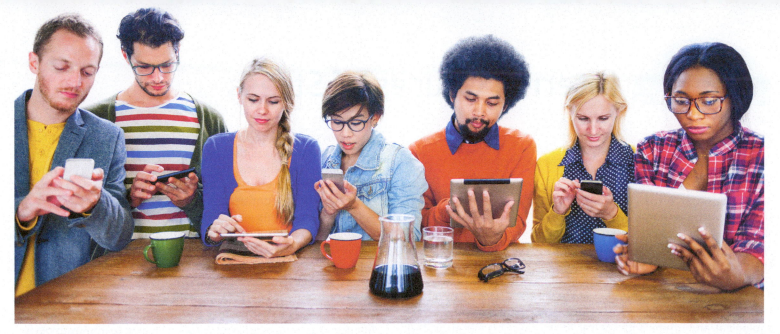

85% of adults are either constant or occasional checkers of email, texts or social media. These individuals experience significantly higher stress levels, particularly when their devices don't work. Unplugging or taking a "digital detox" is an important part of stress management.

American Psychological Association (2017). Stress in America: Coping with Change. Stress in America™ Survey.

internships, and jobs. Challenging classes can be tough enough, but many students must also juggle work in order to pay bills. When economic conditions become strained, the effects on people with limited resources (particularly students) can be significant. An economic downturn can even make student dreams seem unattainable. Increasing reports of mental health problems on college campuses may be one of the results of too much stress.

Frustrations and Conflicts Disparity between our goals (what we hope to obtain in life) and our behaviors (actions that may or may not lead to these goals) can trigger frustration. Conflicts occur when we are forced to decide among competing motives, impulses, desires, and behaviors, or to face demands incompatible with our own values and sense of importance. College students away from their families and familiar communities for the first time may face conflicts among parental values, their own beliefs, and the beliefs of those different from themselves.

Overload We've all experienced times when the combined demands of work, responsibilities, and relationships seem to be pulling us under—and our physical, mental, and emotional reserves are insufficient to deal with it all. Students suffering from **overload** may experience depression, sleeplessness, mood swings, frustration, and anxiety. Unrelenting overload can lead to a state of physical and mental exhaustion known as *burnout*.

Stressful Environments For many students, the environment around them can cause significant stress. Perhaps you cannot afford safe, healthy housing, a bad roommate constantly makes life uncomfortable, or loud neighbors keep you up at night.

Unexpected natural disasters—such as flooding, earthquakes, hurricanes, blizzards, and tornadoes—can cause tremendous stress at the time and for years later. Often equally damaging are environmental **background distressors**—including noise, air, and water pollution; allergy-aggravating pollen and dust; and second-hand smoke—that trigger a constant resistance phase.

Bias and Discrimination Diversity of students, faculty members, and staff enriches everyone's educational experience. It also challenges us to examine our attitudes and biases. Those perceived as dissimilar due to race, ethnicity, religious affiliation, age, or sexual orientation—or differences in viewpoint, appearance, behavior, or background—may become victims of subtle and not-so-subtle bigotry, insensitivity, harassment, or hostility, or may simply be ignored.[53]

Dealing with bigotry and even subtle hostility can lead to heightened vigilance and changes in behavior, which in themselves produce a stress response. In other words, just anticipating discrimination is enough to cause stress. Some adults also report stress from trying to prepare themselves in advance for possible insults from other people.[54]

Research shows a definite connection between discrimination, chronic stress, and impacts on health. For instance, a recent survey shows that among all adults, those who report experiencing extreme levels of stress (a rating of 8, 9, or 10 on the survey's 10-point scale) are twice as likely to report fair or poor health, compared to adults with low stress levels. Nearly half of black adults who rate their stress as extreme (46 percent) report fair or poor health, while only 22 percent who report low stress levels say the same. One in three Hispanics who report having extreme stress (35 percent) also report being in fair or poor health, compared to 19 percent of Hispanics reporting low stress.[55]

Approximately 45 percent of adults who do not report discrimination describe their health as excellent or very good, compared to only 31 percent who report experiencing discrimination. More than one-fourth of American Indian/Alaska Natives (39 percent), Blacks (30 percent), and Hispanics (29 percent) report that they are in fair or poor health, compared to 23 percent of adults overall.[56]

Check Yourself

- **What are five sources of psychosocial stress?**

- **Which psychosocial sources of stress do you encounter most frequently?**

3.6 Internal Causes of Stress

Learning Outcome

3.6 Discuss and classify internal causes of stress.

Although stress can come from the environment and other external sources, it can result from internal factors as well. Internal stressors such as negative appraisal, low self-esteem, and low self-efficacy can cause unsettling thoughts or feelings and can ultimately affect your health. It is important to address and manage these internal stressors.

Appraisal and Stress Throughout life, we encounter many different demands and potential stressors—some biological, some psychological, and others sociological. In any case, it is our **appraisal** of these demands, rather than the demands themselves, that results in our experiencing stress. Appraisal is defined as the interpretation and evaluation of information provided to the brain by the senses. As new information becomes available, appraisal helps us recognize stressors, evaluate them on the basis of past experiences and emotions, and decide whether or not we have the ability to cope with them. When you feel that the stressors of life are overwhelming and you lack control, you are more likely to feel strain and distress.

Self-Esteem and Self-Efficacy *Self-esteem* refers to how you feel about yourself. Research on adolescents and young adults indicates that high stress and low self-esteem significantly predict **suicidal ideation**, a desire to die and thoughts about suicide. Fortunately, research has shown that you can improve your ability to cope with stress by increasing self-esteem.[57]

However, new research also points to a potential dark side of too much self-esteem. Today's college students have the highest level of narcissism ever recorded, and the quest to have thousands of "friends" on Facebook or huge Twitter followings can be severe stressors.[58] Environments in which individuals are always compared to others as indicators of self-worth may contribute to more elitism, more bullying in a quest for power, more prejudice between groups, and more difficulties in working with other people after graduation.[59]

Self-efficacy—confidence in one's skills and ability to cope with life's challenges—is considered one of the most important personality traits that influence psychological and physiological stress responses.[60] Developing self-efficacy is also vital to coping with and overcoming academic pressures and worries.[61] High test anxiety has been shown to account for up to 15 percent of the variance in student performance on exams.[62] Research suggests that by learning to handle test anxiety, you will increase your confidence and improve your test scores, leading to improved performance overall.[63]

Type A and Type B Personalities In 1974, physicians Meyer Friedman and Ray Rosenman published a book indicating that type A individuals had a greatly increased risk of heart disease.[64] *Type A* personalities are defined as hard-driving, competitive, time-driven perfectionists. In contrast, *type B* personalities are described as being relaxed, noncompetitive, and more tolerant of others.

Today, most researchers recognize that none of us will be wholly type A or type B all of the time, and we may exhibit either type in selected situations. In addition, recent research indicates that not all type A people experience negative health

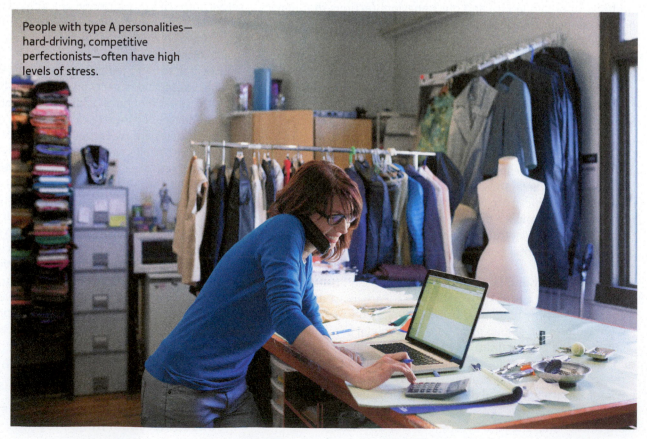

People with type A personalities—hard-driving, competitive perfectionists—often have high levels of stress.

consequences; in fact, some hard-driving individuals seem to thrive on their super-charged lifestyles. Only those type A individuals who exhibit a "toxic core"—who have disproportionate amounts of anger, are distrustful of others, and have a cynical, glass-half-empty approach to life; in total, a set of characteristics referred to as **hostility**—are at increased risk for heart disease.[65]

Type C and Type D Personalities
In addition to CVD risks, personality types have been linked to increased risk for a variety of illnesses ranging from asthma to cancer. *Type C*

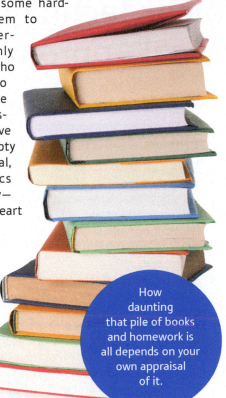

How daunting that pile of books and homework is all depends on your own appraisal of it.

personality is one such type, characterized as stoic, with a tendency to stuff feelings down and conform to the wishes of others (or be "pleasers"). Preliminary research suggests that type C individuals may be more susceptible to illnesses such as asthma, multiple sclerosis, autoimmune disorders, and cancer; however, more research is necessary to support this relationship.[66]

A more recently identified personality type is *type D* (distressed), characterized by a tendency toward excessive negative worry, irritability, gloom, and social inhibition. Several recent studies have shown that type D people may be up to eight times more likely to die of a heart attack or sudden cardiac death.[67]

Psychological Hardiness and Resilience
According to psychologist Susanne Kobasa, **psychological hardiness** may negate self-imposed stress associated with type A behavior. Psychologically hardy people are characterized by control, commitment, and willingness to embrace challenge.[68] People with a sense of control are able to accept responsibility for their behaviors and change those that they discover to be debilitating. People with a sense of commitment have good self-esteem and understand their purpose in life. Those who embrace challenge see change as a stimulating opportunity for personal growth.[69] These individuals are described as being **psychologically resilient**—a dynamic process in which people exposed to sustained adversity or traumatic challenges adapt positively.

Shift and Persist
An emerging body of research proposes that in the midst of extreme, persistent adversity, youth—often with the help of positive role models in their lives—are able to reframe appraisals of current stressors more positively (*shifting*), while *persisting* in focusing on a positive future. These youth are able to endure the present by adapting, holding on to meaningful things in their lives, and staying optimistic and positive. These "**shift-and-persist**" strategies are among the most recently identified factors that protect against the negative effects of too much stress in our lives.[70]

Skills for Behavior Change
Overcoming Test Taking Anxiety

Here are helpful hints to increase your self-efficacy and reduce your stress levels in a familiar situation: an academic exam.

Before the Exam

- **Manage your study time.** Start studying at least a week before your test to reduce anxiety. Do a limited review the night before, get a good night's sleep, and arrive for the exam early.
- **On an index card, write down three reasons you will pass the exam.** Keep the card with you and review it whenever you study. When you get the test, write your three reasons on the test or on a piece of scrap paper.
- **Eat a balanced meal before the exam.** Avoid sugar and rich or heavy foods, as well as foods that might upset your stomach. You want to feel your best.
- **Think about how much time you might need to answer different types of test questions.** Make a general strategy before the test to efficiently use the time allotted. Wear a watch to class on the day of the test.

During the Test

- **Manage your time during the test.** Look at how many questions there are and what each is worth. Prioritize the high-point questions, allow a certain amount of time for each, and make sure that you leave some time for the rest. Hold to this schedule.
- **Slow down and pay attention.** Focus on one question at a time. Check off each part of multipart questions to make sure your answers are complete.

Check Yourself

- What are five causes of internal stress?
- Which internal causes of stress do you experience most frequently?

3.7 Stress Management Techniques: Mental and Physical Approaches

3.7 **Examine mental and physical approaches to stress management.**

Being on your own in college may pose challenges, but it also lets you take control of and responsibility for your life and take steps to reduce negative stressors. **Coping** is the act of managing events or conditions to lessen the physical or psychological effects of excess stress.[71] One of the most effective ways to combat stressors is to build coping strategies and skills, known collectively as *stress-management techniques*.

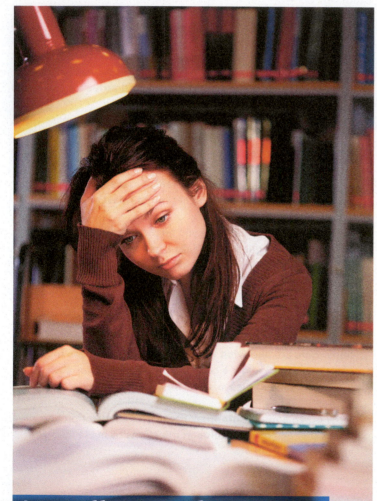

Are college students more stressed out than other groups?

The combination of a new environment, peer and parental pressure, and the demands of course work, campus activities, and social life contribute to above average stress levels in college students.

Practicing Mental Work to Reduce Stress

Your perceptions often contribute to your stress, so assessing your "self-talk," beliefs, and actions are good first steps. Here's how:

- Make a list of things you're worried about.
- Examine the causes of your problems and worries.
- Consider the size of each problem. What are the consequences of doing nothing versus taking action?
- List your options, including ones you may not like much.
- Outline a plan, then act. Even little things can make a big difference.
- After you act, evaluate. How did you do? Do you need to change your actions to achieve a better outcome next time? How?

One way to anticipate and prepare for specific stressors is a technique known as **stress inoculation**. Suppose speaking in front of a class scares you. To prevent freezing up during a presentation, practice in front of friends or a video camera.

Negative self-talk can take the form of *pessimism*, or focusing on the negative; *perfectionism*, or expecting superhuman standards; *should-ing*, or reprimanding yourself for things you should have done; *blaming* yourself or others for circumstances and events; and *dichotomous thinking*, in which everything is seen as either entirely good or bad. To combat negative self-talk, become aware of an irrational or overreactive thought, interrupt it by saying "stop" (under your breath or out loud), then replace it with positive thoughts—a process called **cognitive restructuring**.

People fall into patterns and ways of thinking that can cause stress and increase their levels of anxiety. The fact is, your thought patterns can be your own worst enemy. If you can become aware of the internal messages you are giving yourself, you can recognize them and work to change them. Some strategies for doing this include the following:

- **Reframe a distressing event from a positive perspective.** For example, if you feel perpetually frustrated that you can't be the best in every class, reframe the issue to highlight your strengths.
- **Break the worry habit.** If you are preoccupied with "what if's" and worst case scenarios, doubts and fears can sap your strength and send your stress levels soaring.
  - If you must worry, create a "worry period"—a 20-minute time period each day when you can journal or talk about it. After that, move on.
  - Focus on the many things that are going right, rather than the one thing that might go wrong.
- **Look at life as being fluid.** If you accept that change is a natural part of living and growing, the jolt of changes will become less stressful.
- **Moderate your expectations.** Aim high, but be realistic about your circumstances and motivation.

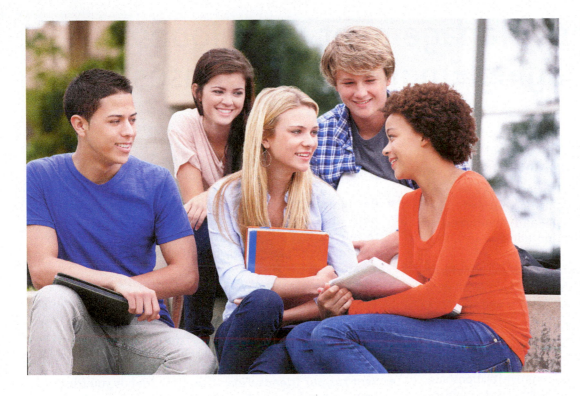

Achievement. Consider the steps to achieve your goals in life, and view failure along the way as an opportunity. Celebrate accomplishments, both your own and those of others, and readily give praise.

The Action for Happiness movement has developed a ten-step set of recommendations for actions that will lead to a more positive society.

- Do things for others.
- Connect with people.
- Take care of your body.
- Notice the world around you.
- Keep learning new things.
- Have goals to look forward to.
- Find ways to bounce back.
- Take a positive approach.
- Be comfortable with who you are.
- Be part of something bigger.[73]

- **Weed out trivia.** Cardiologist Robert Eliot offers two rules for coping with life's challenges: "Don't sweat the small stuff," and remember, "It's all small stuff."
- **Tolerate mistakes by yourself and others.** Rather than getting angry or frustrated by mishaps, evaluate what happened and learn from it.

Cultivating Happiness

For decades, noted psychologist Martin Seligman has conducted research focused on positive psychology and authentic happiness. His work has been the framework for a new way of looking at life with a glass-half-full perspective. Research supports the idea that people who are optimistic and happier have fewer mental and physical problems.[72] Today, Seligman takes happiness a step further, focusing on the concept of *flourishing*. Flourishing consists of five elements, which positive psychologists believe will help you flourish in life, avoid stress, and be healthier:

- **Positive emotion.** Take time to get to know people's names. Share highs of the day rather than lows. Be active in complimenting others and verbalize their strengths.
- **Engagement.** Practice mindfulness: see, hear, touch, and feel the present moment. Make time to fully engage in the activities that bring you joy.
- **Relationships.** Listen to others and ask questions. Connect in person. Empower others to see their strengths, and check in to show that you care.
- **Meaning.** Think about how you want to be remembered. Read and explore new things. Learn about different cultures and history. Work to help others and to improve the world.

Taking Physical Action

Physical activities can complement your strategies of stress management.

- **Exercise regularly.** The human stress response is intended to end in physical activity; exercise "burns off" stress hormones by directing them toward their intended metabolic function and can combat stress by raising levels of endorphins—mood-elevating, painkilling hormones—in the bloodstream.[74]
- **Get enough sleep.** Adequate sleep allows you to cope with multiple stressors more effectively and to be more productive.
- **Practice self-nurturing.** Find time each day for something fun—something that you enjoy and that calms you. Like exercise, relaxation can help you cope with stressful feelings, as well as preserve and refocus your energies.
- **Eat healthfully.** A balanced, healthy diet will help provide the stamina you need to get through problems while stress-proofing you in ways not yet fully understood. Undereating, overeating, and eating the wrong foods can create distress in the body. In particular, avoid **sympathomimetics**, foods that produce (or mimic) stresslike responses, such as caffeine.

Check Yourself

- What are four effective mental or physical approaches to managing stress? Which might be best for you?

3.8 Stress Management Techniques: Managing Emotional Responses

Learning Outcome

3.8 Explain how management of emotional responses contributes to stress management.

We often get upset not by realities, but by our faulty perceptions. Stress management requires examining your emotional responses to interactions with others—and remembering that you are responsible for the emotion and the resulting behaviors.

Learning to identify emotions based on irrational beliefs, or expressed and interpreted in an over-the-top manner, can help you stop such emotions or express them in healthy and appropriate ways.

Learn to Laugh, Be Joyful, and Cry Smiling, laughing, and even crying can elevate mood, relieve stress, and improve relationships. In the moment, laughter and joy raise endorphin levels, increase blood oxygen, decrease stress, relieve pain, and enhance productivity. Additional evidence for long-term effects on immune function and protection against disease is only starting to be understood.[75]

Fight the Anger Urge Anger usually results when we feel we have lost control of a situation or are frustrated by events we can do little about. Major sources of anger include (1) perceived *threats* to self or others we care about; (2) *reactions to injustice*; (3) *fear*; (4) *faulty emotional reasoning* or misinterpretation of normal events; (5) *low frustration tolerance*, often fueled by stress, drugs, or lack of sleep; (6) *unreasonable expectations* for ourselves and others; and (7) *people rating*, or applying derogatory ratings to others.

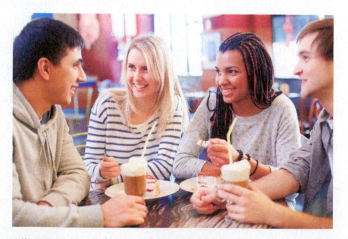

Spending time communicating and socializing can be an important part of building a support network and reducing your stress level.

To deal with anger, you can express, suppress, or calm it. Surprisingly, expressing anger is probably the healthiest option, if you do so assertively rather than aggressively. Several strategies can help redirect aggression into assertion:[76]

- **Recognize anger patterns and learn to de-escalate them.** Note what angers you. What thoughts or feelings led up to your boiling point? Try changing your self-talk or interrupting anger patterns by counting to ten or taking deep breaths.
- **Verbally de-escalate.** When conflict arises, be respectful and state your needs or feelings rather than shooting zingers. Avoid "you always" or "you never" and instead say, "I feel__ when you__" or "I would really appreciate it if you could__."
- **Plan ahead.** Explore ways to minimize your exposure to anger triggers, such as traffic jams.
- **Vent to your friends.** Find a few close friends you trust and who can be honest with you about your situation. Allow them to listen to provide perspective. Don't wear down supporters with continual rants.
- **Develop realistic expectations.** Anger is often the result of unmet expectations, frustrations, resentments, and impatience. Are your expectations of yourself and others realistic?
- **Turn complaints into requests.** Try reworking a problem into a request. Instead of screaming because your neighbors' music woke you up at 2 a.m., talk with them. Try to reach an agreement.
- **Leave past anger in the past.** Learn to resolve issues that have caused pain, frustration, or stress. If necessary, seek professional counsel.

Invest in Loved Ones Too often, we don't make time for the people most important to us: friends and family. Cultivate and nurture social relationships built on trust, mutual acceptance and understanding, honesty, and caring. Treating others empathically provides them with a measure of emotional security and reduces *their* anxiety.

Cultivate Your Spiritual Side Spiritual health and spiritual practice can link you to a community and offer perspective on the things that truly matter.

Check Yourself

- How can emotions affect your stress levels?
- List three strategies to express anger assertively rather than aggressively.

Stress Management Techniques: Managing Your Time and Your Finances

Learning Outcome

3.9 Describe strategies for managing your time and your finances.

Managing Your Time

Ever put off writing a paper until the night before it was due? We all **procrastinate**—voluntarily delay doing some task despite expecting to be worse off for it. Procrastination results in academic difficulties, financial problems, relationship problems, and stress-related ailments.

One key to beating procrastination is to set clear "implementation intentions."[77] Having a plan that includes specific deadlines (and rewards for meeting deadlines) can help you stay on task. Start with a simple plan and be flexible.

What else can you do to make better use of your time? Try logging your activities for 2 days—everything from going to class to doing laundry to texting friends—and the amount of time you spend doing each. Assess your results and make changes accordingly. Use these time-management tips to help you:

- **Do one thing at a time.** Don't try to watch television, wash clothes, and write your term paper all at once.
- **Clear your desk.** Toss unnecessary papers; file those you'll need later. Read your mail, recycle what you don't need, and file the rest for later action.
- **Prioritize tasks.** Make a daily "to do" list and stick to it. Categorize things you must do today, things you must do but not immediately, and "nice to dos" that you can take on if you finish the others or if they include something fun.
- **Find a clean, comfortable place to work, and avoid interruptions.** For a project that requires concentration, schedule uninterrupted time. Close your door and turn off your phone—or go to a quiet room in the library or student union.
- **Reward yourself.** Did you finish a task? Do something nice for yourself. Breaks give you time to recharge.
- **Work when you're at your best.** If you're a morning person, study in the morning. Take breaks when you start to slow down.

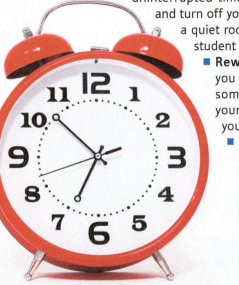

- **Learn to say no.** Avoid overcommitment by scheduling your time wisely. Don't give in to guilt or pressure when others request your time. Avoid spontaneous "yes" responses to new projects.

Managing Your Finances

Higher education can impose a huge financial burden on parents and students—and consequently become a major stressor. Worries over finding a job after graduation coupled with student loans underscore the fact that finances are a major source of stress for most students.[78] These helpful tips can create a less stressful financial situation:

- **Create a budget.** Set a goal to avoid debt as much as possible. Track expenses such as tuition, books, rent, food, and entertainment. List your income to see if what you're spending is equitable to what you're earning or if it's putting you on the debt track.
- **Use credit cards wisely.** Resist credit card offers; racking up debt in school can affect your finances for years to come. Reserve credit cards you do have for less frequent, big-ticket buying, and carry cash whenever possible.
- **Complete a financial inventory.** How much money will you need to do the things you want to do in the future? Will you live alone or share costs with roommates? Do you need to buy a car, or can you rely on public transportation? Consider options for saving money; you need to prepare for emergencies and for future plans.

Consider Downshifting Many people, questioning whether "having it all" is worth it, are taking a step back and simplifying their lives. This trend has been labeled **downshifting**, or **voluntary simplicity**. Moving from a large urban area to a smaller town or leaving a high-stress job for one that makes you happy are examples of downshifting.

Downshifting involves a fundamental alteration in values and honest introspection about what is important in life. It means cutting down on shopping habits, buying only what you need to get by, and living within modest means. When you contemplate any form of downshift, move slowly by planning attainable goals to simplify your life.

- What are some time management strategies that could help reduce your stress levels?

- What are some strategies to improve your financial situation?

3.10 Relaxation Techniques for Stress Management

Learning Outcome

3.10 **Discuss relaxation techniques that can reduce stress.**

Relaxation techniques to reduce stress have been practiced for centuries, and there is a wide array of practices from which to choose. Common techniques include yoga, qigong, tai chi, deep breathing, meditation, visualization, progressive muscle relaxation, massage therapy, biofeedback, and hypnosis.

Yoga Yoga is an ancient practice that combines meditation, stretching, and breathing exercises designed to relax, refresh, and rejuvenate. It began about 5,000 years ago in India and has been evolving ever since. In the United States today, over 80 million Americans (24 percent of the population) say that, over the next year, they are very likely or somewhat likely to practice yoga.[79]

Classical yoga is the ancestor of nearly all modern forms of yoga. Breathing, poses, and verbal mantras are often part of classical yoga. Of the many branches of classical yoga, *Hatha yoga* is the most well known because it is the most body focused. This style of yoga involves the practice of breath control and *asanas*—held postures and choreographed movements that enhance strength and flexibility. Research shows increased evidence of benefits of Hatha yoga in reducing inflammation, boosting mood, increasing relaxation, and reducing stress among those who practice regularly.[80]

Qigong *Qigong* (pronounced "chee-gong"), one of the fastest-growing and most widely accepted forms of mind-body health exercises, is used by some of the country's largest health care organizations, particularly for people suffering from chronic pain or stress. Qigong is an ancient Chinese practice that involves becoming aware of and learning to control *qi* (or *chi*, pronounced "chee"), or vital energy in your body. According to Chinese medicine, a complex system of internal pathways called *meridians* carry *qi* throughout your body. If your *qi* becomes stagnant or blocked, you'll feel sluggish or powerless. Qigong incorporates a series of flowing movements, breath techniques, mental visualization exercises, and vocalizations of healing sounds designed to restore balance and integrate and refresh the mind and body.

Tai Chi *Tai chi* (pronounced "ty-chee") is sometimes described as "meditation in motion." Originally developed in China as a form of self-defense, this graceful form of exercise has existed for about 2,000 years. Tai chi is noncompetitive and self-paced. To do tai chi, you perform a defined series of postures or movements in a

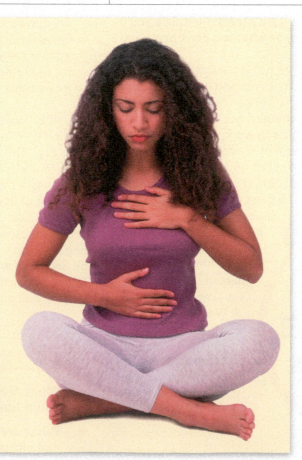

1 Assume a natural, comfortable position either sitting up straight with your head, neck, and shoulders relaxed or lying on your back with your knees bent and your head supported. Close your eyes and loosen binding clothes.

2 In order to feel your abdomen moving as you breathe, place one hand on your upper chest and the other just below your rib cage.

3 Breathe in slowly and deeply through your nose. Feel your stomach expanding into your hand. The hand on your chest should move as little as possible.

4 Exhale slowly through your mouth. Feel the fall of your stomach away from your hand. Again, the hand on your chest should move as little as possible.

5 Concentrate on the act of breathing. Shut out external noise. Focus on inhaling and exhaling, the route the air is following, and the rise and fall of your stomach.

Figure 3.6 Diaphragmatic Breathing
This exercise will help you learn to breathe deeply as a way to relieve stress. Practice this for 5 to 10 minutes several times a day and soon diaphragmatic breathing will become natural for you.

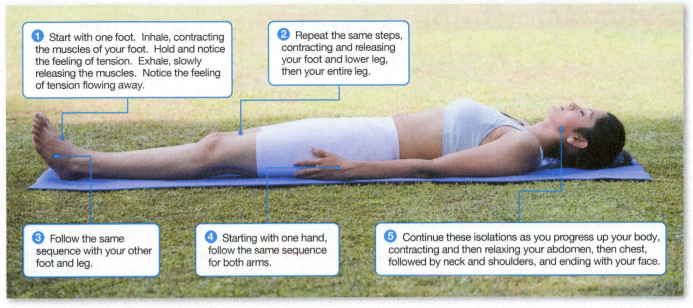

1 Start with one foot. Inhale, contracting the muscles of your foot. Hold and notice the feeling of tension. Exhale, slowly releasing the muscles. Notice the feeling of tension flowing away.

2 Repeat the same steps, contracting and releasing your foot and lower leg, then your entire leg.

3 Follow the same sequence with your other foot and leg.

4 Starting with one hand, follow the same sequence for both arms.

5 Continue these isolations as you progress up your body, contracting and then relaxing your abdomen, then chest, followed by neck and shoulders, and ending with your face.

Figure 3.7 Progressive Muscle Relaxation
Sit or lie down in a comfortable position and follow the steps described to increase your awareness of tension in your body.

slow, graceful manner. Each movement or posture flows into the next without pause. Tai chi has been widely practiced in China for centuries and is becoming increasingly popular around the world, both as a basic exercise program and as a complement to other health care methods. Health benefits include stress reduction, improved balance, and increased flexibility.

Diaphragmatic or Deep Breathing Typically, we breathe using only the upper chest and thoracic region rather than involving the abdominal region. Simply stated, diaphragmatic breathing is deep breathing that maximally fills the lungs by involving the movement of the diaphragm and lower abdomen. This technique is commonly used in yoga exercises and in other meditative practices. Try the diaphragmatic breathing exercise in **Figure 3.6** right now and see if you feel more relaxed!

Meditation There are many different forms of **meditation**. Most involve sitting quietly for 15 minutes or longer, focusing on a particular word or symbol or observing one's thoughts, and controlling breathing. Practiced by Eastern religions for centuries, meditation is seen as an important form of introspection and personal renewal. Recent research found that one form of meditation, *transcendental meditation*, appeared to be most effective in lowering blood pressure, overall mortality, and cardiovascular events.[81]

Visualization Often it is our own thoughts and imagination that provoke distress by conjuring up worst-case scenarios. Our imagination, however, can also be tapped to reduce stress. In **visualization**, you create mental scenes using your imagination. The choice of mental images is unlimited, but natural settings such as ocean beaches and mountain lakes are often used to represent stress-free environments. Recalling specific physical senses of sight, sound, smell, taste, and touch can replace stressful stimuli with peaceful or pleasurable thoughts.

Progressive Muscle Relaxation Progressive muscle relaxation involves systematically contracting and relaxing different muscle

groups in your body. The standard pattern is to begin with the feet and work your way up your body, contracting and releasing as you go (**Figure 3.7**). The process is designed to teach awareness of the different feelings of muscle tension and muscle release. With practice, you can quickly identify tension in your body when you are facing stressful situations, then consciously release that tension to calm yourself.

Massage Therapy If you have ever had someone massage your stiff neck or aching feet, you know that massage is an excellent way to relax. Techniques vary from deep-tissue massage to gentler acupressure.

Biofeedback Biofeedback is a technique in which a person learns to use the mind to consciously control body functions like heart rate, body temperature, and breathing rate. Using machines from those as simple as stress dots that change color with body temperature variation to sophisticated electrical sensors, individuals learn to listen to their bodies and make necessary adjustments, such as relaxing certain muscles, changing breathing, or concentrating to slow heart rate and relax. Eventually, you develop the ability to recognize and lower stress responses without the help of the machine.

Hypnosis Hypnosis requires a person to focus on one thought, object, or voice, thereby freeing the right hemisphere of the brain to become more active. The person then becomes unusually responsive to suggestion. Whether self-induced or induced by someone else, hypnosis can reduce certain types of stress.

Check Yourself

- What are three potential benefits to learning a variety of relaxation techniques?

- Which relaxation technique is the most effective for you? Why?

3.11 Mindfulness Strategies to Relax and Reduce Stress

3.11 Describe mindfulness strategies that can help you reduce stress.

We thrive under a certain amount of stress; however, excessive stress can leave us overwhelmed and unable to cope. Recent studies of college students indicate that the emotional health self-rating of first-year college students compared to their peers is at an all-time low. In fact, researchers report that the emotional health of students has fallen precipitously since surveys were first conducted in 1985, with increasing numbers frequently feeling overwhelmed.[82] Students spend more time studying and less time socializing with friends, and nearly 10 percent report that they are driven to succeed and are frequently depressed.[83] In contrast, sophomores and juniors reported fewer problems with these issues, and seniors reported the fewest problems. This may indicate students' progressive emotional growth through experience, maturity, increased awareness of support services, and more social connections.[84]

A Mindful Approach to Stress

Although you can't eliminate all life stressors, you can train yourself to recognize the events that cause stress and anticipate your reactions to them. Training in mindfulness strategies, particularly **dispositional mindfulness**—an acute "tuning in" and awareness of your thoughts, feelings, and reactions focused on working on nonjudgmental views of situations—may significantly improve your overall stress responses.[85] Studies have shown that stress management and mindfulness training can help people develop resilience and grit, particularly if they have strong social support, healthy family environments, and community supports during the stress-management programming.[86]

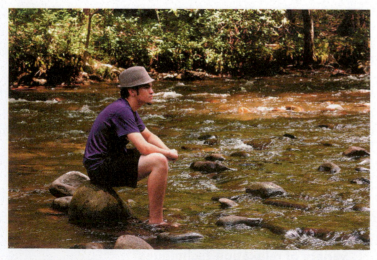

Practicing mindfulness means tuning in to the present, such as taking time to contemplate a scenic view. When you pay attention to the present, you can begin to let go of the stressful distractions in your life.

Stress management isn't something that just happens. It calls for getting a handle on what is going on in your life, taking a careful look at yourself, and coming up with a personal plan of action. Because your perceptions are often part of the problem, assessing your self-talk, beliefs, and actions is a good first step.

Assess Your Stressors to Solve Problems Mindfully Before you can prevent or control your life stressors, you must first analyze them. Several quick mindfulness assessments, which can help you look at your daily experiences and determine whether you are tuned in or merely reacting to circumstances, are available online. Beyond self-assessments, here are some more suggestions for ways to destress:

- **Start a journal.** Track your worries and the factors that seem to trigger stress every day for a week. Think about when your stress is greatest, who is around you, and how you respond. Do you move on, or do you dwell on things?
- **Examine the causes of your stress.** Which causes are tangible? Which are intangible?
- **Think about what is going on with you right now.** Are you wound up and edgy? Tired? A bit ticked at someone? Focus on your body. Are you tense? Sweating? Exhausted? Breathe deeply several times, and focus on your breath. Take a moment that is all about you. Tune in on you, and tune out whatever is bothering you.
- **Take a 10-minute break.** Go for a walk. Focus on the smells in the air, the colors of the landscape, or anything that takes you away from your worries. If you sense yourself being judgmental, stop. Focus on one good thing about someone near you. Smile at a stranger.
- **Focus on your stressor.** Whether it's unnecessary clutter, conflict with friends and family, or chaotic world events putting you over the edge, jot down 3 things you will change, starting now—and then *act!* Limit unsettling news to 30 minutes a day or less. Take care of clutter. Focus on something positive.

A mindful action plan—in which you increase your self-awareness, tune in to your body and surroundings, and assess your stressors and determine how to avoid them—can help reduce stress. It doesn't take earth-shattering changes to help you cope. Making small changes now—and focusing on your life and reactions—can really make a difference.

Change Your Inner Voice: Be Compassionate Often, we are our own worst enemies—nicer to strangers than we are to ourselves or to people we care about. Remember that *compassion* includes kindness, empathy,

See It! Videos

Looking for ways to relax and reduce stress? Watch **Generation Stress: Tips for Millennials to Reduce Stress** in the Study Area of Mastering Health.

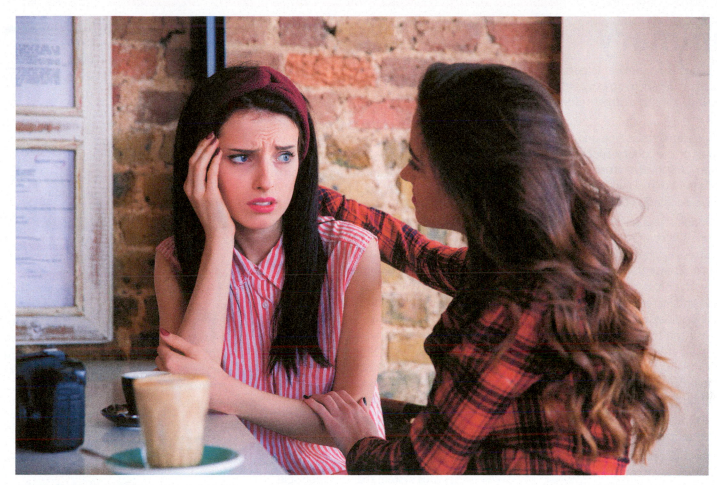

Mindfulness means having compassion and empathy for others.

tolerance, concern for others, sensitivity, and a desire to help someone who needs emotional or tangible help. Unfortunately, many of us grieve for hurt animals and certain other people but walk right past homeless people without looking at them, giving them nonhuman status. Our biases, beliefs, and values can keep us from being compassionate toward certain individuals and groups. We can also be our own worst critics.

A good place to begin is with *self-compassion*. Start each day with two or three things you are thankful for—the good things in your life or something you like about yourself—instead of seeing only faults. Practicing mindfulness can help reduce your stress interactions, help you become less sensitive to potential criticisms, and let you look at your day in a more positive light.

Check Yourself

- Describe five mindfulness strategies that can help you manage stress.

- What is self-compassion? List three things in your life for which you are thankful.

Summary

LO 3.1 Stress is an inevitable part of our lives. *Eustress* refers to stress associated with positive events; *distress* refers to negative events.

LO 3.2 The alarm, resistance, and exhaustion phases of the general adaptation syndrome (GAS) involve physiological responses to both real and imagined stressors and cause complex hormonal reactions.

LO 3.3 Undue stress for extended periods of time can compromise the immune system. Stress has been linked to cardiovascular disease (CVD), weight gain, headaches, hair loss, diabetes, digestive problems, and increased susceptibility to infectious diseases. Psychoneuroimmunology is the science that analyzes the relationship between the mind's reaction to stress and immune function. Stress can affect intellectual and psychological health and contribute to depression and anxiety.

LO 3.4 Sleep conserves body energy and restores physical and mental functioning.

LO 3.5 Psychosocial factors contributing to stress include change, hassles, relationships, pressure, conflict, overload, and environmental stressors. Persons subjected to discrimination or bias may face unusually high levels of stress.

LO 3.6 Some sources of stress are internal and related to appraisal, self-esteem, self-efficacy, personality, and psychological hardiness and resilience.

LO 3.7–3.11 College can be stressful. Recognizing the signs of stress is the first step toward better health. To manage stress, find coping skills that work for you—probably some combination of managing emotional responses, taking mental or physical action, downshifting, time management, managing finances, relaxation techniques, and mindfulness strategies.

Pop Quiz

Visit Mastering Health to personalize your study plan with Chapter Review Quizzes and Dynamic Study Modules.

LO 3.1 1. Even though Andre experienced stress when he graduated from college and moved to a new city, he viewed these changes as an opportunity for growth. What is Andre's stress called?
a. Strain
b. Distress
c. Eustress
d. Adaptive response

LO 3.1 2. Which of the following is an example of a chronic stressor?
a. Giving a talk in public
b. Meeting a deadline for a big project
c. Dealing with a permanent disability
d. Preparing for a job interview

LO 3.2 3. During what phase of the general adaptation syndrome has the physical and psychological energy used to fight the stressor been depleted?
a. Alarm phase
b. Resistance phase
c. Endurance phase
d. Exhaustion phase

LO 3.2 4. In which stage of the general adaptation syndrome does the fight or flight response occur?
a. Exhaustion stage
b. Alarm stage
c. Resistance stage
d. Response stage

LO 3.2 5. The branch of the autonomic nervous system that is responsible for energizing the body for either fight or flight and for triggering many other stress responses is the
a. central nervous system.
b. parasympathetic nervous system.
c. sympathetic nervous system.
d. endocrine system.

LO 3.5 6. A state of physical and mental exhaustion caused by excessive stress is called
a. conflict.   c. hassles.
b. overload.   d. burnout.

LO 3.5 7. Losing your keys is an example of what psychosocial source of stress?
a. Pressure
b. Inconsistent behaviors
c. Hassles
d. Conflict

LO 3.6 8. Which of the following test-taking techniques is not recommended to reduce test-taking stress?
a. Plan ahead and study over a period of time for the test.
b. Eat a balanced meal before the exam.
c. Do all your studying the night before the exam so it is fresh in your mind.
d. Remind yourself of three reasons you will pass the exam.

LO 3.9 9. After 5 years of 70-hour work-weeks, Tom decided to leave his high-paying, high-stress law firm and lead a simpler lifestyle. What is this trend called?
a. Adaptation
b. Conflict resolution
c. Burnout reduction
d. Downshifting

LO 3.9 10. Which of the following is not an example of a time-management technique?
a. Doing one thing at a time
b. Rewarding yourself for finishing a task
c. Practicing procrastination in completing homework assignments
d. Breaking tasks into smaller pieces

Answers to these questions can be found on page A-1. If you answered a question incorrectly, review the module identified by the Learning Outcome. For even more study tools, visit Mastering Health.

Think About It!

LO 3.1 1. Define stress. What are some examples of scenarios in which you might feel distress? Eustress?

LO 3.1 2. Why are the college years often high-stress times for many students?

LO 3.2 3. Describe the alarm, resistance, and exhaustion phases of the general adaptation syndrome and the body's physiological response to stress. Does stress lead to more irritability or emotionality, or does irritability or emotionality lead to stress? Provide examples.

LO 3.3 4. What are some of the health risks that result from chronic stress?

LO 3.8 5. How does anger affect the body? Discuss how mindfulness strategies could help you control your anger and remain calm as you think about things that are bugging you right now.

LO 3.9 6. How much of a procrastinator are you? What sorts of situations make you the most likely to procrastinate? What could you do to reduce the likelihood of procrastinating in these situations?

LO 3.7–3.11 7. What are three important actions you can take right now to help manage your stressors?

Relationships and Sexuality

Humans are social animals—we have a basic need to belong and to feel loved. We can't live without interacting with other people in some way. We build **social capital**, or networks of friends, family, and significant others, who help us feel connected and cope with life's challenges. Numerous studies have shown that supportive interpersonal relationships are beneficial to health.[1]

All relationships involve a degree of risk. However, only by taking risks can we grow and experience all life has to offer. This chapter examines healthy relationships and the communication skills necessary to create and maintain them. Expressing ourselves well

and knowing how to listen to and understand what other people are saying are essential for healthy relationships.

Sexuality is a component of some of our most important relationships—and of our understanding of ourselves. How you experience yourself as a sexual person affects everything from your self-image to your identity, happiness, fertility, and health. Sexuality begins with a person's biological sex, gender, anatomy and physiology, and sexual functions, but it also encompasses values, beliefs, and attitudes about how people see themselves as sexual beings and how they relate to others.

4.1 Characteristics and Types of Intimate Relationships

Learning Outcome

4.1 **List characteristics of intimate relationships, and compare and contrast different theories of love.**

Intimate relationships can be defined in terms of four characteristics: *behavioral interdependence, need fulfillment, emotional attachment,* and *emotional availability.*

Behavioral interdependence refers to the mutual impact that people have on each other as their lives intertwine. Interdependence may become stronger over time, such that each person would feel a great void if the other were gone.

Intimate relationships also provide *need fulfillment.* Through relationships with others, we fulfill our needs for *intimacy* (someone with whom we can share our feelings freely), *social integration* (someone with whom we can share worries and concerns), *nurturance* (someone we can take care of and who will take care of us), *assistance* (someone to help us in times of need), and *affirmation* (someone who will reassure us of our own worth and tell us that we matter).

Intimate relationships also involve strong bonds of *emotional attachment,* or feelings of love. When we hear the word *intimacy,* we often think of a sexual relationship. Although sex can play an important role in emotional attachment, a relationship can be very intimate and yet not sexual. Two people can be emotionally or spiritually intimate, or they can be intimate friends.

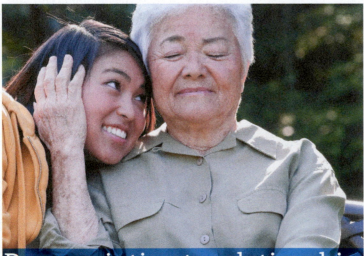

Does an intimate relationship have to be sexual?

We may be accustomed to hearing the word *intimacy* used to describe romantic or sexual relationships, but intimate relationships can take many forms. The emotional bonds that characterize intimate relationships often span generations and give insight into each other's worlds.

Emotional availability is the ability to give to and receive from others emotionally without fear of being hurt or rejected. At times, we may limit our emotional availability—for example, after a painful breakup, holding back can offer time for healing. Some people who have experienced intense trauma find it difficult to ever be available emotionally.[2]

Relating to Yourself

You have probably heard that you must love yourself before you can honestly love someone else. But how do you learn to value and accept who you are? People with high self-esteem show respect for themselves by remaining true to their values and beliefs. They feel worthy of success in love, relationships, and life in general.

Two qualities important to any good relationship are *accountability* and *self-nurturance.* **Accountability** entails recognizing that you are responsible for your own decisions, choices, and actions. **Self-nurturance** means developing individual potential through a balanced and realistic appreciation of self-worth and ability. Individuals who are on a path of accountability and self-nurturance have a much better chance of maintaining satisfying relationships with others.

Self-Esteem and Self-Acceptance Factors that affect your ability to nurture yourself and maintain healthy relationships include how you define yourself (*self-concept*) and how you evaluate yourself (*self-esteem*).

Your perception of yourself influences your relationship choices. If you feel unattractive or inferior to others, you may choose not to interact with them. Or you may unconsciously seek out individuals who confirm your view of yourself by treating you poorly. Conversely, a positive self-concept makes it easier to form relationships with people who nurture you and to interact with others in a healthy, balanced way.

Family Relationships A family is a group whose central focus is to care for, love, and socialize with one another. The family is a dynamic institution that changes as society changes, and the definition of *family* changes over time. Historically, most families have been made up of people related by blood, marriage or long-term committed relationships, or adoption. Yet today, many other groups are recognized and functioning as family units. It is from our **family of origin,** those in our household during our first years, that we initially learn about feelings, problem solving, love, intimacy, and gender roles. We learn to negotiate relationships and have opportunities to communicate, develop attitudes and values, and explore spiritual beliefs. When we establish relationships outside the family, we often rely on experiences and skills modeled by our family of origin.

Friendships

Friendships are often the first relationships we form outside our immediate families, and they can be some of our most stable and enduring. Being able to establish and maintain strong friendships may be a good predictor of success in establishing love relationships because both types of relationship require shared interests and values, mutual acceptance, trust, and respect.

Developing meaningful friendships is more than merely "friending" someone on Facebook. Getting to know someone well requires time, effort, and commitment. A good friend can be an honest and trustworthy companion, someone who honors and respects your strengths and weaknesses, who can share your joys and sorrows, and whom you can count on for support.

Romantic Relationships

Most people choose at some point to enter into an intimate romantic and sexual relationship with another person. Romantic relationships typically include all the characteristics of friendship as well as the following:

- **Fascination.** Lovers are often preoccupied by each other and want to think about, talk to, or be with each other.
- **Exclusiveness.** Lovers have a relationship that usually precludes having the same relationship with a third party. The love relationship often takes priority over all others.
- **Sexual desire.** Lovers desire physical intimacy and want to touch, hold, and engage in sexual activities with each other.
- **Giving the utmost.** Lovers care enough to give the utmost when the other is in need.
- **Being an advocate.** Lovers actively champion each other's interests and attempt to ensure that the other succeeds.

Theories of Love Love may mean different things to different people, depending on cultural values, age, gender, and situation. Although we may not know how to put our feelings into words, we know it when the "lightning bolt" of love strikes. In his Triangular Theory of Love, psychologist Robert Sternberg proposes three key components to loving relationships (**Figure 4.1**):[3]

- **Intimacy.** The emotional component, which involves closeness, sharing, and mutual support.
- **Passion.** The motivational component, which includes lust, attraction, sexual arousal, and sharing.
- **Commitment.** The cognitive component, which includes the decision to be open to love in the short term and commitment to the relationship in the long term.

Sternberg uses the term **consummate love** to describe a combination of intimacy, passion, and commitment.

Quite different from Sternberg's approach are theories of love and attraction based on brain circuitry and chemistry. Anthropologist Helen Fisher, among others, has hypothesized that attraction and love follow a fairly predictable pattern based on (1) *imprinting*,

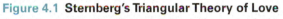

Figure 4.1 Sternberg's Triangular Theory of Love
According to Sternberg's model, three elements—intimacy, passion, and commitment—existing alone or in combination, form different types of love. The most complete, ideal type of love in the model is consummate love, which combines balanced amounts of all three elements.

in which our evolutionary patterns, genetic predispositions, and past experiences trigger a romantic reaction; (2) *attraction*, in which neurochemicals produce feelings of euphoria and elation; (3) *attachment*, in which endorphins—natural opiates—cause lovers to feel peaceful, secure, and calm; and (4) production of a *cuddle chemical*, in which the brain secretes the hormone oxytocin, stimulating sensations during lovemaking and eliciting feelings of satisfaction and attachment.[4]

A love-smitten person's endocrine system secretes chemical substances such as *dopamine, norepinephrine,* and *phenylethylamine (PEA)*, which are chemical cousins of amphetamines. Attraction may in fact be a "natural high." However, this passion "buzz" loses effectiveness over time as the body builds up a tolerance. Fisher suggests that the significant drop in PEA levels over a 3- to 4-year period leads to the "4-year itch" that manifests in peaking fourth-year divorce rates. Romances that last beyond the 4-year mark are influenced by endorphins that give lovers a sense of security, peace, and calm.[5]

Check Yourself

- **What are the common characteristics of intimate relationships?**
- **What are the most important characteristics you look for in a friend? In a romantic relationship?**
- **What are the strengths and weaknesses of the proposed theories of love?**

4.2 Strategies for Success in Relationships

Learning Outcome

4.2 Compare characteristics of healthy and unhealthy relationships, and identify factors that affect the choice of a romantic partner and the achievement of a healthy relationship.

Although success in a relationship is often defined by the number of years together, respect, friendship, enjoyment of each other's company, and communication are the true measures of success.

What Makes a Healthy Relationship?

Satisfying and stable relationships share traits such as good communication, intimacy, and friendship (**Figure 4.2**). A key ingredient is trust, the degree of confidence each person feels in a relationship. Trust includes three fundamental elements:

1. **Predictability.** You can predict your partner's behavior on the basis of past actions.
2. **Dependability.** You can rely on your partner for emotional support, particularly in situations in which you feel threatened with hurt or rejection.
3. **Faith.** You feel certain about your partner's intentions and behavior.

How do you know whether you're in a healthy relationship? Answering some basic questions can help you determine whether a relationship is working.

- Do you love and care for yourself to the same extent that you did before the relationship? Can you be yourself in the relationship? Do you feel that you are equals in the relationship?
- Do you share interests, values, and opinions? Is there mutual respect for, and civil discussion of, differences?
- Are there genuine caring and goodwill? Are there mutual encouragement and emotional support?
- Do you trust each other? Are you honest with each other? Can you comfortably express feelings, needs, and desires?
- Is there room for growth as you both evolve and mature?

Choosing a Romantic Partner

The choice of partner is influenced by more than just chemical and psychological processes. One important factor is *proximity*: The more often you see someone, the more likely it is that interaction will occur.

We often choose partners on the basis of *similarities* (in attitudes, values, intellect, interests, education, and socioeconomic status); the adage that "opposites attract" usually isn't true.

Also playing a significant role is *physical attraction*. Attraction is complex and influenced by social, biological, and cultural factors.[6]

Hooking up Hooking up is a vague term that is often used to describe sexual encounters, from kissing to intercourse, without the expectation of the commitment involved in a romantic relationship. Hooking up may feel new, but research tells us that young adults' sexual behavior hasn't changed much in the past few decades in terms of the number of sexual encounters or the number of partners. We may just communicate about it more freely and use different modes of communication.

Sternberg's Triangular Theory of Love would place hooking up in the infatuation category; passion with no commitment or intimacy; far from Sternberg's picture of "ideal." Additionally, according to Fisher, attraction and sex create a chemical reaction in the brain that fosters an emotional response even if we say, "it's just about the sex."

It's important to understand the risks involved in hookups. In a recent study, students reported that they were more likely to hook up if they had been drinking alcohol. Reduced inhibitions due to alcohol along with a lack of communication with a new partner increases the risk of unprotected sex and thus the risk for unintended pregnancy and sexually transmitted infections (STIs).[7]

Confronting Couple Issues

Couples in long-term relationships must confront issues that can either enhance or diminish their chances of success.

Jealousy Jealousy is an unhappy or angry feeling caused by the belief that someone you love likes or is liked by someone else or that someone is coming between the two of you in some way. Jealousy often indicates underlying problems such as insecurity or possessiveness. Often, jealousy is rooted in past deception and loss. Other common causes include the following:

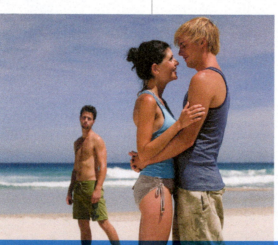

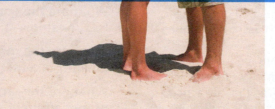

Is it normal to be **jealous?**

Most of us have insecurities, and as a result, many relationships include a certain amount of jealousy. If you communicate about your jealous feelings, your relationship shouldn't suffer. However, if jealousy is ignored or becomes extreme, it can undermine and threaten a relationship.

In an unhealthy relationship...	In a healthy relationship...
You care for and focus on another person only and neglect yourself, or you focus only on yourself and neglect the other person.	You both love and take care of yourselves before and while in a relationship.
One of you feels pressure to change to meet the other person's standards and is afraid to disagree or voice ideas.	You respect each other's individuality, embrace your differences, and allow each other to be yourselves.
One of you has to justify what you do, where you go, and whom you see.	You both do things with friends and family and have activities independent of each other.
One of you makes all the decisions and controls everything without listening to the other's input.	You discuss things with each other, allow for differences of opinion, and compromise equally.
One of you feels unheard and is unable to communicate what you want.	You express and listen to each other's feelings, needs, and desires.
You don't have any personal space and have to share everything with the other person.	You respect each other's need for privacy.
Your partner keeps his or her sexual history a secret or hides a sexually transmitted infection from you, or you do not disclose your history to your partner.	You share sexual histories and information about sexual health with each other.
You feel stifled, trapped, and stagnant. You are unable to escape the pressures of the relationship.	You both have room for positive growth, and you both learn more about each other as you develop and mature.

Figure 4.2 Healthy versus Unhealthy Relationships

Source: Adapted from Advocates for Youth, Washington, DC, www .advocatesforyouth.org. Copyright © 2000. Reprinted with permission.

- **Overdependence.** People with few social ties who rely exclusively on their significant others tend to be fearful of losing them.
- **Severity of the threat.** People may feel uneasy if someone with stunning good looks and a great personality appears to be interested in their partner or makes what appear to be "come-on" communications.
- **High value on sexual exclusivity.** People who believe that sexual exclusivity is a crucial indicator of love are more likely to become jealous.
- **Low self-esteem.** People who think poorly of themselves are more likely to fear someone will gain their partner's affection.
- **Fear of losing control.** Feeling one may lose attachment to or control over a partner can cause jealousy.

Although a certain amount of jealousy can be expected in any relationship, it doesn't have to threaten a relationship as long as partners communicate openly about it.[8]

Changing Gender Roles Throughout history, women and men have taken on various roles in relationships. Modern American society has very few gender-specific roles; many couples find that it makes more sense to divide tasks according to convenience and preference. Others still believe that there are women's roles and men's roles. Problems arise when couples do not share the same view. Regardless of what the perception of modern roles may be, facts show a different picture. While many women work as many hours outside the home as men, the division of labor at home is rarely equal. The Bureau of Labor Statistics estimates that on a typical day, 50 percent of women do household chores such as cleaning or laundry, where the same is true of only 22 percent of men; while 70 percent of women prepare food or clean up afterward, only 43 percent of men do those tasks.[9] Over time, if couples can't communicate about this, the relationship may suffer.

Sharing Power Power can be defined as the ability to make and implement decisions. In traditional relationships, men were the wage earners and consequently had decision-making power. As women have become earners, the dynamics have shifted considerably. In general, successful couples share responsibilities, power, and control.

Unmet Expectations We all have expectations of ourselves and our partners—how we'll spend our time and money, express love, and grow as a couple. If we can't communicate our expectations, we set ourselves up for disappointment, frustration, and anger. Partners in healthy relationships communicate wants and needs and have honest discussions when problems occur.

Check Yourself

- What three characteristics do you think are most important in a healthy relationship? Which one do you consider the most important?
- What factors are involved in the choice of a romantic partner?
- What are common obstacles to achieving a successful relationship?

4.3 Relationships and Social Media

Learning Outcome

4.3 Discuss appropriate uses for social media in establishing and maintaining relationships.

Technology has revolutionized our access to information and the ways we communicate. Couples can meet on a site such as Match.com, keep in constant contact via texting, and inform the world of their relationship highs and lows via Facebook, Twitter, Instagram, and Snapchat. With all these tools available, it can be easy to share *TMI* (*too much information*). At their best, social media can bring people closer together; at their worst, social media can be used intentionally or unintentionally to embarrass, damage reputations or worse. Fake news, uncivil behavior, and other negative communications have prompted many sources to call for changes in existing social media activities. In a recent national meeting, Mark Zuckerberg, Facebook CEO, outlined Facebook's new mission: *To bring the world closer together and to build community . . . to help create a more civil and productive debate on bigger issues.*[10]

Dating and Social Media

With the growing trend in online dating, you may be just as likely to meet your future life partner through a website or app than at school or work. In a 2016 study, 27 percent of 18- to 24-year-olds had used online dating—triple the rate of just 2 years previously.[11]

When you join an online dating site or use social networks to meet others, it's important to be honest about yourself and your background. State your own interests and characteristics fairly, including things that you think might be less attractive than stereotypes and cultural norms dictate. Show a recent photo of yourself; not a photoshop creation.

If you meet someone online and want to meet in person, put safety first. Plan something brief, preferably during daylight hours. Meet in a public place, such as a coffee shop. Do not meet with anyone who wants to keep the time and location a secret. Tell a friend or family member the details of when and where you are meeting and any information you have on the person you are meeting (including his or her name and contact information).

Whether or not you meet romantic partners online, use social media responsibly while dating:

- Discuss limits with your partner on the type of information each of you wants shared online. Agree to share only within those limits.
- Be aware that your partner might not be as comfortable with posting information to social media as you are. Be mindful, and ask permission, before posting any pictures of you as a couple or information about your activities or whereabouts.
- Recognize that constant electronic updates throughout the day can leave little to share when you are together. Save some information for face-to-face talks.
- Sober up before you click "submit." Things that seem funny under the influence might not seem funny the next morning.
- Remember that the Internet is forever. Once a picture or a post has been sent, it can never be completely erased. Never post anything that would embarrass someone if it were seen by a family member or potential employer.
- Respect your partner's privacy. Logging onto his or her e-mail or social media account to look at private messages is a breach of trust.
- Know that the GPS in a phone can be used to track your location and that cell phone spyware can be installed that allows e-mail and texts to be read from another device. If you think you may be a victim of *cyberstalking* by a current (or former) partner, get a new phone or ask the phone company to reinstall the phone's operating system to wipe out the software.
- Do not break up with someone via text, e-mail, tweet, Facebook, or chat. People deserve the respect of a more personal break up.
- If you break up, be sure to change any passwords you might have confided in your partner. The temptation to use those for ill may be too strong to resist.

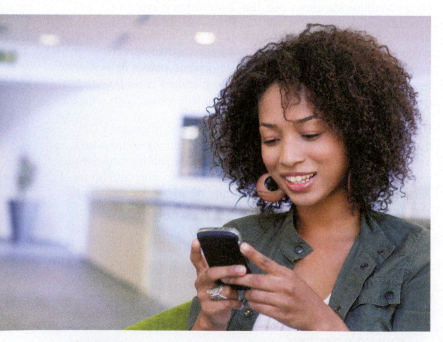

Chatting with potential romantic partners online? Be honest about yourself and your interests, and stay away from people who don't seem like they're being honest with you.

Check Yourself

- **What are three safety measures to take when dating online?**

- **How can social media be used responsibly when dating?**

4.4 Skills for Better Communication: Appropriate Self-Disclosure

Learning Outcome

4.4 **Discuss the role of appropriate self-disclosure in good communication.**

From the moment of birth, we struggle to be understood. We flail our arms, cry, scream, smile, frown, and make sounds and gestures to attract attention or to communicate what we want or need. By the time we enter adulthood, each of us has developed a unique way of communicating with gestures, words, expressions, and body language. No two people communicate in the exact same way or have the same need for connecting. Some of us are outgoing and quick to express our emotions and thoughts. Others are quiet and reluctant to talk about feelings.

Different cultures have different ways of expressing feelings and using body language. Men and women also tend to have different styles of communication, largely dictated by culture and socialization.

Although people differ in how they communicate, no one sex, culture, or group is better at it than another. We must be willing to accept differences and work to keep communication open and fluid. Remaining interested, engaged, and willing to exchange ideas and thoughts are skills typically learned with practice.

When two people begin a relationship, they bring their communication styles with them. How often have you heard someone say, "We just can't communicate" or "You're sending mixed messages"? Communication is a process; our every action, word, expression, gesture, and posture become part of our shared experience and part of the evolving impression we make on others. If we are angry in our responses, others will be reluctant to interact with us. If we bring "baggage" from past bad interactions to new relationships, we may be cynical, distrustful, and guarded. If we are positive, happy, and share openly, other people may be more likely to communicate openly with us. The ability to communicate appropriately and openly is an important skill in relationships. Effective communicators are in touch with their feelings and values and can communicate their needs directly, appropriately, and honestly.

Sharing personal information with others is called **self-disclosure**. If you want to learn more about someone, you have to be willing to share parts of yourself with that person. Self-disclosure is not storytelling or deep, dark, secrets; rather, it is revealing how you are reacting to the present situation in a comfortable setting and giving any information about the past that is relevant to the other person's understanding of your current reactions and that you feel safe in sharing.

If you sense that sharing feelings and thoughts will result in a closer relationship, you will likely take such a risk. But if you believe that the disclosure may result in rejection or alienation, you might not open up so easily. If the confidentiality of shared information has been violated, you might hesitate to disclose yourself in the future. However, the risk in not disclosing yourself to others is that you will lack intimacy in relationships.[12]

If self-disclosure is such a key to creating healthy communication but fear is a barrier to that process, what can you do? The following suggestions can help:

- **Get to know yourself.** The more you know about your feelings, beliefs, thoughts, and concerns, the more likely it is that you'll be able to communicate with other people about yourself.
- **Become more accepting of yourself.** No one is perfect or has to be.
- **Be willing to discuss your sexual history.** The U.S. culture puts many taboos on discussions of sex, so it's no wonder we find it hard to disclose our sexual feelings. However, with the triple threat of unintended pregnancy, STIs, and HIV/AIDS, it is important to discuss your sexual history with a partner. Time and positive interactions help build trust. Where there is trust, sharing may be easier.
- **Choose a safe context for self-disclosure.** When and where you make such disclosures and to whom may greatly influence the response. Choose a setting in which you feel safe to let yourself be known.

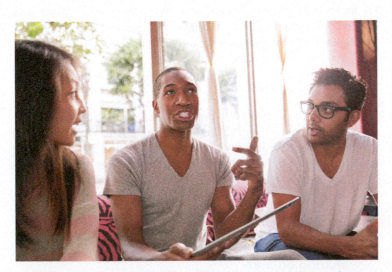

While everyone's communication style is unique, cultural norms have a big impact. Members of some cultures gesture broadly; others maintain a closed body posture. Some are offended by direct eye contact; others welcome a steady gaze.

Check Yourself

- How can appropriate self-disclosure contribute to healthy communication?

- Describe two ways to help get over fear of self-disclosure and create healthy communication.

Skills for Better Communication: Using Technology Responsibly

4.5 Identify what is appropriate and inappropriate to share online.

Self-disclosure can be an effective method of building intimacy with another person but not with large groups. While it may seem tempting or funny, sharing highly personal information via social media can make you vulnerable or embarrassed later.

Headlines such as "Gay students accidentally outed to parents via Facebook" remind us that we can no longer expect privacy. We are all a photo tag away from a family member or potential employer seeing us in less than flattering circumstances or knowing information that we would prefer be kept secret.

Social media screening, the practice of searching out all possible information on a prospective employee (sometimes to the point of asking for a Facebook password at an interview) is practiced by about a third of employers. Their biggest concerns: inappropriate photos; evidence of drug or alcohol use or abuse; biased, illegal behaviors; and poor writing skills.

Posting negative comments online about employers, your peers, and anyone else you interact with can also spell trouble. It's not uncommon for employees to get fired for posting rants against their employers on blogs and social media. University administrators may also check your social network feeds. Early In 2017, several prospective new students were rejected for university admission when their online posts were deemed inappropriate by university administrators. Things you post to peers may quickly circulate and be shared, making you vulnerable to lawsuits and legal interventions. Increasing numbers of lawsuits for slander and

In a survey,

34%

of hiring managers who currently research candidates via social media said they have found information that has caused them not to hire a candidate.

defamation have been filed against people who post hateful, false, or damaging information about others online.

Take measures to protect your privacy online and spare yourself from the damaging repercussions that can follow misuse of social media:[13]

- Make sure your publicly available information is what you want prospective employers, community members, and family to see. Assume that potential employers will look you up on Facebook, Twitter, and other social media sites.
- Anything you posted in the past has the potential to resurface and damage your reputation now or in the future. Tighten your privacy settings, and untag yourself in photos and videos you don't want others to see.
- Know your rights if someone posts photos or other information about you as a means of damaging your reputation.
- Don't post damaging or hurtful comments about anyone online, even if you feel that you have been wronged or you are angry about something the other person has said or done. This includes employers, housemates, professors, and anyone else you're tempted to gripe about.
- Remember that even if you post comments on social networking sites "anonymously," someone who is determined enough could still track you down. Be cautious even when you think you're incognito.

Because of cached sites and reposts, you can't erase everything, so you might need to prepare an explanation for past posts, photos, and other information. As our "private" lives get more public, we may have to accept Facebook founder Mark Zuckerberg's philosophy, that "privacy is no longer a social norm."[14]

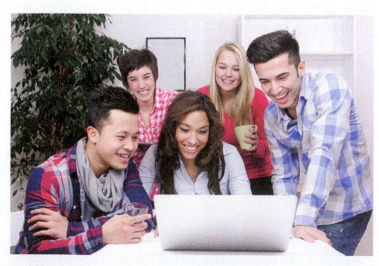

Avoid having your private life become the life of the party. Whenever you share information online—whether it's positive or negative—remember that it can easily be seen and shared beyond your intended audience.

- What types of information should you avoid sharing online?

- Do you think people have the right to say what they want about a person or a business online? Why or why not?

4.6 Skills for Better Communication: Understanding Gender Tendencies

Learning Outcome

4.6 Describe differences and similarities in communication tendencies between men and women.

Men and women tend to differ in communication styles (Figure 4.3), largely as a result of culture and gender socialization—though it is important to note that there may be significant variation within groups of men and women, depending on culture, age, geography, and other factors.

Recognizing these tendencies can help us avoid frustrations and irritations. For example, a man communicating with a woman might make an effort to provide opportunities for the woman to jump into the conversation, since women tend to be less willing to interrupt.

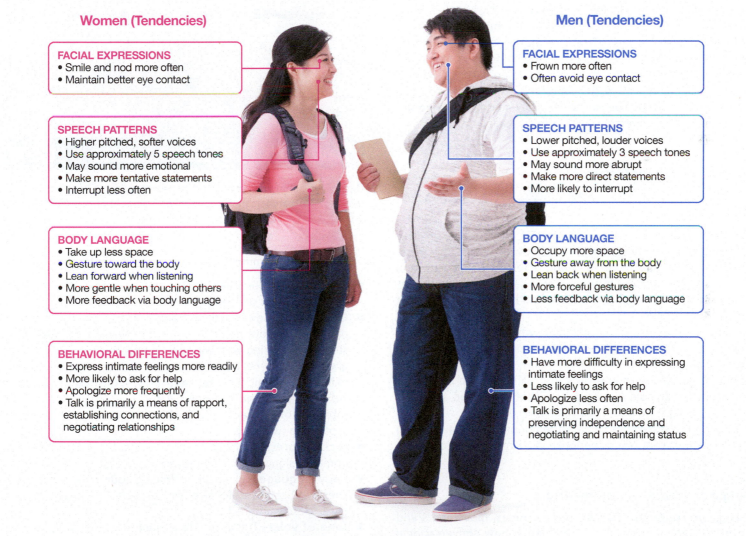

Women (Tendencies)

FACIAL EXPRESSIONS
• Smile and nod more often
• Maintain better eye contact

SPEECH PATTERNS
• Higher pitched, softer voices
• Use approximately 5 speech tones
• May sound more emotional
• Make more tentative statements
• Interrupt less often

BODY LANGUAGE
• Take up less space
• Gesture toward the body
• Lean forward when listening
• More gentle when touching others
• More feedback via body language

BEHAVIORAL DIFFERENCES
• Express intimate feelings more readily
• More likely to ask for help
• Apologize more frequently
• Talk is primarily a means of rapport, establishing connections, and negotiating relationships

Men (Tendencies)

FACIAL EXPRESSIONS
• Frown more often
• Often avoid eye contact

SPEECH PATTERNS
• Lower pitched, louder voices
• Use approximately 3 speech tones
• May sound more abrupt
• Make more direct statements
• More likely to interrupt

BODY LANGUAGE
• Occupy more space
• Gesture away from the body
• Lean back when listening
• More forceful gestures
• Less feedback via body language

BEHAVIORAL DIFFERENCES
• Have more difficulty in expressing intimate feelings
• Less likely to ask for help
• Apologize less often
• Talk is primarily a means of preserving independence and negotiating and maintaining status

Figure 4.3 Tendencies in Verbal and Nonverbal Communication by Gender
Sources: Tannen, D. (2007). *You just don't understand: Women and men in conversation.* New York: Harper Collins; Torppa, C.B. (2010). *Gender issues: Communication differences in interpersonal relationships.* Retrieved from https://ohioline.osu.edu/factsheet/FLM-FS-4-02-R10; Wood, J. and Fixmer-Oraiz, N. (2017). *Gendered lives.* Boston: Cengage.

Check Yourself

■ How would you describe communication tendencies among men and women?

4.7 Skills for Better Communication: Mindful Listening and Nonverbal Skills

Learning Outcome

4.7 Explain the importance of mindful listening, and list and describe forms of nonverbal communication.

Listening allows us to share feelings, express concerns, communicate wants and needs and to make our thoughts and opinions known. When we listen mindfully, we focus on the speaker's words and also on their tone of voice, facial expressions, and body language. We are aware, fully listening, and receptive to their message. We avoid interrupting, except to encourage or ask for clarification. This allows us to hear the "meta-message"—the message underlying the words that tells the whole story the speaker is trying to convey. It takes discipline to listen without judging, arguing, or being defensive, but mindful listening helps to avoid conflict and allows the speaker to feel fully heard, improving our relationships and connections with other people.

Becoming a Better Listener

To become a more mindful listener, practice these skills on a daily basis:[15]

- To avoid distractions, turn off the TV and shut down your laptop. Turn off your phone and put it away.
- Be present in the moment. Good listeners participate and acknowledge what the other person is saying through nonverbal cues such as nodding or smiling and by asking questions at appropriate times.
- Ask for clarification. If you aren't sure what the speaker means, say that you don't completely understand or paraphrase what you think you heard.
- Control the desire to interrupt. Try taking a deep breath for 2 seconds, then hold your breath for another second, and really listen to what is being said as you slowly exhale.
- Focus on the speaker. Hold back the temptation to launch into a story about your own experience in a similar situation.

Using Nonverbal Communication

Smiling, eye contact or its lack, making faces, movements and gestures—these nonverbal clues influence how conversational partners interpret messages. **Nonverbal communication** includes all unwritten and unspoken messages, intentional and unintentional. Ideally, nonverbal communication matches and supports verbal communication. Research shows that when verbal and nonverbal communications don't match, we are more likely to believe the nonverbal cues.[16] It's important to be aware of the nonverbal cues we use and understand how other people might interpret them.

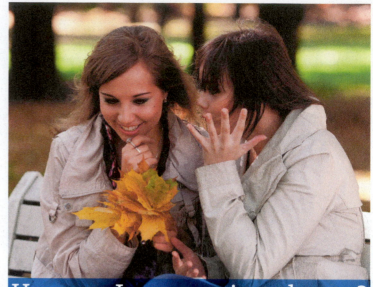

How can I communicate better?

One way to communicate better is to pay attention to your body language. Researchers have found that 93 percent of communication effectiveness is determined by nonverbal cues.

Nonverbal communication can include the following:[17]

- **Touch.** This can be a handshake, a hug, a hand on the shoulder or arm, or a kiss on the cheek.
- **Gestures.** These can include mannerisms such as a thumbs-up or a wave or movements that augment verbal communication, such as indicating with your hands how big the fish was that got away. Gestures can also be rude, such as rolling one's eyes to indicate disdain for what has been said or shaking your head 'no' when someone is talking.
- **Interpersonal space.** This is the amount of physical space separating two people.
- **Facial expressions.** Expressions such as frowns, smiles, and grimaces signal moods and emotions.
- **Body language.** This includes folding your arms across your chest, indicating defensiveness, or leaning forward in your chair to show interest.
- **Tone of voice.** This refers to elements of speaking such as pitch, volume, and speed.

Check Yourself

- **Why is mindful listening an important part of communication?**
- **How do nonverbal cues affect interactions?**

Learning Outcome

4.8 Identify strategies for managing and resolving conflict.

A **conflict** is an emotional state that arises when one person's behavior interferes with that of another. Some conflict is inevitable, and not all conflict is bad; airing feelings and resolving differences can strengthen relationships. **Conflict resolution** and conflict management form a systematic approach to resolving differences fairly and constructively.

Prolonged conflict can destroy relationships unless the parties agree to resolve points of contention. As two people learn to negotiate and compromise, the number and intensity of conflicts should diminish.

During a heated conflict, try to pause before responding, consider the possible impact of your comments or actions, and state your point constructively. You can also say, "I can see we aren't going to resolve this right now. Let's talk when we've both cooled off."

E-mail messages are easily misunderstood because the recipient can't see or hear the person talking. In general, when you're tempted to send a nasty response to an e-mail, stop. Observe the 24-hour rule: Don't hit Send until the next day. Usually, you'll find that it's better to hit Delete and move on or to talk in person.

Rudeness or inconsiderate behavior usually develops when one person fails to recognize the feelings or rights of another. Try to see the other person's point of view, listen actively, avoid interrupting, and avoid gestures such as head-shaking or finger-pointing. Key elements of conflict management include validating others' opinions and treating others as you would like to be treated.

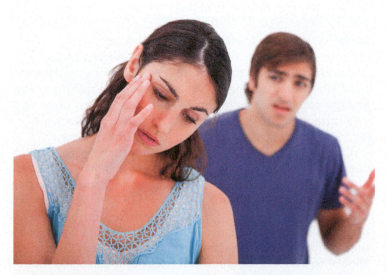

All couples have conflicts. Learning to handle them maturely is vital to relationship success.

Here are some strategies for conflict resolution:

1. **Identify the problem.** Talk together to clarify the conflict or problem. Say what you want, and listen to what the other person wants. Use "I" messages; avoid blaming "you" messages. Be an active listener: Repeat what the other person has said and ask questions for clarification or information.
2. **Generate possible solutions.** Brainstorm ways to address the problem. Base your search on goals and interests that were identified in the first step. Come up with several alternatives, but avoid evaluating them for now.
3. **Evaluate solutions.** Review the possible solutions. Narrow your list to one or two that work for both parties. Focus on finding a solution that you both feel is satisfactory.
4. **Decide on the best solution.** Choose an alternative that is acceptable to both parties. You must both commit to the decision for it to be effective.
5. **Implement the solution.** Discuss how the decision will be carried out. Establish who is responsible to do what and when.
6. **Follow up.** Check in and evaluate whether a solution is working. If it's not working as planned or if circumstances have changed, revise your plan. Remember that both parties must agree to any changes to the original idea.

Skills for **Behavior Change**

Communicating When Emotions Run High

These guidelines can help you express your feelings more effectively in an emotionally charged situation:

- Try to be specific rather than general about how you feel.
- When expressing anger or irritation, describe the specific behavior you don't like, then your feelings.
- If you have mixed feelings, say so; express and explain each feeling.
- Use "I" messages, rather than "you" statements that can cast blame or imply fault. With "I" messages, the speaker takes responsibility for communicating his or her feelings, thoughts, and beliefs.
- When you ask for feedback, be prepared for an honest answer.
- Be careful when trying to communicate or interpret emotionally charged messages via e-mail or text. It can be hard to interpret their intended meaning without the nonverbal support of tone of voice and body language.

Check Yourself

- **Which strategy for conflict resolution do you find most effective? Why?**

4.9 Committed Relationships

Commitment in a relationship means an intent to act over time in a way that perpetuates the well-being of the other person, oneself, and the relationship. Polls show that the vast majority of Americans strive to develop a committed relationship whether in the form of marriage, cohabitation, or partnerships, but an increasing number of young Americans remain single by choice.[18]

Marriage

In many societies, traditional committed relationships take the form of marriage. In the United States, marriage means entering into a legal agreement that includes shared finances and responsibility for raising children. Many Americans also view marriage as a religious commitment.

Approximately 50 percent of U.S. adults are married (**Figure 4.4**). However, the percentage of Americans who are married is at its lowest point since 1920. Half of people aged 18 and over were married in 2015, compared with 72 percent in 1960.[19] This decrease is due to a combination of a delay of first marriages, a substitution of cohabitation for marriage, and concerns over

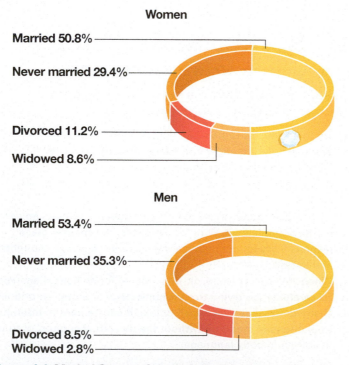

Women

Married 50.8%

Never married 29.4%

Divorced 11.2%

Widowed 8.6%

Men

Married 53.4%

Never married 35.3%

Divorced 8.5%
Widowed 2.8%

Figure 4.4 **Marital Status of the U.S. Population by Sex**
Note: The figure does not list the percentages for married men and women with a spouse absent and separated.
Source: U.S. Census Bureau, "Table MS-1, Marital Status of People 15 Years and Over, by Sex, Race, and Hispanic Origin: 1950 to Present," America's Families and Living Arrangements, 2016, www.census.gov.

88% of Americans list love as the most important reason to marry.

finances. When people do marry, they do so later than ever before. In 1960, the median age for first marriage was 22.8 years for men and 20.3 years for women; today, the median age for first marriage has risen to 29.5 years for men and 27.4 years for women.[20]

Many Americans believe that marriage involves **monogamy**, or exclusive sexual involvement with one partner. However, the lifetime pattern for many Americans appears to be **serial monogamy**, that is, a person has a monogamous sexual relationship with one partner while contemplating or actually moving on to another.[21] Some people prefer **open relationships**, in which partners agree that each may be sexually involved with others outside their relationship.

Considerable research indicates that married people live longer, feel happier, remain mentally alert longer, and suffer fewer physical and mental health problems.[22] A new study by the National Bureau of Economic Research confirms the long-lasting benefits of marriage, indicating that friendship is the critical element of these benefits.[23] A healthy marriage contributes to lower stress levels in three important ways: fewer risky personal behaviors, expanded support networks, and financial stability. Rates of risky personal behaviors, including smoking and heavy alcohol use, are lower in married adults, who are about half as likely to be smokers as are cohabitating, divorced, separated, or widowed adults.[24] The one negative health indicator for married people is body weight in men. Married men are far more likely than never-married men to be overweight; however, they are also more likely to visit a doctor at early stages of disease than their unmarried counterparts.[25]

Choosing Whether to Have Children Choosing to raise children changes a marriage or other relationship. Children can bring joy and meaning to their parents' lives. However, raising children is also highly stressful. Time, energy, and money are split many ways, and the parents will no longer be able to give each other undivided attention. Having a child does not save a bad relationship; in fact, it seems to compound problems that already exist.

Changing patterns in family life affect the way children are raised. Now, either partner may provide primary child care. The blended family is the most common family unit, creating instant families for stepparents and stepchildren. In addition, many individuals have children in a family structure other than heterosexual marriage. Single women and lesbian couples can choose adoption or alternative insemination; single men and gay couples can choose to adopt or obtain the services of a surrogate mother. According to the U.S. Census Bureau, over 28 percent of all children under age 18 are living in families headed by a man or woman raising a child alone.[26] Regardless of structure, certain factors remain important to a family's well-being: consistency, communication, affection, and respect. Good parenting does not necessarily come naturally. Many people parent as they were parented, using strategies that may or may not follow sound childrearing principles. A positive, respectful parenting style sets the stage for healthy family growth and development.

Finally, potential parents must consider the financial implications of having a child. It is estimated that a family with a child will spend more than $240,000 on the child over the next 17 years, not including the cost of college.[27] Prospective parents should think about how they will handle childrearing both financially and practically. For instance, which parent will work less or not at all, or how will they pay for child care?

Cohabitation

Cohabitation is a relationship in which two unmarried people with an intimate connection live together. In some states, cohabitation lasting a designated number of years (usually 7) legally constitutes a **common-law marriage** for purposes of sharing many financial obligations. Cohabitation can offer many of the same emotional benefits as marriage. Some people may also cohabit for financial reasons. More than 9 million couples, about 7 percent of American adults 18 and older—are choosing cohabitation.[28] Cohabitation is increasingly the first co-residential partnership formed by young adults.[29]

Cohabitation before marriage has been a controversial issue for decades. While some critics voiced moral objections, other concerns were related to higher divorce rates among couples who cohabited before marriage. However, according to recent research, cohabitation before marriage is no longer a predictor for divorce.[30]

Cohabitation can be a prelude to marriage, but for some couples, it is an alternative. It is more common among people of lower socioeconomic status, those who are less religious, those who have been divorced, marry later in life, and those who have experienced parental divorce or high parental conflict during childhood. Cohabitation has both advantages and drawbacks. Perhaps the greatest disadvantage is the lack of societal validation for the relationship, especially if the couple subsequently has children. Many cohabitants also deal with difficulties obtaining insurance and tax benefits and legal issues over shared property if there is a divorce.

Gay and Lesbian Partnerships

Lesbians and gay men seek the same things in committed relationships that heterosexuals do: love, friendship, communication, validation, and stability. There are 783,100 reported same-sex couples in the United States, 25 percent of whom are legally married.[31]

Challenges to successful lesbian and gay relationships often stem from discrimination and difficulties dealing with social, legal, and religious doctrines. For lesbian and gay couples, obtaining benefits such as tax deductions, power-of-attorney rights, partner health insurance, and child custody rights has been challenging. Now, however, with the 5-to-4 Supreme Court ruling in

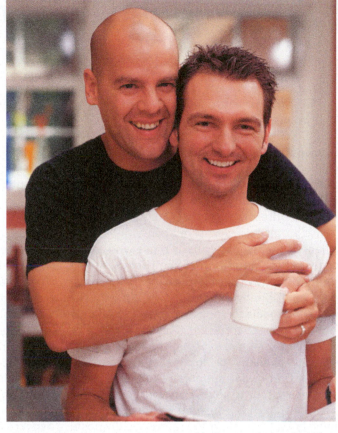

The desire to form lasting and committed intimate relationships is shared by most adults, regardless of sexual orientation.

the *Obergefell v. Hodges* case, same-sex marriage is legal in all 50 states.[32] Supreme Court Justice Anthony Kennedy said that the Court's decision was based on the acknowledgment of four fundamental principles: that marriage is inherent to the concept of individual autonomy, that marriage is of unparalleled importance to committed couples, that marriage is crucial for safeguarding the rights of the children of couples in committed relationships, and that marriage has long been a keystone of social order.[33]

Staying Single

Increasing numbers of adults of all ages are choosing to marry later or remain single altogether. According to the most recent U.S. Census, 57 percent of women and 67 percent of men age 20 to 34 are single.[34] Over a lifetime, 29 percent of females and 35 percent of males remain single, having never married.[35] Contrary to old stereotypes, many single people live rewarding lives and maintain a network of close friends and families.

Check Yourself

- **What forms can committed relationships take? What are the advantages and disadvantages of different types of committed relationships?**

When Relationships Falter

4.10 Discuss common reasons that relationships end, and provide examples of how to cope with a failed relationship.

Breakdowns in relationships usually begin with a change in communication, however subtle. Either partner may stop listening and cease to be emotionally present for the other. In turn, the other feels ignored, unappreciated, or unwanted and may withdraw emotionally. Unresolved conflicts increase, and unresolved anger can cause problems in sexual relations.

College students, particularly those who are socially isolated or far from family and hometown friends, may be particularly vulnerable to staying in unhealthy relationships. They may become emotionally dependent on a partner for everything from sharing meals to spending recreational time. Mutual obligations, such as shared rental arrangements, transportation, and child care, can make it tough to leave. It's also easy to mistake sexual advances for physical attraction or love. Without a network of friends and supporters to talk with, to obtain validation for feelings, or to share concerns, a student may feel stuck in a relationship that is headed nowhere.

Honesty and verbal affection are usually positive aspects of a relationship. In a troubled relationship, however, they can be used to cover up irresponsible or hurtful behavior. "At least I was honest" is not an acceptable substitute for acting in a trustworthy way. "But I really do love you" is not a license for being inconsiderate or rude. Relationships that are lacking in mutual respect and consideration can become physically or emotionally abusive.

Recognizing a Potential Abuser

Is that new person in your life really what he or she appears to be? Your new love interest may appear sensitive, gentle, caring, respectful, and considerate in the beginning—all the things you've been looking for. It can be hard to tell what someone is really like early on, as each person tries to make a good impression on the other. To avoid getting into a long-term relationship with an abuser, watch carefully over time, and trust your instincts. Ask other people about the person, and find out about his or her history with partners, friends, and family. Be immediately wary if your partner demonstrates any of the following red flags:

- Gets extremely angry and swears at you or others.
- Hurts you by making fun of you or putting you down.
- Takes too much control. In a healthy relationship, partners share decision making.
- Displays excessive jealousy.
- Tries to shut out people you want to see and wants to spend more and more time alone with you.

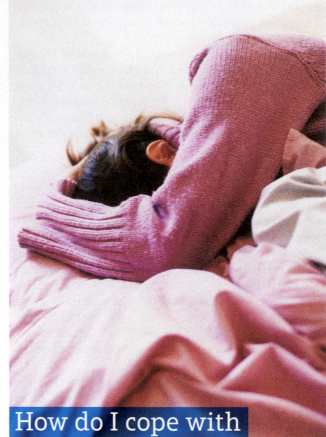

How do I cope with a bad breakup?

It might feel as if there is no end to the sorrow, anger, and guilt that often are the result of a difficult breakup or cheating partner, but time is a miraculous healer. Acknowledging your feelings, finding healthy ways to express them, spending time with friends, and allowing yourself to take as much time as you need to recover are all helpful strategies for dealing with the end of a romantic relationship.

- Expresses continual negativity—sulks, angers easily, throws tantrums when things don't go his or her way.
- Pressures you verbally or physically to have unwanted sex or intimacy.
- Threatens you.
- Is often in trouble or fighting with someone; is alienated from family and criticizes your family/friends.

This list is not exhaustive, and there are degrees of seriousness for each. However, if someone you have known for only a short time displays any sign of physical anger or threatens you early on, it's time to walk away.

When and Why Relationships End

Some estimates indicate that approximately 50 percent of first marriages end in divorce, with even higher divorce rates for second and third marriages.[36] However, other studies suggest that the divorce rate for new marriages is only 30 percent and that it has been declining since the early 1980s.[37] This decrease is related to an increase in the number of couples who cohabit instead of marry, an increase in the age at which people first marry, and a higher level of education among those who do marry.[38] The risk of divorce is lower for college-educated people marrying for the first time; it is lower still for people who wait to marry until their mid-twenties and who haven't cohabited with multiple partners prior to marriage.[39]

Why do relationships end? There are many reasons and many factors, including illness, financial concerns, and career problems. Other breakups arise from unmet expectations. Many people enter a relationship with certain expectations about how they and their partner will behave. Failure to communicate these beliefs can lead to resentment and disappointment. Differences in sexual needs may also contribute to the demise of a relationship. Under stress, communication and cooperation between partners can break down. Conflict, negative interactions, and a general lack of respect between partners can erode even the most loving relationship.

What behaviors signal that trouble is coming? On the basis of 35 years of research and couples therapy, John Gottman has identified four behavior patterns in couples that predict future divorce with better than 90 percent accuracy.[40]

- **Criticism.** Phrasing complaints in terms of a partner's defect, for example: "You never talk about anyone but yourself. You are self-centered."
- **Defensiveness.** Righteous indignation as a form of self-protection, for example: "It's not my fault we missed the flight. You always make us late."
- **Stonewalling.** Withdrawing emotionally from a given interaction, for example: The listener seems to ignore the speaker as he or she speaks, giving no indication that the speaker was heard.
- **Contempt.** Talking down to a person, for example: "How could you be so stupid?" Contempt is the biggest predictor of divorce.

While these behaviors do not guarantee that an individual couple will divorce, they are red flags for relationships that are at great risk for failure.

Coping with Failed Relationships

No relationship comes with a guarantee, no matter how many promises partners make to be together forever. Losing a love is as much a part of life as falling in love. Even so, the uncoupling process can be very painful. Whenever we risk getting close to another person, we also risk being hurt if things don't work out. Remember that knowing, understanding, and feeling good about oneself before entering a relationship is very important. Consider these tips for coping with a failed relationship:

- **Acknowledge that you've gone through a rough spot.** You may feel grief, loneliness, rejection, anger, guilt, relief, and sadness. Seek out trusted friends and, if needed, professional help. Just as you would see a doctor for a broken leg, it makes sense to see a therapist or counselor for a broken heart if it isn't healing by itself.
- **Let go of negative thought patterns and habits and engage in activities that make you happy.** Go for a walk, talk to friends, listen to music, work out at the gym, volunteer with a community organization, or write in a journal.
- **Spend time with current friends, or reconnect with old friends.** Get reacquainted with yourself, what you enjoy doing, and the people whose company you enjoy.
- **Don't rush into a "rebound" relationship.** You need time to resolve your past experience rather than escaping from it. You can't be trusting and intimate in a new relationship if you are still working on getting over a past relationship.

Skills for Behavior Change

How Do You End It?

Relationship endings are just as important as their beginnings. Healthy closure affords both parties the opportunity to move on without wondering or worrying about what went wrong and whose fault it was. If you choose to end a relationship, do so in a manner that preserves and respects the dignity of both partners. If you are the person initiating the breakup, you have probably had time to think about the process and may be at a different stage from your partner.

Here are some tips for ending a relationship in a respectful and caring way:

- Arrange a time and quiet place where you can talk without interruption.
- Say in advance that there is something important you want to discuss.
- Accept that your partner may express strong feelings, and be prepared to listen quietly.
- Consider in advance whether you might also become upset and what support you might need.
- Communicate honestly using "I" messages, rather than "you" messages that often convey a personal criticism or attack. Explain your reasons as much as you can without being cruel or insensitive.
- Don't let things escalate into a fight, even if you have very strong feelings.
- Offer another opportunity to talk about the end of the relationship when you both have had time to reflect.

4.10 Relationships and Sexuality

Check Yourself

- What are some common reasons that relationships end?
- What are three ways to cope with a failed relationship?

Your Sexual Identity: More than Biology

4.11 Define and discuss the major components of sexual identity.

Sexual identity, the recognition and acknowledgment of oneself as a sexual being, is determined by the interaction of genetic, physiological, environmental, and social factors.

The beginning of sexual identity occurs at conception with the combining of chromosomes. Each egg (ovum) carries an X chromosome; a sperm cell may carry either an X or a Y chromosome. Thus, it is the sperm that determines sex. If a sperm carrying an X fertilizes an egg, the resulting combination of chromosomes (XX) produces a female. If a sperm carrying a Y fertilizes an egg, the XY combination produces a male.

The genetic instructions included in the sex chromosomes lead to the differential development of male and female **gonads** (reproductive organs). Once the male gonads (testes) and the female gonads (ovaries) develop, they play a key role in all future sexual development, being responsible for production of sex hormones. The primary female sex hormones are estrogen and progesterone; the primary male sex hormone is testosterone. The release of testosterone in a maturing fetus stimulates the development of a penis and other male genitals. If no testosterone is produced, female genitals form.

At the time of **puberty**, hormones released by the **pituitary gland**, the gonadotropins, stimulate the testes and ovaries to make appropriate sex hormones. The increase of estrogen production in females and testosterone production in males leads to the development of **secondary sex characteristics**, features that distinguish the sexes but have no direct reproductive function. For males, these include deepening of the voice, development of facial and body hair, and growth of the skeleton and musculature. For females, they include growth of breasts, widening of hips, and development of pubic and underarm hair.[41]

Another important component of sexual identity is **gender**, which refers to characteristics and actions typically associated with men or women (masculine or feminine) as defined by culture. Our sense of masculine and feminine traits is largely a result of **socialization** during childhood. **Gender roles** are the behaviors and activities we use to express maleness or femaleness in ways that conform to our society's expectations. For example, as a child, you might have learned to play with dolls or trucks according to how your parents influenced your actions.[42]

Gender roles can be confining when they lead to stereotyping. Boundaries established by **gender-role stereotypes** can make it difficult to express one's identity. In the United States, men are traditionally expected to be independent, aggressive, logical, and in control of their emotions. Women are traditionally expected to be passive, nurturing, intuitive, and emotional.[43] **Androgyny** refers to the combination of traditional masculine and feminine traits in a single person; each of us is in small or large ways androgynous. Highly androgynous people do not always follow traditional sex roles.

Whereas gender roles are an expression of cultural expectations for behavior, **gender identity** is a sense or awareness of being male or female. There are many emerging variations of gender and gender identity that do not fit the traditional gender role norms or sexual orientation roles. One example might be when the sex assigned at birth (male or female) does not match a person's gender identity according to cultural expectations of gender, the person is **transgender**.[44] There is a broad spectrum of expression among transgendered people that reflects their degree of dissatisfaction with their sexual anatomy or their gender roles. Some transgendered people are comfortable with their bodies and content simply to dress and live as the other gender; others feel trapped in their bodies and may opt for interventions such as sex reassignment surgery.

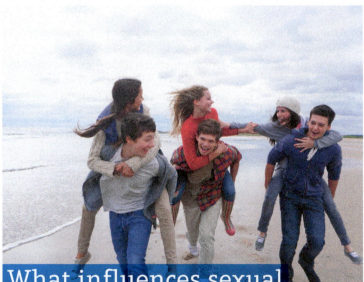

What influences sexual identity besides biology?

How you perceive yourself as a sexual being is influenced by your socialization and personal experience. Your understanding of gender roles, your contact with people of various gender identities or sexual orientations, and your own degree of emotional maturity can all affect your sense of sexual identity.

See It! Videos

What terms are used in talking about gender and sexuality? Watch **Transgender Terms: Breaking Down Definitions and Dos & Don'ts** in the Study Area of Mastering Health.

Sexual Orientation

Sexual orientation is a person's enduring emotional, romantic, sexual, or affectionate attraction to others. You may be primarily attracted to members of the opposite sex (**heterosexual**), the same sex (**homosexual**), or both sexes (**bisexual**). Many prefer the term **gay**, queer, or **lesbian** to describe their

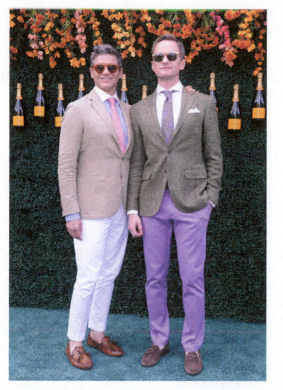

The presence of gay and lesbian celebrities in the media—such as actor Neil Patrick Harris and his husband David Burtka or Ellen DeGeneres and her wife Portia de Rossi—contributes to the increasing acceptance of gay relationships in everyday life.

sexual orientation. *Gay* and *queer* can apply to both men and women; *lesbian* refers specifically to women.[45]

Most researchers agree that sexual orientation is best understood by using a model that incorporates biological, psychological, and socioenvironmental factors. Biological explanations focus on research into genetics, hormones, and differences in brain anatomy, whereas psychological and socioenvironmental explanations examine parent–child interactions, sex roles, and early sexual and interpersonal interactions. Collectively, this growing body of research suggests that the origins of homosexuality, like those of heterosexuality, are complex. To diminish the complexity of sexual orientation to "a choice" is a clear misrepresentation of current research.

Gay, lesbian, and bisexual people are often the targets of **sexual prejudice** (or *sexual bias*). Prejudice refers to negative attitudes and hostile actions directed at a social group. Hate crimes, discrimination, and hostility toward sexual minorities are evidence of ongoing sexual prejudice. Bias regarding sexual orientation is the motivation for approximately 19 percent of all hate crimes reported in the United States.[46]

Sexual orientation is often viewed as based entirely on whom one has sex with, but this is inaccurate and overly simplistic. It depends not only on whom you are sexually attracted to, fantasize about, and have sex with, but also factors such as whom you feel close to emotionally and socialize with and in which "community" you feel comfortable. From this viewpoint, there are not just three orientations (homosexual, heterosexual, and bisexual), but a range of complex, interacting, and fluid factors that influence sexuality over time.

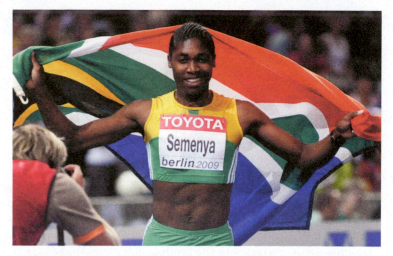

After South African middle-distance runner Caster Semenya won the gold medal in the 800-meter race at the 2009 World Championships, she was required to undergo gender testing and was subsequently barred from competition. Officials wanted to determine whether Semenya has a disorder of sexual development resulting in testosterone levels that were giving her an unfair athletic advantage over other women competitors. After 11 months, a panel of medical experts announced that Semenya was again eligible to compete against other women. Her case highlights the challenges facing athletes and other people with both male and female characteristics.

Disorders of Sexual Development

Sometimes chromosomes are added, lost, or rearranged at conception, and the sex of the offspring is unclear, a condition known as **intersexuality.** Many professional groups use the term **disorders of sexual development (DSDs)**, a less confusing term, to describe intersex conditions, which may occur as often as 1 in 1,500 live births.[47]

People with DSDs are born with various levels of male and female biological characteristics, ranging from different chromosomal arrangements to altered hormone production to variation in primary and secondary sex characteristics. Whereas most people are born with either XX or XY chromosomes, some are born with XXY or XO chromosomes (where O signifies a missing or damaged chromosome). In some people, gonads do not develop fully into ovaries or testicles, although there may be no external signs to indicate this; in others, external genitalia may be ambiguous.

Many, but not all, DSDs require some degree of hormonal or surgical intervention to ensure physical health. It is also necessary to "assign" a gender to children with DSDs as early as possible to ensure good psychological health. If this assignment is later found to be inconsistent with the person's own sense of gender, he or she may adopt a different gender identity. Most people born with DSDs can choose as adults whether to have additional surgeries to alter any sexual tissues they feel are incongruent with their gender.

Check Yourself

- **What is sexual identity?**

- **How is sexual identity similar and/or different from sexual orientation?**

Female Sexual Anatomy and Physiology

4.12 Identify the major features and functions of female sexual anatomy and physiology.

The female reproductive system includes two major groups of structures: the external genitals and the internal organs (Figure 4.5).

The external female genitals are collectively known as the **vulva**. The **mons pubis** is a pad of fatty tissue covering and protecting the pubic bone; after the onset of puberty, it becomes covered with coarse hair. The **labia majora** are folds of skin and erectile tissue that enclose the urethral and vaginal openings; the **labia minora**, or inner lips, are folds of mucous membrane found just inside the labia majora.

The **clitoris** is located at the upper end of the labia minora and beneath the mons pubis; its only known function is to provide sexual pleasure, and it is the most sensitive part of the genital area. Directly below the clitoris is the **urethral opening**, through which urine is expelled from the body; below it is the vaginal opening. In some women, the vaginal opening is covered by a thin membrane called the **hymen.** The hymen can be stretched or torn by physical activity and is not present in all women to begin with. The **perineum** is the area of smooth tissue between the vulva and the anus. The tissue in this area has many nerve endings and is sensitive to touch; it can play a part in sexual excitement.

The internal female genitals include the vagina, uterus, fallopian tubes, and ovaries. The **vagina** is a tubular organ that serves as a passageway from the uterus to the outside of the body. It allows menstrual flow to exit from the uterus during a woman's monthly cycle, it receives the penis during intercourse, and it serves as the birth canal during childbirth. The **uterus (womb)** is a hollow, muscular, pear-shaped organ. Hormones acting on the inner lining of the uterus (the **endometrium**) either prepare the uterus for implantation and development of a fertilized egg or signal that no fertilization has taken place, in which case the endometrium deteriorates and becomes menstrual flow.

The lower end of the uterus, the **cervix**, extends down into the vagina. The **ovaries**, almond-sized organs on either side of the uterus, produce the hormones estrogen and progesterone and are the reservoir for immature eggs. (All the eggs a woman will ever have are present in her ovaries at birth.) Extending from the upper end of the uterus are two thin, flexible tubes called the **fallopian tubes** (or **oviducts**). The fallopian tubes capture eggs as they are released from the ovaries during ovulation and are the site where sperm and egg meet and fertilization takes place. They then serve as the passageway to the uterus, where the fertilized egg becomes implanted.

The Onset of Puberty and the Menstrual Cycle

With the onset of puberty, the female reproductive system matures, and secondary sex characteristics develop, including breasts, widened hips, and underarm and pubic hair. The first sign of puberty is the beginning of breast development, around age 11.

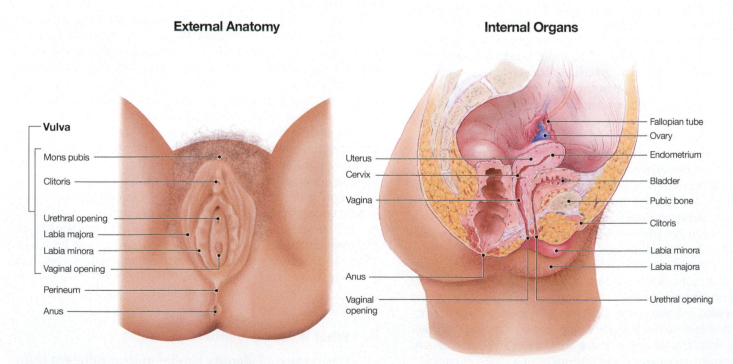

External Anatomy

Internal Organs

Vulva
- Mons pubis
- Clitoris
- Urethral opening
- Labia majora
- Labia minora
- Vaginal opening

Perineum

Anus

Uterus
Cervix
Vagina
Anus
Vaginal opening

Fallopian tube
Ovary
Endometrium
Bladder
Pubic bone
Clitoris
Labia minora
Labia majora
Urethral opening

Figure 4.5 Female Reproductive System

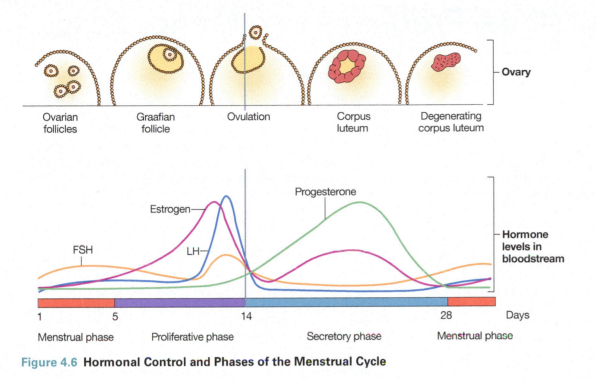

Ovary

Ovarian follicles | Graafian follicle | Ovulation | Corpus luteum | Degenerating corpus luteum

Progesterone

Estrogen

FSH | LH

Hormone levels in bloodstream

1 | 5 | 14 | 28 | Days

Menstrual phase | Proliferative phase | Secretory phase | Menstrual phase

Figure 4.6 Hormonal Control and Phases of the Menstrual Cycle

The pituitary gland, **hypothalamus**, and ovaries all secrete hormones that act as chemical messengers among them.

Around the same time, the hypothalamus receives a message to begin secreting *gonadotropin-releasing hormone (GnRH)*. This, in turn, signals the pituitary gland to release hormones called *gonadotropins*. Two specific gonadotropins, *follicle-stimulating hormone (FSH)* and *luteinizing hormone (LH)*, signal the ovaries to start producing **estrogens** and **progesterone**. The normal age range for the onset of the first menstrual period, or **menarche**, is 10 to 18 years, with the average age falling between 12 and 13 years.[48]

The average menstrual cycle lasts 28 days and consists of the proliferative, secretory, and menstrual phases (**Figure 4.6**). The *proliferative phase* begins with the end of menstruation. During this time, the endometrium develops, or proliferates. The hypothalamus, sensing low levels of estrogen and progesterone in the blood, increases its secretions of GnRH, which in turn triggers the pituitary gland to release FSH. When FSH reaches the ovaries, it signals several **ovarian follicles** to begin maturing. Normally, only one of the follicles, the **Graafian follicle**, reaches full maturity in the days preceding ovulation. While the follicles mature, they begin producing estrogen, which in turn signals the endometrial lining of the uterus to proliferate. High estrogen levels signal the pituitary to slow down FSH production and increase release of LH. Under the influence of LH, the Graafian follicle ruptures and releases a mature **ovum** (plural: *ova*), a single egg cell, near a fallopian tube. This event, which usually occurs around day 14 of the cycle, is referred to as **ovulation.** The other ripening follicles degenerate and are reabsorbed by the body. Occasionally, two ova mature and are released during ovulation. If both are fertilized, fraternal (nonidentical) twins develop. Identical twins develop when

one fertilized ovum (called a *zygote*) divides into two separate zygotes.

The phase following ovulation is called the *secretory phase*. The ruptured Graafian follicle, which has remained in the ovary, is transformed into the **corpus luteum** and begins secreting large amounts of estrogen and progesterone. These secretions peak around the twentieth day of the cycle and cause the endometrium to thicken. If fertilization and implantation take place, cells surrounding the developing embryo release *human chorionic gonadotropin (HCG)*, increasing estrogen and progesterone secretions that maintain the endometrium and signal the pituitary not to start a new menstrual cycle. If no implantation occurs, the hypothalamus signals the pituitary to stop producing FSH and LH, thus causing the levels of progesterone in the blood to peak. The corpus luteum begins to decompose, leading to rapid declines in estrogen and progesterone, the hormones needed to sustain the uterine lining. Without them, the endometrium is sloughed off in the menstrual flow, beginning the *menstrual phase*. Low estrogen levels signal the hypothalamus to release GnRH, which acts on the pituitary to secrete FSH—and the cycle begins again.

Check Yourself

- What are the major features and functions of female sexual anatomy and physiology?

- Describe the phases of a 28-day menstrual cycle. When is pregnancy most likely?

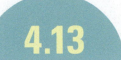

4.13 Menstrual Problems and Menopause

4.13 **Discuss possible menstrual problems.**

Premenstrual Syndrome

Premenstrual syndrome (PMS) is a term used for a collection of physical, emotional, and behavioral symptoms that many women experience 7 to 14 days before the beginning of their menstrual period. The most common symptoms are tender breasts, food cravings, fatigue, irritability, and depression. It is estimated that 85 percent of menstruating women experience at least one symptom of PMS each month.[49] For the majority of women, these disappear as their period begins, but for a small subset of women (3 to 5 percent), symptoms are severe enough to affect daily routines and activities to the point of being disabling. This severe form of PMS has its own designation, **premenstrual dysphoric disorder (PMDD)**, with symptoms that include severe depression, hopelessness, anger, anxiety, low self-esteem, difficulty concentrating, irritability, and tension.[50]

Several natural approaches to managing PMS can also help PMDD. These include eating more carbohydrates (grains, fruits, and vegetables), reducing caffeine and salt intake, exercising regularly, and taking measures to reduce stress. Recent investigation into methods of controlling severe emotional swings has led to the use of antidepressants for treating PMDD.[51]

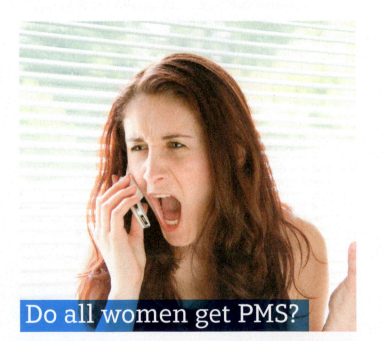

Do all women get PMS?

About 85 percent of menstruating women experience some PMS symptoms every month, but for most women, these symptoms are mild and short-lived. Stress reduction, regular exercise, and a healthy diet are all good strategies for coping with PMS symptoms, which can include irritability and moodiness, fatigue, breast tenderness, and food cravings.

Dysmenorrhea

Dysmenorrhea is a medical term for menstrual cramps, the pain or discomfort in the lower abdomen that many women experience just before or after menstruation. Along with cramps, some women can experience nausea and vomiting, loose stools, sweating, and dizziness. Primary dysmenorrhea doesn't involve any physical abnormality and usually begins 6 months to a year after a woman's first period; secondary dysmenorrhea has an underlying physical cause such as endometriosis or uterine fibroids.[52] If you experience primary dysmenorrhea, you can reduce discomfort by using over-the-counter nonsteroidal anti-inflammatory drugs (NSAIDs) such as aspirin, ibuprofen (Advil or Motrin), or naproxen (Aleve). Soaking in a hot bath or using a heating pad on your abdomen may also ease cramps. For severe cramping, your health care provider may recommend a low-dose oral contraceptive to prevent ovulation, which, in turn, may reduce the production of prostaglandins and therefore the severity of cramps. Managing secondary dysmenorrhea involves treating the underlying cause.

Toxic shock syndrome (*TSS*), although rare today, is still something women should be aware of. It is caused by a bacterial infection facilitated by tampon or diaphragm use. Symptoms, which occur during one's period or a few days afterward, can be hard to recognize because they mimic the flu and include sudden high fever, vomiting, diarrhea, dizziness, fainting, or a rash that looks like sunburn. Proper treatment usually ensures recovery in 2 to 3 weeks.[53]

Changes in the Menstrual Cycle: Menopause

Just as menarche signals the beginning of a woman's potential reproductive years, **menopause**—the permanent cessation of menstruation—signals the end. Generally occurring between the ages of 45 and 55, menopause results in decreased estrogen levels, which may produce symptoms such as decreased vaginal lubrication, hot flashes, headaches, dizziness, and joint pain.[54]

Synthetic forms of estrogen and progesterone have long been prescribed as **hormone replacement therapy**, also known as **menopausal hormone therapy**. This treatment was intended to relieve menopausal symptoms and reduce the risk of heart disease and osteoporosis. However, research later revealed that menopausal hormone therapy increased the risk for heart disease, stroke, blood clots, and breast cancer in some women.[55] Today, doctors prescribe this therapy only when menopause symptoms are severe, the woman is under age 60, and the woman is free of heart disease, diabetes, high cholesterol, high blood pressure, and a history of breast, ovarian, or uterine cancer.[56] Women are now encouraged to manage mild symptoms by changing lifestyle habits such as exercising regularly, sleeping in a cooler room, and limiting caffeine and alcohol intake.[57]

Check Yourself

- **What are some common problems associated with menstruation?**

4.14 Identify major features and functions of male sexual anatomy and physiology.

The structures of the male reproductive system are divided into external and internal genitals (**Figure 4.7**).

The external genitals are the penis and the scrotum. The **penis** is the organ that deposits sperm in the vagina during intercourse. The urethra, which passes through the center of the penis, acts as the passageway for both semen and urine to exit the body. During sexual arousal, the spongy tissue in the penis becomes filled with blood, making the organ stiff (erect). Further sexual excitement leads to **ejaculation**, a series of rapid, spasmodic contractions that propels semen out of the penis.

Situated behind the penis and also outside the body is a sac called the **scrotum**. The scrotum encases the testes, protecting them and helping to control their internal temperature, which is vital to proper sperm production. The **testes** (singular: *testis*) manufacture sperm and **testosterone**, the hormone responsible for development of male secondary sex characteristics, including deepening of the voice and growth of facial, body, and pubic hair.

The development of sperm is referred to as **spermatogenesis**. Like the maturation of eggs in the female, this process is governed by the pituitary gland. Follicle-stimulating hormone (FSH) is secreted into the bloodstream to stimulate the testes to manufacture sperm. Immature sperm are released into a comma-shaped structure on the back of each testis called the **epididymis** (plural: *epididymides*), where they ripen and reach full maturity.

Each epididymis contains coiled tubules that gradually "unwind" to become the **vas deferens**. The two vasa deferentia make up the tubes whose sole function is to store and move sperm. Along the way, the **seminal vesicles** provide sperm with nutrients and other fluids that compose **semen**.

The vasa deferentia eventually connect each epididymis to the **ejaculatory ducts**, which pass through the prostate gland and empty into the urethra. The **prostate gland** contributes more fluids to the semen, including chemicals that help the sperm fertilize an ovum and neutralize the acidic environment of the vagina to make it more conducive to sperm motility and potency. Just below the prostate gland are two pea-shaped nodules called the **Cowper's glands**. The Cowper's glands secrete a fluid that lubricates the urethra and neutralizes any acid that may remain in the urethra after urination. During ejaculation of semen, a small valve closes off the tube to the urinary bladder.

Circumcision

Debate continues over the practice of *circumcision*, the surgical removal of the *foreskin*, a fold of skin that covers the end of the penis. In the United States, approximately 60 percent of all newborn boys are circumcised. Circumcision can be a controversial issue for parents, who must balance personal, cultural, and health issues in deciding whether to circumcise a son.[58]

Arguments for circumcision include religious or cultural reasons (Jewish and Muslim cultures have historically circumcised) and easier genital hygiene. There is also a lower risk of penile cancer, urinary tract infections during infancy, and foreskin infections.

Arguments against circumcision include the possibility of pain during the surgery and potential complications such as infection or improper healing. Families may feel the foreskin is needed for reasons of identity, culture, or sexual pleasure.

Andropause

Men do not experience a rapid hormone decline in middle age as women do during menopause. Instead, men typically experience a gradual decline in testosterone levels throughout adulthood, averaging 1 percent a year after age 30.[59] Many doctors use the term *andropause* to describe age-related hormone changes in some men, with symptoms including reduced sexual desire, infertility, changes in sleep patterns or insomnia, increased body fat, reduced muscle bulk, decreased bone density, and hair loss. Men may also experience emotional changes such as decreased motivation, depression, or memory problems.[60] For some men, testosterone therapy relieves bothersome symptoms. For others, especially older men, the benefits aren't clear.

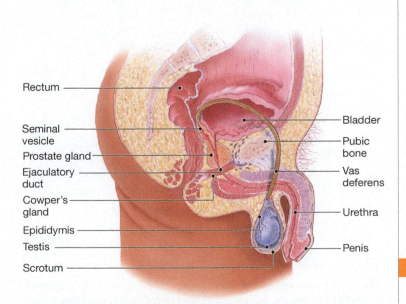

Rectum
Seminal vesicle
Prostate gland
Ejaculatory duct
Cowper's gland
Epididymis
Testis
Scrotum
Bladder
Pubic bone
Vas deferens
Urethra
Penis

Figure 4.7 **Male Reproductive System**

- What are the major features and functions of male sexual anatomy and physiology?

Human Sexual Response and Expression

4.15 Discuss the human sexual response, and give examples of human sexual expression.

For both men and women, sexual response is a physiological process of four stages: excitement/arousal, plateau, orgasm, and resolution. Of course, individuals can vary in their experiences of this pattern.

During *excitement/arousal*, **vasocongestion** (increased blood flow causing swelling in the genitals) stimulates genital responses. The vagina begins to lubricate, and the penis becomes partially erect.

During the *plateau phase*, initial responses intensify. Voluntary and involuntary muscle tensions increase. The woman's nipples and the man's penis become erect. The penis secretes a few drops of pre-ejaculatory fluid, which may contain sperm.

During the *orgasmic phase*, vasocongestion and muscle tension reach their peak, and rhythmic contractions occur through the genital regions. In women, these contractions are centered in the uterus, outer vagina, and anal sphincter. In men, the contractions occur in two stages. First, contractions within the prostate gland begin propelling semen through the urethra. In the second stage, the muscles of the pelvic floor, urethra, and anal sphincter contract. Semen usually, but not always, is ejaculated from the penis.

Muscle tension and congested blood subside in the *resolution phase* as the genital organs return to pre-arousal states. Both sexes usually experience feelings of well-being and profound relaxation. Many women can become re-aroused and experience additional orgasms; most men experience a refractory period of a few minutes to a few hours, during which they are incapable of subsequent arousal.

Although men and women experience the same stages in the sexual response cycle, time spent in any one stage varies; one partner may be in the plateau phase while the other is in the excitement/arousal or orgasmic phase. Such variations are entirely normal.

Sexual Responses among Older Adults

Older adults are commonly stereotyped as being incapable of or uninterested in sex. In truth, although we do experience physical changes as we age, they generally do not cause us to stop enjoying sex.

In women, the most significant physical changes follow menopause. Skin becomes less elastic; vaginal lubrication may decrease. (Use of artificial lubricants usually resolves this problem.) Men's bodies also change; they require more direct and prolonged stimulation to achieve erection and are slower to reach orgasm, with less intense ejaculation.

Sexual Behavior: What Is "Normal"?

Which sexual behaviors are considered normal? Whose criteria should we use? Every society sets standards and attempts to regulate sexual behavior. Some common sociocultural standards for sexual behavior in Western culture today include the following:[61]

- **The coital standard.** Penile–vaginal intercourse (coitus) is viewed as the ultimate sex act.
- **The orgasmic standard.** Sexual interaction should lead to orgasm.
- **The two-person standard.** Sex is an activity to be experienced by two people.
- **The romantic standard.** Sex should be related to love.
- **The safer-sex standard.** If we choose to be sexually active, we should act to prevent unintended pregnancy or disease transmission.

These are not rules, but social scripts. Sexual standards often shift over time, and many people choose not to follow them. Rather than making blanket judgments about normal versus abnormal, we might ask: Is a sexual behavior healthy and fulfilling for a particular person? Is it safe? Does it involve exploitation of others? Does it take place between responsible, consenting adults?[62]

In this way, we can view behavior along a continuum that takes into account many individual factors.

Options for Sexual Expression

The range of human sexual expression is virtually infinite. What you find enjoyable might not be an option for someone else. How you meet your sexual needs may change over time. Accepting yourself as a sexual person with individual desires and preferences is the first step in achieving sexual satisfaction.

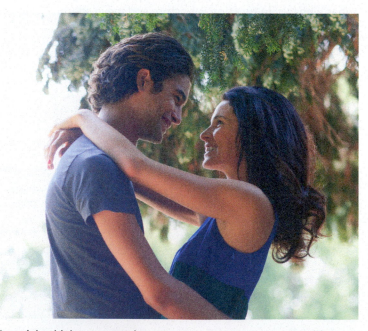

You might think everyone else on campus is having more sex with more partners than you are, but generally speaking, the actual numbers don't measure up to college students' perceptions.

Celibacy **Celibacy** is avoidance of or abstention from sexual activities. Some people choose celibacy for religious or moral reasons. Others may be celibate for a period of time because of illness, the breakup of a long-term relationship, or lack of an acceptable partner. For some, celibacy is lonely, but others find it an opportunity for introspection and personal growth.

Autoerotic Behaviors **Autoerotic behaviors** involve sexual self-stimulation. **Masturbation**, or self-stimulation of the genitals, is one of the most common ways humans seek sexual pleasure. **Sexual fantasies** are sexually arousing thoughts and dreams. Fantasies may reflect real-life experiences, forbidden desires, or the opportunity to mentally practice new or anticipated sexual experiences. The fact that you fantasize about a particular experience does not mean that you want to, or have to, act it out.

Kissing and Erotic Touching Kissing and erotic touching are two common forms of nonverbal sexual communication. Both men and women have **erogenous zones**, areas of the body where touching leads to sexual arousal. These may include genitals as well as areas such as the earlobes, mouth, breasts, and inner thighs. Spending time with your partner to explore and learn about his or her erogenous areas is a pleasurable and safe means of sexual expression.

Manual Stimulation Both men and women can be sexually aroused and achieve orgasm through manual stimulation of the genitals. For many women, orgasm is more likely through manual stimulation than through intercourse. *Sex toys* (such as vibrators and dildos) can be used alone or with a partner. Toys must be cleaned after each use.

Oral–Genital Stimulation **Cunnilingus** is oral stimulation of a woman's genitals, and **fellatio** is oral stimulation of a man's genitals. Many partners find oral stimulation intensely pleasurable. Forty-three percent of college students reported having had oral sex in the past month.[63] Note that HIV and other sexually transmitted infections (STIs) can be transmitted via unprotected oral–genital sex just as through intercourse. Use of an appropriate barrier device is strongly recommended if either partner's disease status is unknown.

Vaginal Intercourse The term *intercourse* generally refers to **vaginal intercourse** (*coitus*, or insertion of the penis into the vagina), the most frequently practiced form of sexual expression. Forty-six percent of college students reported having had vaginal intercourse in the past month.[64] Whatever your circumstances, you should practice safer sex to avoid disease and unintended pregnancy.

Anal Intercourse The anal area is highly sensitive to touch, and some couples find pleasure in stimulation there. **Anal intercourse** is insertion of the penis into the anus. Research indicates that 5 percent of college-aged men and women had anal sex in the past month.[65] Stimulation of the anus by the mouth, fingers, or sex toys is also practiced. If you enjoy this form of sexual expression, use condoms and/or dental dams to avoid transmitting disease. Also, any body part or other item that is inserted into the anus should not then be directly inserted into the vagina without cleaning, as bacteria commonly found in the anus can cause vaginal infections.

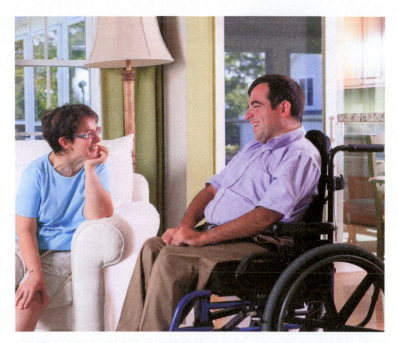

Whether able-bodied or disabled, we are all sexual beings deserving of intimacy and fulfilling sexual relationships.

Variant Sexual Behavior

Although attitudes toward sexuality have changed substantially over time, some people still believe that any sexual behavior other than heterosexual intercourse is abnormal. People who study sexuality prefer to use the neutral term **variant sexual behavior** to describe sexual behaviors that most people do not engage in. Examples include group sex (sexual activity involving more than two people), swinging (partner swapping), fetishism (sexual arousal achieved by looking at or touching inanimate objects, such as underclothing or shoes), and BDSM (a catch-all term for bondage, discipline, domination, submission, sadism, and masochism) as portrayed in popular media, such as "50 Shades of Grey". These activities are all legal when they involve consenting adults.

Some variant sexual behaviors can be harmful to the individual, to other people, or to both. Examples include *exhibitionism* (exposing one's genitals to strangers in public places), *voyeurism* (observing other people for sexual gratification), and *pedophilia* (sexual activity or attraction between an adult and a child). *Autoerotic asphyxiation* is the practice of reducing oxygen to the brain, usually by tying a cord around one's neck while masturbating to orgasm. This can be very dangerous, and some individuals accidentally strangle themselves in the process.

Check Yourself

- **What are the steps of the typical human sexual response?**

- **What are three examples of sexual expression?**

4.16 Sexual Dysfunction

Learning Outcome

4.16 Classify types and causes of sexual dysfunction disorders.

Sexual dysfunction, problems that can hinder sexual functioning, is common. A person can have a breakdown in sexual function just as in any other bodily function. Sexual dysfunction can be divided into four major categories: desire disorders, arousal disorders, orgasmic disorders, and pain disorders. All can be treated successfully.

Libido is a person's sexual drive or desire. A common reason people seek out a sex therapist is **inhibited sexual desire**, a lack of interest and pleasure in sexual activity. A low sex drive (decreased libido) may be caused by a drop in estrogen in women or testosterone in men and women or by fatigue, stress, depression, or anxiety. Antidepressant medications (e.g., Prozac, Zoloft, Paxil) can often reduce sexual desire.[66] **Sexual aversion disorder** is characterized by sexual phobias (unreasonable fears) and anxiety about sexual contact. Causes may include the psychological stress of a punitive upbringing, a rigid religious background, or a history of physical or sexual abuse.

The most common sexual arousal disorder is **erectile dysfunction (ED)**—difficulty achieving or maintaining a penile erection sufficient for intercourse. At some time, every man experiences ED. Risk factors include many medical conditions, medications, and treatments; being overweight; injuries; psychological conditions, drug, alcohol, or tobacco use; and prolonged bicycling.[67] Some 30 million men in the United States, half under age 65, suffer from ED. The condition generally becomes more common with age, affecting 1 in 5 men in their sixties.[68] Drugs treat ED by relaxing the smooth muscle cells in the penis, allowing increased blood flow to erectile tissues.

Premature ejaculation—ejaculation that occurs before or very soon after insertion of the penis into the vagina—affects up to 70 percent of men at some time.[69] Treatment first involves physical examination to rule out organic causes. If the cause is not physiological, therapy can help a man learn how to control the timing of his ejaculation. Fatigue, stress, performance pressure, and alcohol use can all contribute to this problem.

In a woman, the inability to achieve orgasm is called **female orgasmic disorder**. A woman with this disorder often blames herself and learns to fake orgasm to avoid embarrassment or to preserve her partner's ego. The first step is a physical examination to rule out organic causes. However, the problem is often solved by self-exploration to learn more about self-stimulation. Once a woman has become orgasmic through masturbation, she can communicate her needs to her partner.

Both men and women can experience **sexual performance anxiety**. A man may become anxious and unable to maintain an erection or may experience premature ejaculation. A woman may be unable to achieve orgasm or to allow penetration because of involuntary contraction of vaginal muscles. Both men and women

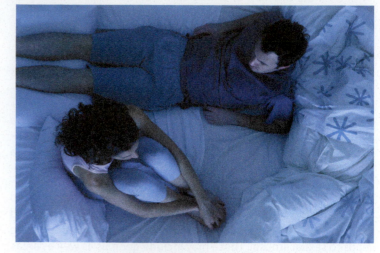

Sexual dysfunction can have both physical and psychological roots. Interpersonal problems can contribute to dysfunction as well.

can overcome performance anxiety by learning to focus on immediate sensations rather than orgasm.

Dyspareunia is pain experienced by a woman during intercourse, which may be caused by endometriosis, uterine tumors, chlamydia, gonorrhea, or urinary tract infections. Damage to tissues during childbirth and insufficient lubrication during intercourse may also cause discomfort. Dyspareunia can also be psychological in origin. As with other sexual problems, dyspareunia can be treated with good results.

Vaginismus is the involuntary contraction of vaginal muscles, making penile insertion painful or impossible. Most cases are related to fear of intercourse or to unresolved sexual conflicts. Treatment involves teaching a woman to achieve orgasm through nonvaginal stimulation.

While sexual dysfunction can happen at any age, the incidence of dysfunction increases during the menopause years in women and after age 50 in men.[70] Don't be afraid to talk to a counselor or medical professional; most colleges and universities have services available. The American Association of Sex Educators, Counselors, and Therapists (AASECT) also lists highly trained and certified counselors, sex therapists, and clinics that treat sexual dysfunctions at www.aasect.org.

Check Yourself

- What are some types and causes of sexual dysfunction?

- Would you consider physical or psychological causes of sexual dysfunction easier to treat? Why?

4.17 Alcohol, Drugs, and Sex

Learning Outcome

4.17 Examine the negative outcomes associated with combining sex with drugs or alcohol.

Because psychoactive drugs and alcohol affect the body's entire physiological functioning, it is only logical that they affect sexual behavior. Promises of increased pleasure make drugs very

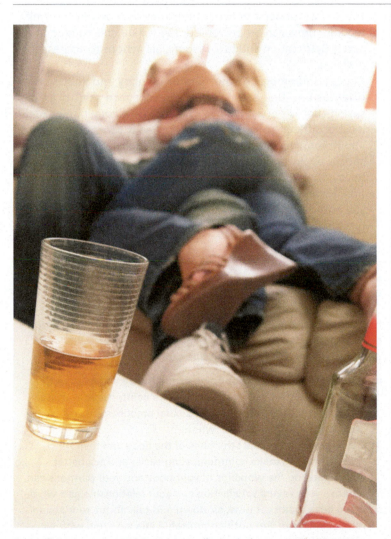

According to a survey of American college students, nearly 22 percent of college men and 21.2 percent of college women who drank alcohol in the past year reported having unprotected sex as a consequence of their drinking.

Source: Data from American College Health Association, *American College Health Association—National College Health Assessment II (ACHA-NCHA II): Reference Group Data Report, Fall 2016* (Baltimore: American College Health Association, 2017).

tempting to people seeking greater sexual satisfaction. Too often, however, drugs and alcohol become central to sexual activities and damage the relationship and sometimes the body.

Drug and alcohol use can also lead to undesired sexual activity as well as a tendency to blame the drug for negative behavior or unsafe sexual activities. "I can't help what I did last night because I was drunk" is a statement that demonstrates immaturity. A mature person carefully examines risks and benefits and makes decisions accordingly. If drugs are necessary to increase erotic feelings, it is likely that the partners are being dishonest about their feelings for each other. Good sex should not depend on chemical substances.

Alcohol is notorious for reducing inhibitions and promoting feelings of well-being and desirability. At the same time, alcohol inhibits sexual response—the mind may be willing, but not the body.

In addition to alcohol use, an increasing number of young men have begun experimenting with recreational use of drugs intended to treat erectile dysfunction or low "T", such as Viagra. Young men who take this type of medication are hoping to increase their sexual stamina or counteract sexual performance anxiety or the effects of alcohol or other drugs.[71] However, these drugs probably have only a placebo effect in men with the ability to have normal erections, and combining them with other drugs, such as ketamine, amyl nitrate (poppers), or methamphetamine, can lead to potentially fatal drug interactions.[72]

"Date rape" drugs have been a growing concern in recent decades. They have become prevalent on college campuses, where they are often used in combination with alcohol. *Rohypnol* ("roofies," "rope," "forget pill"), *GHB* (gamma hydroxybutyrate, or "liquid X," "Grievous Bodily Harm," "easy lay," "Mickey Finn"), and *ketamine* ("K," "Special K," "cat valium") have all been used to facilitate rape. Rohypnol and *GHB* are difficult-to-detect drugs that depress the central nervous system. Ketamine can cause dreamlike states, hallucinations, delirium, amnesia, and impaired motor function. These drugs are often introduced to unsuspecting women through alcoholic drinks to render them unconscious and vulnerable to rape. Victims often wake with little or no memory of what occurred.[73] This problem is so serious that the U.S. Congress passed the Drug-Induced Rape Prevention and Punishment Act to increase federal penalties for using drugs to facilitate sexual assault.

Check Yourself

- **Give three potential negative outcomes from combining sex with drugs or alcohol.**

4.18 Responsible and Satisfying Sexual Behavior

Learning Outcome

4.18 Discuss components of healthy and responsible sexuality.

Sexuality is a fascinating, complex, contradictory, and sometimes frustrating aspect of our lives. Healthy sexuality doesn't happen by chance. It is a product of assimilating information and skills, of exploring values and beliefs, and of making responsible and informed choices. Healthy and responsible sexuality includes the following:[74]

- **Good communication as the foundation.** Open and honest communication with your partner is the basis for establishing respect, trust, and intimacy. Do you communicate with your partner in caring and respectful ways? Can you share your thoughts and emotions freely with your partner? Do you talk about being sexually active and what that means? Can you share your sexual history with your partner? Do you discuss contraception and disease prevention? Are you able to communicate what you like and don't like? All of these are components of the open communication that accompanies healthy, responsible sexuality.

- **Acknowledge that you are a sexual person.** People who can see and accept themselves as sexual beings are more likely to make informed decisions and take responsible actions. If you see yourself as a potentially sexual person, you will plan ahead for contraception and disease prevention. If you are comfortable being a sexually active person, you will not need or want your sexual experiences clouded by alcohol or other drug use. If you choose not to be sexually active, you do so

consciously, as a personal decision based on your convictions. Even if you are not sexually active, it is important to acknowledge that sex is a natural aspect of life and to recognize that you are in charge of your own decisions about your sexuality.

- **Understand sexual structures and their functions.** If you understand how your body works, sexual pleasure and response will not be mysterious events. You will be able to pleasure yourself as well as communicate to your partner how best to please you. You will understand how pregnancy and sexually transmitted infections can be prevented. You will be able to recognize sexual dysfunction and take responsible actions to address the problem.

- **Accept and embrace your gender identity and your sexual orientation.** "Being comfortable in your own skin" is an old saying that is particularly relevant when it comes to sexuality. It is difficult to feel sexually satisfied if you are conflicted about your gender identity or your sexual orientation. You should explore and address questions and feelings you may have about your gender identity and/or your sexual orientation. Having good communication skills, acknowledging that you are a sexual person, and understanding your sexual structures and their functions will allow you to do so.

Skills for **Behavior Change**

Taking Steps Toward Healthy Sexuality

Healthy and responsible sexuality means having information and skills, exploring values and beliefs, and making responsible and informed choices. The following tips can help you:

- **Give some thought to your own sexuality. Do you choose to be sexually active now, or are you more comfortable waiting? If you are sexually active, which sexual practices are you comfortable with, and with whom?**

- **Get to know the sexual structures of the body and their functions in order to make communicating easier and sex better. Understanding the workings of your body and your partner's can improve your sexual satisfaction and your relationship as a whole.**

- **If you have a partner now, sit down and talk about your sexual relationship. Are you both comfortable and satisfied with all aspects of the relationship? Discuss what you like and don't like and what you might like to change.**

- **Explore and address any questions and feelings you may have about your gender identity and/or your sexual orientation.**

Check Yourself

- **What are three components of healthy and responsible sexuality?**

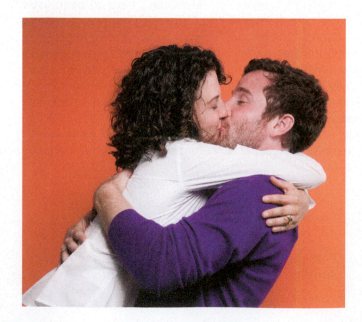

Summary

LO 4.1-4.2 Characteristics of intimate relationships include behavioral interdependence, need fulfillment, emotional attachment, and emotional availability. Issues that can cause problems in relationships include jealousy, differences over gender roles, and unmet expectations.

LO 4.3 It's important to use social media appropriately when dating.

LO 4.4 To improve our ability to communicate, we need to listen effectively, convey and interpret nonverbal communication, practice self-disclosure, and establish a proper climate for communicating.

LO 4.5 Be cautious when sharing personal information on social networking sites.

LO 4.6-4.8 Being a mindful listener and communicator enhances relationships and allows us to manage and resolve conflicts.

LO 4.9 For most people, commitment is an important ingredient in successful relationships.

LO 4.10 Relationships end for many reasons, and the uncoupling process can be very painful.

LO 4.11 Biological sex, gender identity, gender roles, and sexual orientation are all blended into our sexual identity.

LO 4.12-4.13 The major structures of the female sexual anatomy include the mons pubis, labia minora and majora, clitoris, vagina, uterus, cervix, fallopian tubes, and ovaries.

LO 4.14 The major structures of the male sexual anatomy are the penis, scrotum, testes, epididymides, vasa deferentia, ejaculatory ducts, urethra, and the accessory glands.

LO 4.15 Physiologically, both males and females experience four stages of sexual response: excitement/arousal, plateau, orgasm, and resolution.

LO 4.16 Problems with sexual dysfunction are common and can be treated successfully.

LO 4.17 Alcohol and drug use can lead to undesired and/or unsafe sexual activity.

LO 4.18 Responsible and satisfying sexuality involves good communication, understanding of sexual functions, and acceptance of your gender identity and sexual orientation.

Pop Quiz

*Visit **Mastering Health** to personalize your study plan with Chapter Review Quizzes and Dynamic Study Modules.*

LO 4.1 1. Intimate relationships fulfill our psychological need for someone to listen to our worries and concerns. This is known as our need for
a. dependence.
b. social integration.
c. enjoyment.
d. spontaneity.

LO 4.1 2. Lovers tend to pay attention to the other person even when they should be involved in other activities. This is called
a. inclusion.
b. exclusivity.
c. fascination.
d. authentic intimacy.

LO 4.1 3. Terms such as *behavioral interdependence*, *need fulfillment*, and *emotional availability* describe which type of relationship?
a. Dysfunctional
b. Sexual
c. Intimate
d. Behavioral

LO 4.2 4. All of the following are typical causes of jealousy *except*
a. overdependence on the relationship.
b. low self-esteem.
c. a past relationship that involved deception.
d. the belief that relationships can easily be replaced.

LO 4.10 5. Jamie has just broken up with her boyfriend. What is a recommended way to cope with the breakup?
a. Initiate a new relationship as soon as possible to recover.
b. Cut off contact with friends, who will be painful reminders of the relationship.
c. Avoid dwelling on sad feelings.
d. Find ways to express emotions through exercise or listening to music.

LO 4.11 6. Your personal inner sense of maleness or femaleness is known as your
a. sexual identity.
b. sexual orientation.
c. gender identity.
d. gender.

LO 4.12 7. The most sensitive or erotic spot in the female genital region is the
a. mons pubis.
b. vagina.
c. clitoris.
d. labia.

LO 4.12 8. When a woman is ovulating,
a. she has released an egg cell.
b. she has menstrual bleeding.
c. an egg has been fertilized.
d. the lining of her uterus thins.

LO 4.13 9. A condition in which a woman experiences pain when menstruating is known as
a. premenstrual syndrome.
b. dysmenorrhea.
c. premenstrual dysphoric disorder.
d. amenorrhea.

LO 4.14 10. What is the role of testosterone in the male reproductive system?
a. It is used to produce sperm for reproduction.
b. It is the hormone that stimulates development of secondary male sex characteristics.
c. It allows the penis to harden during sexual arousal.
d. It secretes the seminal fluid preceding ejaculation.

Answers to the above questions can be found on page A-1. If you answered a question incorrectly, review the module identified by the Learning Outcome. For even more study tools, visit Mastering Health.

Think About It!

LO 4.1 **1.** What are the four characteristics of intimate relationships? Why is each important in relationship development?

LO 4.3–4.5 **2.** How can social media affect communication and relationships?

LO 4.7 **3.** What is nonverbal communication, and why is it important to develop skills in this area? Give examples of some things you do to communicate without words.

LO 4.9–4.10 **4.** What are common elements of good relationships? What are some warning signs of trouble? What actions can you take to improve your own interpersonal relationships?

LO 4.9–4.10 **5.** What are the different types of committed relationships? How are they different? What does it take for any kind of committed relationship to succeed?

LO 4.15 **6.** How would you describe a "normal" sexual relationship for someone your age? What options are open to you if you and your sexual partner have different ideas about what "normal" looks like?

LO 4.17 **7.** If a close friend confided that he or she was having difficulty with a partner's drug, alcohol, or sexual behavior, what advice might you give?

LO 4.18 **8.** What are the key components that you would want in a healthy and satisfying committed relationship?

Reproductive Choices

Today, we understand the intimate details of reproduction and possess technologies to control **fertility**. Along with information come choice and responsibility, and one measure of maturity is the ability to discuss birth control with one's sex partner. Too often, neither person brings up the topic, and unprotected sex is the result. Only 55 percent of sexually active college women and 50 percent of sexually active college men reported having used a method of contraception the last time they had vaginal intercourse.[1] The sad outcome is too many unwanted pregnancies and the spread of **sexually transmitted infections (STIs)**. If you're thinking about becoming sexually active or you are already sexually active but haven't used birth control, visit your campus or local health clinic to discuss contraceptives and the best methods for preventing an STI.

Birth control (or **contraception**) refers to methods of preventing **conception**, which occurs when a sperm fertilizes an egg. To evaluate a contraceptive method's effectiveness, look at its **perfect use failure rate**, or percentage of pregnancies likely in the first year of use if the method is used entirely without error. Even more important and more useful is its **typical use failure rate**, the percentage of pregnancies likely in the first year with *typical* use— that is, with the normal number of errors, memory lapses, and so on.

5.1 Barrier Methods: Male and Female Condoms

5.1 List the advantages, disadvantages, and effectiveness of the male and female condoms in preventing pregnancy and STIs.

Barrier methods of contraception work on the principle of preventing sperm from reaching the egg by use of a physical or chemical barrier during intercourse. Some barrier methods prevent semen from having contact with the woman's body; others prevent sperm from going past the cervix. In addition, many barrier methods contain, or are used in combination with, a substance that kills sperm.

The Male Condom

The **male condom** is a thin sheath designed to cover the erect penis and catch semen before it enters the vagina. Most male condoms are made of latex, though polyurethane and lambskin condoms are also available. Condoms in a wide variety of styles may be purchased in pharmacies, supermarkets, public bathrooms, and many health clinics. A new condom must be used for each act of vaginal, oral, or anal intercourse.

A condom must be rolled onto the penis before the penis touches the vagina and must be held in place when the penis is removed from the vagina after ejaculation (see **Figure 5.1**). Condoms come with or without **spermicide** and with or without lubrication. If desired, users can lubricate their own condoms with contraceptive foams, creams, jellies, or other water-based lubricants. Never use products such as baby oil, cold cream, petroleum jelly, vaginal yeast infection medications, or body lotion with a condom. These products contain substances that will cause the latex to disintegrate.

Condoms are less effective and more likely to break during intercourse if they are old or improperly stored. To maintain their effectiveness, store them in a cool place (not in a wallet or pocket), and inspect them for small tears before use. Lightly squeeze the package before opening to feel that air is trapped inside and the package has not been punctured. Discard all condoms that have passed their expiration date.

Advantages The condom is the only temporary means of birth control available for men, and latex and polyurethane condoms are the only barriers that effectively prevent the spread of some STIs and HIV. (Skin condoms, made from lamb intestines, are not effective against STIs.) Condoms are a popular choice for birth control because they are inexpensive and readily available without a prescription, and their use is limited to times of sexual activity, with no negative health effects. Some men find that condoms help them stay erect longer or help to prevent premature ejaculation. When used consistently and correctly, condoms can be up to 98 percent effective.[2]

Disadvantages The easy availability of condoms is accompanied by considerable potential for user error; the typical use effectiveness of condoms in preventing pregnancy is around 82 percent.[3] Improper use of a condom can lead to breakage, leakage, or slipping, potentially exposing users to STIs or an unintended pregnancy. Even when used perfectly, a condom doesn't protect against some STIs (e.g., herpes). Some people feel that condoms ruin the spontaneity of sex because stopping to put one on may break the mood. Others report that condoms decrease sensation. Because a new condom is required for each act of intercourse, some users find it difficult to be sure to have a condom available when needed. These inconveniences

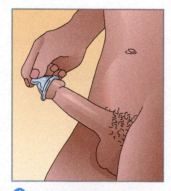 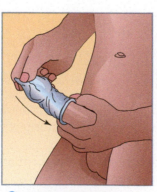 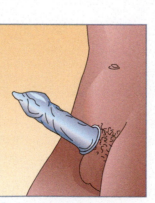 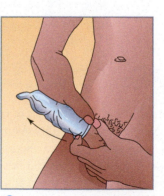

❶ Pinch the air out of the top half-inch of the condom to allow room for semen.

❷ Holding the tip of the condom with one hand, use the other hand to unroll it onto the penis.

❸ Unroll the condom all the way to the base of the penis, smoothing out any air bubbles.

❹ After ejaculation, hold the condom around the base until the penis is totally withdrawn to avoid spilling any semen.

Figure 5.1 How to Use a Male Condom

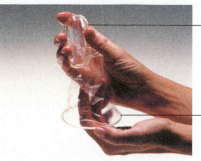

Inner ring is used for insertion and to help hold the sheath in place during intercourse.

Outer ring covers the area around the opening of the vagina.

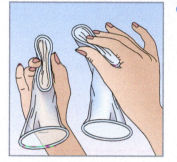

❶ Grasp the flexible inner ring at the closed end of the condom, and squeeze it between your thumb and second or middle finger so it becomes long and narrow.

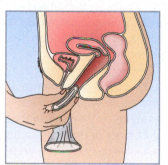

❷ Choose a comfortable position for insertion: squatting, with one leg raised, or sitting or lying down. While squeezing the ring, insert the closed end of the condom into your vagina.

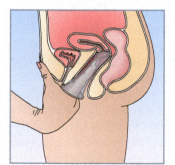

❸ Placing your index finger inside of the condom, gently push the inner ring up as far as it will go. Be sure the sheath is not twisted. The outer ring should remain outside of the vagina.

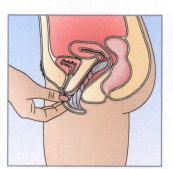

❹ During intercourse, be sure that the penis is not entering on the side, between the sheath and the vaginal wall. When removing the condom, twist the outer ring so that no semen leaks out.

Figure 5.2 **How to Use a Female Condom**

and perceptions contribute to improper use or avoidance of condoms altogether. Partners who apply a condom as part of foreplay are generally more successful with this form of birth control

The Female Condom

The **female condom (FC2)** is a single-use, soft, loose-fitting sheath for internal vaginal use. The newest versions are made from nitrile rather than polyurethane. The sheath has a flexible ring at each end. One ring lies inside the sheath and serves as an insertion mechanism and internal anchor. The other remains outside the vagina once the device has been inserted and protects the labia and the base of the penis from infection. **Figure 5.2** shows proper use of the female condom.

Advantages The female condom can be inserted in advance, so its use doesn't have to interrupt lovemaking. Some women choose the female condom because it gives them more personal control over prevention of pregnancy and STIs or because they cannot rely on their partner to use the male condom. Because the nitrile is thin and pliable, there is less loss of sensation with the female condom than with the latex male condom. The female condom can be used with or without lubrication. The female condom is relatively inexpensive, readily available without a prescription, and causes no negative health effects. Used consistently and correctly, female condoms are 95 percent effective at preventing pregnancy.[4] They also can help to prevent the spread of HIV and other STIs.

Disadvantages As with the male condom, there is potential for user error with the female condom, including possible breaking, slipping, or leaking, all of which could lead to STI transmission or an unintended pregnancy. Because of the potential problems, the typical use effectiveness of the female condom is 79 percent.[5] Some people dislike using the female condom because they find it disruptive, noisy, odd looking, or difficult to use. Some women have reported external or vaginal irritation from using the female condom. As with the male condom, a new condom is required for each act of intercourse, so users may not always have one available when needed. Remember that male and female condoms should never be used simultaneously.

Check Yourself

- What are the advantages and disadvantages of the male and female condoms?

- How effective are the male and female condoms in preventing pregnancy and STIs?

- What are some reasons you might give to persuade a partner to use a condom?

5.2 Other Barrier Methods

Learning Outcome

5.2 List the advantages, disadvantages, and effectiveness of different types of barrier methods in preventing pregnancy and STIs.

There are options beyond the male and female condoms for people who wish to use other barrier methods. These options include spermicides, the sponge, the diaphragm, and the cervical cap.

Spermicides

Some barrier methods—jellies, creams, foams, suppositories, and film—require no prescription. These are spermicides, substances designed to kill sperm.

Jellies and creams come in tubes, and **foams** come in aerosol cans with applicators for vaginal insertion. These substances must be inserted far enough to cover the cervix, providing both a chemical barrier that kills sperm and a physical barrier that stops sperm from continuing toward an egg.

Suppositories are capsules inserted into the vagina, where they melt. They must be inserted 10 to 20 minutes before intercourse but no more than 1 hour before or they lose their effectiveness. Additional contraceptive chemicals must be applied for each subsequent act of intercourse.

With **vaginal contraceptive film**, a thin film infused with spermicidal gel is inserted into the vagina so that it covers the cervix. The film dissolves into a spermicidal gel effective for up to 3 hours. As with other spermicides, a new film must be inserted for each act of intercourse.

Advantages Spermicides are inexpensive, require no prescription or pelvic examination, and are available over the counter. They are simple to use, and use is limited to the time of sexual activity.

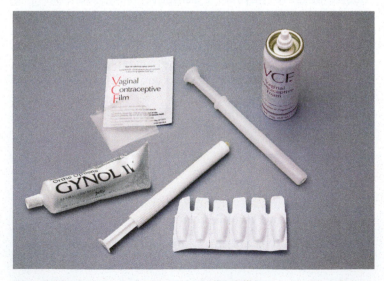

Spermicides come in many forms, including jellies, creams, films, foam, and suppositories.

Spermicides are most effective when used with another barrier method (condom, diaphragm, etc.). When used alone, they offer only 72 percent (typical use) to 82 percent (perfect use) effectiveness at preventing pregnancy.[6]

Disadvantages Spermicides can be messy and must be reapplied for each act of intercourse. A small number of people experience irritation or allergic reactions to spermicides. The most commonly used spermicide, *nonoxynol-9* (N-9), can cause irritation and increase the likelihood of infection, including HIV infection, when used multiple times per day. However, N-9 can be used safely by women who are at low risk for HIV and STIs and who do not use N-9 more than once a day.[7]

Contraceptive Sponge

The **contraceptive sponge** (sold in the United States as *the Today Sponge*) is made of polyurethane foam. Before insertion, it is moistened with water to activate the infused spermicide. It is then folded and inserted into the vagina, where it fits over the cervix and creates a barrier against sperm.

Advantages A main advantage of the sponge is convenience. it requires no doctor's fitting. Protection begins on insertion and lasts for up to 24 hours. It is not necessary to reapply spermicide or insert a new sponge within the same 24-hour period; it must be left in place for at least 6 hours after last intercourse. The sponge is fairly effective (91 percent perfect use; 88 percent typical use) when used consistently and correctly.[8] Like the diaphragm and cervical cap, the sponge offers limited protection from some STIs.

Disadvantages The sponge is less effective for women who have given birth (80 percent perfect use; 76 percent typical use).[9] Allergic reactions, such as irritation of the vagina, are more common than with other barrier methods. If the vaginal lining becomes irritated, the risk of yeast infections and other STIs may increase. Some cases of **toxic shock syndrome (TSS)** have been reported in women using the sponge; precautions should be taken as with

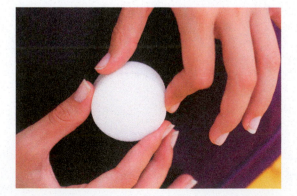

The Today Sponge is a combination barrier method and spermicide that is most effective when used in conjunction with male condoms.

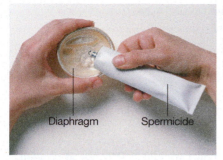

1 Place spermicidal jelly or cream inside the diaphragm and all around the rim.

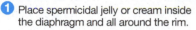
Diaphragm   Spermicide

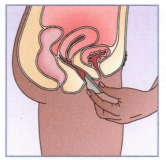

2 Fold the diaphragm in half and insert dome-side down (spermicide-side up) into the vagina, pushing it along the back wall as far as it will go.

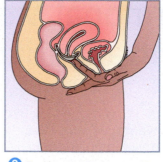

3 Position the diaphragm with the cervix completely covered and the front rim tucked up against your pubic bone; you should be able to feel your cervix through the rubber dome.

Figure 5.3 The Proper Use and Placement of a Diaphragm

the diaphragm and cervical cap. Some women find the sponge difficult or messy to remove.

The Diaphragm

Invented in the mid-nineteenth century, the **diaphragm** was the first widely used birth control method for women. The device is a soft, shallow cup made of thin latex rubber. Its flexible, rubber-coated ring is designed to fit behind the pubic bone in front of the cervix and over the back of the cervix on the other side. Diaphragms must be used with spermicidal cream or jelly that is applied to the inside of the diaphragm before insertion. A diaphragm may be inserted up to 6 hours before intercourse. The diaphragm holds the spermicide in place, creating a physical and chemical barrier against sperm (**Figure 5.3**). Diaphragms come in different sizes and must be fitted by a trained practitioner, who should ensure that the user knows how to insert her diaphragm correctly before she leaves the practitioner's office.

The U.S. Food and Drug Administration (FDA) has approved a new one-size-fits-most diaphragm, *Caya*. One-size-fits-most means that women will not have to be fitted to use it or refitted for a different size if they gain or lose weight.[10]

Advantages After the initial prescription and fitting, the only ongoing expense is spermicide. Because the diaphragm can be inserted up to 6 hours in advance and used for multiple acts of intercourse, some users find it less disruptive than other barrier methods. If used consistently and correctly, diaphragms can be 94 percent effective in preventing pregnancy.[11] When used with spermicidal jelly or cream, the diaphragm also offers protection against gonorrhea and possibly chlamydia and human papillomavirus (HPV).

Disadvantages Although the diaphragm can be left in place for multiple acts of intercourse, additional spermicide must be applied each time, and the diaphragm must then stay in place for 6 to 8 hours afterward to allow the chemical to kill any sperm remaining in the vagina. Some women find insertion awkward. When inserted incorrectly, diaphragms are much less effective. A diaphragm may also slip out of place, be difficult to remove, or require refitting (e.g., after pregnancy).

The Cervical Cap

One of the oldest methods used to prevent pregnancy, early **cervical caps** were made from beeswax, silver, or copper. The currently available *FemCap* is a clear silicone cup that fits over the cervix. It comes in three sizes and must be fitted by a practitioner. The FemCap is designed for use with spermicidal jelly or cream. It is held in place by suction created during application and works by blocking sperm from the uterus.

Advantages Cervical caps are relatively inexpensive; the only ongoing cost is for spermicide. The FemCap can be inserted up to 6 hours before intercourse, making it potentially less disruptive than other barrier methods. The device must be left in place for 6 to 8 hours afterward; after that, if removed and cleaned, it can be reinserted immediately. Because the FemCap is made of surgical-grade silicone, it is a suitable alternative for people allergic to latex. Cervical caps can be reasonably effective (up to 86 percent) with typical use.[12] They may also offer some protection against transmission of gonorrhea, HPV, and possibly chlamydia.

Disadvantages The FemCap is somewhat more difficult to insert than a diaphragm because of its size. Like a diaphragm, it requires a fitting by a trained healthcare provider and may require subsequent refitting if a woman's cervix size changes, as after giving birth. Because the FemCap can become dislodged during intercourse, placement must be checked frequently. It cannot be used during the menstrual period or for longer than 48 hours because of the risk of TSS. Some women report unpleasant vaginal odors after use.

Check Yourself

- **What are the advantages and disadvantages of different types of barrier methods of birth control?**

- **What factors influence effectiveness and proper use of different types of barrier methods?**

Hormonal Methods: Oral Contraceptives

5.3 List the advantages, disadvantages, and effectiveness of oral contraceptives in preventing pregnancy and STIs.

The term *hormonal contraception* refers to birth control containing synthetic estrogen, progestin, or both. These ingredients are similar to the hormones estrogen and progesterone, which a woman's ovaries produce naturally for the process of ovulation and the menstrual cycle. In recent years, hormonal contraception has become available in a variety of forms (transdermal, injection, and oral). All forms require a prescription from a health care provider.

Hormonal contraception alters a woman's biochemistry, preventing ovulation (release of the egg) from taking place and producing changes that make it more difficult for the sperm to reach the egg if ovulation does occur. Synthetic estrogen works to prevent the ovaries from releasing an egg. If no egg is released, there is nothing to be fertilized by sperm, and pregnancy cannot occur. Progestin, too, can prevent ovulation. It also thickens cervical mucus, which hinders sperm movement, inhibits the egg's ability to travel through the fallopian tubes, and suppresses sperm's ability to unite with the egg. Progestin also thins the uterine lining, rendering the egg unlikely to implant in the uterine wall.

Oral Contraceptives

Oral contraceptive pills were first marketed in the United States in 1960. Their convenience quickly made them the most widely used reversible method of fertility control. Most modern pills are more than 99 percent effective at preventing pregnancy with perfect use.[13] Today, oral contraceptives are a commonly used birth control method among college women (Table 5.1).[14]

Most oral contraceptives work through the combined effects of synthetic estrogen and progesterone (*combination pills*). Combination pills are taken in a cycle. At the end of each 3-week cycle, the user discontinues the drug or takes placebo pills for 1 week. The resultant drop in hormones causes the uterine lining to disintegrate; the user then has a menstrual period, usually within 1 to 3 days. Menstrual flow is generally lighter than for women who don't use the pill, because the hormones in the pill prevent thick endometrial buildup.

Several newer brands of pills have extended cycles, such as the 91-day *Seasonale* and *Seasonique*. A woman using this type of regimen takes active pills for 12 weeks, followed by 1 week of placebos. On this cycle, women can expect to have a menstrual period every 3 months. *Lybrel*, another extended-cycle pill, is taken continuously for 1 year, eliminating menstruation completely. While the idea of never having a period may be unsettling to some women, there is no physiological need for a woman to have a monthly period, and there are no known risks associated with its avoidance.

Advantages Combination pills are highly effective at preventing pregnancy: more than 99 percent with perfect use and 91 percent with typical use.[15] It is easier to achieve perfect use with pills than with barrier contraceptives because there is less opportunity for user error. Aside from its effectiveness, much of the pill's popularity is due to convenience and discreetness. Users like the fact that it does not interfere with lovemaking.

In addition to effectively preventing pregnancy, the combination pill may lessen menstrual difficulties such as cramps and premenstrual syndrome (PMS) and lower the risk of several health conditions, including endometrial and ovarian cancers, noncancerous breast disease, osteoporosis, ovarian cysts, pelvic inflammatory disease, and iron-deficiency anemia.[16] Many different brands of combination pills are on the market, some of which contain progestin, which offer benefits such as reducing acne or minimizing fluid retention. Less-expensive generic versions are also available for many brands. With the extended-cycle pills, the major additional benefit is reduction in or absence of menstruation and associated cramps or PMS symptoms. Users of these pills also like that they don't need to remember when to stop or start a cycle of pills or when to use placebos.

TABLE

5.1 Top Reported Means of Contraception Used by College Students or Their Partners the Last Time They Had Sex

Method	Male	Female	Total
Male condom	69%	60%	63%
Birth control pills (monthly or extended-cycle)	61%	58%	59%
Withdrawal	29%	35%	34%
Intrauterine device	9%	10%	9%
Nexplanon/implant	6%	6%	6%
Depo-Provera/shot	5%	4%	4%
Spermicide (foam, jelly, cream)	6%	3%	4%
Sterilization	2%	2%	2%
Xulane/patch	1%	1%	1%
Female condom	1%	0%	1%
Diaphragm or cervical cap	0.5%	0.3	0.3%
Sponge	0.5%	0.1%	0.2%

Note: Survey respondents could select more than one method.

Source: Data from American College Health Association, *American College Health Association—National College Health Assessment II: Reference Group Data, Fall, 2016* (Hanover, MD: American College Health Association, 2017).

Disadvantages Estrogen in combination pills is associated with increased risk of several serious health problems among older women, but the risk is low for most healthy women under 35 who do not smoke. Problems include increased risk for blood clots and higher risk for increased blood pressure, stroke, and heart attack. These risks increase with age and cigarette smoking. Early warning signs of complications associated with oral contraceptives include severe abdominal, chest, or leg pain; severe headache; and eye problems.[17]

Different brands of pills can cause varying minor side effects. Some of the most common are spotting between periods (particularly with extended-cycle regimens), breast tenderness, and nausea. With most pills, these side effects clear up within a few months. Other potential side effects include change in sexual desire, acne, weight gain, and hair loss or growth. Because so many brands are available, most women who wish to use the pill are able to find one that works for them with few side effects.

The pill's other major disadvantage is that it must be taken every day. If a woman misses one pill, she should use an alternative form of contraception for the remainder of that cycle. A backup method of birth control is also necessary during the first week of use. After a woman discontinues the pill, return of fertility may be delayed, though the pill is not known to cause infertility. Another drawback is that the pill does not protect against STIs.

The costs associated with the pill (and all other hormonal contraceptives) have long been reported as a barrier to use. However, in the United States, the Affordable Care Act currently makes contraceptives more accessible by requiring new private health insurance plans to cover "preventive services," including birth control and yearly physicals without co-payments or deductibles. Whether these provisions will continue in the current administration remains in question.

Progestin-Only Pills

Progestin-only pills (or *minipills*) contain small doses of progesterone and no estrogen. These pills are available in 28-day packs of active pills. (Menstruation usually occurs during the fourth week even though the active dose continues through the entire month.)

Advantages Progestin-only pills are a good choice for women who are at high risk for estrogen-related side effects or who cannot take estrogen-containing pills because of diabetes, high blood pressure, or other cardiovascular conditions. They can also be used safely by women over age 35 and breast-feeding mothers. Progestin-only pills share some health benefits associated with combination pills and carry no estrogen-related cardiovascular risks.

In addition, some typical side effects of combination pills, including nausea and breast tenderness, seldom occur with progestin-only pills. With progestin-only pills, menstrual periods

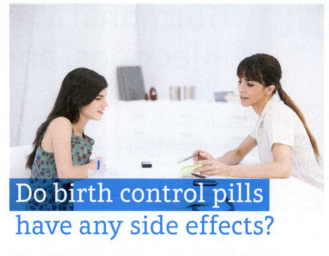

Do birth control pills have any side effects?

Many different brands and regimens of oral contraceptives are available to women today, and some of these are associated with health benefits such as acne reduction or lessening of PMS symptoms. Some women experience minor side effects from pill use—the most common being headaches, breast tenderness, nausea, and breakthrough bleeding—but these usually clear up within 2 to 3 months.

generally become lighter or stop altogether. The effectiveness rate of these pills is more than 99 percent with perfect use and 91 percent with typical use.[18]

Disadvantages Because of the lower dose of hormones in progestin-only pills, it is especially important that they be taken at the same time each day. If a woman takes a pill 3 or more hours later than usual, she will need to use a backup method of contraception for the next 48 hours.

The most common side effect of progestin-only pills is irregular menstrual bleeding or spotting. Less common side effects include mood changes, changes in sex drive, and headaches. As with all oral contraceptives, progestin-only pills do not protect against STI transmission.

Check Yourself

- **What are the advantages and disadvantages of oral contraceptives?**

- **How effective are oral contraceptives in preventing pregnancy and STIs?**

- **What are the differences between combination pills and progestin-only pills (minipills)? Who should take progestin-only pills?**

Hormonal Methods: The Patch, Ring, Injections, and Implants

5.4 List the advantages, disadvantages, and effectiveness of various hormonal methods of contraception in preventing pregnancy and STIs.

Some hormonal methods, such as oral contraceptives, require the user to remember to take the pill every day. Others, such as the skin patch, ring, injections, and implants, do not require daily action.

Contraceptive Skin Patch

Xulane (a generic form of *Ortho Evra*, which has been removed from the market) is a square transdermal (through the skin) adhesive patch less than 2 inches wide, as thin as a plastic bandage. It is worn for 1 week and replaced on the same day of the week for 3 consecutive weeks; during the fourth week, no patch is worn. *Xulane* works by delivering continuous levels of estrogen and progestin into the bloodstream. The patch can be worn on the buttocks, abdomen, upper torso (front or back, excluding the breasts), or upper outer arm. It should not be used by women over age 35 who smoke cigarettes and is less effective in women who weigh more than 198 pounds.[19]

Advantages Women who choose to use the patch often do so because they find it easier to remember than taking a daily pill, and they like the fact that they need to change the patch only once a week. *Xulane* probably offers potential health benefits similar to those of combination pills (reduction in risk of certain cancers and diseases, lessening of PMS symptoms, etc.). Like other hormonal methods, the patch regulates a woman's menstrual cycle. *Xulane* is 99.7 percent effective with perfect use and 91 percent with typical use.[20] As with other hormonal methods, there is less room for user error than with barrier methods.

Disadvantages Using the patch requires an initial exam and prescription, weekly patch changes, and the ongoing monthly expense of patch purchase. Like other hormonal methods of birth control, the patch offers no protection against HIV or other STIs. Some women experience minor side effects, such as those associated with combination pills. The estrogen in the patch is associated with cardiovascular risks, particularly in women who smoke and women over the age of 35.[21] Amid evidence that the patch may increase the risk of life-threatening blood clots, the FDA mandated an additional warning label explaining that patch use exposes women to about 60 percent more estrogen than a typical combination pill.[22]

Vaginal Contraceptive Ring

NuvaRing is a soft, flexible plastic hormonal contraceptive ring about 2 inches in diameter. The user inserts the ring into her vagina, leaves it in place for 3 weeks, and removes it for 1 week for her menstrual period. Once the ring has been inserted, it releases a steady flow of estrogen and progestin.

Advantages Advantages of *NuvaRing* include less likelihood of user error, protection against pregnancy for 1 month, no pill to take daily or patch to change weekly, no need to be fitted by a clinician, no requirement to use spermicide, and rapid return of fertility when use is stopped. It also exposes the user to a lower dosage of estrogen than do the patch and some combination pills, so it may have fewer estrogen-related side effects. It probably offers some of the same potential health benefits as combination pills, and like other hormonal contraceptives, it regulates the menstrual cycle. The ring is 99.7 percent effective with perfect use and 91 percent effective with typical use.[23]

Disadvantages *NuvaRing* requires an initial exam and prescription, monthly ring changes, and the ongoing monthly expense of purchasing the ring (a generic version is not currently available). A backup method must be used during the first week, and the ring provides no protection against STIs. Like combination pills, the ring has possible minor side effects and potentially more serious health risks for some women. Possible side effects unique to the ring include increased vaginal discharge and vaginal irritation or infection. Oil-based vaginal medicines to treat yeast infections cannot be used when the ring is in place, and a woman using *NuvaRing* cannot use a diaphragm or cervical cap as a backup method for contraception.

Xulane is an adhesive patch that delivers estrogen and progestin through the skin for 1 week. Patches are changed weekly and worn for 3 out of 4 weeks.

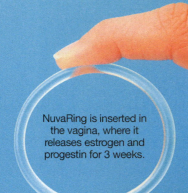

NuvaRing is inserted in the vagina, where it releases estrogen and progestin for 3 weeks.

Nexplanon is inserted by a clinician beneath the skin of a woman's arm, where it releases progestin for up to 3 years.

Contraceptive Injections

Depo-Provera (injected intra-muscularly) and the newer **Depo-SubQ Provera** (injected just below the skin in a lower dose) are long-acting synthetic progesterones that are injected every 3 months by a health care provider. Both prevent ovulation, thicken cervical mucus, and thin the uterine lining, all of which prevent pregnancy.

Advantages *Depo-Provera* takes effect within 24 hours of the first shot, so there is usually no need to use a backup method. Some women feel that *Depo-Provera* encourages sexual spontaneity because they do not have to remember to take a pill or insert a device. With continued use of this method, a woman's menstrual periods become lighter and may eventually stop altogether. No estrogen-related health risks are associated with *Depo-Provera*, and it offers the same potential health benefits as progestin-only pills. Unlike estrogen-containing hormonal methods, *Depo-Provera* can be used by women who are breastfeeding. There is little chance of user error with the shot because it is administered by a clinician every 3 months. With perfect use, the shot is 99.8 percent effective; and with typical use, it is 94 percent effective.[24]

Disadvantages Using *Depo-Provera* requires an initial exam and prescription, as well as follow-up visits every 3 months to have the shot administered. It offers no protection against STIs. The main disadvantage of *Depo-Provera* use is irregular bleeding, which can be troublesome at first, but within a year most women are amenorrheic (have no menstrual periods). Weight gain is commonly reported. Prolonged use of *Depo-Provera* has been linked to loss of bone density.[25] Other possible side effects include dizziness, nervousness, and headache. Unlike other methods of contraception, this method cannot be stopped immediately if problems arise, and the drug and its side effects may linger for up to 6 months after the last shot. A disadvantage for women who want to get pregnant is that fertility might not return for up to 1 year after the final injection.

Contraceptive Implants

A single-rod implantable contraceptive, **Nexplanon** (formerly called **Implanon**) is a small (about the size of a matchstick), soft plastic capsule that is inserted just beneath the skin on the inner side of a woman's upper underarm by a health care provider. *Nexplanon* continually releases a low, steady dose of progestin for up to 3 years, suppressing ovulation during that time.

Advantages After insertion, *Nexplanon* is generally not visible, making it a discreet method of birth control. The main advantages of *Nexplanon* are that it is highly effective (99.95 percent), it is not subject to user error, and it needs to be replaced only every 3 years.[26] It has benefits similar to those of other progestin-only forms of contraception, including the lightening or cessation of menstrual periods, the lack of estrogen-related side effects, and safety for use by breast-feeding women. Fertility usually returns quickly after removal of the implant.

Disadvantages Insertion and removal of *Nexplanon* must be performed by a clinician. The initial cost is higher for this method, and it may not be covered by all health plans. Potential minor side effects include irritation, allergic reaction, swelling, or scarring around the area of insertion; there is also a possibility of infection or complications with removal. As with other progestin-only contraceptives, users can experience irregular bleeding. *Nexplanon* offers no protection against transmission of STIs, and it may require a backup method during the first week of use.

Check Yourself

- What are the advantages and disadvantages of the various hormonal methods of contraception?

- How effective are various hormonal methods of contraception in preventing pregnancy and STIs?

- What are the benefits and drawbacks of methods of contraception that remain in place for days or weeks?

5.5 List the advantages, disadvantages, and effectiveness of intrauterine contraceptives in preventing pregnancy and STIs.

The **intrauterine device (IUD)** is a small, plastic, flexible device with a nylon string attached that is placed in the uterus through the cervix and left there for 3 to 10 years. The exact mechanism by which it works is not clearly understood, but researchers believe that IUDs affect the way sperm and egg move, thereby preventing fertilization, and/or affect the lining of the uterus to prevent a fertilized ovum from implanting.

The IUD was once extremely popular in the United States; however, in the 1970s most brands were removed from the market because the design of the most popular type caused serious complications in some women, including pelvic inflammatory disease and infertility. Redesigned for safe use, the IUD is again very popular with women around the world and is experiencing a resurgence of popularity among U.S. women.[27]

Brands of IUDs

Five IUDs are currently available in the United States. *ParaGard* is a T-shaped plastic device with copper wrapped around the shaft. It does not contain any hormones and can be left in place for 10 years before replacement. *Mirena* is effective for 5 years and releases small amounts of progestin. *Skyla* and *Kyleena*

are smaller-sized versions of *Mirena*, specifically designed for women who have not yet had a baby. *Skyla* is effective for 3 years, and *Kyleena* is effective for 5 years. *Liletta*, also smaller-sized and effective for 3 years, was designed to be a more affordable choice.

A health care provider must fit and insert an IUD. One or two strings extend from the IUD into the vagina so the user can check to make sure that her IUD is in place.

Advantages The IUD is a safe, discreet, and highly effective method of birth control. It is over 99 percent effective both in perfect use and typical use.[28] It is effective immediately and needs to be replaced only every 3 to 10 years. *ParaGard* has the benefit of containing no hormones at all, and so has none of the potential negative health impacts of hormonal contraceptives. *Skyla*, *Mirena*, *Kyleena*, and *Liletta*, on the other hand, likely offer some of the same potential health benefits as other progestin-only methods. With *Mirena*, periods become lighter or stop altogether.

IUDs are fully reversible; that is, after removal there is usually no delay in return of fertility. Although IUDs are effective for 3 to 12 years, a health care provider can remove the IUD at any time if the woman decides to become pregnant. (If a woman does become pregnant while using the IUD, the device can be safely removed after pregnancy begins.) All of these methods offer sexual spontaneity, because there is no need to keep supplies on hand or to interrupt lovemaking.

Disadvantages Some disadvantages of IUDs include possible discomfort during insertion and removal and potential complications, such as expulsion. Also, the IUD does not protect against HIV and STIs. In some women, *ParaGard* can cause heavy menstrual flow and severe cramps for the first few months. Other negative side effects of *ParaGard* include acne, headaches, mood changes, uterine cramps, and backache, which seem to occur most often in women who have never been pregnant. These side effects typically go away after the first few months.

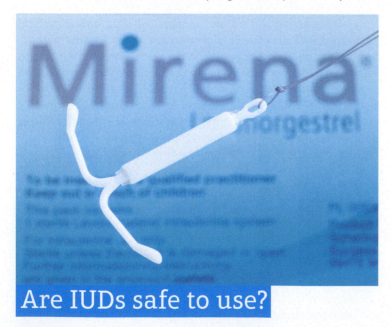

Are IUDs safe to use?

Mirena IUD is a flexible plastic device inserted by a clinician into a woman's uterus, where it releases progestin for up to 5 years.

Check Yourself

- **What are the advantages and disadvantages of intrauterine contraceptives?**

- **How effective are intrauterine contraceptives in preventing pregnancy and STIs?**

- **Why do you think the IUD is gaining popularity in the United States and worldwide?**

5.6 **Describe how emergency contraception prevents pregnancy.**

Emergency contraception is the use of a contraceptive to prevent pregnancy after unprotected intercourse, a sexual assault, or the failure of another birth control method. Combination estrogen-progestin pills and progestin-only pills are two common types of **emergency contraceptive pills (ECPs)**, sometimes referred to as "morning-after pills." ECPs contain the same type of hormones as regular birth control pills and are used after unprotected intercourse but before the woman misses her period. A woman taking ECPs does so to prevent pregnancy; the method will not work if she is already pregnant, nor will it harm an existing pregnancy.

Multiple types of ECPs are available in the United States with no prescription. Most types must be taken within 72 hours (3 days) of intercourse. The FDA has more recently approved *ella*, which is available only by prescription, and can prevent pregnancy when taken up to 120 hours (5 days) after unprotected intercourse.

ECPs prevent pregnancy in the same way as other hormonal contraceptives: by delaying or inhibiting ovulation, inhibiting fertilization, or blocking implantation of a fertilized egg, depending on the phase of the woman's menstrual cycle. When taken within 24 hours, ECPs reduce the risk of pregnancy by up to 95 percent; when taken 2 to 5 days later, ECPs reduce the risk of pregnancy by 88 percent.[29]

Women can also take two additional doses (12 hours apart) of their regular birth control pills as emergency contraception if the pills are the combination (progestin and estrogen) type. However, the exact number of pills to take varies depending on the brand. Women should never combine types of emergency contraception. Today, ECPs are kept on the regular store shelves, usually near other family planning supplies. According to a recent national survey, about 1 in 11 sexually active college students reported using (or their partner using) emergency contraception within the past year.[30]

Although ECPs are no substitute for taking proper precautions (such as using a condom) before having sex, widespread availability of emergency contraception has the potential to significantly reduce the rates of unintended pregnancies and abortions, particularly among young women.

Advantages

Because most types of emergency contraceptive pills are available without a prescription, they are a convenient and easily-obtained solution when other forms of contraception fail (or are not used in the first place). Emergency contraceptive pills are safe to use for

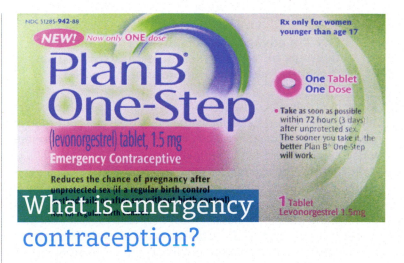

What is emergency contraception?

Emergency contraception is hormone-containing pills used after an act of unprotected intercourse. When taken within 24 hours of unprotected intercourse, ECPs reduce the risk of pregnancy by up to 95 percent. In the United States, *Plan B One Dose*, *Take Action*, *Next Choice One Dose*, and *My Way* are all available without a prescription; *ella*, which can prevent pregnancy up to 5 days after unprotected intercourse, requires a prescription.

nearly every woman. In cases of sexual assault, emergency contraception can protect the victim from an unwanted pregnancy or the ordeal of an abortion.

Disadvantages

Emergency contraception does not protect against STIs and is not as effective as some other forms of birth control. Although emergency contraception has no known serious side effects, some women report short-term feelings of nausea and/or vomiting after taking the pills. Other potential short-term side effects are headache, tenderness in the breasts, lower abdominal pain, dizziness, and fatigue. In addition, emergency contraception is more expensive than other forms of contraception (typically $35 or more per dose).

- How does emergency contraception prevent pregnancy?

- What restrictions, if any, do you think there should be on providing emergency contraception?

- What are the disadvantages of using emergency contraception as a form of birth control?

5.7 Behavioral Methods and Fertility Awareness Methods

Learning Outcome

5.7 List the advantages, disadvantages, and effectiveness of behavioral and fertility awareness methods in preventing pregnancy and STIs.

Some methods of contraception rely on one or both partners altering their sexual behavior. In general, these methods require more self-control, diligence, and commitment, making them more prone to user error than other methods.

Withdrawal, or *coitus interruptus*, involves removing the penis from the vagina just before ejaculation. In a recent survey, 32 percent of respondents reported that withdrawal was the method of birth control (or one of the methods) they used the last time they had sexual intercourse.[31] This statistic is startlingly high, considering the high risk of both STI transmission and pregnancy (only 78 percent effective with typical use) associated with this method of birth control.[32] Withdrawal is highly unreliable, even with "perfect" use; there can be up to half a million sperm in the drop of fluid at the tip of the penis *before* ejaculation. Timing withdrawal is also difficult. Withdrawal offers no protection against transmission of STIs.

Strictly defined, **abstinence** means deliberately avoiding intercourse, which would allow one to engage in such forms of intimacy as massage, kissing, and masturbation. Couples who go beyond fondling and kissing to activities such as oral sex and mutual masturbation, but not vaginal or anal sex, are sometimes said to be engaging in "outercourse."

Abstinence is the only method of avoiding pregnancy that is 100 percent effective. It is also the only one that is 100 percent effective against transmitting disease. Outercourse can be 100 percent effective for birth control as long as the male does not ejaculate near the vaginal opening, though it is not 100 percent effective against STIs. Oral–genital contact can transmit disease, although the practice can be made safer by using a condom on the penis or a latex barrier, such as a dental dam, on the vaginal opening. Both abstinence and outercourse require discipline and commitment for couples to sustain over long periods of time. Thirty-three percent of college students report being abstinent for the past 12 months. Nearly 35 percent report having never engaged in vaginal sex, 31.1 percent never in oral sex, and 76 percent never in anal sex.[33]

Fertility awareness methods (FAMs) of birth control rely on altering sexual behavior during certain times of the month (**Figure 5.4**); they are based on the facts that an ovum can survive for up to 48 hours after ovulation and sperm can live for up to 5 days in the vagina. Strategies include the *cervical mucus method*, which requires tracking changes in vaginal secretions; the *body temperature method*, which requires tracking subtle changes in a woman's basal body temperature; and the *calendar method*, which involves recording the menstrual cycle for 12 months and assuming that ovulation occurs during the midpoint of the cycle. All these methods require abstaining from penis–vagina contact during fertile times.

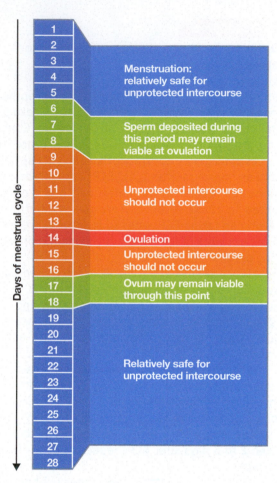

Figure 5.4 The Fertility Cycle
It is important to remember that most women do not have a consistent 28-day cycle.

Fertility awareness methods are the only types of birth control that comply with certain religious teachings, including those of the Roman Catholic Church. They require no medical visit or prescription and have no negative health effects. Their effectiveness depends on diligence and self-discipline; they have a 76 percent effectiveness rate with typical use.[34] Women who attempt to use these methods without proper training run a high risk of unintended pregnancy. Anyone interested in using them is advised to take a class, often offered for free by health centers and churches.

Check Yourself

- **What are the advantages and disadvantages of behavioral and fertility awareness methods?**
- **How effective are these methods in preventing pregnancy and STIs?**
- **Why do many people use highly ineffective methods of birth control, such as withdrawal? What do you think it will take to change these behaviors?**

5.8 Sterilization Methods

5.8 List the advantages, disadvantages, and effectiveness of sterilization methods in preventing pregnancy and STIs.

In the United States, **sterilization** has become the second leading method of contraception for women of all ages and the leading method of contraception among women over age 35.[35] Because sterilization is usually permanent, anyone who Is considering it should think through possibilities such as divorce and remarriage or improvement in financial status that might make a pregnancy desirable at some later point.

Female Sterilization

In **tubal ligation**, the woman's fallopian tubes are sealed to block sperm's access to released eggs (**Figure 5.5**). The operation is usually done laparoscopically on an outpatient basis and takes less than an hour. Tubal ligation does not affect ovarian and uterine function. The menstrual cycle continues; released eggs disintegrate and are absorbed by the lymphatic system. As soon as her incision heals, the woman may resume intercourse with no fear of pregnancy.

A newer procedure, *Essure*, involves placement of microcoils into the fallopian tubes via the vagina. The microcoils expand, promoting growth of scar tissue that blocks the tubes. Essure is recommended for women who cannot have a tubal ligation because of health conditions such as obesity or heart disease. Essure has been under review by the FDA because of concerns about its safety and effectiveness, so anyone interested in this method should be informed of all potential risks.[36]

A **hysterectomy**, or removal of the uterus, is a method of sterilization requiring major surgery. It is usually done only when a woman's uterus is diseased or damaged.

The main advantage to female sterilization is that it is highly effective (less than a 1 percent failure rate) and permanent.[37] Afterward, no other cost or action is required. Sterilization has no negative effect on sex drive. The Essure method requires no incision. As with any surgery, there are risks involved. Furthermore, sterilization offers no protection against STIs and is initially expensive.

Male Sterilization

Sterilization in men is less complicated. A **vasectomy** is frequently done on an outpatient basis, using a local anesthetic (see **Figure 5.6**). It involves making a small incision in each side of the scrotum to expose the vasa deferentia, cutting and either tying or cauterizing the ends. Because sperm constitute only a small percentage of semen, the amount of ejaculate is not changed significantly. The testes continue to produce sperm, which disintegrate and are absorbed into the lymphatic system.

A vasectomy is a highly effective and permanent means of preventing pregnancy; typical effectiveness rates are more than 99 percent.[38] The procedure requires minimal recovery time, and no cost or action is required afterward. Vasectomy has no effect on sex drive or sexual performance.

Male sterilization offers no protection against STI transmission. Also, a vasectomy is not immediately effective; because sperm are stored in other areas besides the vasa deferentia, couples must use alternative birth control for at least 1 month afterward. A physician's semen analysis determines when unprotected intercourse can take place. As with any surgery, there are some risks. Very infrequently the vas deferens may create a new path, negating the procedure.

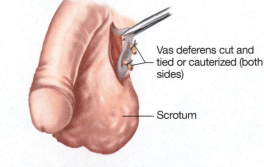

Figure 5.6 **Male Sterilization: Vasectomy**

Vas deferens cut and tied or cauterized (both sides)

Scrotum

■ What are the advantages, disadvantages, and effectiveness of sterilization methods in preventing pregnancy?

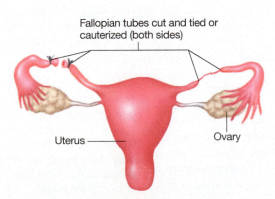

Fallopian tubes cut and tied or cauterized (both sides)

Uterus

Ovary

Figure 5.5 **Female Sterilization: Tubal Ligation**

Learning Outcome

5.9 Explore questions to consider when choosing a method of contraception and strategies for discussing contraception with a partner.

With all the options available, how does a person or a couple decide what method of contraception is best? Take some time to research the various methods, ask questions of your health care provider, and be honest with yourself and your partner about your own preferences. Questions to ask yourself include the following:

- **How comfortable would I be using a particular method?** If you aren't at ease with a method, you might not use it consistently, and it probably will not be a reliable choice for you. Think about whether the method may cause discomfort for you or your partner, and consider your own comfort level with touching your body. For women, methods such as the diaphragm, sponge, and NuvaRing require inserting an apparatus into the vagina and taking it out. For men, using a condom requires rolling it onto the penis.

- **Will this method be convenient for me and my partner?** Some methods require more effort than do others. Be honest with yourself about how likely you are to use the method consistently. Are you willing to interrupt lovemaking, to abstain from sex during certain times of the month, or to take a pill every day? You might feel that condoms are easy and convenient to use, or you might prefer something that requires little ongoing thought, such as Nexplanon or an IUD.

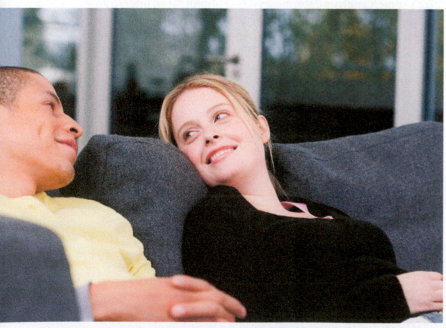

Don't let embarrassment put your health at risk! Talking about safer sex may be tough, but it is worth the effort.

- **Am I at risk for the transmission of STIs?** If you have multiple sex partners or are uncertain about the sexual history or disease status of your current sex partner, then you are at risk for transmission of STIs and HIV (the virus that causes AIDS). Condoms (both male and female) are the *only* birth control methods, apart from abstinence, that protect against STIs and HIV (although some other barrier methods offer limited protection).

- **Do I want to have a biological child in the future?** If you are unsure about your plans for future childbearing, you should use a temporary birth control method rather than a permanent one such as sterilization. Keep in mind that you might regret choosing a permanent method if you are young, if you have few or no children, if you are choosing this method because your partner wants you to, or if you believe that this option will fix relationship problems. If you know that you want to have children in the future, consider how soon that will be, because some methods, such as Depo-Provera, cause a delay in return to fertility.

- **How would an unplanned pregnancy affect my life?** If an unplanned pregnancy would be a potentially devastating event for you or would have a serious impact on your plans for the future, then you should choose a highly effective birth control method, such as the pill, patch, ring, implant, or IUD. However, if you are in a stable relationship, have a reliable source of income, are planning to have children in the future, and would embrace a pregnancy if it happened to occur now, then you may be comfortable with a less reliable method such as condoms, fertility awareness, the diaphragm, cervical cap, or spermicides.

- **What are my religious and moral values in relation to contraception?** If your beliefs prevent you from considering other birth control methods, fertility awareness methods are a good option. When both partners are motivated to use these methods, they can be successful at preventing unintended pregnancy. If you are considering this option, sign up for a class to get specific training in using the method effectively.

- **How much will the birth control method cost?** Some contraceptive methods involve an initial outlay of money and few continuing costs (e.g., sterilization, IUD), whereas others are fairly inexpensive but must be purchased repeatedly (e.g., condoms, spermicides, monthly pill prescriptions). Remember that any prescription method requires routine checkups, which may involve some cost to you. Be sure to check your health insurance to determine whether hormonal contraceptives are available to you at little or no cost.

See It! Videos

Concerned about health effects of contraception? Watch **Newer Birth Control Pills May Have Increased Risks of Blood Clots** in the Study Area of Mastering Health.

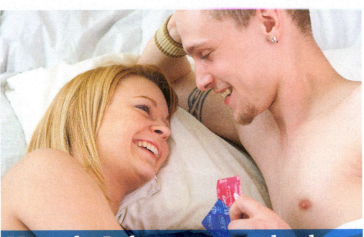

How do I choose a method of birth control?

Many different methods of birth control are on the market: barrier methods, hormonal methods, surgical methods, and other options. When you choose a method, you'll need to consider several factors, including cost, comfort level, convenience, and health risks. All of these factors together will influence your ability to consistently and correctly use the contraceptive and prevent unwanted pregnancy.

- **Do I have any health factors that could limit my choice?** Hormonal birth control methods can pose health risks to women with certain preexisting conditions, such as high blood pressure, a history of stroke or blood clots, liver disease, migraines, or diabetes. You should discuss this issue with your health care provider when considering birth control methods. In addition, women who smoke or are over the age of 35 are at risk from complications of combination hormonal contraceptives. Breast-feeding women can use progestin-only methods but should avoid methods containing estrogen. Men and women with latex allergies can use barrier methods made of polyurethane, silicone, or other materials rather than latex condoms.
- **Are there any additional benefits I would like to get from my contraceptive?** Hormonal birth control methods may have desirable secondary effects, such as the reduction of acne or the lessening of premenstrual symptoms. Certain pills are marketed as having specific effects, so it is possible to choose one that is known to clear skin or reduce mood changes caused by menstruation. Hormonal birth control methods are also associated with reduced risks of certain cancers. Extended-cycle pills and some progestin-only methods cause menstrual periods to be less frequent or to stop altogether, which some women find desirable. Condoms also have the potential to reduce the risk of contracting an STI.

Communicating about Contraception

Communication is key to a healthy relationship, and it is especially so between people who are sexually intimate. Communication is a sign of care and respect for your own body and your partner's, and it empowers both of you to be assertive about your individual needs, likes, limits, and desires in the sexual relationship. Open communication also creates a safe environment to ask about your partner's sexual history, STI testing, and sexual expectations.

You might feel awkward or uncomfortable discussing sex, and you might believe that talking beforehand ruins the naturalness or spontaneity of sex. Some people are concerned that their partner will misinterpret the conversation and feel accused of infidelity, distrust, promiscuity, or lack of love in the relationship. Try to address these concerns in an honest and open manner. And remember: Sexual communication is about protecting both of your bodies and ensuring that you are clear about the needs and concerns of both people.

If you are afraid that talking about sex beforehand is going to make your partner think you don't trust him or her, take some time to examine the strength of your relationship. Trust is about being open and honest. If you're afraid to talk with your partner, the chances are that you actually don't trust your partner, and you might be better off with a partner you do trust.

Before you talk with your partner, it's a good idea to talk with your health care provider about your options for practicing safer sex. Remember that you need to think about pregnancy and avoiding STIs.

With your partner, try to find a time and place where you are both comfortable and free of distractions and you have time to have a full conversation. It's generally better to have this conversation outside of the bedroom so that you're not pressured by the heat of the moment to do things you don't want to do.

Some tips to boost your confidence in negotiating safer sex include the following:

- It can be helpful to have condoms and/or dental dams around so that when things start to really heat up, you will be ready.
- Talk to your partner about using protection before getting intimate. This will help both of you be more comfortable and prepared to use a condom or dental dam when the time comes.
- Practice makes perfect. The best way to learn how to use condoms correctly and guarantee their effectiveness is to practice putting them on yourself or your partner.
- If you are concerned about the interruption of using either condoms or dental dams, try to incorporate them into your foreplay. By helping your partner put on protection together, you both will stay aroused and in the moment.
- If your partner complains that sex "doesn't feel as good with a condom/dental dam," remind him or her that it will make you feel more relaxed to worry less about the risk of STIs and pregnancy. You can also use lubricants to increase sensation.

Check Yourself

- What are some questions to consider when you are choosing a method of contraception? How might these considerations change during different stages of your life?
- What are some potential obstacles to communicating about contraception, and how can you overcome them?

5.10 Abortion

5.10 Summarize the various types of abortion procedures.

The vast majority of abortions occur because of unintended pregnancies,[39] as even the best birth control methods can fail. Other pregnancies are terminated because they are a consequence of rape or incest or because of health risks to the mother. Other reasons commonly cited are not being ready financially or emotionally to care for a child.[40]

In 1973, the landmark U.S. Supreme Court decision in *Roe v. Wade* stated that the "right to privacy . . . founded on the Fourteenth Amendment's concept of personal liberty . . . is broad enough to encompass a woman's decision whether or not to terminate her pregnancy."[41] The decision maintained that during the first trimester of pregnancy, a woman and her health care practitioner have the right to terminate the pregnancy through **abortion** without legal restrictions. It allowed individual states to set conditions for second-trimester abortions. Third-trimester abortions were ruled illegal unless the mother's life or health was in danger. Before this, women who wanted to terminate a pregnancy had to travel to a country where the procedure was legal, consult an illegal abortionist, or perform their own abortions. These procedures sometimes led to death from hemorrhage or infection or infertility from internal scarring.

The Debate over Abortion

Abortion is a highly charged issue in America. In a recent national poll, 47 percent of Americans described themselves as pro-choice, while 46 percent described themselves as pro-life.[42] Pro-choice individuals believe that it is a woman's right to make decisions about her own body and health, including the decision to continue or terminate a pregnancy. On the other side of the issue, pro-life, or anti-abortion, individuals believe that the embryo or fetus is a human being with rights that must be protected. Pro-life groups lobby for laws prohibiting the use of public funds for abortion and abortion counseling at the same time that pro-choice groups lobby for laws that make abortions more widely available. At times, violence has arisen as a result of this controversy in the form of attacks on clinics or on individual physicians who perform abortions.

In the 40-plus years since *Roe v. Wade* legalized abortion nationwide, hundreds of laws have been passed at the state and federal levels to narrow or expand limits on abortion. In 2016 alone, more than 60 new abortion-related laws were passed in the United States, most of which focused on regulation of abortion providers or facilities or limitations on the provision of abortions.[43] These types of laws make abortions more difficult and costly to provide, consequently reducing the number of clinics and providers willing and able to provide safe abortion services. Thus, while abortion remains legal in all 50 states, abortion availability is severely limited for many women, owing to difficulty accessing abortion services.

Abortion in the Developing World

Unintended pregnancy is the primary reason why over 50 million women globally each year choose abortions. Eighty-one percent of these abortions occur In developing countries where contraceptives are unavailable. Between 8 percent and 18 percent of maternal deaths worldwide are due to unsafe abortions in developing regions of the world such as Africa, Asia, Latin America and the Caribbean. Although death rates are high, millions of additional women suffer serious complications, and over 40 percent of these at-risk women never receive treatment.[44] When abortion is legal, risks to the mother are significantly lower.[45]

Emotional Aspects of Abortion

The best scientific evidence published indicates that among adult women who have an unplanned pregnancy, the risk of mental health problems is no greater if they have an abortion than if they deliver a baby. Although a variety of feelings such as regret, guilt, sadness, relief, and happiness are normal, evidence does not show that having an abortion causes an increase in anxiety, depression, or suicidal ideation.[46] Researchers have found that the best predictor of a woman's emotional well-being after an abortion was her emotional well-being before the procedure.[47] Factors that place a woman at higher risk for negative psychological responses after an abortion include perception of stigma, need for secrecy, low levels of social support for the abortion decision, prior history of mental health issues, low self-esteem, and avoidance and denial coping strategies.[48] Certainly, a support network is helpful to any woman who is struggling with the emotional aspects of her abortion decision.

Methods of Abortion

The choice of abortion procedure is determined by how many weeks the woman has been pregnant. Length of pregnancy is calculated from the first day of her last menstrual period.

Surgical Abortions The majority of abortions performed in the United States today are surgical. If performed during the first trimester of pregnancy, abortion presents a relatively low health risk to the mother. About 89 percent of abortions occur during the first 12 weeks of pregnancy (see **Figure 5.7**).[49] The most commonly used method of first-trimester abortion is **suction curettage**, also called vacuum aspiration or dilation and curettage (D&C) (**Figure 5.8**). The vast majority of abortions in the United States are done by using this procedure, usually under local anesthetic. The cervix is dilated with instruments or by placing laminaria, a sterile seaweed product, into the cervical canal, where it slowly dilates the cervix. After the laminaria is removed, a long tube is inserted through the cervix and into the uterus, and gentle suction removes fetal tissue from the uterine walls.

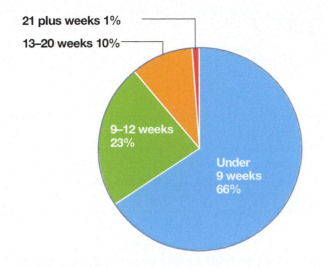

Figure 5.7 When Women Have Abortions (in weeks from the last menstrual period)

21 plus weeks 1%
13–20 weeks 10%
9–12 weeks 23%
Under 9 weeks 66%

Source: T.C. Jatlaoi et al., "Abortion Surveillance—United States 2013," *Morbidity and Mortality Weekly Report* 65, no. SS12 (2016).

Pregnancies in the second trimester (after week 12) can be terminated through **dilation and evacuation (D&E)**. For this procedure, the cervix is dilated for 1 to 2 days, and a combination of instruments and vacuum aspiration is used to empty the uterus. Second-trimester abortions may be done under general anesthetic. The D&E can be performed on an outpatient basis, with or without pain medication. Generally, however, the woman is given a mild tranquilizer to help her relax. This procedure may cause moderate to severe uterine cramping and blood loss. After a D&E, a return visit to the clinic is an important follow-up.

Abortions during the third trimester are very rare (fewer than 2 percent of abortions in the United States).[50] When they are performed, a D&E or saline **induction abortion** can be performed. The much debated, **intact dilation and extraction (D&X)**, often referred to as "partial birth abortion," is illegal in the United States. However, several states do not enforce the law and allow the procedure when a mother's life or health is at risk.[51]

The risks associated with surgical abortion include infection, incomplete abortion (when parts of the placenta remain in the uterus), missed abortion, excessive bleeding, and cervical and uterine trauma. Follow-up and attention to danger signs decrease the chances of long-term problems.

The mortality rate for women undergoing first-trimester abortions in the United States averages 3 deaths for every 1 million procedures at 8 or fewer weeks.[52] The risk of death increases with the length of pregnancy. At 18 weeks or later, the mortality rate is 7 per 100,000.[53] This higher rate later in the pregnancy is due to the increased risk of uterine perforation, bleeding, infection, and incomplete abortion; these complications occur because the uterine wall becomes thinner as the pregnancy progresses. As a comparison, for every 100,000 live births, nearly 24 women die during or within 42 days of birth.[54]

Medical Abortions Unlike surgical abortions, **medical abortions** are performed without entering the uterus. *Mifepristone,* formerly called *RU-486* and currently sold in the United States under the name *Mifeprex,* is a steroid hormone that induces abortion by blocking the action of progesterone, which maintains the lining of the uterus. As a result, the uterine lining and embryo are expelled from the uterus, terminating the pregnancy.

Mifepristone's nickname, "the abortion pill," might seem to imply an easy process; however, this treatment actually involves more steps than a suction curettage abortion. With mifepristone, a first visit involves a physical exam and a dose of three tablets, which may cause minor side effects, such as nausea, headaches, weakness, and fatigue. The patient returns 2 to 3 days later for a dose of prostaglandins (misoprostol), which causes uterine contractions that expel the fertilized egg. The patient is required to stay under observation at the clinic for 4 hours and to make a follow-up visit within 2 weeks.[55]

More than 99 percent of women who use mifepristone early in pregnancy will experience a complete abortion.[56] The side effects are similar to those reported during heavy menstruation and include cramping, minor pain, and nausea. Fewer than 1 percent of women have more serious outcomes requiring a blood transfusion because of severe bleeding or the administration of intravenous antibiotics.[57]

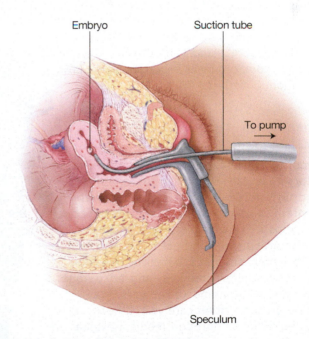

Embryo   Suction tube
                To pump
Speculum

Figure 5.8 Suction Curettage Abortion
This procedure, in which a long tube with gentle suction is used to remove fetal tissue from the uterine walls, can be performed up to the twelfth week of pregnancy.

Check Yourself

- What is the current legal status of abortion?

- What are the various types of abortion procedures?

The many methods available to control fertility give you choices that did not exist when your parents—and even you—were born. If you are in the process of deciding whether, or when, to have children, take the time to evaluate your emotions, finances, and physical health.

Emotional Health

First and foremost, consider why you may want to have a child. To fulfill an inner need to carry on the family? To share love? To give your parents grandchildren? Because it's expected? Then consider the responsibilities involved with becoming a parent. Are you ready to make all the sacrifices necessary to bear and raise a child? Can you care for this new human being in a loving and nurturing manner? Do you have a strong social support system? This emotional preparation for parenthood can be as important as the physical preparation.

Maternal Health

The birth of a healthy baby depends in part on the mother's **preconception care**. Maternal factors that can affect a fetus or infant include drug use (illicit, prescription, or over-the-counter), alcohol consumption, tobacco use and exposure to tobacco smoke, or obesity. To promote preconception health, get the best medical care you can, practice healthy behaviors, build a strong support network, and encourage safe environments at home and at work.[58]

During a preconception care visit, a health care provider performs a thorough medical evaluation and talks with the woman about any conditions she might have, such as diabetes or high blood pressure. The health care provider will also determine whether the woman has had any problems with prior pregnancies, whether any genetic disorders run in the family, and whether the woman's immunizations are up to date. For example, if the woman has never had rubella (German measles), she needs to be immunized before becoming pregnant. A rubella infection can kill the fetus or cause blindness or hearing disorders in the infant. The health care provider will encourage the woman to eliminate alcohol consumption and tobacco use and may adjust some medications, such as antidepressants, to safer levels.

Nutrition counseling is another important part of preconception care. Among the many important nutrition issues is folic acid (folate) intake. When consumed the month before conception and during early pregnancy, folate reduces the risk of spina bifida, a congenital birth defect resulting from failure of the spinal column to close.

Why is preconception care so important? Beginning prenatal care at week 11 or 12 of a pregnancy is often late to prevent a variety of health problems for both child and mother. The fetus is most susceptible to developing certain problems in the first 4 to 10 weeks after conception, before prenatal care is normally initiated. Because many women don't realize they are pregnant until later, they often can't reduce health risks unless intervention begins before conception.[59]

Additional suggestions for preparing for a healthy pregnancy can be found in the Skills for Behavior Change feature.

Maternal Age The average age at which a woman has her first child has risen (from age 21 in 1970 to almost 26 today), so a woman who becomes pregnant in her thirties has plenty of company.[60] In fact, births to women in their twenties are declining, while the rate of first births to women between the ages of 30 and 39 is the highest reported in four decades. Births to women over age 39 have continued to increase slightly over the years.[61]

The chances of miscarriage or of having a baby with birth defects, including Down syndrome, rise after the age of 35.[62] However, many doctors note that older mothers tend to be more conscientious about self-care during pregnancy and are more psychologically mature and ready to include an infant in their family than are some younger women.

Being in good physical shape will help prepare you for the demands of pregnancy

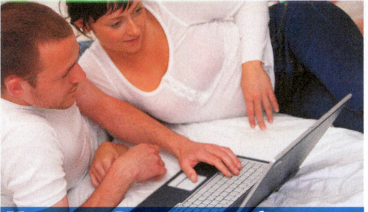

How can I prepare to be a parent?

Following a doctor-approved exercise program during pregnancy is just one aspect of healthy preparation for parenthood. Even before they conceive, prospective mothers and fathers should evaluate their emotional, physical, social, and financial well-being and implement healthy change where needed to better ready themselves for bringing a child into the world.

Paternal Health

Fathers-to-be are encouraged to practice the same healthy habits as mothers-to-be because, by one route or another, dozens of chemicals studied so far (from occupational exposures to by-products of cigarette smoke to hormones) appear to harm sperm.[63] A father's age may also play a role; research shows a relationship between older fathers and autism, ADHD, bipolar disorder, and schizophrenia.[64]

Financial Evaluation

Finances are an important consideration. Can you afford to give your child the life you would like for him or her? The U.S. Department of Agriculture estimates that it will cost an average of $233,610 to raise a child born today to age 18, not including college tuition.[65] Balancing the economics of successful childrearing with the realities of your financial resources and desired lifestyle should be an important part of family planning.

It is important to check whether your medical insurance provides maternity benefits. If not, you can expect to pay, on average, $8,775 for a normal delivery and $11,525 for a cesarean section, not including prenatal care.[66] Both partners should investigate their employers' policies on parental leave, including length of leave available and conditions for returning to work.

Contingency Planning

A final consideration is how to provide for your child if something dire should happen to you and/or your partner. If you both die at early ages, do you have relatives or close friends who could raise your child? Will there be financial resources to ease the burden on these guardians? If you have more than one child, would they have to be split up or could they be kept together? Although these things are unpleasant to think about, contingency planning is crucial. Children who lose their parents are heartbroken and confused. A prearranged plan of action can smooth their transition into new families; without one, a judge will usually decide who will raise them.

Skills for **Behavior Change**

Preparing For Pregnancy

Before conceiving a child, parents-to-be should take stock of, and possibly improve, their own health to help ensure the health of their child. Among the most important factors to consider are the following.

FOR WOMEN:

- If you smoke, drink alcohol, or use drugs, stop.
- Reduce or eliminate your caffeine intake.
- Get checked for sexually transmitted infections and seek treatment if you have one
- Maintain a healthy weight; lose or gain weight if necessary.
- Avoid X-rays and environmental chemicals, such as lawn and garden herbicides and pesticides.
- Take prenatal vitamins, which are especially important in providing adequate folic acid.
- Get immunized for rubella, if you have not already been vaccinated.

FOR MEN:

- If you smoke, quit.
- Drink alcohol only in moderation, and avoid drug use.
- Get checked for sexually transmitted infections and seek treatment if you have one.
- Avoid exposure to toxic chemicals in your work or home environment.
- Maintain a healthy weight; lose or gain weight if necessary.

Check Yourself

- What are key issues to consider in planning a pregnancy?

- Of the issues discussed, which do you think are the most important?

- When considering the lifestyle changes needed for a successful pregnancy, which do you think would be the most challenging to implement?

The Process of Pregnancy

5.12 Describe the process of pregnancy, from ovulation to implantation.

Pregnancy is an important event in a woman's life. Actions taken before, as well as behaviors engaged in during, pregnancy can significantly affect the health of both infant and mother.

The process of pregnancy begins the moment a sperm fertilizes an ovum in the fallopian tubes (**Figure 5.9**). From there, the single fertilized cell, now called a *zygote*, multiplies and becomes a sphere-shaped cluster of cells called a *blastocyst*, which travels toward the uterus, a journey that may take 3 to 4 days. Upon arrival, the embryo burrows into the thick, spongy endometrium—in a process called implantation—and is nourished from this carefully prepared lining.

Pregnancy Testing A pregnancy test scheduled in a medical office or birth control clinic will confirm a pregnancy. Some home pregnancy test kits, sold over the counter in drugstores, can be used as early as a week after conception, and many are 99 percent reliable.[67] A positive test is based on the secretion of **human chorionic gonadotropin (HCG)**, which is found in the woman's urine. If the test is done too early in the pregnancy, it may show a false negative. Other causes of false negatives are unclean testing devices, ingestion of certain drugs, and vaginal or urinary tract infections. A blood test administered and analyzed by your health care provider at your first prenatal appointment will officially confirm a pregnancy.

Early Signs of Pregnancy A woman's body undergoes substantial changes during the course of a pregnancy (**Figure 5.10**). The first sign of pregnancy is usually a missed menstrual period (although some women spot in early pregnancy, which may be mistaken for a period). Other signs include breast tenderness, emotional upset, extreme fatigue, and sleeplessness, as well as nausea and vomiting, especially in the morning.

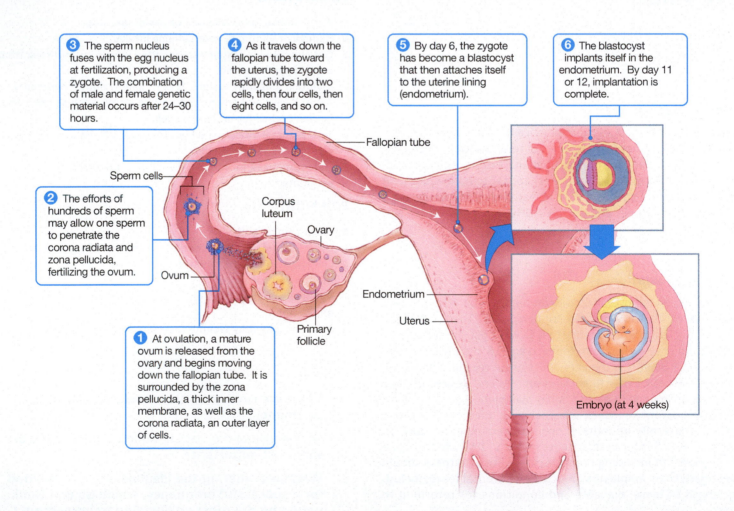

❸ The sperm nucleus fuses with the egg nucleus at fertilization, producing a zygote. The combination of male and female genetic material occurs after 24–30 hours.

❹ As it travels down the fallopian tube toward the uterus, the zygote rapidly divides into two cells, then four cells, then eight cells, and so on.

❺ By day 6, the zygote has become a blastocyst that then attaches itself to the uterine lining (endometrium).

❻ The blastocyst implants itself in the endometrium. By day 11 or 12, implantation is complete.

❷ The efforts of hundreds of sperm may allow one sperm to penetrate the corona radiata and zona pellucida, fertilizing the ovum.

❶ At ovulation, a mature ovum is released from the ovary and begins moving down the fallopian tube. It is surrounded by the zona pellucida, a thick inner membrane, as well as the corona radiata, an outer layer of cells.

Fallopian tube

Sperm cells

Corpus luteum

Ovary

Ovum

Endometrium

Primary follicle

Uterus

Embryo (at 4 weeks)

Figure 5.9 Fertilization
Fertilization usually occurs in the upper third of the fallopian tube, and implantation in the uterus takes place about 6 days later.

Pregnancy typically lasts 40 weeks and is divided into three phases, or **trimesters**, of approximately 3 months each. The due date is calculated from the expectant mother's last menstrual period.

The First Trimester During the first trimester, few visible changes occur in the mother's body. She may urinate more frequently and may experience morning sickness, swollen breasts, or fatigue. These symptoms may or may not be frequent or severe, so she might not even realize she is pregnant unless she takes a pregnancy test.

During the first 2 months after conception, the **embryo** differentiates and develops its various organ systems, beginning with the nervous and circulatory systems. At the start of the third month, the embryo is called a **fetus**, a term indicating that all organ systems are in place. For the rest of the pregnancy, growth and refinement occur in each major body system so that each can function independently yet in coordination with all the others.

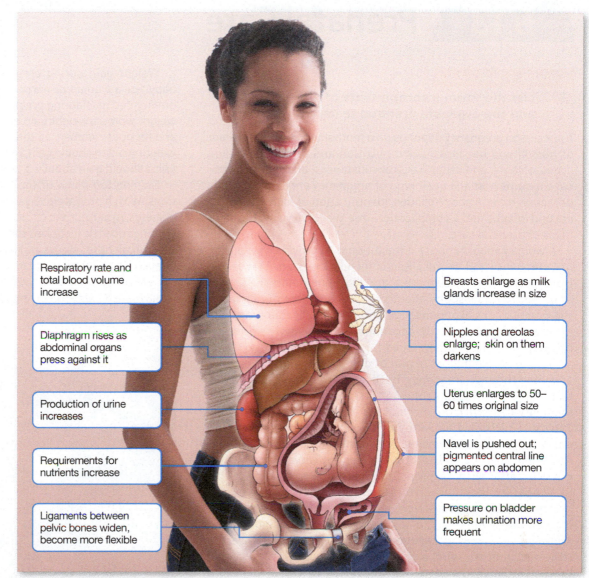

Respiratory rate and total blood volume increase

Diaphragm rises as abdominal organs press against it

Production of urine increases

Requirements for nutrients increase

Ligaments between pelvic bones widen, become more flexible

Breasts enlarge as milk glands increase in size

Nipples and areolas enlarge; skin on them darkens

Uterus enlarges to 50–60 times original size

Navel is pushed out; pigmented central line appears on abdomen

Pressure on bladder makes urination more frequent

Figure 5.10 **Changes in a Woman's Body during Pregnancy**

The Second Trimester At the beginning of the second trimester, physical changes in the mother become more visible. Her breasts swell, and her waistline thickens. During this time, the fetus makes greater demands on the mother's body. In particular, the **placenta**, the network of blood vessels that carries nutrients and oxygen to the fetus and fetal waste products to the mother, becomes well established.

The Third Trimester From the end of the sixth month through the ninth month is the third trimester. This is the period of greatest fetal growth, when the fetus gains most of its weight. The growing fetus depends entirely on the mother for nutrition and must receive large amounts of calcium, iron, and protein from the mother's diet.

Although the fetus may survive if it is born during the seventh month, it needs the layer of fat it acquires during the eighth month and time for the organs (especially respiratory and digestive organs) to develop fully. Infants born prematurely usually require intensive medical care.

Emotional Changes Of course, the process of pregnancy involves much more than the changes in a woman's body and the developing fetus. Many important emotional changes occur from the time a woman learns she is pregnant through the *postpartum period* (the first 6 weeks after her baby is born). Throughout pregnancy, women may experience fear of complications, anxiety about becoming a parent, and wonder and excitement over the developing baby.

Check Yourself

- **What is the process of pregnancy, from ovulation to implantation?**

- **What are some physical changes experienced by a mother during the three trimesters of pregnancy?**

5.13 Prenatal Care

5.13 List the various components of prenatal care and the available prenatal tests.

A successful pregnancy depends on a mother who takes good care of herself and her fetus. Good nutrition and exercise; avoiding drugs, alcohol, and other harmful substances; and regular medical checkups from the beginning of pregnancy are essential. Early detection of fetal abnormalities, identification of high-risk mothers and infants, and a complication-free pregnancy are the major goals of prenatal care.

A woman should choose a practitioner to provide care during her pregnancy and delivery. Recommendations from friends and from her family physician are a good starting point; she should also consider philosophy about pain management during labor, the practitioner's experience in handling complications, and the practitioner's willingness to accommodate the woman's personal beliefs on these and other issues.

Several different types of practitioners are qualified to care for a woman through pregnancy, birth, and the postpartum period, including obstetrician-gynecologists, family practitioners, and midwives. *Obstetrician-gynecologists* are medical doctors (MDs). They are specialists trained to handle all types of pregnancy- and delivery-related emergencies. They generally can perform deliveries only in a hospital setting and cannot serve as the baby's physician after birth. Family practitioners provide care for people of all ages, so they can serve as the baby's physician after birth. However, they may provide pregnancy care only to women having low-risk pregnancies, and they rarely perform home births. *Midwives* can be lay or certified. *Certified midwives* can oversee deliveries in nonhospital settings and have access to traditional medical facilities. They cannot provide any medication and might need to refer high-risk pregnancies to a clinician. *Lay midwives* are educated through informal routes such as apprenticeship and might not have training to handle an emergency.

Ideally, a woman should begin prenatal appointments within the first 3 months after becoming pregnant. This early care reduces infant mortality and the likelihood of low birth weight. On the first visit, the practitioner should obtain a complete medical history of the mother and her family and note any hereditary conditions that could put a woman or her fetus at risk. Regular checkups to measure weight gain and blood pressure and to monitor the fetus's size and position should continue throughout the pregnancy. The American Congress of Obstetricians and Gynecologists recommends seven or eight prenatal visits for women with low-risk pregnancies.

Nutrition and Exercise Despite "eating for two," pregnant woman need only about 300 additional calories a day. Special attention should be paid to getting enough folic acid (found in dark leafy greens), iron (dried fruits, meats, legumes, liver, egg yolks), calcium (nonfat or low-fat dairy products and some canned fish), and fluids. Babies born to poorly nourished mothers run high risks of substandard mental and physical development.

Weight gain during pregnancy helps to nourish a growing baby. For a woman of normal weight before pregnancy, the recommended gain during pregnancy is 25 to 35 pounds.[68] For overweight women, weight gain of 15 to 25 pounds is recommended, and for obese women, 11 to 20 pounds is recommended.[69] Underweight women should gain 28 to 40 pounds, and women carrying twins should gain about 35 to 45 pounds.[70]

Gaining too much or too little weight can lead to complications. With higher weight gains, women may develop gestational diabetes, hypertension, or increased risk of delivery complications. Gaining too little increases the chance of a low birth weight baby.

As in all other stages of life, exercise is an important factor in overall health during pregnancy. Regular exercise is recommended for pregnant women; however, they should consult with their health care provider before starting any exercise program. Exercise

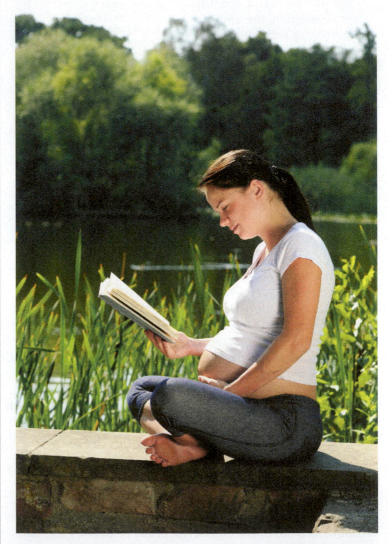

A pregnant woman who exercises, eats well, avoids harmful substances, and has regular medical checkups is more likely to have a successful pregnancy.

can help control weight, make labor easier, and help with a faster recovery because of increased strength and endurance. Women can usually maintain their customary level of activity during most of the pregnancy, although there are some cautions: Pregnant women should avoid exercise that puts them at risk of falling or having an abdominal injury, such as horseback riding, soccer, or skiing, and in the third trimester, exercises that involve lying on the back should be avoided, as they can restrict blood flow to the uterus.

Drugs and Alcohol A woman should consult with a health care provider about the safety of any drugs she might use during pregnancy. Even too much of common over-the-counter medications such as aspirin can damage a developing fetus. During the first 3 months of pregnancy, the fetus is especially subject to the **teratogenic** (birth defect–causing) effects of drugs, environmental chemicals, X-rays, and diseases. The fetus can also develop an addiction to or tolerance for drugs that the mother uses.

Maternal consumption of alcohol is detrimental to a growing fetus. Symptoms of **fetal alcohol syndrome (FAS)** include mental retardation, slowed nerve reflexes, and small head size. The exact amount of alcohol that causes FAS is not known; therefore, the American Congress of Obstetricians and Gynecologists recommends completely avoiding alcohol during pregnancy.[71]

Smoking Tobacco use, and smoking in particular, causes harm during every phase of reproduction. Women who smoke have more difficulty becoming pregnant and a higher risk of infertility. Women who smoke during pregnancy have a greater chance of miscarriage, complications, premature births, low birth weight infants, stillbirth, and infant mortality specifically due to sudden infant death syndrome.[72] Smoking restricts the blood supply to the developing fetus and thus limits oxygen and nutrition delivery and waste removal. Tobacco use also appears to be a significant factor in the development of cleft lip and palate.[73]

Other Teratogens A pregnant woman should avoid exposure to X-rays, toxic chemicals, heavy metals, pesticides, gases, and other hazardous compounds. She shouldn't clean cat litter boxes; cat feces can contain organisms that cause **toxoplasmosis**, a disease that can cause a baby to be stillborn or suffer mental disabilities or other birth defects.

Prenatal Testing and Screening Modern technology enables detection of fetal health defects as early as the fourteenth week of pregnancy. One common test is **ultrasonography**, or **ultrasound**, which uses high-frequency sound waves to create a *sonogram* of the fetus in the uterus—a visual image used to determine the fetus's size and position. Sonograms can also detect birth defects in the central nervous and digestive systems.

Chorionic villus sampling (CVS) involves snipping tissue from the developing fetal sac. It can be used at 10 to 12 weeks of pregnancy and is an attractive option for couples at high risk for having a baby with Down syndrome or a debilitating hereditary disease.

The **triple marker screen (TMS)** is a maternal blood test done at 16 to 18 weeks. TMS can detect susceptibility to a birth defect or genetic abnormality but is not meant to diagnose any condition. A *quad screen test* screens for an additional protein in

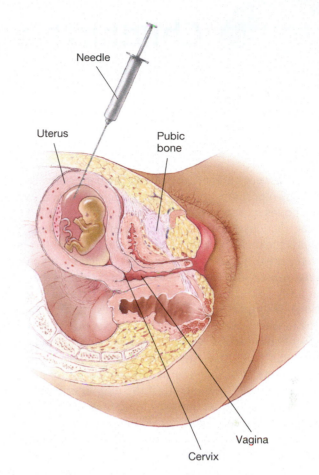

Figure 5.11 Amniocentesis
The process of amniocentesis, in which a long needle is used to withdraw a small amount of amniotic fluid for genetic analysis, can detect certain congenital problems as well as the fetus's sex.

maternal blood; it is more accurate than the triple marker screen. Even more precise is the *integrated screen*, which uses the quad screen, results from an earlier blood test, and ultrasound to screen for abnormalities.

Amniocentesis, a common test recommended for women over age 35, involves inserting a needle through the abdominal and uterine walls into the **amniotic sac** surrounding the fetus (**Figure 5.11**). The needle draws out 3 to 4 teaspoons of fluid, which is analyzed for genetic information. Amniocentesis can be performed between weeks 14 and 18.

If a test reveals a serious birth defect, the parents are advised to undergo genetic counseling. In the case of a chromosomal abnormality such as Down syndrome, the parents are usually offered the option of a therapeutic abortion. Some parents choose this option; others research the disability and decide to go ahead with the pregnancy.

Check Yourself

- **What are the key components of prenatal care?**

- **Which, if any, prenatal tests would you choose if you or your partner were pregnant? Why?**

5.14 Childbirth and the Postpartum Period

Learning Outcome

5.14 Describe the stages of labor and the postpartum period.

Childbirth

During the few weeks preceding delivery, the baby normally shifts to a head-down position, and the cervix begins to dilate (widen). The pubic bones loosen to permit expansion during birth. Strong uterine contractions signal the beginning of labor. Another common signal is the breaking of the amniotic sac (commonly referred to as "water breaking"). The birth process, which occurs in three stages (Figure 5.12), can last from several hours to more than a day.

If the baby is in physiological distress, a **cesarean section (C-section)**—a surgical procedure that involves making an incision across the mother's abdomen and through the uterus to remove the baby—may be used. A C-section may also be performed if labor is extremely difficult, maternal blood pressure falls rapidly, the placenta separates from the uterus too soon, or other problems occur. A C-section can be traumatic if the mother is not prepared for it. Risks for Casarean section are higher than for vaginal delivery and recovery typically takes considerably longer.

The rate of delivery by C-section in the United States has increased from 5 percent in the mid-1960s to nearly one-third of all births today.[74] Although this procedure is necessary in certain cases, some doctors and critics, including the Centers for Disease Control and Prevention (CDC), think that C-sections are performed too frequently in this country. Natural birth advocates suggest that hospitals, driven by profits and worried about malpractice, are too quick to intervene in the birth process. Some doctors say that the increase is due to maternal demand: Busy mothers want to schedule their deliveries.[75]

Complications of Pregnancy and Childbirth

Pregnancy carries the risk of complications that can interfere with fetal development or threaten the health of mother and child.

Preeclampsia and Eclampsia **Preeclampsia** is characterized by high blood pressure, protein in the urine, edema, and swelling in the hands and face. Symptoms may include sudden weight gain, headache, nausea or vomiting, changes in vision, racing pulse, mental confusion, and stomach or right shoulder pain. If untreated, preeclampsia can cause *eclampsia*, with outcomes including seizures, liver and kidney damage, internal bleeding, stroke, poor fetal growth, and fetal and maternal death. Preeclampsia tends to occur in the late second trimester or the third trimester. The cause is unknown. However, the incidence is higher in first-time mothers; women over 40 or under 18 years of age; women carrying multiple fetuses; and women with a history of chronic hypertension, diabetes, kidney disorder, or previous history of preeclampsia.[76]

Ectopic Pregnancy Implantation of a fertilized egg in the fallopian tube or pelvic cavity is called an **ectopic pregnancy**. If an

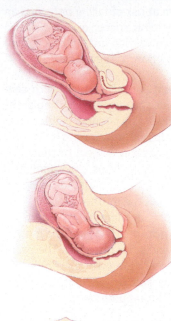

1 **Stage I: Dilation of the cervix** Contractions in the abdomen and lower back push the baby downward, putting pressure on the cervix and dilating it. The first stage of labor may last from a couple of hours to more than a day for a first birth, but it is usually much shorter during subsequent births.

2 **End of Stage I: Transition** The cervix becomes fully dilated, and the baby's head begins to move into the vagina (birth canal). Contractions usually come quickly during transition, which generally lasts 30 minutes or less.

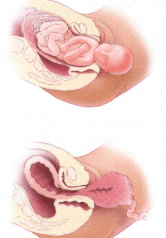

3 **Stage II: Expulsion** Once the cervix has become fully dilated, contractions become rhythmic, strong, and more intense as the uterus pushes the baby headfirst through the birth canal. The expulsion stage lasts 1 to 4 hours and concludes when the infant is finally pushed out of the mother's body.

4 **Stage III: Delivery of the placenta** In the third stage, the placenta detaches from the uterus and is expelled through the birth canal. This stage is usually completed within 30 minutes after delivery.

Figure 5.12 The Birth Process
The entire process of labor and delivery usually takes from 2 to 36 hours. Labor is generally longer for a woman's first delivery and shorter for subsequent births.

ectopic pregnancy goes undiagnosed and untreated, the fallopian tube can rupture, putting the woman at risk of hemorrhage, peritonitis (abdominal infection), and even death. Ectopic pregnancy occurs in about 2 percent of pregnancies in North America and is a leading cause of maternal mortality in the first trimester.[77]

Miscarriage Even when a woman does everything "right," not every pregnancy ends in delivery. In fact, in the United States, between 10 to 15 percent of known pregnancies end in **miscarriage** (also referred to as *spontaneous abortion*).[78] Most miscarriages occur during the first trimester. Reasons for miscarriage vary. In some cases, the fertilized egg has failed to divide correctly. In others, genetic abnormalities, maternal illness, or infections are responsible. In most cases, the cause is not known.

Stillbirth One of the most traumatic events a couple can face is a **stillbirth**, the death of a fetus *after* the twentieth week of pregnancy but before delivery. Each year in the United States, there is about 1 stillbirth in every 160 births.[79] Birth defects, placental problems, poor fetal growth, infections, and umbilical cord accidents all may contribute to stillbirth.

The Postpartum Period

The postpartum period typically lasts 6 weeks after delivery. During this period, many women experience fluctuating emotions and physical challenges.

For many new mothers, the physical stress of labor, dehydration and blood loss, and other stresses challenge their stamina. Many experience the "baby blues," characterized by sadness, anxiety, headache, sleep disturbances, and irritability. For most women, these symptoms disappear after a short while. About 1 in 7 new mothers experience **postpartum depression**, a more disabling syndrome characterized by mood swings, lack of energy, crying, guilt, and depression any time within the first year after childbirth.[80] Mothers who experience postpartum depression should seek professional treatment. Counseling is the most common type of treatment, but sometimes medication is recommended.[81]

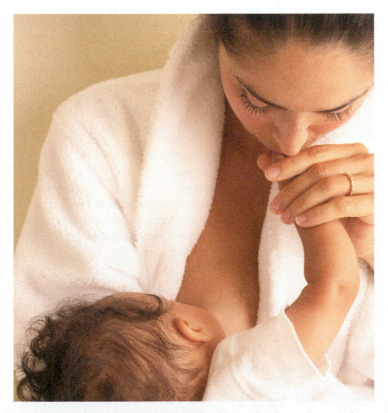

In addition to numerous health benefits, breast-feeding enhances the development of intimate bonds between mother and child.

Breastfeeding Although the new mother's milk will not begin to flow for 2 or more days after delivery, her breasts secrete a yellow fluid called *colostrum*. Because colostrum contains vital antibodies to help fight infection, the newborn should be allowed to suckle.

The American Academy of Pediatrics strongly recommends that infants be exclusively breast-fed for 6 months and should be breast-fed as a supplement until 12 months of age.[82] Scientific findings indicate there are many advantages to breastfeeding. Breast milk is perfectly matched to babies' nutritional needs as they grow. Breast-fed babies have fewer illnesses and much lower hospitalization rates because breast milk contains maternal antibodies and immunological cells that stimulate the infant's immune system. When breast-fed babies do get sick, they recover more quickly. They are also less likely to be obese later in life than are babies fed formula, and they have fewer allergies. They may even be more intelligent; a recent study found that the longer a baby was breast-fed, the higher the IQ in adulthood.[83] Breastfeeding also has the added benefit of helping mothers lose weight after birth because the production of milk burns hundreds of calories a day. Breastfeeding also causes the hormone oxytocin to be released, which makes the uterus return to its normal size faster.

Some women are unable or unwilling to breast-feed; women with certain medical conditions or taking certain medications are advised not to breast-feed. Prepared formulas can provide nourishment that allows a baby to grow and thrive. Both feeding methods can supply the physical and emotional closeness that is essential to fostering a close parent–child relationship.

Infant Mortality After birth, infant death can be caused by birth defects, low birth weight, injuries, or unknown causes. In the United States, the unexpected death of a child under 1 year of age for no apparent reason is called **sudden infant death syndrome (SIDS)**. SIDS is responsible for about 1,500 deaths a year.[84] It is the leading cause of death for children age 1 month to 1 year and most commonly occurs in babies younger than 6 months old.[85] It is not a specific disease; rather, it is ruled a cause of death after all other possibilities are ruled out. A SIDS death is sudden and silent; death occurs quickly, often during sleep, with no signs of suffering.

The exact cause of SIDS is unknown, but a few risk factors are known. For example, babies placed to sleep on their stomachs are more likely to die from SIDS than those placed on their backs, as are babies who are placed on or covered by soft bedding; however, breastfeeding and avoiding exposure to tobacco smoke are known protective factors.[86]

Check Yourself

- What are the stages of labor, from Stage I to Stage III?

- What are the advantages and drawbacks of breastfeeding?

- What steps can be taken to reduce the risk of SIDS?

5.15 Infertility

An estimated 1 in 10 American couples experiences **infertility**, usually defined as the inability to conceive after trying for a year or more.[87] Although the focus is often on women, in about one-third of cases, infertility is due to a cause involving only the male partner, and in another third of cases, infertility is due to causes involving both partners or an unknown origin.[88]

Reasons for high levels of infertility in the United States include the trend toward delaying childbirth (older women are less likely to conceive), endometriosis, pelvic inflammatory disease, and low sperm count. Environmental contaminants known as *endocrine disrupters*, such as some pesticides and emissions from burning plastics, appear to affect fertility in both men and women. Stress, anxiety, obesity, and diabetes also have reproductive implications.

Most infertility in women results from problems with ovulation. The most common is *polycystic ovary syndrome (PCOS)*. When an egg is mature, its follicle breaks open, releasing the egg to travel to the uterus for fertilization. In women with PCOS, follicles bunch together, forming cysts. The eggs mature, but the follicles don't open to release them. Researchers estimate that 5 to 10 percent of women of child-bearing age—as many as 5 million women in the United States—have PCOS.[89] Although obesity doesn't cause infertility, it is a risk factor for PCOS. It also increases the level of estrogen in the body and can cause ovulatory disorders, both of which interfere with getting pregnant.[90]

In *premature ovarian failure*, the ovaries stop functioning before natural menopause. In **endometriosis**, parts of the endometrial lining of the uterus block the fallopian tubes. In **pelvic inflammatory disease (PID)**, chlamydia, or gonorrhea, bacteria invade the fallopian tubes, forming scar tissue that blocks the movement of eggs into the uterus. About 1 in 10 women with PID becomes infertile, and if a woman has multiple episodes of PID, her chance of becoming infertile increases.[91]

Among men, the single largest fertility problem is **low sperm count**.[92] Although only one viable sperm is needed for fertilization, research has shown that all the other sperm in the ejaculate aid in the fertilization process. There are normally at least 40 million sperm per milliliter of semen. When the count drops below 20 million, fertility declines.[93]

Low sperm count may be attributable to environmental factors (such as exposure of the scrotum to intense heat or cold, radiation, certain chemicals, or altitude), being overweight, or excessively tight underwear or clothing. The mumps virus can damage the cells

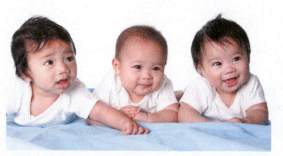

that make sperm, or varicocele (enlarged veins on a man's testicle) can heat the testicles and damage sperm.[94]

Infertility Treatments

Medical procedures can identify the cause of infertility in about 90 percent of cases.[95] Once an appropriate treatment has been instituted, the chances of becoming pregnant range from 30 to 70 percent, depending on the reason for infertility.[96]

Fertility drugs stimulate ovulation in 60 to 80 percent of women who are not ovulating; of those who ovulate, about half will conceive.[97] The drugs sometimes trigger the release of more than one egg. As many as 1 in 3 women treated with fertility drugs will become pregnant with more than one child.[98]

Other treatment options include **alternative insemination** (or *artificial insemination*) of a woman with her partner's sperm or that of a donor. In **in vitro fertilization (IVF)**, the most common type of *assisted reproductive technology (ART)*, eggs and sperm are combined in a laboratory dish to fertilize; fertilized eggs (zygotes) are then transferred to the uterus. Other ART techniques may combine an egg and sperm at different points, inside or outside the body.

In *nonsurgical embryo transfer*, a donor egg is fertilized by the man's sperm and implanted in the woman's uterus. In *embryo transfer*, an egg donor is artificially inseminated by the man's sperm, and the resulting embryo is transplanted into the birth mother's uterus. Another alternative—embryo adoption—allows infertile couples to adopt excess fertilized eggs generated by treatments such as IVF.

Surrogate Motherhood

Some infertile couples pursue surrogate motherhood. With **surrogacy**, a woman is hired to carry another person's pregnancy to term, at which point the intended parents gain custody. In *traditional surrogacy*, the gestational carrier is also the biological mother of the child. In *gestational surrogacy*, the surrogate is not the biological mother; instead an embryo is created via IVF using the couple's own (or donor) egg and sperm.[99]

Adoption

Approximately 2 percent of U.S. children are adopted.[100] In *confidential adoption*, the birth parents and adoptive parents never know each other. In *open adoption*, birth parents and adoptive parents know some things about each other and may have a defined ongoing relationship.

Summary

LO 5.1–5.9 Latex or polyurethane male condoms and female condoms, when used correctly for oral sex or intercourse, provide the most effective protection against sexually transmitted infections (STIs). Other contraceptive methods include spermicides, the diaphragm, cervical cap, Today Sponge, oral contraceptives, Xulane, NuvaRing, Depo-Provera, Nexplanon, and intrauterine devices. Emergency contraception may be used within 72 hours of unprotected intercourse or failure of another contraceptive method. Fertility awareness methods rely on altering sexual practices to avoid pregnancy, as do abstinence, outercourse, and withdrawal. All these methods of contraception are reversible; sterilization is usually permanent.

LO 5.10 Abortion is legal in the United States but is strongly opposed by many Americans. Abortion methods include suction curettage, dilation and evacuation (D&E), and medical abortions. Intact dilation and extraction (D&X) is no longer legal in the United States.

LO 5.11 Parenting is a demanding job. Prospective parents must consider their emotional and physical health and financial plans.

LO 5.12–5.13 Full-term pregnancy covers three trimesters. Prenatal care includes a complete physical exam within the first trimester, follow-up checkups throughout the pregnancy, nutrition and exercise, and avoidance of substances that could have teratogenic effects on the fetus. Prenatal tests can be used to detect birth defects during pregnancy.

LO 5.14 Childbirth occurs in three stages. Two-thirds of births in the United States are vaginal. The number of C-sections has risen since the 1960s. Possible complications of childbirth include pre-eclampsia/eclampsia, ectopic pregnancy, miscarriage, and stillbirth.

LO 5.15 Infertility in women may be caused by pelvic inflammatory disease (PID) or endometriosis. In men, it may be caused by low sperm count. Treatments may include fertility drugs, alternative insemination, in vitro fertilization (IVF), and assisted reproductive technology (ART).

Pop Quiz

Visit **Mastering Health** *to personalize your study plan with Chapter Review Quizzes and Dynamic Study Modules.*

LO 5.1 1. What lubricant could you safely use with a latex condom?
a. Mineral oil
b. Water-based lubricant
c. Body lotion
d. Petroleum jelly

LO 5.1 2. Why is the use of lambskin condoms not recommended?
a. They are less elastic than latex condoms.
b. They cannot be stored for as long as latex condoms.
c. They don't protect against transmission of STIs.
d. They're likely to cause allergic reactions.

LO 5.1 3. What is meant by the failure rate of contraceptive use?
a. The number of times a woman fails to get pregnant when she wants to
b. The number of times a woman gets pregnant when she doesn't want to
c. The number of pregnancies that occur for women using a particular method of birth control
d. The reliability of alternative methods of birth control that do not use condoms

LO 5.2 4. Which of the following is a barrier contraceptive?
a. Seasonale
b. FemCap
c. Xulane
d. Contraceptive patch

LO 5.9 5. Twenty-year-old Lani is in a monogamous relationship with her boyfriend. She has a hard time remembering to take the pill or to carry her diaphragm with her. Which form of contraception would you recommend that she try?
a. Female condom
b. Tubal ligation
c. Nexplanon
d. FemCap

LO 5.10 6. What is the most commonly used method of first-trimester abortion?
a. Suction curettage
b. Dilation and evacuation (D&E)
c. Medical abortion
d. Induction abortion

LO 5.13 7. Toxic chemicals, pesticides, X-rays, and other hazardous compounds causing birth defects are called
a. carcinogens.
b. teratogens.
c. mutants.
d. environmental assaults.

LO 5.13 8. What prenatal test involves snipping tissue from the developing fetal sac?
a. Fetoscopy
b. Ultrasound
c. Amniocentesis
d. Chorionic villus sampling

LO 5.14 9. In an ectopic pregnancy, the fertilized egg implants itself in the
a. fallopian tube.
b. uterus.
c. vagina.
d. ovaries.

LO 5.15 10. The number of American couples who experience infertility is
a. 1 in 10.
b. 1 in 24.
c. 1 in 60.
d. 1 in 100.

Answers to these questions can be found on page A-1. If you answered a question incorrectly, review the module identified by the Learning Outcome. For even more study tools, visit Mastering Health.

Think About It!

LO 5.1 **1.** How, in general, do contraceptives work? What is the difference between perfect use and typical-use failure rates? Which do you think is a better predictor of effectiveness?

LO 5.1–5.9 **2.** What are the options for birth control methods? What are their major advantages and disadvantages?

LO 5.1–5.9 **3.** List the most effective contraceptive methods. What are their drawbacks? What medical conditions would keep a person from using each one? Which methods do you think would be most effective for you? Why?

LO 5.10 **4.** What are the various methods of abortion? What are the two opposing viewpoints concerning abortion? What is *Roe v. Wade*, and what impact has it had on the abortion debate in the United States?

LO 5.11–5.13 **5.** Discuss the growth of the fetus through the three trimesters.

What medical checkups or tests should be done during each trimester?

LO 5.14 **6.** What are some of the complications that can occur during pregnancy and childbirth? What actions can we take to prevent these complications?

LO 5.15 **7.** If you and your partner are unable to have children, what alternative methods of conception would you consider? Would you consider adoption?

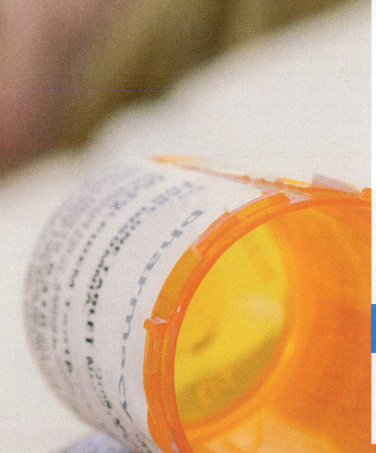

Addiction and Drug Abuse

It's easy to find high-profile cases of compulsive and destructive behavior. Stories of celebrities, athletes, and politicians struggling with addictions to drugs, sex, and alcohol are often splashed in the headlines. However, the rich and famous are not the only ones struggling with addictions. In fact, millions of people, from all ages, races, socioeconomic, education, religions, and geographic locations are waging their own, often hidden, battles with addiction.

Drug misuse and abuse are potentially devastating problems, and drug addiction wreaks havoc on individuals, families, businesses, and society. An American dies every 19 minutes from an opioid overdose.[1] Drug misuse and abuse can cause problems ranging from deterioration of relationships to mental illness and violence, major health issues, financial crises, loss of employment, and even death. It's impossible to put a dollar amount on the pain, suffering, and dysfunction that drugs cause in our everyday lives. However, the cost to our struggling mental health and health care services is staggering.

Why do people abuse drugs? Human beings appear to have a need to alter their consciousness, or mental state and to feel good when times aren't so good. Some abuse drugs out of peer pressure or trying to fit in—to be cool. Others abuse to avoid thinking about or feeling pain: to self-medicate their stresses or anxieties away. Because drugs are increasingly more available, and there are so many options, they get used to the "highs" and get hooked on the experience in much the same way that some engage in extreme sports or other high risk behaviors. Some opt to listen to music, skydive, meditate, pray, or have sex for their feel-good, "take-me away" moments. Others turn to drugs.

6.1 What Is Addiction?

Learning Outcome

6.1 List the characteristics of addiction.

Addiction is a persistent, compulsive dependence on a behavior or substance, despite ongoing negative consequences. Some researchers speak of two types of addictions: *substance addictions* (e.g. alcoholism, drug abuse, and smoking) and *process addictions* (e.g. gambling, shopping, gaming, eating, and sex). Regardless of the addictive behavior, the person experiencing it usually feels a sense of pleasure or control that is beyond the addict's power to achieve in other ways. Eventually, the addicted person needs to do the behavior to feel normal.

Physiological dependence, the adaptive state that occurs with regular addictive behavior and results in withdrawal syndrome, is one indicator of addiction. Chemicals are responsible for the most profound addictions because they cause cellular changes to which the body adapts so well that it eventually requires the chemical to function normally.

Psychological dynamics also play an important role, which explains why behaviors not related to chemicals may also be addictive. Addictive behaviors have the potential to produce a positive mood change; some behaviors, such as gambling, shopping, working, and sex, also create changes at the cellular level.[2] A person with an intense, uncontrollable urge to continue engaging in a particular activity is said to have developed a *psychological dependence(or behavioral dependence)*. Psychological and physiological dependence are intertwined and nearly impossible to separate; all forms of addiction probably reflect dysfunction of certain biochemical systems in the brain.[3]

Five symptoms are present in addictions: (1) **compulsion** characterized by **obsession**, or excessive preoccupation, with the behavior and an overwhelming need to perform it; (2) **loss of control**, or inability to reliably predict whether any occurrence of the behavior will be healthy or damaging; (3) **negative consequences**, such as physical damage, financial problems, academic failure, and family dissolution, that don't occur with healthy involvement in the behavior; (4) **denial**, the inability to perceive the behavior as self-destructive; and (5) an **inability to abstain**.[4]

Addiction evolves over time, beginning when a person repeatedly seeks the illusion of relief to avoid unpleasant feelings or situations. This pattern, known as *nurturing through avoidance*, is a maladaptive way of taking care of emotional needs. As a person becomes increasingly dependent on the addictive behavior, relationships with family, friends, and coworkers deteriorate, as do performance at work or school and the person's personal life. Eventually, addicts do not find the addictive behavior pleasurable but consider it preferable to the unhappy realities they are seeking to escape. **Figure 6.1** illustrates the cycle of psychological addiction.

The Physiology of Addiction

Virtually all intellectual, emotional, and behavioral functions occur as a result of biochemical interactions in the body. Biochemical

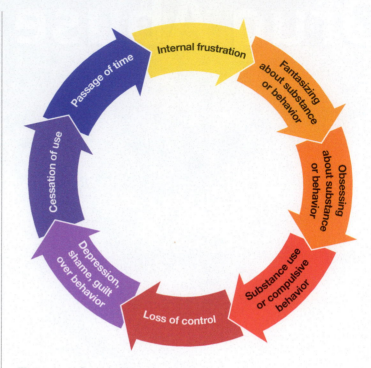

Figure 6.1 Cycle of Psychological Addiction

Source: Adapted from Recovery Connection, Cycle of Addiction, 2016, www.recoveryconnection.org.

Mastering Health & Nutrition Addiction Cycle

messengers called **neurotransmitters** exert their influence at specific receptor sites on nerve cells. Drug use and chronic stress can alter these receptor sites, leading to either production or breakdown of neurotransmitters. Some people's bodies naturally produce insufficient quantities of these neurotransmitters, predisposing them to seek out chemicals, such as alcohol, as substitutes and making them more susceptible to addiction.

Mood-altering substances and experiences produce **tolerance**—when progressively larger doses or more intense involvement are needed to obtain the desired effects. Addicts tend to seek more intense mood-altering experiences and eventually increase the amount and intensity to the point of negative effects.

An addictive substance or activity replaces an effect that the body normally provides on its own. If the experience is repeated often enough, the body adjusts by requiring the drug or experience to obtain the effect. Stopping causes a **withdrawal** syndrome. Mood-altering chemicals, for example, fill receptor sites for the body's "feel-good" neurotransmitters (endorphins), and nerve cells shut down production of these substances temporarily. When drug use stops, those receptor sites sit empty, resulting in uncomfortable feelings that remain until the body resumes normal neurotransmitter production or the person consumes more of the drug.

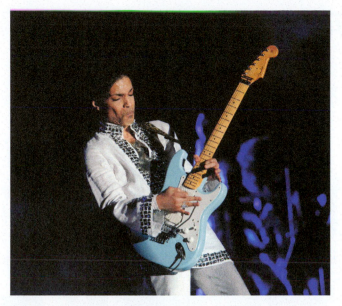

Abusing prescription drugs is no safer than abusing illicit drugs. The death of pop star Prince stemmed from an overdose of fentanyl, a narcotic prescribed to treat pain.

Withdrawal symptoms of chemical dependencies are generally the opposite of the effects of the drugs. Addicts who feel a high from cocaine will experience a "crash" (depression and lethargy) when they stop taking it. Withdrawal symptoms for addictive behaviors usually involve psychological discomfort and preoccupation with or craving for the behavior.

The Biopsychosocial Model of Addiction

The most effective treatment today is based on the **biopsychosocial model of addiction**, which proposes that addiction is caused not by a single influence but by multiple biological, psychological, social, and environmental factors operating in complex interaction.

Psychological Factors People with low self-esteem, tendencies for risk-taking behavior, or poor coping skills are more likely to develop addictive behavior. Individuals who consistently look outside themselves for solutions and explanations for life events (who have an external locus of control) are more likely to experience addiction.

Biological or Disease Influences Brain processes controlling memory, motivation, and emotional state are subjects for genetic research into risk for addiction, particularly to mood-altering substances. Studies show that drug addicts metabolize these substances differently than do others. For example, genes affecting activity of the neurotransmitters serotonin and GABA (gamma-aminobutyric acid) are likely involved in the risk for alcoholism.[5]

Research also supports a genetic influence on addiction. Identical twins, who share the same genes, are about twice as likely as fraternal twins, who share an average of 50 percent of genes, to resemble each other in terms of alcoholism. Approximately half of the risk for alcoholism is genetically determined.[6]

Environmental Influences Cultural expectations and mores help determine whether people engage in certain behaviors. Low rates of alcoholism typically exist in countries, such as Italy, where children are gradually introduced to alcohol in diluted amounts, on special occasions, and within a strong family group; intoxication is not viewed as socially acceptable, stylish, or funny.[7] Such traditions and values are less widespread in the United States, where the incidence of alcohol addiction is very high.

Societal attitudes and messages also influence addictive behavior. Media emphasis on appearance and the ideal body plays a significant role in exercise addiction. Societal changes, in turn, influence individual norms. People living in cities characterized by rapid social change or social disorganization often feel disenfranchised and disconnected, leading to increased addiction rates.[8]

Social learning theory proposes that people learn behaviors by watching role models—parents, caregivers, and significant others. Many studies show that modeling by parents and by idolized celebrities exerts a profound influence on young people.[9]

On an individual level, major life events such as marriage, divorce, change in work status, or death of a loved one may trigger addictive behaviors. One thing that makes addictive behaviors so attractive is that they reliably alleviate personal pain, at least for a while—though in the long term, they cause more pain than they relieve.

Family members whose needs for love, security, and affirmation are not consistently met; who are refused permission to express feelings or needs; and who frequently submerge their personalities to "keep the peace" are prone to addiction. Children whose parents are not consistently available (physically or emotionally); who are subjected to abuse; or who receive inconsistent or disparaging messages about their self-worth may experience addiction in adulthood.

Effect on Family and Friends

Family and friends of an addicted person often struggle with **codependence**. Codependents find it hard to set healthy boundaries and often live in the chaotic, crisis-oriented mode occurring around the addict, the result being that they actually help or support the addiction. They assume responsibility for meeting other peoples' needs to the point that they subordinate, or even cease being aware of, their own. Family and friends can also become **enablers**, knowingly or unknowingly protecting addicts from the consequences of their behavior. Both addicts and those around them must learn to see how addicts' behavior affects others and work to establish healthier relationships and boundaries.

Check Yourself

- What are the characteristics of addiction?
- How does addiction affect the family and friends of the addict?
- According to the biopsychosocial model of addiction, what types of factors combine to cause addiction?

6.2 Addictive Behaviors

6.2 Give examples of process addictions.

Process addictions are behaviors known to be addictive because they are mood altering. Traditionally, the word *addiction* was used mainly with regard to psychoactive substances. However, new knowledge suggests that, as far as the brain is concerned, a reward is a reward, whether brought on by a chemical or a behavior.[10]

Gambling Disorder

In the United States, more than 5 million people meet the criteria for having a gambling addiction; many others are directly or indirectly affected by the gambling behavior of friends or relatives.[11] Characteristic behaviors include preoccupation with gambling, unsuccessful efforts to quit, and lying to conceal the extent of one's involvement.[12]

There is strong evidence that disordered gambling has a biological component. A study of individuals with gambling disorder found the participants to have decreased blood flow to a key section of the brain's reward system. Individuals with gambling disorder, like people who abuse drugs, compensate for this deficiency in their brain's reward system by overdoing it and getting hooked.[13] Most compulsive gamblers seek excitement even more than money. Their cravings can be as intense as those of drug abusers; they show tolerance in their need to increase the amount of bets; and they experience intense highs. Up to half show withdrawal symptoms, including sleep disturbance, sweating, irritability, and craving.

It is estimated that 6 percent of college students in the United States have a serious gambling problem, which can result in psychological difficulties, debt, and failing grades.[14]

Compulsive Buying Disorder

Compulsive buying is estimated to affect 6 percent of the U.S. population, mostly women.[15] Individuals with **compulsive buying disorder** are preoccupied with shopping and spending, and they exercise little control over impulses to buy. Signs that a person

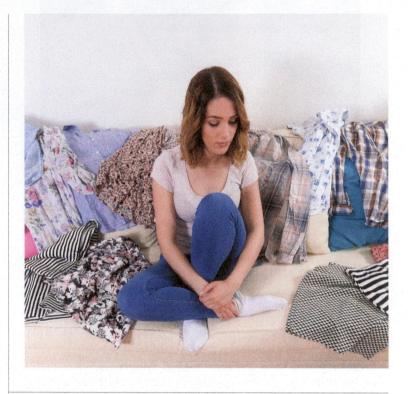

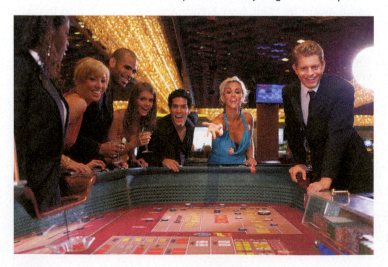

has crossed the line into compulsive buying include buying more than one of the same item, repeatedly buying much more than one needs or can afford, and buying to the point that it interferes with social activities or work and creates financial problems. Compulsive buying frequently results in depression and feelings of guilt, as well as conflict with friends and between couples.[16]

Compulsive buying disorders most often begin in the late teens and early twenties, coinciding with establishment of credit and independence from parents. It can be seasonal (shopping during the winter to alleviate seasonal anxiety and depression) and can occur when people feel depressed, lonely, or angry. Both compulsive gambling and compulsive buying frequently lead to repeated borrowing to help support the addiction.

Technology Addictions

Do you have friends who seem more concerned with checking their smart phones and social media, texting, or Web surfing than with eating, going out, or studying? These attitudes and behaviors are not unusual. An estimated 1 in 8 Internet users will likely experience **Internet addiction**.[17] Approximately 9 percent of college students report that Internet use and computer games have interfered with their academic performance.[18]

What you do online may be as important as how long

$25,000 is the average amount of debt that a compulsive shopper owes.

you spend doing it; some activities, such as gaming and cybersex, seem to be more potentially addictive than others. Technology addicts typically exhibit symptoms such as general disregard for their health, sleep deprivation, depression, neglecting family and friends, lack of physical activity, euphoria when online, uncomfortable feelings when not online, and poor grades or job performance. Addicts may be compensating for loneliness, marital or work problems, a poor social life, or financial problems. If you can't put your smartphone down, you may be *nomophobic*, the emerging name for a cell phone junkie.

Work Addiction

To understand work addiction, we must understand the concept of healthy work. Healthy work provides a sense of identity, helps develop our strengths, and is a means of satisfaction and mastery. Although work may occasionally keep them from family, friends, and personal interests, healthy workers generally maintain balance in their lives.

Conversely, **work addiction**, commonly referred to as "*workaholism*" is the compulsive or uncontrollable need to work incessantly, using work to fulfill needs of intimacy, power, and success. Work addicts usually fail to set boundaries regarding work and feel driven to work even when away from the workplace.[19]

Work addicts may feel too busy to take care of their health, and there is some evidence that work addiction may cause physical symptoms such as sleep problems and exhaustion, high blood pressure, anxiety and depression, weight gain, ulcers, and chest pain, or more chronic health conditions such as heart disease and asthmatic attacks.[20] While work addiction can bring admiration, as the addicts often excel in their professions, the negative effects on individuals and those around them may be far-reaching.[21]

Exercise Addiction

Exercise addicts use exercise compulsively to try to meet needs—for nurturance, intimacy, self-esteem, and self-competency—that an object or activity cannot truly meet. Consequently, addictive or compulsive exercise results in negative consequences similar to those of other addictions: alienation of family and friends, injuries from overdoing it, and craving for more.

Warning signs of exercise addiction include injuring and reinjuring the body through excess exercise or lack of proper rest; difficulty concentrating; feeling restless; adhering to a rigid workout plan; becoming fixated on burning calories or losing weight; canceling social plans, skipping work, or missing class to exercise; or working out beyond the point of pain.[22]

Compulsive Sexual Behavior

Sexual addiction is compulsive involvement in sexual activity. Compulsive sexual behavior may involve a normally enjoyable

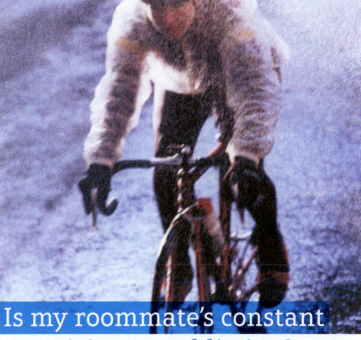

Is my roommate's constant exercising an addiction?

Obsession with a substance or behavior, even a generally positive activity such as exercise, can eventually develop into an addiction. If there are negative consequences from exercising, such as overuse injuries or withdrawal from friends and other activities, then addiction is a possibility.

sexual experience that becomes an obsession, or it may involve fantasies or activities outside the bounds of culturally, legally, or morally acceptable sexual behavior.[23] In fact, people with sexual addictions may be satisfied by masturbation, whether alone or during phone sex or while reading or watching erotica. They may participate in affairs, sex with strangers, prostitution, voyeurism, exhibitionism, rape, incest, or pedophilia. People who are addicted to sex frequently experience depression and anxiety fueled by fear of discovery. The toll that sexual addiction exacts is seen in loss of intimacy with loved ones, which frequently leads to family disintegration. Sexual addictions affect men and women of all ages, married and single people, and people of any sexual preference. Most had dysfunctional childhood families, often characterized by addiction. Many were physically, emotionally, and/or sexually abused.

Multiple Addictions

Although addicts tend to have a "favorite" drug or behavior, 55 percent of people in treatment have problems with more than one addiction.[24] For example, alcohol addiction and eating disorders are commonly paired in women, whereas individuals who are trying to break a chemical dependency frequently resort to compulsive eating. Multiple addictions complicate recovery but don't make it impossible.

Check Yourself

- What is an example of a process addiction?
- How can a positive behavior such as exercise become addictive?

6.3 Describe the six major categories of drugs and the interactions that can result from polydrug use.

Most bodily processes result from chemical reactions or changes in electrical charge. Drugs have an electrical charge and chemical structure similar to those of chemicals occurring naturally in the body and thus can affect physical functions in many ways.

How Drugs Affect the Brain

Pleasure, which scientists call *reward*, is a powerful biological force for survival. If you do something that you experience as pleasurable, the brain is wired so that you tend to do it again. Life-sustaining activities, such as eating, activate a circuit of specialized nerve cells devoted to producing and regulating pleasure. One important set of these cells, which uses a chemical neurotransmitter called *dopamine*, sits at the top of the brain stem in the *ventral tegmental area (VTA)*. Here, dopamine-containing neurons relay messages about pleasure to nerve cells in the limbic system—brain structures that regulate emotions. Still other fibers connect to a related part of the frontal region of the cerebral cortex, the area of the brain that plays a key role in memory, perception, thought, and consciousness. So this "pleasure circuit," the *mesolimbic dopamine* system, spans the survival-oriented brain stem, the emotional limbic system, and the thinking frontal cerebral cortex.

All drugs that are addicting can activate the brain's pleasure circuit. Drug addiction is a biological, pathological process that alters how the pleasure center and other parts of the brain function. Almost all **psychoactive drugs** (those that change the way the brain works) do so by affecting chemical neurotransmission—enhancing, suppressing, or interfering with it. Some drugs, such as heroin and lysergic acid diethylamide (LSD), mimic the effects of natural neurotransmitters. Others, such as phencyclidine (PCP), block receptors, preventing neuronal messages from getting through. Still others, such as cocaine, block neurons' reuptake of neurotransmitters, increasing neurotransmitter concentration in the synaptic gap between individual neurons. Finally, some drugs, such as methamphetamine, act by causing neurotransmitters to be released in greater than normal amounts.

Categories of Drugs

Scientists divide drugs into six categories. Each includes some drugs that stimulate the body, some that depress body functions, and others that produce hallucinations (sensory perceptions that are not real). Each category also includes psychoactive drugs.

- *Prescription drugs* can be obtained only with a prescription from a licensed health care practitioner. Approximately 49 percent of Americans have reported using at least one prescription medication in the past month.[25]
- *Over-the-counter (OTC) drugs* can be purchased without a prescription. They treat everything from headaches to pain, colds, stomach upsets, and athlete's foot, and they provide an important access to medicine. They create substantial savings for the health care system through decreased visits to health care providers and decreased use of prescription medications.[26] However, there is a risk of OTC drugs being used improperly or misused.[27]
- *Recreational drugs* belong to a category whose boundaries depend on how the term *recreation* is defined. Generally, recreational drugs contain chemicals that help people relax or socialize. Most of these drugs, like alcohol, tobacco, and caffeine, are legal even though they are psychoactive.
- *Herbal preparations* encompass approximately 750 substances, including herbal teas and other products of botanical (plant) origin, that are believed to have medicinal properties.
- *Illicit (illegal) drugs* are the most notorious type of drug. Although laws governing their use, possession, cultivation, manufacture, and sale differ from state to state, illicit drugs are generally recognized as harmful. All are psychoactive.
- *Commercial preparations* are the most universally used, yet least commonly recognized, chemical substances. More than 1,000 exist, including seemingly benign items such as perfumes, cosmetics, household cleansers, paints, glues, inks, dyes, and pesticides.

Routes of Drug Administration

Route of administration refers to how a drug is taken into the body. The route of administration largely determines the rapidity of a drug's effect (**Figure 6.2**). The most common route is **oral ingestion**—swallowing a tablet, capsule, or liquid. A drug taken orally may not reach the bloodstream for 30 minutes.

Drugs can also enter the body through the respiratory tract via sniffing, smoking, or **inhalation**. Drugs inhaled and absorbed by the lungs travel the most rapidly of all routes of drug administration. Another rapid form of drug administration is **injection** directly into the bloodstream (intravenously), muscles (intramuscularly), or just under the skin (subcutaneously). Intravenous injection, which involves inserting a hypodermic needle directly into a vein, is the most common method of injection for drug users because of the speed of effect (within seconds in most cases). It is also the most dangerous, due to the risk of damaging blood vessels and contracting HIV (human immunodeficiency virus) and hepatitis (a severe liver disease). Drugs can also be absorbed through the skin or tissue lining (**transdermal**)—the nicotine patch is a common example of a drug administered in this manner—or through the mucous membranes, such as those in the nose (snorting) or the vagina or anus (**suppositories**, typically

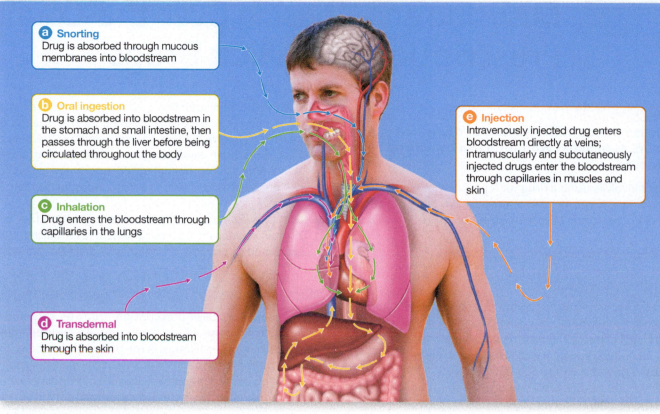

Figure 6.2 Routes of Drug Administration
Drugs are most commonly swallowed, inhaled, or injected. They can also be absorbed through the skin or mucous membranes by snorting and via suppository (not shown here).

Mastering Health & Nutrition Psychoactive Drugs Acting on the Brain

mixed with a waxy medium that melts at body temperature, releasing the drug into the bloodstream).

However a drug enters the system, it eventually finds its way to the bloodstream and is circulated throughout the body to **receptor sites** where chemicals, enzymes, and other substances interact. Psychoactive drugs can cross the blood–brain barrier to reach receptor sites in the brain, where they can affect cognition, emotion, and physiological functioning. Once a drug reaches receptor sites in the brain and other organs, it may remain active for several hours before it dissipates and is carried by the blood to the liver, where it is metabolized (broken down by enzymes). The products of enzymatic breakdown, called *metabolites*, are then excreted, primarily through the kidneys (in urine) or bowels (in feces) but also through the skin (in sweat) or lungs (in expired air).

Drug Interactions

Polydrug use—taking several drugs simultaneously—can lead to dangerous health problems. Alcohol in particular frequently has dangerous interactions with other drugs.

Synergism, also called *potentiation*, is an interaction of two or more drugs in which the effects of the individual drugs are multiplied beyond what would normally be expected if they were taken alone. You might think of synergism as 2 + 2 = 10. A synergistic reaction can be very dangerous and even deadly.

Antagonism, though usually less serious than synergism, can also produce unwanted and unpleasant effects. In an antagonistic reaction, drugs work at the same receptor site; one blocks the action of the other. The blocking drug occupies the receptor site and prevents the other drug from attaching, altering its absorption and action.

With **inhibition**, the effects of one drug are eliminated or reduced by the presence of another drug at the receptor site. **Intolerance** occurs when drugs combine in the body to produce extremely uncomfortable reactions. The drug *Antabuse* (disulfiram), used to help alcoholics give up alcohol, works by producing this type of interaction. A final type of interaction, **cross-tolerance**, occurs when a person develops a physiological tolerance to one drug and shows a similar tolerance to certain other drugs as a result.

Check Yourself

- What are the six major categories of drugs and what is unique about each?

- What is polydrug use, and what are its risks?

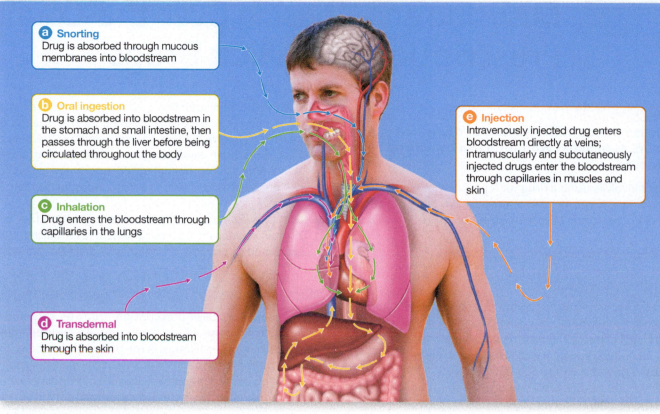

a Snorting
Drug is absorbed through mucous membranes into bloodstream

b Oral ingestion
Drug is absorbed into bloodstream in the stomach and small intestine, then passes through the liver before being circulated throughout the body

c Inhalation
Drug enters the bloodstream through capillaries in the lungs

d Transdermal
Drug is absorbed into bloodstream through the skin

e Injection
Intravenously injected drug enters bloodstream directly at veins; intramuscularly and subcutaneously injected drugs enter the bloodstream through capillaries in muscles and skin

6.4 Misusing and Abusing Over-the-Counter, Prescription, and Illicit Drugs

Learning Outcome

6.4 **Discuss trends in the misuse of drugs and factors associated with drug use by college students.**

Drug misuse involves using a drug for a purpose for which it was not intended. This is not too far removed from **drug abuse**, or excessive use of any drug. Misuse or abuse of any drug may lead to addiction.

Abuse of Over-the-Counter Drugs

Over-the-counter medications come in many different forms, including pills, liquids, nasal sprays, and topical creams. Abusing OTC medications can result in health complications and potential addiction. Teenagers, young adults, and people over 65 years of age are most vulnerable to abusing OTC drugs.

Over-the-counter drugs are abused when the drug is taken in more than the recommended dosage, combined with other drugs, or taken over a longer time than recommended. Tolerance from continued use can create unintended dependence. Teenagers and young adults sometimes abuse OTC medications in search of a cheap high—by drinking large amounts of cough medicine, for instance. Several types of OTC drugs are subject to misuse and abuse:

- **Sleep aids.** In excess, these drugs can cause sleep problems, weaken areas of the body, or induce narcolepsy (excessive, intrusive sleepiness). Continued use can lead to tolerance and dependence.
- **Cold medicines (cough syrups and tablets).** *Dextromethorphan (DXM)* is present in many OTC medications; approximately 5 percent of high school seniors report having taken drugs containing DXM to get high.[28] Large doses can cause hallucinations, loss of motor control, and "out-of-body" sensations.

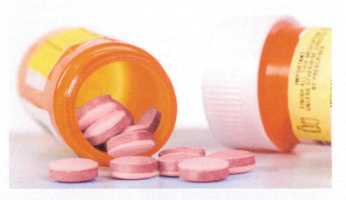

Prescription painkillers such as Percocet, Percodan, Vicodin, and OxyContin are highly addictive.

Other effects include impaired judgment, blurred vision, dizziness, paranoia, excessive sweating, slurred speech, irregular heartbeat, and numbness of fingers and toes. Abuse can lead to seizures, brain damage, and death. Some states have passed laws limiting the amount of products containing DXM a person can purchase or prohibiting sale to individuals under 18 years of age.[29]

- **Diet pills.** Some teens use diet pills to get high. Diet pills often contain a stimulant such as caffeine or a herbal ingredient that is claimed to promote weight loss such as *Hoodia gordonii*.

Nonmedical Use or Abuse of Prescription Drugs

Many people perceive prescription drugs as safe and socially acceptable. However, when these drugs are misused, they can be as dangerous as illegal drugs. In the United States today, the abuse of prescription medications is at an all-time high; only marijuana is more widely abused.[30] Approximately 6.4 million Americans age 12 and older have used prescription drugs for nonmedical reasons in the past month.[31] In 2015, 2 percent of teenagers age 12 to 17 and 5 percent of people 18 to 25 reported having abused prescription drugs in the past month.[32] The problem may be getting worse, with approximately 13 percent of twelfth-graders reporting abuse of prescription drugs by the time they graduate from high school.[33]

Abusing opioids, narcotics, and pain relievers can result in life-threatening respiratory depression (reduced breathing). Individuals who abuse depressants place themselves at risk of seizures, respiratory depression, and decreased heart rate. Stimulant abuse can cause elevated body temperature, irregular heart rate, cardiovascular system failure, and fatal seizures. Individuals who abuse prescription drugs by injecting them expose themselves to additional risks, including contracting HIV, hepatitis B and C, and other bloodborne viruses.

Prescription drugs are often easier to obtain than illegal ones. In some cases, unscrupulous pharmacists or other medical professionals steal the drugs or sell fraudulent prescriptions. Abusers visit several doctors to obtain multiple prescriptions, fake or exaggerate symptoms to get prescriptions, or call pharmacies with fraudulent prescriptions. Some teenagers and college students who have legitimate prescriptions sell or give away their medications to other students or trade them for others.

College Students and Prescription Drug Abuse Approximately 12 percent of college students reported illegally using prescription drugs in the last year.[34] The most commonly abused prescription drugs on college campuses are stimulants—drugs intended to treat attention deficit/hyperactivity disorder (ADHD) such as Ritalin or Adderall, followed by painkillers (e.g., OxyContin and Vicodin).[35] Approximately 7 percent of students report having used stimulants not prescribed to them in the past 12 months,

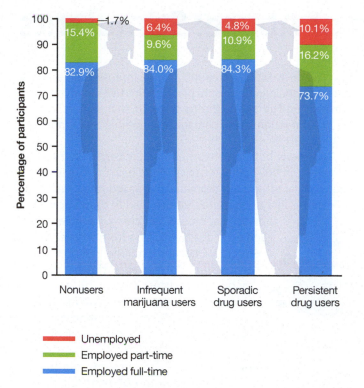

Legend:
- ■ Unemployed (red)
- ■ Employed part-time (green)
- ■ Employed full-time (blue)

Chart data (Percentage of participants):

Category	Unemployed	Employed part-time	Employed full-time
Nonusers	1.7%	15.4%	82.9%
Infrequent marijuana users	6.4%	9.6%	84.0%
Sporadic drug users	4.8%	10.9%	84.3%
Persistent drug users	10.1%	16.2%	73.7%

Figure 6.3 Employment after College Based on College Drug Use
Even periodic use of drugs increases the chances of unemployment after college.

Source: A. M. Arria, "Drug Use Patterns in Young Adulthood and Post-College Employment," Drug and Alcohol Dependence 1, no. 127 (2013): 23–30, DOI: 10.1016/j.drugalcdep.2012.06.001.

while 5 percent of students report having used painkillers that were not prescribed to them in the past 12 months.[36] Taking prescription painkillers daily for several weeks is enough time to develop an addiction.

According to a recent study, students indicate that it is easy or very easy to get prescription medications. Friends with prescriptions were the most commonly reported source.[37]

Illicit Drugs

The problem of illicit drug use touches us all. We may use illicit substances ourselves, watch someone we love struggle with drug abuse, or become the victim of a drug-related crime or accident. At the very least, we are forced to pay increasing taxes for law enforcement and drug rehabilitation. Illicit drug use spans ages, genders, ethnicities, occupations, and socio-economic groups.

Use of illicit drugs in the United States peaked between 1979 and 1986 and then declined until 1992, and it has since remained stable at around 27 million users per year.[38] Illicit drug use has been increasing in youth overall in recent years with first-time marijuana use in college students at the highest level in over three decades. One in every 5 college students will become a first-time user during the first year on campus, compared to 1 in 10 young adults who do not go to college.[39]

Illicit Drug Use on Campus

Overall, illicit drug use has seen a resurgence on college campuses. Close to 50 percent of college-aged students nationwide have tried an illicit drug at some point; the vast majority of them reported having used marijuana.[40] Of those who try marijuana and keep using, 1 in 17 college students smokes pot at least 20 times a month.[41] College administrators, faculty, and staff are concerned about the link between substance abuse and poor academic performance, depression, anxiety, suicide, vandalism, fights, serious medical problems, and death. Students who use marijuana and/or other illicit drugs are at increased risk for disruptions in college attendance.[42] A longer-term consequence of illicit drug use among college students is a significantly increased chance of unemployment after college (**Figure 6.3**).[43]

Research has identified factors in a student's life that increase the risk of substance abuse. The more factors, the greater the risk:

- **Positive expectations.** Some students take drugs such as Adderall and Ritalin believing that the drugs will improve their ability to study. Many students say they take drugs to relax or reduce stress.[44]
- **Genetics and family history.** These play a significant role in risk for addiction.
- **Substance use in high school.** Two-thirds of college students who use illicit drugs began doing so in high school.[45]
- **Social Norms.** College students often overestimate the amount of drug use on campus. Surveys conducted on college campuses found that students perceived that 85 percent of their peers had used marijuana within the last 30 days, when actually 19 percent had.[46]
- **Sorority and fraternity membership.** Being a member of a sorority or fraternity increases the likelihood of abusing alcohol and drugs.[47] A few factors that may contribute to more drinking and use of drugs in sororities and fraternities include group living, hazing or initiation rituals, lack of supervision, and social pressure.[48]
- **Stress.** For some students who are under academic and social stress, seemingly easy relief comes in the form of drugs or alcohol.

See It! Videos
What are the recent rates of overdose by heroin? Watch **New Report Shows Surge in Heroin Deaths** in the Study Area of Mastering Health.

Check Yourself

- **What are recent trends in how college students misuse and abuse drugs?**
- **What factors increase or decrease a college student's risk of substance abuse?**
- **Just because a drug is legal, does that guarantee that it's safe? Explain your answer.**

6.4

Addiction and Drug Abuse

Learning Outcome

6.5 Discuss the effects and health risks of stimulants that are commonly misused or abused.

Hundreds of drugs are subject to abuse—some are legal, such as recreational drugs and prescription medications, whereas many others are illegal and classified as "controlled substances." Some of the drugs of most concern are stimulants, marijuana, depressants, hallucinogens, inhalants, and anabolic steroids.

Stimulants

A **stimulant** is a drug that increases activity of the central nervous system. Its effects usually involve increased activity, anxiety, and agitation; users often seem jittery or nervous while high. Commonly used illegal stimulants include cocaine, amphetamines, methamphetamine, and cathinones. Legal stimulants include caffeine and nicotine.

Cocaine A white crystalline powder derived from the leaves of the South American coca shrub (not related to cocoa plants), cocaine ("coke") has been described as one of the most powerful naturally occurring stimulants.

Cocaine can be taken in several ways, including snorting, smoking, and injecting. The powdered form is snorted through the nose, which can damage mucous membranes and cause sinusitis. It can destroy the user's sense of smell, and occasionally it even eats a hole through the septum. When snorted, the drug enters the bloodstream through the lungs in less than 1 minute and reaches the brain in less than 3 minutes. It binds at receptor sites in the central nervous system, producing an intense high that usually disappears quickly, leaving a powerful craving for more.

Cocaine alkaloid, or *freebase*, is obtained by removing the hydrochloride salt from cocaine powder. *Freebasing* refers to smoking freebase by placing it at the end of a pipe and holding a flame near it to produce a vapor, which is then inhaled. *Crack* is identical pharmacologically to freebase, but the hydrochloride salt is still present and is processed with baking soda and water. It is a cheap, widely available drug that is smokable and very potent. Crack is commonly smoked in the same manner as freebase. Because crack is such a pure drug, it takes little time to achieve the desired high, and a crack user can become addicted quickly.

Some cocaine users inject the drug intravenously, which introduces large amounts

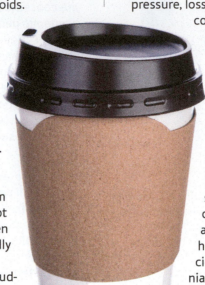

Caffeine is a legal stimulant.

into the body rapidly, creating a brief, intense high and a subsequent crash. Injecting users place themselves at risk not only for contracting HIV and hepatitis through shared needles, but also for skin infections, vein damage, inflamed arteries, and infection of the heart lining.

Cocaine is both an anesthetic and a central nervous system stimulant. In tiny doses, it can slow the heart rate. In larger doses, the physical effects are dramatic: increased heart rate and blood pressure, loss of appetite that can lead to dramatic weight loss, convulsions, muscle twitching, irregular heartbeat, and even death resulting from an overdose. Other effects of cocaine include temporary relief of depression, decreased fatigue, talkativeness, increased alertness, and heightened self-confidence. However, as the dose increases, users become irritable and apprehensive, and their behavior may turn paranoid or violent.

Amphetamines The **amphetamines** include a large and varied group of synthetic agents that stimulate the central nervous system. Small doses of amphetamines improve alertness, lessen fatigue, and generally elevate mood. With repeated use, however, physical and psychological dependencies develop. Sleep patterns are affected (insomnia); heart rate, breathing rate, and blood pressure increase; and restlessness, anxiety, appetite suppression, and vision problems are common. High doses over long periods of time can produce hallucinations, delusions, and disorganized behavior.

Certain types of amphetamines or amphetamine-like drugs are used for medicinal purposes. As was discussed earlier, drugs prescribed to treat ADHD are stimulants and are increasingly abused on campus.

Methamphetamine An increasingly common form of amphetamine, methamphetamine (commonly called "meth") is a potent,

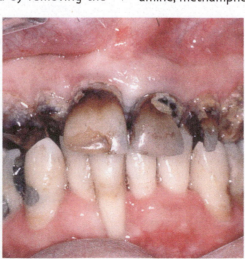

long-acting, addictive drug that strongly activates the brain's reward center by producing a sense of euphoria. Over 897,000 Americans are regular users. People over the age of 18 make up the largest proportion of people using methamphetamine.[49] In 2015, about 1 percent of high school seniors reported having used methamphetamine in their lifetime.[50] The rate of methamphetamine use may be increasing because the drug is relatively easy to make.

Methamphetamine users often damage their teeth beyond repair because of the toxic chemicals in the substance. This condition is commonly referred to as "meth mouth."

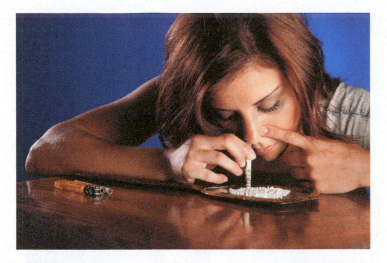

Although cocaine use has declined from its peak in the 1980s, it continues to be a commonly abused illicit drug.

Recipes often include common OTC ingredients such as ephedrine and pseudoephedrine.

In the short term, methamphetamine produces increased physical activity, alertness, euphoria, rapid breathing, increased body temperature, insomnia, tremors, anxiety, confusion, and decreased appetite; the drug's effects quickly wear off, leaving the user seeking more.

Methamphetamine can be snorted, smoked, injected, or orally ingested. When snorted, the effects can be felt in 3 to 5 minutes; if orally ingested, effects occur within 15 to 20 minutes. The pleasurable effects of methamphetamine are typically an intense rush lasting only a few minutes when snorted; in contrast, smoking the drug can produce a high lasting more than 8 hours. Users often experience tolerance after the first use, making methamphetamine a highly addictive drug.

Methamphetamine increases the release and blocks the reuptake of the neurotransmitter dopamine, leading to high levels of the chemical in the brain. This action occurs rapidly and produces the intense euphoria, or "rush," that many users feel. Over time, methamphetamine destroys dopamine receptors, making it impossible to feel pleasure. Because of the destruction of dopamine receptors, people who abuse methamphetamine (or cocaine) are at increased risk for developing Parkinson's disease later in life.[51]

Other long-term effects of methamphetamine can include severe weight loss, cardiovascular damage, increased risk of heart attack and stroke, hallucinations, extensive tooth decay and tooth loss, violence, paranoia, psychotic behavior, and even death. Recent studies of chronic methamphetamine abusers have revealed severe structural and functional changes in areas of the brain associated with emotion and memory, which may account for the emotional and cognitive problems observed in chronic methamphetamine abusers. Some of these changes persist after the methamphetamine abuse has stopped. Other changes reverse after sustained periods of abstinence from methamphetamine, typically longer than a year, but problems often remain.[52]

Cathinones (Bath Salts) "**Bath salts**" are synthetic (human-made) cathinones—drugs chemically related to the stimulant cathinone, occurring naturally in the *khat plant*.[53] The designer drug is synthetic powder sold legally online and in corner stores and truck stops. These packages contain various amphetamine or cocaine-like substances, such as *methylene-dioxypyrovalerone (MPDV)*, which act much like cocaine does but are at least ten times stronger.[54] The powder can be smoked, snorted, injected, and wrapped in pieces of paper and ingested or "bombed."

Cathinones can have significant effects on the cardiovascular system, resulting in rapid heart rate, increased blood pressure, and chest pain. Psychiatric effects at higher doses consist of anxiety, agitation, hallucinations, paranoia, and erratic behavior. Depression and suicide have also been reported.[55]

Caffeine Unlike the drugs previously discussed, **caffeine** is a legal stimulant. More than 85 percent of Americans drink at least one caffeinated beverage per day,[56] such as coffee, tea, soft drinks, chocolate, and energy drinks. Caffeine may be commonplace, but excessive consumption is associated with addiction and certain health problems.

Caffeine is derived from the chemical family called *xanthines*, which are found in plants. The xanthines are mild central nervous system stimulants that enhance mental alertness and reduce feelings of fatigue. Other stimulant effects include increased heart muscle contractions, oxygen consumption, metabolism, and urinary output. A person feels these effects within 15 to 45 minutes of ingesting a caffeinated product. It takes 4 to 6 hours for the body to metabolize half of the caffeine ingested, so, depending on the amount of caffeine taken in, it may continue to exert effects for a day or longer.

As the effects of caffeine wear off, frequent users may feel let down—mentally or physically depressed, exhausted, and weak. To counteract this, they commonly choose to drink another cup of coffee. Habitually engaging in this practice leads to tolerance and psychological dependence. Symptoms of excessive caffeine consumption include chronic insomnia, jitters, irritability, nervousness, anxiety, and involuntary muscle twitches. Withdrawing from caffeine may compound the effects and produce headaches, fatigue, and nausea. Because caffeine meets the requirements for addiction—tolerance, psychological dependence, and withdrawal symptoms—it can be classified as addictive.

Heavy caffeine use has been suspected of being linked to several serious health problems such as high blood pressure, arrhythmias, increased risk of heart attacks among young adults, and increased anxiety and depression.[57] However, no strong evidence exists that moderate caffeine use (less than 300 mg, or approximately 3 cups or less of regular coffee, a day) produces harmful effects in healthy, nonpregnant people. For most people, caffeine poses few health risks and may actually have some benefits, such as increased memory, improved reaction time, reducing chronic inflammation, and possibly preventing skin cancer.[58]

Check Yourself

- What is a stimulant?

- What are the effects and health risks of commonly abused stimulants?

- Compare caffeine to illicit stimulants.

6.6 Common Drugs of Abuse: Marijuana

Although archaeological evidence indicates that **marijuana** ("grass," "weed," "pot") was used as long as 6,000 years ago, the drug did not become popular in the United States until the 1960s. Today, marijuana is the most commonly used illicit drug in the country. Some 33 million Americans have reported using marijuana in the past year, and more than 22 million have reported using marijuana within the past month.[59] Marijuana use is on the rise on college campuses, following the trend of increased use in the general population.[60]

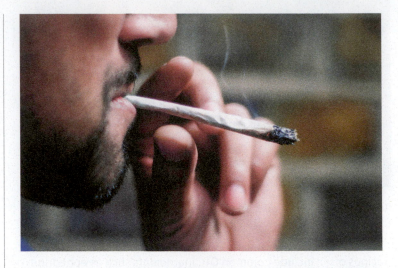

Methods of Use and Physical Effects

Marijuana is derived from either the *Cannabis sativa* or *Cannabis indica* (hemp) plant. Most of the time, marijuana is smoked, although it can also be ingested, as in brownies baked with marijuana in them. When marijuana is smoked, it is usually rolled into cigarettes (joints) or placed in a pipe or water pipe (bong).

Tetrahydrocannabinol (THC) is the psychoactive substance in marijuana and the key to determining how powerful a high it will produce. More potent forms of the drug can contain up to 27 percent THC, but most forms average 15 percent.[61] *Hashish*, a potent cannabis preparation derived mainly from the plant's thick, sticky resin, contains high THC concentrations. Hash oil, a substance produced by percolating a solvent such as ether through dried marijuana to extract the THC, is a tar-like liquid that may contain up to 300 mg of THC in a dose. Smoking THC-rich resin extracts, called *dabbing*, is becoming much more common among marijuana users. These extracts contain high levels of THC and have resulted in people ending up in the emergency room. Another danger is the extraction process, which involves butane lighter fluid; a number of people have suffered burns and explosions or fires in their homes.[62]

The effects of smoking marijuana are generally felt within 10 to 30 minutes and usually wear off within 3 hours. The most noticeable visible effect of THC is dilation of the eyes' blood vessels, which gives the smoker bloodshot eyes. Marijuana smokers also exhibit coughing; dry mouth and throat; increased thirst and appetite; lowered blood pressure; and mild muscular weakness, primarily exhibited in drooping eyelids. Users can also experience severe anxiety, panic, paranoia, and psychosis and may have intensified reactions to various stimuli; for example, colors, sounds, and the speed at which things move may seem altered. High doses of hashish may produce vivid visual hallucinations.

Marijuana and Driving

Marijuana use presents clear hazards for drivers who are under its influence and other people who are on the road with them. The drug's effects substantially reduce a driver's ability to react and make quick decisions. Perceptual and other performance deficits may persist for some time after the high subsides. Users who attempt to drive, fly, or operate heavy machinery often fail to recognize their impairment. In the state of Washington, where recreational use of marijuana is legal, 1 in 6 drivers involved in fatal car crashes had recently used marijuana.[63] Recent research indicates you are two and a half times more likely to be involved in a motor vehicle accident if you drive under the influence of marijuana.[64] Combining even a low dose of marijuana with alcohol enhances the impairing effects of both drugs.

Effects of Chronic Marijuana Use

Smoke from marijuana has been shown to contain many of the same toxins, irritants, and carcinogens as tobacco smoke.[65] Because marijuana smokers typically inhale more deeply and hold the smoke in their lungs longer than do tobacco smokers, the lungs are exposed to more tar per breath. Likewise, effects from irritation similar to those experienced by tobacco smokers can occur.[66] Lung conditions such as chronic bronchitis, emphysema, and other lung disorders are also associated with smoking marijuana.

Some marijuana users believe that "vaping" marijuana poses fewer health risks than smoking. However, studies report a very minimal difference for lungs from vaping instead of smoking.[67]

Inhaling marijuana smoke introduces carbon monoxide into the bloodstream. Because the blood has a greater affinity for carbon monoxide than it does for oxygen, its oxygen-carrying capacity is diminished; the heart must work harder to pump oxygen to oxygen-starved tissues. Furthermore, the tar from cannabis contains higher levels of carcinogens than does tobacco smoke.

Frequent and/or long-term marijuana use may significantly increase a man's risk of developing testicular cancer. The risk is particularly elevated (about twice that of those who never smoked marijuana) for those who use marijuana at least weekly or who have long-term exposure to the substance beginning in adolescence.[68]

The link between marijuana and common mental health disorders is somewhat conflicting. A recent study found that using marijuana as an adult is not associated with mood and anxiety disorders, including depression and bipolar disorder, challenging some previous research.[69] However, use of marijuana is associated with a higher likelihood of drug dependence.[70]

The American Academy of Pediatrics has stated that marijuana is harmful to adolescent health and development.[71] For adolescents, marijuana use can disrupt concentration and memory. It can also cause problems with learning, and it is linked to lower rates of high school and college completion.[72] It can also affect motor control, coordination, and judgment, which increase the risk of unintentional deaths and injuries.[73]

Other risks associated with marijuana use include suppression of the immune system, blood pressure changes, impaired memory function, and disrupted sleep. Recent studies suggest that pregnant women who smoke marijuana may have children who have subtle brain changes that can cause difficulties with problem-solving skills, memory, and attention.[74]

Legalization of Marijuana and Medicinal Uses

Although classified as a dangerous drug by the U.S. government, marijuana has been legalized for medicinal uses in 28 states and the District of Columbia and is legal for recreational use in eight states. Marijuana's legal status for medicinal purposes continues to be hotly debated. Following are some arguments for legalization:[75]

- There are medical benefits. Marijuana helps to control such side effects as the severe nausea and vomiting produced by chemotherapy, the chemical treatment for cancer. Marijuana improves appetite and forestalls the loss of lean muscle mass associated with AIDS-wasting syndrome. Marijuana reduces the muscle pain and spasticity caused by diseases such as multiple sclerosis and is an alternative to highly addictive prescription pain killers.
- Legalizing marijuana and taxing its sale could bring in millions of dollars in revenue for the government and create thousands of jobs in production, sales, and distribution.
- Legal government and U.S. Food and Drug Administration (FDA) oversight would allow for standardization of marijuana

cultivation and production and could promote more responsible cultivation methods.

- Legalizing marijuana would result in more effective law enforcement and criminal justice, since police officers would have more time and money to pursue criminals for other, more serious crimes.
- Having legal outlets for drugs such as marijuana could reduce illegal drug trafficking from offshore criminal elements and reduce the risk of harmful drug additives.

Arguments against legalization include the following:[76]

- Some individuals believe that using marijuana is morally wrong.
- Research indicates that marijuana use affects young users the most in the long term.
- Research has found that people who used marijuana heavily as teenagers lose an average of 8 IQ points that are not recovered with quitting or aging.
- Marijuana use can cause or worsen respiratory symptoms or conditions such as bronchitis, alter mood and judgment, damage the immune system, and impair short-term memory and motor coordination. These side effects make it inappropriate for FDA approval.
- Marijuana is known to be addictive; approximately 9 percent of people who experiment with marijuana become addicted.
- Legalization could make marijuana more available to children and teenagers.

Synthetic Marijuana (Spice or K2)

The term *synthetic marijuana* is used to describe a diverse family of herbal blends marketed under many names, including K2, spice, fake marijuana, Yucatan Fire, Skunk, and Moon Rocks. These products contain dried, shredded plant material and one or more synthetic cannabinoids, with results that mimic those of marijuana intoxication but with longer duration and poor detection on urine drug screens. K2 is sold legally as herbal blend incense. However, spice is smoked to gain effects similar to other forms of cannabis.[77]

K2 is used by nearly 1 in 7 college students.[78] Students who reported using K2 were more likely to have smoked cigarettes, marijuana, and hookahs.[79] K2 is also gaining more attention among high school seniors, with reports that 1 in every 9 high school seniors are using this drug.[80]

People who smoke K2 may experience several adverse health effects such as hallucinations, severe agitation, extremely elevated heart rate and blood pressure, coma, suicide attempts, and drug dependence, which is not common among cannabis users.[81] Emergency departments are also reporting a significant increase in the numbers of people being treated for K2 use.[82]

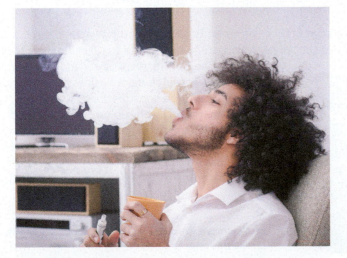

One common way of smoking marijuana is vaping.

Check Yourself

- **What are the effects and health risks of marijuana?**

- **How is marijuana used for medicinal purposes?**

- **What are the differences between marijuana and synthetic marijuana?**

Common Drugs of Abuse: Depressants and Narcotics

Learning Outcome

6.7 Discuss the effects and health risks of depressants and narcotics that are commonly misused or abused.

Whereas central nervous system stimulants increase muscular and nervous system activity, **depressants** have the opposite effect. These drugs slow down neuromuscular activity and cause sleepiness or calmness. If the dose is high enough, brain function can stop, causing death. Alcohol is the most widely used central nervous system depressant. Others include opioids, benzodiazepines, and barbiturates.

Benzodiazepines and Barbiturates

A *sedative* drug promotes mental calmness and reduces anxiety, whereas a *hypnotic* drug promotes sleep or drowsiness. The most common sedative-hypnotic drugs are **benzodiazepines**, more commonly known as *tranquilizers*.[83] These include prescription drugs such as Valium, Ativan, and Xanax. Benzodiazepines are most commonly prescribed for tension, muscular strain, sleep problems, anxiety, panic attacks, and alcohol withdrawal. **Barbiturates** are sedative-hypnotic drugs that include Amytal and Seconal. Today, benzodiazepines have largely replaced barbiturates, which were used medically in the past for relieving tension and inducing relaxation and sleep.

Sedative-hypnotics have a synergistic effect when combined with alcohol. Taken together, these drugs can lead to respiratory failure and death. All sedative or hypnotic drugs can produce physical and psychological dependence in several weeks. A complication specific to sedatives is cross-tolerance, which occurs when users develop tolerance for one sedative or become dependent on it and develop tolerance for others as well. Withdrawal from sedative or hypnotic drugs may have effects ranging from mild discomfort to severe symptoms, depending on the degree of dependence.[84]

Rohypnol One benzodiazepine of concern is Rohypnol, a potent tranquilizer that is similar to Valium but many times stronger. The drug produces a sedative effect, amnesia, muscle relaxation, and slowed psychomotor responses. The most publicized "date rape" drug, Rohypnol has gained notoriety as a growing problem on college campuses. The drug has been added to punch and other drinks at parties, where it is reportedly given to women in hopes of lowering their inhibitions and facilitating potential sexual conquests.

GHB

Gamma-hydroxybutyrate (GHB) is a central nervous system depressant known to have euphoric, sedative, and anabolic (bodybuilding) effects. It was originally sold over the counter to bodybuilders to help reduce body fat and build muscle. The FDA banned OTC sales of GHB in 1992, and it is now a Schedule I controlled substance.[85] GHB is an odorless, tasteless fluid that can be made easily at home or in a chemistry lab. Like Rohypnol, GHB has been slipped into drinks without being detected, resulting in loss of memory, unconsciousness, amnesia, and even death. Other dangerous side effects include nausea, vomiting, seizures, hallucinations, coma, and respiratory distress.

Opioids (Narcotics)

Opioids cause drowsiness, relieve pain, and produce euphoria. Also called *narcotics*, opioids are derived from the parent drug **opium**, a dark, resinous substance made from the milky juice of the opium poppy seedpod. All opioids are highly addictive. Opium and heroin are both illegal in the United States, but some opioids are available by prescription for medical purposes: Morphine is sometimes prescribed for severe pain, and codeine is found in prescription cough syrups and other painkillers.

Several prescription drugs, including Vicodin, Percodan, OxyContin, Demerol, and Dilaudid, contain synthetic opioids. These prescription painkillers are highly addictive. OxyContin, in particular, can be highly addictive with long-term use and is a dangerous narcotic when abused. The "rush" is similar to that of heroin. In fact, it's common for people who are addicted to OxyContin to turn to heroin when they can't afford to buy OxyContin; unfortunately, pain medications such as OxyContin are believed to be a major contributor to the soaring heroin epidemic in the United States. Chronic use can also result in increasing tolerance, as more of the drug is needed to achieve the desired effect.

Physical Effects of Opioids Opioids are powerful depressants of the central nervous system. In addition to relieving pain, these drugs lower heart rate, respiration, and blood pressure. Side effects include drowsiness, mental confusion, nausea, and constipation.[86]

The human body's physiology could be said to make us particularly susceptible to opioid addiction. Opioid-like hormones called **endorphins** are manufactured in the body and have multiple receptor sites, particularly in the central

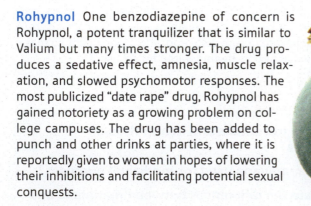

Opium is extracted from opium poppy seedpods like this one.

Why is it so hard to quit using heroin?

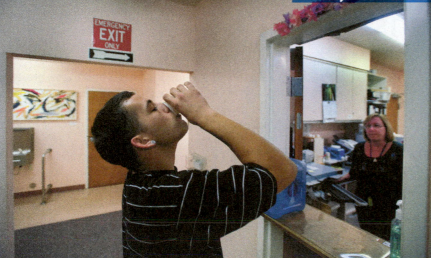

Heroin's effect on the body is similar to the painless well-being created by endorphins. Stopping heroin use causes withdrawal symptoms that are very difficult to withstand or tolerate, which keeps many addicts from attempting to quit. Methadone is a synthetic narcotic that blocks the effects of withdrawal. Although it is still a narcotic and must be administered under the supervision of clinic or pharmacy staff, methadone allows many heroin addicts to lead somewhat normal lives.

nervous system. When endorphins attach themselves at these sites, they create feelings of painless well-being; medical researchers refer to them as "the body's own opioids." When endorphin levels are high, people feel euphoric. The same euphoria occurs when opioids or related chemicals are active at the endorphin receptor sites. Of all the opioids, heroin has the greatest notoriety as an addictive drug. The following section discusses the progression of heroin addiction; addiction to any opioid follows a similar path.

Heroin Use *Heroin* is a white powder derived from morphine. *Black tar heroin* is a sticky, dark brown, foul-smelling form of heroin that is relatively pure and inexpensive. Once considered a cure for morphine dependence, heroin was later discovered to be even more addictive and potent than morphine. Today, heroin has no medical use.

Heroin is a depressant that produces drowsiness and a dreamy, mentally slow feeling. It can cause drastic mood swings, with euphoric highs followed by depressive lows. Heroin slows respiration and urinary output and constricts the pupils of the eyes. Symptoms of tolerance and withdrawal can appear within 3 weeks of first use.[87]

In 2015, 591,000 Americans reported having used heroin in the past year, a considerable increase since 2002.[88] This trend appears to be driven largely by 18- to 25-year-olds, among whom there have been the largest increases. Young and older adults hooked on painkillers are finding that heroin is cheaper and easier to obtain than prescription opioids.[89]

While heroin is usually injected intravenously ("mainlined"), the contemporary version of heroin is so potent that users can get high by snorting or smoking the drug. This has attracted a more affluent group of users who may not want to inject, for reasons such as the increased risk of contracting diseases such as HIV.

Many users describe the "rush" they feel when injecting themselves as intensely pleasurable; others report unpredictable and unpleasant side effects. The temporary nature of the rush contributes to the drug's high potential for addiction—many addicts shoot

10.3 million people reported driving under the influence of illicit drugs in the past year.

up four or five times a day. Mainlining can cause veins to scar and eventually collapse. Once a vein has collapsed, it can no longer be used to introduce heroin into the bloodstream. Addicts become expert at locating new veins to use in the feet, in the legs, in the temples, under the tongue, or in the groin.

Heroin addicts experience a distinct pattern of withdrawal. Symptoms of withdrawal include intense desire for the drug, sleep disturbance, dilated pupils, loss of appetite, irritability, goose bumps, and muscle tremors. The most difficult time in the withdrawal process occurs 24 to 72 hours after last use. All of the preceding symptoms continue, along with nausea, abdominal cramps, restlessness, insomnia, vomiting, diarrhea, extreme anxiety, hot and cold flashes, elevated blood pressure, and rapid heartbeat and respiration. Once the peak of withdrawal has passed, all these symptoms begin to subside.[90]

Check Yourself

- **What is a depressant?**

- **What are the effects and health risks of commonly abused depressants?**

- **Why has use of heroin increased so dramatically in recent years?**

Common Drugs of Abuse: Hallucinogens

Hallucinogens, or *psychedelics*, are substances capable of creating auditory or visual hallucinations and unusual changes in mood, thoughts, and feelings. Major receptor sites for hallucinogens are in the reticular formation (located in the brainstem at the upper end of the spinal cord), which is responsible for interpreting outside stimuli before allowing these signals to travel to other parts of the brain. When a hallucinogen is present at a reticular formation site, messages become scrambled. The user may see wavy walls instead of straight ones or, in a mixing of sensory messages known as *synesthesia*, may "smell" colors and "hear" tastes. Users may also become less inhibited or recall events long buried in the subconscious mind.

LSD

First synthesized in the late 1930s, *lysergic acid diethylamide (LSD)* received media attention in the 1960s when young people used it to "turn on and tune out." In 1970, federal authorities placed LSD on the list of controlled substances (Schedule I).

It is estimated that 9.5 percent of Americans aged 12 or older have used LSD at least once in their lifetime.[91] A national survey of college students showed that fewer than 4.5 percent had used the drug in their lives.[92]

The most popular form is blotter acid—small squares of paper impregnated with LSD that are swallowed or chewed. LSD also comes in gelatin squares called *windowpane* and tiny tablets called *microdots*.

One of the most powerful drugs known to science, LSD can produce strong effects in doses as low as 20 micrograms (μg). (A postage stamp weighs 60,000 μg.) The potency of a typical dose currently ranges from 20 to 80 μg, compared to doses of 150 to 300 μg that were commonly used in the 1960s.

Depending on the quantity users have eaten, LSD usually takes 20 to 60 minutes to take effect and can last 6 to 8 hours. Psychological effects of LSD vary. Euphoria is common, but dysphoria (a sense of evil and foreboding) may also be experienced. LSD also causes distortions of perception and auditory or visual hallucinations. Thoughts may be interposed so the user experiences several thoughts simultaneously. Users become introspective, and suppressed memories may surface. Other possible effects include decreased aggressiveness and enhanced sensory experiences.[93]

Physical effects of LSD include increased heart rate, elevated blood pressure, muscle twitches, perspiration, chills, headaches, and mild nausea. Because the drug also stimulates uterine muscle contractions, it can lead to premature labor and miscarriage in pregnant women. Research into long-term effects has been inconclusive.

Although there is no evidence that LSD is addictive, it does produce tolerance, so users may need to take more of the drug to get the same effect. This is a dangerous practice, as the drug is unpredictable.[94]

Ecstasy

Ecstasy is the most common name for the drug *methylene-dioxymethamphetamine (MDMA)*, a synthetic compound with stimulant and mildly hallucinogenic effects. It is one of the most well-known **club drugs** or "designer drugs," synthetic analogs of illicit drugs that are popular at nightclubs and all-night parties. Ecstasy creates feelings of extreme euphoria, increased willingness to communicate, feelings of warmth and empathy, and heightened appreciation for music. Like other hallucinogenics, Ecstasy can enhance sensory experience and distort perceptions, but it does not create visual hallucinations. Effects begin within 20 to 90 minutes and can last for 3 to 5 hours.[95]

Some of the risks associated with Ecstasy use are similar to those of other stimulants. Because of the nature of the drug, Ecstasy users are at greater risk of inappropriate or unintended emotional bonding. Physical consequences may include jaw clenching, short-term memory loss or confusion, increased body temperature as a result of dehydration and heat stroke, and increased heart rate and blood pressure. Combined with alcohol, Ecstasy can be extremely dangerous and sometimes fatal. As the effects begin to wear off, the user can experience mild depression, fatigue, and a hangover that can last from days to weeks. Chronic use appears to damage the brain's ability to think and to regulate emotion, memory, sleep, and pain. Some studies indicate that the drug may cause long-lasting neurotoxic effects by damaging brain cells that produce serotonin.[96]

MDMA in powder or crystal form—called "Molly"—has become a popular festival drug. Unlike Ecstasy, which tends to be laced with ingredients such as caffeine or methamphetamine, Molly is considered pure MDMA. However, many powders sold as Molly contain zero actual MDMA. Typical side effects include grinding ones teeth, becoming dehydrated, feeling anxious, having trouble sleeping, fever, losing one's

Psilocybe mushrooms produce hallucinogenic effects when ingested.

Just how risky are club drugs?

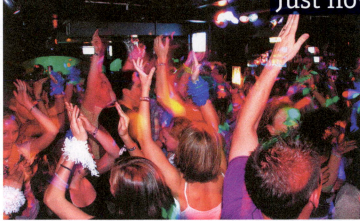

So-called club drugs are a varied group of synthetic drugs, including Ecstasy, GHB, ketamine, Rohypnol, and methamphetamine, that are often abused by teens and young adults at nightclubs, bars, or all-night dances. The sources and chemicals used to make these drugs vary, so dosages are unpredictable, and the drugs may not be "pure." Although users may think them relatively harmless, research has shown that club drugs can produce hallucinations, paranoia, amnesia, dangerous increases in heart rate and blood pressure, coma, and, in some cases, death. Some club drugs work on the same brain mechanisms as alcohol and can be particularly dangerous when used in combination with alcohol. In addition, some club drugs can be easily slipped into unsuspecting partygoers' drinks, facilitating sexual assault and other crimes.

appetite, uncontrollable seizures, elevated blood pressure, high body temperature, and depression.[97]

Mescaline

Mescaline is both a powerful hallucinogen and a central nervous system stimulant. Products sold on the street as mescaline are likely to be synthetic relatives of the true drug.

Mescaline comes from the "buttons" of the peyote cactus. Users typically swallow 10 to 12 buttons. These taste bitter and generally induce immediate nausea or vomiting. Users who are able to keep the drug down feel its effects within 30 to 90 minutes. Effects may persist for up to 12 hours.[98]

Psilocybin

Psilocybin and *psilocin* are the active chemicals in a group of mushrooms sometimes called "magic mushrooms." Psilocybe mushrooms, which grow throughout the world, can be cultivated from spores or harvested wild. When consumed, they can cause hallucinations. Because many mushrooms resemble the psilocybe variety, people who harvest wild mushrooms for any purpose should be certain of what they are doing. Mushroom varieties can be easily misidentified, and mistakes can be fatal. Psilocybin is similar to LSD in its physical effects, which generally wear off in 4 to 6 hours.[99]

PCP

Phencyclidine (PCP) was originally developed as a dissociative anesthetic; patients could keep their eyes open, apparently remain conscious, and feel no pain during a medical procedure. Afterward, they would experience amnesia for the time that the drug was in their system. The unpredictability and drastic effects (postoperative delirium, confusion, and agitation) caused it to be withdrawn from the legal market.[100]

On the illegal market, PCP is a white, crystalline powder that users often sprinkle onto marijuana cigarettes. It is dangerous and unpredictable regardless of method of administration. Effects depend on dosage. A small dose can produce effects similar to those of strong central nervous system depressants: slurred speech, impaired coordination, reduced sensitivity to pain, and

reduced heart and respiratory rate. Large doses can cause fever, salivation, nausea, vomiting, and total loss of sensitivity to pain. PCP can also cause a rise in blood pressure, seizures, violent outbursts, coma and possibly death.[101]

Psychologically, PCP may produce either euphoria or dysphoria. It is also known to produce hallucinations, delusions, and overall delirium. Long-term effects of PCP use are unknown.

Ketamine

The liquid form of *ketamine* ("Special K") is used as an anesthetic in hospital and veterinary clinics. After stealing it from hospitals or medical suppliers, dealers typically dry the liquid (usually by cooking it) and grind the residue into powder. Special K inhibits the relay of sensory input, triggering hallucinations as the brain fills the resulting void with visions, memories, and sensory distortions. Effects are similar to those of PCP—confusion, agitation, aggression, and lack of coordination—and less predictable. The aftereffects are less severe than those of Ecstasy, so ketamine has grown in popularity as a club drug.[102]

Salvia

Native to Southern Mexico, *salvia* is an herb from the mint family.[103] Its main active ingredient, salvinorin A, causes hallucinations by changing brain chemistry.[104] Although associated hallucinatory episodes have been described as intense, they are relatively short lasting, often beginning after a minute and fading after 30 minutes.[105] These brief but extreme hallucinations often include changes in mood, unusual body sensations, changes to visual perception, emotional swings, feeling detached, and an altered sense of self and reality.[106] Salvia's long-term effects have not been studied.

Check Yourself

- **What is a hallucinogen?**
- **What are the effects and health risks of commonly abused hallucinogens?**
- **Why do you think some users mistakenly consider hallucinogens to be less harmful than other types of drugs?**

6.9 Discuss the effects and health risks of inhalants that are commonly misused or abused.

Inhalants are chemicals whose vapors, when inhaled, can cause hallucinations and create intoxicating and euphoric effects. Not commonly recognized as drugs, inhalants are legal to purchase and universally available but dangerous. They generally appeal to young people who can't afford or obtain illicit substances. Some misused products include rubber cement, model glue, paint thinner, aerosol sprays, lighter fluid, varnish, wax, spot removers, and gasoline. Most of these substances are sniffed or "huffed" by users in search of a quick, cheap high.

Because they are inhaled, the volatile chemicals in these products reach the bloodstream and then the brain within seconds. This characteristic, along with the fact that dosages are extremely difficult to control because everyone has unique lung and breathing capacities, makes inhalants particularly dangerous. The effects of inhalants usually last for fewer than 15 minutes and resemble those of central nervous system depressants. Users may experience dizziness, disorientation, impaired coordination, reduced judgment, and slowed reaction times.[107] Combining inhalants with alcohol produces a synergistic effect and can cause severe and sometimes fatal liver damage.

An overdose of fumes from inhalants can cause unconsciousness and even death. Because the effect only lasts a few minutes, users can continue to inhale readily over several hours; by doing this, users can suffer loss of consciousness and death.[108]

Amyl Nitrite

Sometimes called "poppers" or "rush," *amyl nitrite* is packaged in small, cloth-covered glass capsules that can be crushed to release the active chemical for the user to inhale. The drug is often prescribed to alleviate chest pain in heart patients, because it dilates small blood vessels and reduces blood pressure. Dilation of blood vessels in the genital area is thought to enhance sensations or perceptions of orgasm. Dilation of blood vessels also produces fainting, dizziness, warmth, and skin flushing.

Nitrous Oxide

Nitrous oxide is sometimes used as an adjunct to dental anesthesia or minor surgical anesthesia. It is also a propellant chemical in aerosol products such as whipped toppings. Users who inhale nitrous oxide experience a state of euphoria, floating sensations, and illusions. Effects also include pain relief and a silly feeling, demonstrated by laughing and giggling (hence its nickname "laughing gas"). Regulating dosages of this drug can be difficult. Sustained inhalation can lead to unconsciousness, coma, and death.

Skills for **Behavior Change**

Responding to an Offer of Drugs

No matter what your experience until now, it is likely that you will be invited to use drugs at some point in your life. Here are some questions to consider before you find yourself in a situation in which you have the opportunity or feel pressure to use illicit drugs:

- Why am I considering trying drugs? Am I trying to fit in or impress my friends? What does this say about my friends if I need to take drugs to impress them? Are my friends really looking out for what is best for me?
- Am I using this drug to cope or feel different? Am I depressed?
- What could taking drugs cost me? Will this cost me my career if I am caught using? Could using drugs prevent me from getting a job?
- What are the long-term consequences of using this drug?
- What will this cost me in terms of my friendships and family? How would my close family and friends respond if they knew I was using drugs?

Even when you make the decision not to use drugs, it can be difficult to say no gracefully. Some good ways to turn down an offer include the following:

- "Thanks, but I've got a big test (game, meeting) tomorrow morning."
- "I've already got a great buzz right now. I really don't need anything more."
- "I don't like how (insert drug name here) makes me feel."
- "I'm driving tonight. So I'm not using."
- "I want to go for a run in the morning."
- "No."

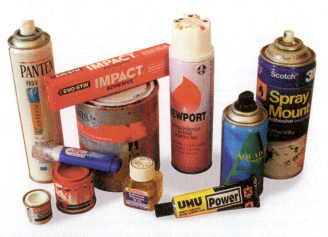

Common household products, such as aerosol sprays, solvents, or glues, can be inhaled for a quick high.

- What is an inhalant?
- What are the effects and health risks of inhalants?

Common Drugs of Abuse: Anabolic Steroids

Learning Outcome

6.10 Discuss the effects and health risks of anabolic steroids.

Anabolic steroids are artificial forms of the male hormone testosterone that promote muscle growth and strength. Steroids are available in two forms: injectable solutions and pills. These **ergogenic drugs** are used primarily by people who believe the drugs will increase their strength, power, bulk (weight), speed, and athletic performance.

It was once estimated that up to 20 percent of college athletes used steroids. Now that stricter drug-testing policies have been instituted by the National Collegiate Athletic Association (NCAA), reported use of anabolic steroids among intercollegiate athletes has decreased. Currently, fewer than half of 1 percent of college athletes surveyed report having used anabolic steroids within the past 12 months.[109] Those who report using anabolic steroids use them less than once per week. Of those, half reported that their first experience with anabolic steroids occurred after the age of 18.[110] The use of anabolic steroids on the college campus is very low; fewer than 1 percent of students report having used them within the past 30 days.[111] The perception of anabolic steroid use on the college campus is much higher than reality.[112]

Physical Effects of Steroids

Although their primary effects are not psychotropic, anabolic steroids can produce a state of euphoria and diminished fatigue in addition to increased bulk and power in both sexes. These qualities give steroids an addictive quality. When users stop using steroids, they can experience psychological withdrawal and sometimes severe depression, in some cases leading to suicide attempts.[113]

Men and women who use steroids experience a variety of adverse effects, including mood swings (aggression and violence, sometimes known as "roid rage"), acne, liver damage, elevated cholesterol levels, kidney damage, and immune system disturbances.[114] There is also a danger of transmitting HIV and hepatitis through shared needles. In women, large doses of anabolic steroids may trigger the development of masculine attributes such as lowered voice, increased facial and body hair, and male-pattern baldness; they may also result in an enlarged clitoris, smaller breasts, and changes in or absence of menstruation. When taken by healthy men, anabolic steroids shut down the body's production of testosterone, causing men's breasts to grow and testicles to atrophy.

Steroid Use and Society

The Anabolic Steroids Control Act (ASCA) of 1990 makes it a crime to possess, prescribe, or distribute anabolic steroids for any use other than the treatment of specific diseases. Penalties for illegal use of anabolic steroids include up to 1 year of imprisonment and/

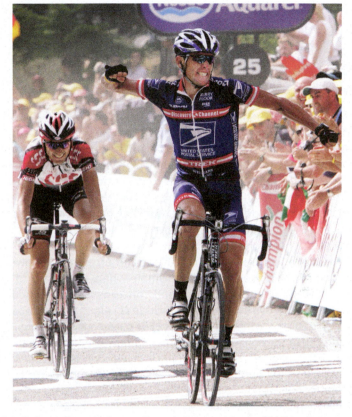

After being stripped of seven Tour de France titles in 2012 and an Olympic medal in 2013, cyclist Lance Armstrong publicly ended his years of denial and admitted to doping. He was banned from cycling for life and has been sued by the U.S. federal government and others for fraud.

or a fine of $1,000 for the first offense and a mandatory 15 days and maximum 2-year imprisonment and a $2,500 fine. Federal punishment for intent to distribute steroids is not more than 5 years of imprisonment, with 2 years of parole and a $250,000 fine for the first offense.[115]

In recent years, high-profile athletes in sports such as cycling, track and field, swimming, and baseball have garnered media attention for suspected use of steroids or other banned performance-enhancing drugs. Over 100 Russian track and field athletes were barred from the 2016 Summer Olympic Games for illegal drug use.

Check Yourself

- **What are anabolic steroids?**
- **What are the effects and health risks of anabolic steroids?**

6.11 Treatment, Recovery, and Mindfulness-Based Relapse Prevention

6.11 Discuss treatment and recovery options for people with an addiction.

Recovery from addiction is a lifelong process, starting with treatment—and, before that, recognition—of the addiction.

Intervention

Intervention is a planned process of confrontation by people who are important to the addict, including spouses, parents, children, bosses, and friends. Its purpose is to break down denial compassionately so that the person can see the addiction's destructive nature. Getting addicts to admit that they have a problem is not enough; they must come to perceive that the behavior is destructive and requires treatment.

Individual confrontation is difficult and often futile. However, an addict's defenses generally crumble when significant others collectively share observations and concerns about the addict's behavior. Effective interventions include (1) emphasizing care and concern for the addicted person; (2) describing the behavior that is the cause for concern; (3) expressing how the behavior affects the addict, each person taking part in the intervention, and other people; and (4) outlining specifically what you would like to see happen.

Participants in the intervention must clarify how they plan to end their enabling. People who are contemplating interventions must also choose consequences they are ready to stick to if the addict refuses treatment—and be ready to give support if the addict is willing to begin a recovery program.

Treatment for Addiction

Treatment and recovery for any addiction generally begin with **abstinence**, that is, refraining from the addictive behavior. For people addicted to behaviors such as work and sex, abstinence means restoring balance to their lives through noncompulsive engagement in the behaviors. An estimated 20.8 million Americans aged 12 and older needed treatment for a substance use disorder in 2015.[116, 117] Only 2.2 million of these individuals (10.4 percent) received treatment.[117]

Detoxification refers to the early period during which an addict adjusts physically and cognitively to being free from the addiction's influence. It occurs in virtually every recovering addict. Detoxification is uncomfortable and can be dangerous. For some addicts, early abstinence may involve profound withdrawal that requires medical supervision.

Abstinence alone does little to change the psychological, biological, and environmental dynamics underlying addictive behavior. Without treatment, an addict is apt to relapse or to change addictions. Treatment involves learning new ways of looking at oneself, other people, and the world. It may require exploring a traumatic past so that psychological wounds can heal. It also involves learning interdependence with significant others and new ways of caring for oneself physically and emotionally.

Finding a Treatment Program

For many addicts, recovery begins with a period of formal treatment. A good treatment program includes the following:

- Staff familiar with the specific addictive disorder for which help is being sought
- Availability of both inpatient and outpatient services
- Medical personnel who can assess the addict's health and treat medical concerns, as needed
- Medical supervision of addicts at risk for complicated detoxification
- Involvement of family members in the treatment process
- A coordinated team approach to treating addictive disorders (e.g., medical personnel, counselors, psychotherapists, clergy, and dietitians)
- Group and individual therapy options
- Peer-led support groups that encourage involvement after treatment ends
- Structured aftercare and relapse-prevention programs
- Accreditation by the Joint Commission (a national organization that accredits and certifies health care organizations and programs) and a license from the state in which it operates.

Treatment Approaches

Outpatient behavioral treatment encompasses a variety of programs for addicts who visit a clinic at regular intervals. Most involve individual or group counseling. *Residential treatment programs* can be effective for those with more severe problems. For example, therapeutic communities are highly structured programs in which addicts remain at a residence, typically for 6 to 12 months. The focus is on resocialization to a drug-free lifestyle.

The first *12-step program*, Alcoholics Anonymous (AA), began in 1935. The 12-step program has since become the most widely used approach to dealing with addictive or dysfunctional behaviors. More than 200 recovery programs are based on the program, including Narcotics Anonymous and Gamblers Anonymous.

The 12-step program is nonjudgmental and based on the idea that its purpose is to work on personal recovery. Working the 12 steps involves admitting to having a problem, recognizing there is an outside power that could help, consciously relying on that power, admitting and listing character defects, seeking deliverance from defects, apologizing to those one has harmed, and helping others with the same problem. Free meetings, held at a variety of times and locations in almost every city, are open to anyone who wishes to attend.[118]

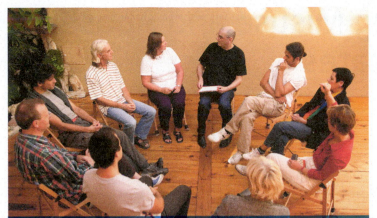

How do people recover from drug addiction?

For most addicts, recovery is a long, difficult process. For some people, it can be a lifelong journey. Treatment and recovery usually begin with detoxification. Once the person's body has adjusted, the addict usually enters therapy to learn how to cope without the drug and avoid relapse. Therapy often takes the form of group meetings, such as those held by 12-step programs.

Medicinal Treatments Methadone maintenance is one treatment available for people addicted to heroin or other opioids. Methadone is chemically similar enough to opioids to control the tremors, chills, vomiting, diarrhea, and severe abdominal pains of withdrawal. Critics of methadone maintenance contend that the program merely substitutes one addiction for another. Proponents argue that people on methadone maintenance are less likely to engage in criminal activities to support their habits than heroin addicts are.

A number of new drug therapies for opioid dependence are emerging as well, such as naltrexone (Trexan), an opioid antagonist. While on naltrexone, recovering addicts do not have the compulsion to use heroin, and if they do use it, they don't get high, so there is no point in using heroin.

Recovery Coaching Recovery coaches are not treatment providers but help individuals being discharged from treatment to connect with community resources. In addition to providing emotional and informational support, recovery coaches facilitate access to health and social services and help those in recovery find healthy social connections and recreational activities.[119]

Social, Recreational, and Social Media Support Systems There are an increasing number of social and recreational programs that provide support for people in recovery. Programs or businesses such as recovery cafes, clubhouses, sports leagues, and arts and theater groups are just a few examples. Social media, mobile health apps, and online recovery programs can also provide social support. Studies show that these emerging tools have positive benefits for preventing relapse and providing support for those in recovery.[120]

Vaccines against Addictive Drugs Two heroin vaccines are advancing towards human clinical trials. The first stimulates the immune system to attack the heroin and eliminate it from the body. The second keeps heroin from reaching the brain and also prevents HIV infection.[121] Also in development are promising new vaccines against cocaine, nicotine, and methamphetamine.[122]

Relapse

Relapse, an isolated occurrence of or full return to addictive behavior, is a defining characteristic of addiction. Addicts are set up to relapse because of their tendency to meet change and other forms of stress with the same kind of denial once used to justify addictive behavior (e.g., "I don't have a problem; I can handle this"). Good treatment programs recognize this tendency and teach clients and significant others how to recognize and respond to signs of imminent relapse. Relapse should not be interpreted as failure to change or lack of desire to stay well. The appropriate response is to remind addicts that they are addicted and redirect them to strategies that have worked for them.

Mindfulness-Based Relapse Prevention Mindfulness can be an effective way to prevent relapse. Similar to mindfulness-based cognitive therapy used to treat depression, **Mindfulness-Based Relapse Prevention (MBRP)** focuses on two major predictors of relapse: negative emotions and cravings. MBRP is a group-based program that typically meets for eight sessions. It was originally created for people coming out of treatment who needed an aftercare program, but it has since evolved to provide continued support throughout the recovery process.

The theoretical framework for the integration of mindfulness and cognitive-behavioral relapse prevention is that mindfulness may help people become less attached to emotions, helping them prevent spiraling thoughts that might lead to relapse. By increasing emotional awareness, redefining how one responds to triggers for relapse such as boredom, and developing coping skills, the person in recovery learns how to interrupt the cycle of substance abuse behavior. If a lapse does occur, mindfulness can help to reduce the feelings of guilt and shame that increase the risk of relapse. It can also help the person to focus on more self-awareness and self-compassion, allowing individuals who slip in their path to recovery to cut themselves some slack and acknowledge the difficulties of their addiction and reasons for the slip, while providing support for getting back on track with positive self-talk and behaviors.

To bring awareness to your own triggers and cravings, try the following activity: Over the next week, pay attention to the way your body responds to pleasant events. Be aware of detailed bodily sensations, thoughts, and emotions that occur when you experience a pleasant event. Record them in as much detail as you can. Do your best to pay attention to at least one pleasant occurrence each day.

Check Yourself

- **What are the steps in treatment and recovery from addiction?**

6.12 Addressing Drug Misuse and Abuse in the United States

Learning Outcome

6.12 Identify strategies to address drug misuse and abuse.

Illegal drug use in the United States costs about $193 billion per year.[123] This estimate includes $11 billion in the cost of health care, $120 billion in lost productivity, and $61 billion in the cost of criminal investigation, prosecution, incarceration, and other associated criminal justice costs.[124]

Preventing Drug Use and Abuse on Campus

College and university campuses should consider multiple strategies to reduce substance use among students:

- Changing student expectations that college is a time to experiment with drugs
- Engaging parents and encouraging them to continue open communication with their children
- Identifying high-risk students through early detection programs
- Providing programs specifically tailored for students needing treatment and recovery support.

The pressure to take drugs is often tremendous, and reasons for use are complex. People who develop drug problems generally believe that they can control their use when they start out. Peer influence is also a strong motivator, especially among adolescents.

Solving the Drug Problem

Americans are alarmed by the persistent problem of illegal drug use. Respondents in public opinion polls say that the government should focus on treatment for people who use illegal drugs such as heroin or cocaine. There is increased support for moving away from mandatory sentences for nonviolent drug crimes. Many strategies include prevention strategies that focus on helping individuals develop the knowledge, attitudes, and skills to make good decisions. Other approaches encourage use of community prevention strategies to make it easier to act in healthy ways. These strategies involve community leaders, parents, and local officials working together to shift individual attitudes and community norms.[125] To address safety concerns, many employers have instituted mandatory drug testing. Despite controversies over the accuracy of urinalysis tests, this practice is becoming more common.

All of these approaches will probably help up to a point, but they do not offer a total solution to the problem. Drug abuse has been a part of human behavior for thousands of years, and it is not

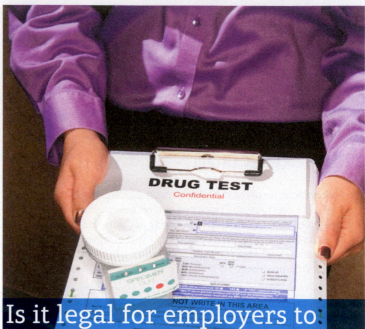

Is it legal for employers to require employees to take a drug test?

Several court decisions have affirmed the right of employers to test their employees for drug use. They ruled that Fourth Amendment rights pertain only to employees of government agencies, not to employees of private businesses. Most Americans apparently support drug testing for certain types of jobs.

likely to disappear in the near future. For this reason, it is necessary to educate ourselves and to develop the self-discipline necessary to avoid dangerous drug dependence.

In general, researchers in the field of drug education agree that a multimodal approach is best. Young people should be taught the difference between drug use, drug misuse, and drug abuse. Factual information that is free of scare tactics must be presented. Lecturing and moralizing have proven not to work.

Check Yourself

- **What are some strategies to address substance abuse? Which, if any, of these are present on your campus?**

Summary

LO 6.1 Addiction is continued use of a substance or activity despite ongoing negative consequences. All addictions share four common symptoms: compulsion, loss of control, negative consequences, and denial.

LO 6.1 Codependents are typically friends or family members who are controlled by an addict's addictive behavior. Enablers are people who protect addicts from consequences of their behavior.

LO 6.1 The biopsychosocial model of addiction takes into account biological (genetic) factors as well as psychological and environmental influences in understanding the addiction process.

LO 6.2 Addictive behaviors include disordered gambling, compulsive buying, compulsive Internet or technology use, work addiction, compulsive exercise, and sexual addiction.

LO 6.3 The six categories of drugs are prescription drugs, over-the-counter (OTC) drugs, recreational drugs, herbal preparations, illicit drugs, and commercial preparations.

LO 6.4 Over-the-counter medications are drugs that do not require a prescription. Some OTC medications can be addictive.

LO 6.4 Prescription drug abuse is at an all-time high, particularly among college students. The most commonly abused prescription drugs are painkillers.

LO 6.4 People from all walks of life use illicit drugs. Drug use declined from the mid-1980s to the early 1990s but has remained steady since then. However, among young people, use of drugs has been rising in recent years.

LO 6.5–6.10 Controlled substances include cocaine and its derivatives, amphetamines, methamphetamine, marijuana, opioids, depressants, hallucinogens/psychedelics, inhalants, and steroids.

LO 6.11 Treatment begins with abstinence from the drug or addictive behavior, usually instituted through intervention by close family, friends, or other loved ones. Treatment programs may include individual, group, or family therapy, 12-step programs, recovery coaching, recreational and social media programs, vaccines, and mindfulness-based relapse prevention.

LO 6.12. Drug abuse is a major problem in many regions of the world and several key problems have escalated in recent years, particularly use of marijuana and opioids, such as heroin. Programs designed to reduce risk by focusing on mental health and mental health services earlier in life, prevention programs that help individuals resist drug use, and treatment programs that are available to larger segments of the population at lower costs are key to stemming the tide of drug abuse from youth through end of life.

Pop Quiz

Visit **Mastering Health** *to personalize your study plan with Chapter Review Quizzes and Dynamic Study Modules.*

LO 6.1 1. Which of the following is *not* a characteristic of addiction?
a. Denial
b. Acknowledgment of self-destructive behavior
c. Loss of control
d. Obsession with a substance or behavior

LO 6.1 2. Aaliyah is addicted to the Internet. She is so preoccupied with it that she is failing her classes. What symptom of addiction does her preoccupation characterize?
a. Denial
b. Compulsion
c. Loss of control
d. Negative consequences

LO 6.1 3. An individual who knowingly tries to protect an addict from natural consequences of the addict's destructive behaviors is
a. enabling.
b. helping the addict to recover.
c. practicing intervention.
d. controlling.

LO 6.3 4. Cross-tolerance occurs when
a. drugs work at the same receptor site so that one blocks the action of the other.
b. the effects of one drug are eliminated or reduced by the presence of another drug at the receptor site.
c. a person develops a physiological tolerance to one drug and shows a similar tolerance to selected other drugs as a result.
d. two or more drugs interact so their effects are multiplied.

LO 6.3 5. Jayden takes Prinivil (an antihypertensive drug), insulin (a diabetic medication), and Claritin (an antihistamine). This is an example of
a. synergism.
b. illegal drug use.
c. polydrug use.
d. antagonism.

LO 6.4 6. The most widely used illicit drug in the United States is
a. alcohol.
b. heroin.
c. marijuana.
d. methamphetamine.

LO 6.5 7. Which of the following is classified as a stimulant drug?
a. Amphetamines
b. Alcohol
c. Marijuana
d. LSD

LO 6.7 8. Drugs that depress the central nervous system are called
a. amphetamines.
b. hallucinogens.
c. depressants.
d. psychedelics.

LO 6.8 9. The psychoactive drug mescaline is found in what plant?
a. Mushrooms
b. Peyote cactus
c. Marijuana
d. Belladonna

LO 6.11 10. Chemical dependency relapse refers to
a. a person experiencing a blackout.
b. a gap in one's drinking or drug-taking patterns.
c. a full return to addictive behavior.
d. failure to change one's behavior.

Answers to these questions can be found on page A-1. If you answered a question incorrectly, review the module identified by the Learning Outcome. For even more study tools, visit Mastering Health.

Think About It!

LO 6.1 1. Discuss how addiction affects family and friends. What role do family and friends play in helping the addict get help and maintain recovery?

LO 6.2 2. What differentiates a process addiction from a substance abuse addiction?

LO 6.3 3. Why and how do drugs work? What are some of the different ways that different types of drugs interact with brain chemistry?

LO 6.4 4. Why do you think so many young people today are abusing prescription drugs? Do you perceive prescription drug abuse as being less dangerous or illegal than illicit drug use? Why? Do you think this is an accurate or biased perception?

LO 6.6 5. Why do you think many people today feel that marijuana use is not dangerous? What are the arguments in favor of legalizing marijuana? What are the arguments against legalization?

LO 6.4–6.9 6. Do you think there is such a thing as responsible use of illicit drugs? Would you change any of the current laws governing drugs? How would you determine what is legitimate and illegitimate use?

LO 6.10 7. Why do you think so many athletes use steroids to improve performance? How big of a problem do you think it is on your campus? Do you know whether they test for steroids among athletes on your campus? What are the penalities for getting caught "using"? Under what circumstances might mindfulness programs be most effective in reducing risks?

LO 6.11 8. What are some of the treatment options for drug abuse and addiction today? Which of these do you think might be most effective for college students? Why? What role do you think Mindfulness-Based Relapse Prevention programs should be a part of campus resources for students who find themselves in trouble with drug abuse?

LO 6.12 9. What types of policies and programs do you think would be effective in preventing drug abuse among high school and college students? How would programs for high school students differ from those for college students? Which types of programs or policies might be most effective in reducing risks?

Alcohol and Tobacco

People throughout history have used alcohol. Alcohol consumption is part of many traditions, and moderate use can enhance special times. Although alcohol can play a positive role in some people's lives, it is a drug and, if used irresponsibly, can become dangerous.

Approximately half of all Americans consume alcohol regularly, while 21 percent abstain altogether.[1] More men are regular drinkers, and men typically drink more than women. Women are more likely to be abstainers, along with Asian Americans, African Americans, and people who are employed. Adults in poor families are more than twice as likely to be lifetime abstainers as adults in nonpoor families.[2]

Although tobacco use has declined overall in the United States in recent decades, approximately 36 million Americans age 18 and older reported having used tobacco products (cigarettes, cigars, smokeless tobacco, and pipe tobacco) at least once in the past month.[3] Tobacco use is the single most preventable cause of death in the United States: Close to half a million Americans die each year of tobacco-related diseases.[4] Another 16 million people suffer from health disorders caused by tobacco. To date, tobacco is known to cause about 20 diseases, and about half of all regular smokers die of smoking-related diseases.[5] Any contention by the tobacco industry that tobacco use is not dangerous completely ignores scientific evidence.

Alcohol and College Students

7.1 Discuss the alcohol use patterns of college students and the factors that make college students vulnerable to alcohol-related problems.

Alcohol is the most popular drug on college campuses, where large numbers of students report having consumed alcoholic beverages in the past 30 days (**Figure 7.1**). In a new trend on college campuses, women's consumption of alcohol has come close to equaling that of men.[6]

Approximately 40 percent of all college students engage in **binge drinking**,[7] consuming five or more drinks (men) or four or more drinks (women) in about 2 hours.[8] Students who drink only once a week are considered binge drinkers if they consume these amounts within 2 hours. Binge drinking can quickly lead to extreme intoxication, unconsciousness, alcohol poisoning, and even death.

For some students, independence is symbolized by alcohol use. Others drink to "have fun," which often means drinking simply to get drunk. This may be a way of coping with stress, boredom, anxiety, or academic and social pressures.

In the past 12 months, a significant number of college students who drank experienced at least one negative consequence of alcohol consumption (**Figure 7.2**). In the last year, nearly 33 percent of college students who drank reported doing something they later regretted; 28 percent forgot where they were or what they did due to intoxication; just over 21 percent had unprotected sex; and 12.4 percent accidentally injured themselves.[9]

Fortunately, many students report always or usually practicing protective sexual behaviors when consuming alcohol. However, some students don't drink responsibly, and the stakes are high. According to one study, 1,825 college students die each year because of alcohol-related unintentional injuries, including car accidents.[10] Alcohol consumption is the top cause of preventable death among U.S. undergraduates.[11]

Alcohol use among college students also has consequences related to academic performance.[12] Alcohol consumption tends to disrupt sleep and decreases REM sleep. Alcohol use is associated with shorter sleep duration, greater sleep irregularity, bedtime delay, weekend oversleeping, and sleep-related impairment.[13] These disruptive effects increase daytime sleepiness and decrease alertness, which can also negatively affect students' academic performance.[14]

Why Do College Students Drink So Much?

College students seem to be particularly vulnerable to alcohol-related problems. In addition to newfound freedom, several factors encourage drinking during college:

- Many student customs (Greek rush), norms (reputation as party schools), and traditional celebrations (St. Patrick's Day) encourage drinking.
- Alcohol advertising and promotions target students.
- College students are particularly vulnerable to peer influence.
- Drink specials enable students to consume large amounts of alcohol cheaply.
- College administrators often deny the extent of alcohol problems on their campuses.

Student Drinking Behavior

College students are more likely than their noncollegiate peers to drink recklessly and to engage in dangerous drinking practices. One such practice, **pregaming** (also known as preloading or frontloading), involves planned heavy drinking before going out to a bar, nightclub, or sporting event. In a recent study, 92 percent of students reported pregaming during the academic year.[15] Students who pregame consume more drinks and have higher blood levels of alcohol. Negative consequences of pregaming include passing out, drunk driving, aggression, alcohol poisoning, and violent acts.[16]

Competitive drinking is also common on college campuses, with students playing drinking games such as beer pong, quarters, and flip cup.[17] People who play drinking games are less likely to monitor or regulate how much they drink and are at risk for extreme intoxication and negative related outcomes.[18] Drinking games are associated with blacking out, regrettable sexual experiences, alcohol-related injuries, and deaths from alcohol poisoning.[19]

Some college students use extreme measures to control their eating and/or exercise excessively so that they can save calories, consume more alcohol, and become intoxicated faster.[20]

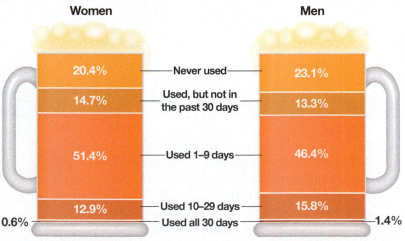

Women		Men
20.4%	Never used	23.1%
14.7%	Used, but not in the past 30 days	13.3%
51.4%	Used 1–9 days	46.4%
12.9%	Used 10–29 days	15.8%
0.6%	Used all 30 days	1.4%

Figure 7.1 **College Students' Patterns of Alcohol Use in the Past 30 Days**

Source: Data from American College Health Association, *American College Health Association—National College Health Assessment II: Reference Group Executive Summary, Fall 2016* (Hanover, MD: American College Health Association, 2017).

Drunkorexia describes the combination of two dangerous behaviors: disordered eating and heavy drinking. Potential risks of drunkorexia include risk of blackouts, forced sexual activity, unintended sexual activity, and alcohol poisoning.

What Is the Impact of Student Drinking?

The more students drink, the more likely they are to miss class, do poorly on tests and papers, have lower grade point averages, and fall behind on assigned work. Some students even drop out of school as a result of their drinking.

In a recent survey, almost 20 percent of undergraduate women and 5 percent of undergraduate men reported having been sexually assaulted by physical force or while incapacitated while in college.[21] Among the women who experienced a sexual assault or unwanted sexual contact, 61 percent had been drinking alcohol, and 88 percent reported not having taken or used any drug other than alcohol before the incident.[22]

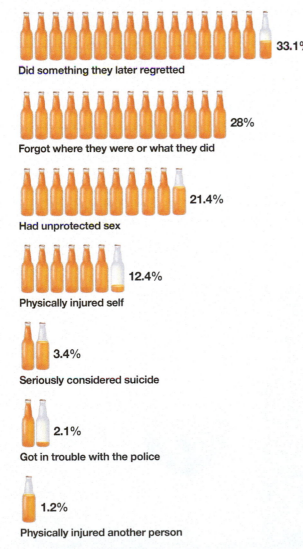

Figure 7.2 Prevalence of Negative Consequences of Drinking among College Students in the Past Year

Source: Data from American College Health Association, *American College Health Association—National College Health Assessment II: Reference Group Executive Summary, Fall 2016* (Hanover, MD: American College Health Association, 2017).

The laws about sexual consent are clear: A person who is drunk or passed out cannot consent to sex. If you have sex with someone who is drunk or unconscious, you are committing rape. Claiming that you were also drunk does not absolve you of legal and moral responsibility for this crime.

Colleges' Efforts to Reduce Student Drinking

Some colleges are instituting strong policies against drinking; at the same time, schools are making more help available to students with drinking problems. The Brief Alcohol Screening and Intervention for College Students (BASICS) is an effective program for students who drink heavily and have experienced alcohol-related problems or are at risk for them.[23] E-interventions—electronically based alcohol education interventions using Web interventions such as the Alcohol EDU® and e-Check Up to Go (e-Chug) have also shown to be highly effective in reducing alcohol-related problems among students.[24]

Web-based education for first-year college students has become an increasingly important intervention. Because first-year students are at particular risk for alcohol-related problems, schools ensure that students are made aware of risks and effects of alcohol, as well as the campus resources available for dealing with issues with alcohol use.

See It! Videos

Heavy drinking during spring break can lead to bad decisions, or worse. Watch **Sloppy Spring Breaker** in the Study Area of Mastering Health.

Skills for **Behavior Change**

Tips For Drinking Responsibly

- Eat before and while you drink.
- Don't drink before the party.
- Avoid drinking if you are angry, anxious, or depressed.
- Drink no more than one alcoholic drink an hour.
- Alternate alcoholic and nonalcoholic drinks.
- Determine ahead of time how many drinks you'll have.
- Avoid drinking games.
- Keep track of how much you drink.
- Don't drink and drive. Volunteer to be the sober driver.
- Avoid parties where you can expect heavy drinking.

Check Yourself

- How does this module's description of college student drinking compare to drinking on your campus?

- What is binge drinking?

- What factors make college students vulnerable to alcohol-related problems? Which of these factors exist on your campus?

7.2 Alcohol Effects in Your Body

7.2 Explain the processes by which alcohol is absorbed and metabolized in the human body and the factors that affect blood alcohol concentration.

Learning about the metabolism and absorption of alcohol can help you understand how it is possible to drink safely—and how to avoid life-threatening circumstances such as alcohol poisoning. This information can be critical for your safety and that of your friends.

The Chemistry and Potency of Alcohol

The intoxicating substance found in beer, wine, liquor, and liqueurs is **ethyl alcohol**, or **ethanol**. It is produced during **fermentation**, in which yeast organisms break down plant sugars, yielding ethanol and carbon dioxide. For beers, ales, and wines, the process ends with fermentation. Hard liquor is produced through further processing called **distillation**, in which alcohol vapors are condensed and mixed with water to make the final product.

The **proof** of an alcoholic drink is a measure of its percentage of alcohol and therefore its strength. Alcohol percentage by volume is half of the given proof; for example, 80 proof whiskey is 40 percent alcohol by volume. Lower-proof drinks produce fewer alcohol effects than do the same amount of higher-proof drinks. Most wines are 12 to 15 percent alcohol, and most beers are 2 to 8 percent.

As defined by the National Institute on Alcohol Abuse and Alcoholism (NIAAA), a **standard drink** contains about 14 grams (0.6 fluid ounce or 1.2 tablespoons) of pure alcohol (**Figure 7.3**). A 12-ounce can of beer, a 5-ounce glass of wine, and a 1.5-ounce shot of vodka are each considered one standard drink—each contains the same amount of alcohol. In estimating blood alcohol concentration using standard drinks as a measure, keep in mind both proof and drink size. You may have bought one beer at the ballpark, but if it came in a 22-ounce cup, you actually consumed two standard drinks.

Absorption and Metabolism

Unlike the molecules in most foods and drugs, alcohol molecules are sufficiently small and fat soluble to be absorbed throughout the gastrointestinal system. Approximately 20 percent of ingested alcohol diffuses through the stomach lining into the bloodstream and nearly 80 percent through the lining of the upper third of the small intestine.

Several factors influence how quickly your body will absorb alcohol: the alcohol concentration in your drink; the amount you consume; the amount of food in your stomach; and your metabolism, weight, body mass index, and mood. The higher the concentration of alcohol in your drink, the more rapidly it will be absorbed in your digestive tract. As a rule, wine and beer are absorbed more slowly than distilled beverages. "Fizzy" alcoholic beverages, carbonated beverages, and drinks served with mixers cause the pyloric valve to relax, emptying stomach contents more rapidly into the small intestine and increasing the rate of absorption.

Students often mix energy drinks with alcohol, and these combinations can be particularly dangerous. Students who consume alcohol mixed with energy drinks often report not noticing signs of intoxication (e.g., dizziness, fatigue, headache, and trouble walking). Caffeine may delay the onset of normal sleepiness, increasing the amount of time a person would normally stay awake and drink. Caffeine also reduces the subjective feeling of drunkenness without reducing alcohol-related impairment. Students who reported drinking alcohol mixed with energy drinks were more likely to consume large amounts of alcohol, have unprotected sex or sex under the influence, be hurt or injured, and meet criteria for alcohol dependency.[25]

The more alcohol you consume, the longer absorption takes. High concentrations of alcohol can cause irritation of the digestive system or vomiting. Alcohol also takes longer to absorb if there is food in your stomach, because the surface area exposed to alcohol is smaller; a full stomach also retards emptying of alcoholic beverages into the small intestine.

Mood also affects how long it takes for the stomach's contents to empty into the intestine. Alcohol is absorbed much more rapidly when people are tense than when they are relaxed.

Once absorbed into the bloodstream, alcohol circulates throughout the body and is metabolized in the liver, where it is converted to *acetaldehyde* by the enzyme *alcohol dehydrogenase*. It is then rapidly oxidized to *acetate*, converted to carbon dioxide and water, and eventually excreted from the body. Acetaldehyde is a toxic chemical that can cause immediate symptoms such as nausea and vomiting, as well as long-term effects such as liver

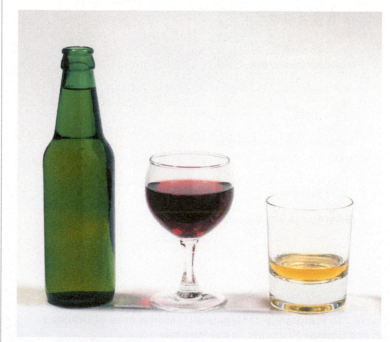

Figure 7.3 What Is a Standard Drink?
One standard drink of beer (12 ounces), wine (5 ounces), or liquor (1.5 ounces) contains the same amount of alcohol.

damage. A very small portion of alcohol is excreted unchanged by the kidneys, lungs, and skin.

Alcohol contains 7 calories (kcal) per gram; the average regular beer contains about 150 calories. Mixed drinks may contain more. The body uses the calories in alcohol in the same manner as it uses those in carbohydrates: for immediate energy or for storage as fat if not immediately needed.

Breakdown of alcohol occurs at a fairly constant rate of 0.5 ounce (slightly less than one standard drink) per hour. Unmetabolized alcohol circulates in the bloodstream until enough time passes for the body to break it down.

Blood Alcohol Concentration

Blood alcohol concentration (BAC), the ratio of alcohol to total blood volume, is the primary method used to measure physiological and behavioral effects of alcohol. Despite individual differences, alcohol produces some general effects, depending on BAC (**Figure 7.4**).

At a BAC of 0.02 percent, a person feels relaxed and in a good mood. At 0.05 percent, relaxation increases, and there is some motor impairment and increased willingness to talk. At 0.08 percent come euphoria and further motor impairment. At 0.10 percent, the depressant effects of alcohol become apparent, drowsiness sets in, and motor skills are further impaired, followed by a loss of judgment. A driver might not be able to estimate distance or speed; some drinkers lose their ability to make value-related decisions and may do things they wouldn't do when sober. As BAC increases, the drinker suffers increased negative physiological and psychological effects.

BAC depends on weight and body fat, concentration of alcohol in a beverage, rate of consumption, and volume of alcohol consumed. Heavier people have more body area through which to diffuse alcohol, so have lower concentrations of blood alcohol than do thin people after drinking the same amount.

Gender also plays a role. Compared to men's bodies, women's bodies contain half as much *alcohol dehydrogenase*. So if a man

Blood Alcohol Concentration (BAC)	Psychological and Physical Effects
Not Impaired	
<0.01%	Negligible
Sometimes Impaired	
0.01–0.04%	Slight muscle relaxation, mild euphoria, slight body warmth, increased sociability and talkativeness
Usually Impaired	
0.05–0.07%	Lowered alertness, impaired judgment, lowered inhibitions, exaggerated behavior, loss of small muscle control
Always Impaired	
0.08–0.14%	Slowed reaction time, poor muscle coordination, short-term memory loss, judgment impaired, inability to focus
0.15–0.24%	Blurred vision, lack of motor skills, sedation, slowed reactions, difficulty standing and walking, passing out
0.25–0.34%	Impaired consciousness, disorientation, loss of motor function, severely impaired or no reflexes, impaired circulation and respiration, uncontrolled urination, slurred speech, possible death
0.35% and up	Unconsciousness, coma, extremely slow heartbeat and respiration, unresponsiveness, probable death

Figure 7.4 The Psychological and Physical Effects of Alcohol

and a woman drink the same amount of alcohol, the woman's BAC will be approximately 30 percent higher than the man's.

Alcohol does not diffuse as rapidly into body fat as into body tissues; BAC is higher in people with more body fat. Because a woman is likely to have proportionately more body fat than a man of the same weight, women will be more intoxicated after drinking the same amount of alcohol.

Breath analysis (breathalyzer tests) and urinalysis are used to determine whether an individual is legally intoxicated, though blood tests are more accurate. An increasing number of states require blood tests for people suspected of driving under the influence of alcohol. In some states, refusal to take a breath, urine, or blood test results in immediate driver's license revocation.

People can develop physical and psychological tolerance of the effects of alcohol through regular use. The nervous system adapts over time, so greater amounts of alcohol are required to produce the same effects. Though BAC may be quite high, the individual has learned to modify his or her behavior to appear sober, an ability called **learned behavioral tolerance**.

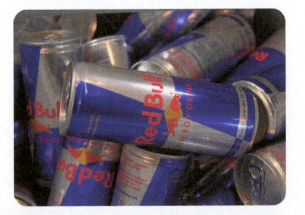

Combining alcohol with energy drinks can have dangerous results.

Sources: J. Verster et al., "Motives for Mixing Alcohol with Energy Drinks and Other Nonalcoholic Beverages and Consequences for Overall Alcohol Consumption," *International Journal of Internal Medicine* 7 (2014): 285–93.

Check Yourself

- What is a standard drink of alcohol?

- How Is alcohol absorbed and metabolized In the body?

- What are some of the factors that increase and decrease blood alcohol concentration?

7.3 Alcohol and Your Health: Short-Term Effects

7.3 **Discuss the short-term health effects of alcohol consumption.**

Immediate and long-term effects of alcohol consumption can vary greatly (**Figure 7.5**). The effects you experience depend on you as an individual, how much alcohol you consume, and your circumstances.

The most dramatic effects produced by ethanol occur within the central nervous system (CNS). Alcohol depresses CNS function, which decreases respiratory rate, pulse rate, and blood pressure. As CNS depression deepens, vital functions become affected. In extreme cases, coma and death can result.

Alcohol is a diuretic that increases urinary output. Although this might be expected to lead to **dehydration** (loss of water), the body actually retains water, most of it in the muscles and cerebral tissues. Because water is pulled out of the *cerebrospinal fluid* (fluid within the brain and spinal cord), drinkers may suffer symptoms that include "morning-after" effects.

Alcohol irritates the gastrointestinal system and may cause indigestion and heartburn if consumed on an empty stomach. People who consume unusually high amounts of alcohol in a short time also put themselves at risk for irregular heartbeat or even total loss of heart rhythm, which can disrupt blood flow and damage the heart muscle.[26]

Hangover

A **hangover** is often experienced the morning after a drinking spree. Its symptoms are familiar to most people who drink: headache, muscle aches, upset stomach, anxiety, depression, diarrhea, and thirst. **Congeners**, forms of alcohol that are metabolized more slowly than ethanol and are more toxic, are thought to play a role in the development of a hangover; the body metabolizes congeners after ethanol is gone from the system, and their toxic by-products may contribute to hangover. Alcohol upsets the body's water balance, resulting in hangover symptoms including excess urination, dehydration, and thirst. Increased production of hydrochloric acid can irritate the stomach lining and cause nausea. Recovery from a hangover usually takes 12 hours. Bedrest, solid food, plenty of water, and aspirin or ibuprofen may help to relieve a hangover's discomforts. The U.S. Food and Drug Administration (FDA) has approved the only over-the-counter hangover drug, called Blowfish. The tablet is a combination of aspirin, an antacid, and caffeine to fight headache, fatigue, and upset stomach after a night of drinking.[27] However, the only way to avoid a hangover completely is to abstain from excessive alcohol use in the first place.

Alcohol and Injuries

The relationship between alcohol and a variety of accidents, such as automobile crashes, falls, and fires, has long been established.

Approximately 70 percent of fatal injuries during activities such as swimming and boating involve alcohol.[28] Drinking affects psychomotor skills and cognitive skills; in other words, drinking can have an adverse effect on a person's reaction time and judgment, so people under the influence of alcohol often set themselves up for injury.[29]

Alcohol use is also a key risk factor for suicide, playing a role in approximately 20 percent of suicides in the United States.[30] Alcohol may increase the risk for suicide by intensifying depressive thoughts or feelings of hopelessness, lowering inhibitions to hurt oneself, and interfering with the ability to assess future consequences of one's actions.[31]

Alcohol and Sexual Decision Making

Alcohol affects your ability to make good decisions about sex because it lowers inhibitions. About 1 in 5 college students reports engaging in sexual activity, after drinking, including having sex with someone they just met and having unprotected sex.[32] The chance of acquiring a sexually transmitted infection or experiencing unplanned pregnancy also increases as students drink more heavily.[33]

Alcohol and Rape and Sexual Assault

More than 30 percent of rape victims reported that their assailant was under the influence of alcohol.[34] Most college assault victims know their attacker, and assaults occur frequently at parties. Alcohol use by women makes them more vulnerable to sexual assault.[35] While men, when drinking, are also at increased risk of victimization, they are also more likely than women to engage in coercive sexual behaviors, including sexual assault.[36]

Alcohol and Weight Gain

Alcohol has 7 calories per gram—nearly as much as fat—and the calories from alcohol provide few nutrients. A standard drink contains 12 to 15 grams of alcohol, so a single drink can add about 100 empty calories to your daily intake. By drinking an extra 150 calories a day more than you need, you can gain 1 pound a month and up to 12 pounds a year.[37]

Alcohol Poisoning

Alcohol poisoning (*acute alcohol intoxication*) occurs much more frequently than people realize and can be fatal. Drinking large amounts of alcohol in a short period of time can cause one's BAC to quickly reach the lethal range. Alcohol, used either alone or in combination with other drugs, is responsible for more toxic overdose deaths than any other substance.

The amount of alcohol that causes loss of consciousness is dangerously close to the lethal dose. Death from alcohol poisoning can be caused either by CNS and respiratory depression or by inhalation of vomit or fluid into the lungs. Alcohol depresses the

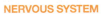

Short-Term Health Effects

NERVOUS SYSTEM
• Slowed reaction time, slurred speech
• Impaired judgment and motor coordination
• High BACs can lead to coma and death

SENSES
• Dulled senses of taste and smell
• Less acute vision and hearing

SKIN
• Broken capillaries
• Flushing, sweating, heat loss

HEART AND LUNGS
• Decreased pulse and respiratory rate
• Lowered blood pressure

STOMACH
• Nausea
• Irritation and inflammation

URINARY SYSTEM
• Increased urination

SEXUAL RESPONSE
• **Women:** decreased vaginal lubrication
• **Men:** erectile dysfunction

Long-Term Health Effects

BRAIN
• Memory impairment
• Damaged/destroyed brain cells

IMMUNE SYSTEM
• Lowered disease resistance

HEART
• Weakened heart muscle
• Elevated blood pressure

LIVER
• Increased risk of liver cancer
• Fatty liver and cirrhosis

DIGESTIVE SYSTEM
• Chronic inflammation of the stomach and pancreas
• Increased risk of cancers of the mouth, esophagus, stomach, pancreas, and colon

BONES
• Increased risk of osteoporosis

REPRODUCTIVE SYSTEM
• **Women:** menstrual irregularities and increased risk of birth defects
• **Men:** impotence and testicular atrophy
• **Both sexes:** increased risk of breast cancer

Figure 7.5 Effects of Alcohol on the Body and Health

Mastering **Health & Nutrition** Long- and Short-Term Effects of Alcohol

nerves that control involuntary actions such as breathing and the gag reflex (which prevents choking). At higher BAC levels, these functions can be completely suppressed. If a drinker becomes unconscious and vomits, there is danger of deadly asphyxiation through choking on one's own vomit. BAC can rise even after a drinker becomes unconscious, because alcohol in the stomach and intestine continues to empty into the bloodstream.

Skills for **Behavior Change**

Dealing With An Alcohol Emergency

Heavy drinking can be life threatening. Anyone who has passed out from drinking should be watched very closely. Roll an unconscious drinker onto his or her side with knees bent to minimize the chance of vomit obstructing the airway. If the drinker vomits, you might need to reach into his or her mouth and clear the airway.

If you suspect that someone has alcohol poisoning, call 9-1-1 immediately to get help. For the safety of yourself and your friends, know the signs of acute alcohol intoxication:

■ Mental confusion, stupor, coma, or inability to be roused
■ Vomiting and/or seizures
■ Slow breathing (fewer than eight breaths per minute)
■ Rapid or irregular pulse (100 beats or more per minute) or irregular breathing (10 seconds or more between breaths)
■ Cool, clammy skin; bluish skin, fingernails, or lips.

Check Yourself

■ What are the short-term health effects of alcohol consumption?

■ What actions should you take if you're with someone who shows symptoms of alcohol poisoning?

7.4 Alcohol and Your Health: Long-Term Effects

Learning Outcome

7.4 **Discuss the long-term health effects of alcohol consumption.**

Alcohol is distributed throughout most of the body and may affect many organs and tissues. Problems associated with long-term, habitual alcohol abuse include diseases of the nervous system, cardiovascular system, and liver, as well as some cancers.

The nervous system is especially sensitive to alcohol. Even moderate drinkers experience shrinkage in brain size and weight and some loss of intellectual ability. Alcohol appears to damage the frontal areas of the adolescent brain—crucial for controlling impulses and thinking through consequences of intended actions.[38]

People who begin drinking at an early age are at much higher risk of experiencing alcohol abuse or dependence, drinking five or more drinks per occasion, and driving under the influence of alcohol at least weekly.[39]

Numerous studies have associated light-to-moderate alcohol consumption (no more than two drinks a day) with reduced risk of coronary artery disease, most likely as a result of an increase in high-density lipoproteins (HDLs), or "good" cholesterol.[40] However, alcohol consumption causes many more cardiovascular health hazards than benefits, contributing to high blood pressure and slightly increased heart rate and cardiac output.

One of the most common diseases related to alcohol abuse is **cirrhosis** of the liver (**Figure 7.6**). With heavy drinking, the liver begins to store fat; fat-filled cells stop functioning. Continued drinking can cause *fibrosis*, in which the liver develops fibrous scar tissue. If the person continues to drink, cirrhosis results—the liver cells die, and the damage becomes permanent. In **alcoholic hepatitis**, another serious condition, chronic inflammation of the liver develops, which may be fatal in itself or may progress to cirrhosis.

Long-term alcohol use has been linked to cancers of the esophagus, colon, rectum, breast, stomach, oral cavity, and liver. The leading alcohol-related cancer in women is breast cancer; in men, the leading alcohol-related cancer is colorectal cancer.[41]

There is substantial evidence to suggest that women who consume even low levels of alcohol have a higher risk of breast cancer than those who abstain. A recent study found that women who consumed 0.5 to 1.5 drinks per day had a 6 percent increased risk of breast cancer compared to those who drank less than half a drink a day.[42] The risk was higher for women with a family history of breast cancer.[43]

The pancreas produces digestive enzymes and insulin. Chronic alcohol abuse reduces enzyme production, inhibiting nutrient absorption. Alcohol may also impair the body's ability to recognize and fight bacteria and viruses. Drinking alcohol can block absorption of calcium, a matter of particular concern to women because of their risk for osteoporosis. Drinking alcohol also significantly increases trouble with both falling asleep and staying asleep.

Alcohol and Pregnancy

Teratogenic substances cause birth defects. Of 30 known teratogens, alcohol is one of the most dangerous. In the United States, more than 1 in 5 pregnant women report alcohol use during early pregnancy.[44]

Consuming four or more drinks a day during pregnancy may significantly increase the baby's risk of childhood mental health and learning problems. Alcohol consumed during the first trimester poses the greatest threat to fetal organ development; exposure during the last trimester, when the brain develops rapidly, is most likely to affect the CNS.

Fetal alcohol syndrome (FAS), which is associated with alcohol consumption during pregnancy, is the third most common birth defect and the second leading cause of mental retardation in the United States, with an estimated incidence of 0.2 to 1.5 cases in every 1,000 live births.[45] Symptoms include mental retardation; small head; tremors; abnormalities of the face, limbs, heart, and brain; poor memory; reduced attention span; and impulsive behavior.

Children with some symptoms of FAS may be diagnosed with partial fetal alcohol syndrome (PFAS) or alcohol-related neurodevelopmental disorder (ARND); these, like FAS, are *fetal alcohol spectrum disorders (FASD)*. Infants whose mothers binge-drink when pregnant are at higher risk for FASD.[46] To avoid any chance of harming her fetus, any woman who is or may become pregnant should not consume alcohol.

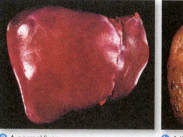 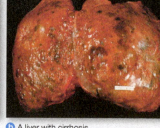

ⓐ A normal liver ⓑ A liver with cirrhosis

Figure 7.6 Comparison of a Healthy Liver with a Cirrhotic Liver

Check Yourself

- **What are some long-term health effects of alcohol consumption?**

- **How does awareness of these effects influence your decision whether to consume alcohol?**

7.5 Drinking and Driving

Learning Outcome

7.5 List effects of alcohol use on the ability to drive safely.

Traffic accidents are the leading cause of accidental death for all age groups from 1 to 25 years old.[47] In the United States, adults drink too much and get behind the wheel approximately 121 million times (based on self-reports) in a year.[48] Alcohol-impaired drivers are involved in about 1 in 3 crash deaths, resulting in nearly 10,000 deaths a year—roughly one traffic fatality every 53 minutes.[49]

Unfortunately, college students are overrepresented in alcohol-related crashes. A recent survey reported that 21 percent of college students have driven after drinking, and about 2 percent said they had driven after drinking five or more drinks in the past 30 days.[50]

Over the past 20 years, the percentage of intoxicated drivers involved in fatal crashes decreased for all age groups (**Figure 7.7**). Several factors probably contributed: laws that raised the drinking age to 21, stricter law enforcement, laws prohibiting anyone under 21 from driving with any detectable BAC, increased automobile safety, and educational programs designed to discourage drinking and driving. Furthermore, all states have zero-tolerance laws for driving while intoxicated, and the penalty is usually suspension of the driver's license.

Despite all these measures, the risk of being involved in an alcohol-related automobile crash remains substantial. Laboratory and test track research shows that the vast majority of drivers are impaired even at 0.08 BAC with regard to critical driving tasks. The likelihood of a driver being involved in a fatal crash rises significantly with a BAC of 0.05 percent and even more rapidly after 0.08 percent.[51]

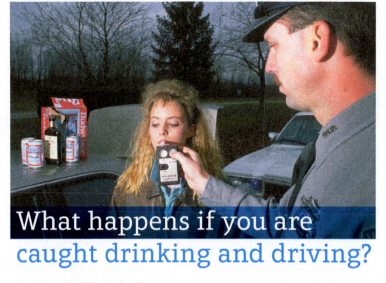

What happens if you are caught drinking and driving?

Getting behind the wheel if you have consumed alcohol is a dangerous choice, with serious legal consequences if you are caught and convicted of driving under the influence (DUI). If you are under age 21 and have any detectable alcohol in your bloodstream, your license can be revoked. Other common penalties for DUI include driver's license restrictions, fines, mandatory counseling, and jail time, even for a first offense. In many states, if you are convicted three times for DUI, you are considered a habitual violator and penalized as a felon, meaning that you lose your right to vote and to own a weapon, among other rights, as well as possibly losing your license permanently. If you are involved in an accident in which someone is injured or killed, the consequences are even more serious. Involvement in such an incident is considered a felony in many states. If a person dies as a result of the accident, the drunk driver may be charged with manslaughter or second-degree murder.

Alcohol-related fatal crashes occur more often at night than during the day, and the hours between 9:00 p.m. and 6:00 a.m. are the most dangerous.[52] Fifty-three percent of fatally injured drivers involved in nighttime single-vehicle crashes had BACs at or above 0.08 percent.[53] The risk of being involved in an alcohol-related crash increases not only with the time of day, but also with the day of the week; 23 percent of all fatal crashes during the week were alcohol related, compared with 42 percent on weekends.[54]

3 in 10 Americans will be involved in an **alcohol-related accident** at some time in their lives.

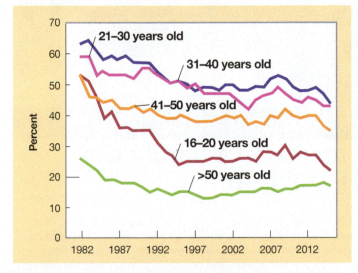

Figure 7.7 Percentage of Fatally Injured Drivers with BACs Greater Than 0.08%, by Driver Age, 1982–2015

Source: Insurance Institute for Highway Safety, "Alcohol Impaired Driving 2015: Alcohol," Copyright 2017. Reprinted with permission.

Check Yourself

■ How does alcohol impact the ability to drive?

Alcohol Use Disorder

7.6 Discuss biological and psychological causes of alcohol use disorder.

The new edition of the *Diagnostic and Statistical Manual of Mental Disorders (DSM-5)* has integrated alcohol abuse and alcohol dependence into a single disorder: **alcohol use disorder (AUD)**. Any person who meets two or more of the new criteria would receive a diagnosis of AUD. The severity of AUD falls along a spectrum from mild to moderate to severe, according to the number of criteria a person meets.

Identifying an Alcoholic

As with other drug addictions, tolerance, psychological dependence, and withdrawal symptoms must be present to qualify a drinker as an addict. Irresponsible and problem drinkers, such as people who get into fights or embarrass themselves or others when they drink, aren't necessarily alcoholics. About 15 percent of people in the United States are problem drinkers, and about 5 to 10 percent of male drinkers and 3 to 5 percent of females would be diagnosed as alcohol dependent.[55]

About 1 in 5 college students meet the criteria for AUD.[56] In a recent study, the progression to alcohol dependency based on college students' drinking patterns when they entered showed that 1.9 percent of nondrinkers, 4.3 percent of light drinkers, 12.8 percent of moderate drinkers, and 19 percent of heavy drinkers developed alcohol dependency.[57]

Causes of Alcohol Abuse and Alcoholism

Biological and Family Factors Children of alcoholics have higher rates of alcoholism than the general population. Alcoholism among individuals with a family history of alcoholism is about four to eight times more common than it is among individuals with no such family history.[58]

Despite such evidence, scientists do not yet understand the precise role of genes in increased risk for alcoholism, nor have they identified a specific "alcoholism" gene. Alcohol use disorders are approximately 60 percent heritable.[59] Adoption studies demonstrate a strong link between biological parents' substance use and their children's risk for addiction.[60]

Research has found that alcohol stimulates the production of dopamine, which activates the pleasure center of the brain. In alcoholics, the dopamine response to alcohol is diminished, leading them to drink more alcohol to feel the same pleasurable effects.[61] No single gene causes addiction, though, and multiple genes can affect the ability to develop addiction.

Social and Cultural Factors Some people begin drinking as a way to dull the pain of an acute loss or an emotional or social problem. Unfortunately, the discomfort that causes many people to turn to alcohol ultimately causes even more discomfort as the drug's depressant effect takes its toll. Eventually, the drinker becomes physically dependent.

Family attitudes also seem to be an influence; people raised in cultures in which alcohol is a part of religious or ceremonial activities or a traditional part of the family meal are less prone to alcohol dependence. In contrast, the tendency for abuse appears greater in societies in which alcohol purchase is carefully controlled and drinking regarded as a rite of passage.

The amount of alcohol a person consumes seems to be directly related to the drinking habits of that individual's social group. People whose friends and relatives drink heavily are more likely to drink heavily themselves—a finding with importance for individuals who need to sever ties with heavy drinkers to maintain abstinence.

AUD in Women

Women tend to become alcoholics at later ages and after fewer years of heavy drinking than do men. Women also get addicted faster with less alcohol use. With greater risks for cirrhosis; excessive memory loss and shrinkage of the brain; heart disease; and cancers of the mouth, throat, esophagus, liver, and colon than male alcoholics, women suffer the consequences of alcoholism more profoundly. The risk of breast cancer increases with alcohol use.[62]

The highest risks for alcoholism occur among women who are unmarried but living with a partner, are in their twenties or early thirties, or have a husband or partner who drinks heavily. Other

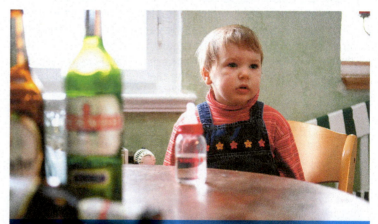

How does it affect you to grow up in a family with alcoholism?

Adult children of alcoholics have unique problems stemming from a lack of parental nurturing during childhood: difficulty developing social attachments, a need to be in control of all emotions and situations, low self-esteem, and depression. Fortunately, not everyone who grows up in an alcoholic family is doomed to lifelong problems. As they mature, many develop resiliency in response to their families' problems and enter adulthood armed with positive strengths and valuable skills.

risks for women include a family history of drinking problems, pressure to drink from a peer or spouse, depression, and stress.

Effects on Family and Friends

An estimated 7.5 million children in the United States live with a parent who has experienced an AUD in the past year. These children are at increased risk for physical illness, emotional disturbances, depression, suicide, behavioral problems, lower educational performance, violence, and susceptibility to alcoholism or other addictions later in life.[63]

In dysfunctional families, children learn certain unspoken rules that allow the family to avoid dealing with real problems: Don't talk, don't trust, and don't feel. Unfortunately, these behaviors enable the alcoholic to keep drinking. Children in such families generally assume at least one of the following roles:

- **Family hero.** Tries to divert attention from the problem by being too good to be true.
- **Scapegoat.** Draws attention from the family's primary problem through delinquency or misbehavior.
- **Lost child.** Becomes passive and withdraws from upsetting situations.
- **Mascot.** Disrupts tense situations with comic relief.

Children in alcoholic homes have to deal with constant stress, anxiety, and embarrassment. The alcoholic is the center of attention; the children's needs are often ignored. It is not uncommon for these children to be victims of violence, abuse, neglect, or incest.

Living with a family member (or friend or roommate) who is an alcoholic can be extremely stressful. People in close proximity to alcoholics can find themselves in codependent relationships that are often emotionally destructive or abusive and that enable the alcoholic's addiction. Codependents try to cover up for the addicted person: They may make excuses for the drinker's behavior or lie to others to cover for him or her.

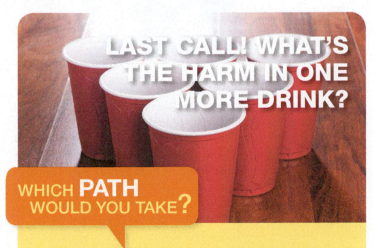

LAST CALL! WHAT'S THE HARM IN ONE MORE DRINK?

WHICH **PATH** WOULD YOU TAKE?

Go to Mastering Health to play "Making Smart Choices about Alcohol Use" and see how your actions today affect your future health.

Costs to Society

Alcohol-related costs to society are estimated to be well over $249 billion when health insurance, criminal justice costs, treatment costs, and lost productivity are considered.[64] These costs break down to 72 percent from loss in workplace productivity, 11 percent related to health care expenses for treating problems caused by excessive drinking, 10 percent for criminal justice costs, and 5 percent related to losses from motor vehicle crashes.[65] Binge drinking alone accounts for the majority (77 percent) of the economic cost. Ultimately, excessive drinking losses cost an estimated $807 per person, or $2.05 for each drink consumed.[66]

Alcoholism is directly or indirectly responsible for more than 25 percent of the nation's medical expenses and lost earnings.[67] Emotional, mental, and physical costs are impossible to measure. However, the toll that alcohol takes from loss of loved ones in drunk-driving accidents, as a result of alcohol-related violence and abuse in homes, and the costs to families and relationships is likely to be huge.

AUD as a Global Issue

Throughout the world, alcohol is a factor in 60 types of diseases and injuries and a component cause in 200 others. Almost 4 percent of all deaths worldwide are attributed to alcohol, more than deaths caused by HIV/AIDS, violence, or tuberculosis. Worldwide, the impact of alcohol use is as follows:[68]

- Alcohol use results in 3.3 million deaths each year.
- * 5.1 percent of the global burden of disease and injury is attributable to alcohol, as measured by disability-adjusted life years.
- 7.6 percent of male deaths and 4.0 percent of female deaths worldwide are attributable to alcohol consumption.
- Early alcohol use (before the age of 14) is positively correlated with harmful behaviors later in life, including alcohol addiction and drunk driving.
- At the same level of alcohol consumption, men are more likely to become injured and women are more likely to experience negative health outcomes such as cancer (particularly breast cancer), cardiovascular disease, and gastrointestinal problems.

A large variation exists in adult per capita alcohol consumption. The highest consumption levels can be found in the developed world, including Europe and the Americas. Intermediate consumption levels can be found in regions of the Western Pacific and Africa. Low consumption levels can be found in Southeast Asia and the Eastern Mediterranean regions. Many factors, including culture, religion, economic development, and socioeconomic status, contribute to these differences.[69]

Check Yourself

- What factors can make a person more likely to abuse alcohol or become an alcoholic?
- How does alcohol use disorder affect the family and friends of the alcoholic?
- What actions can you take to reduce your own risks of alcohol use disorder? What might you do to help a friend or family member who is struggling with AUD?

7.6

Alcohol and Tobacco

7.7 List practical steps for reducing alcohol intake.

Alcohol use disorder is characterized by symptoms including craving, loss of control, physical dependence, and tolerance. People who recognize one or more of these behaviors in themselves may wish to seek professional help to determine whether alcohol has become a controlling factor in their lives.

There are some steps that you can take on your own if you are concerned about the amount of alcohol that you consume. Being worried about your consumption is a strong signal that there may be cause for alarm. If a counselor or health care practitioner advises you to reduce or eliminate alcohol intake, you should follow their suggestions and guidance. There are also ways for you to cut down your drinking on your own, depending on their recommendations.

Skills for **Behavior Change**

How To Cut Down On Your Drinking

If you suspect that you drink too much, talk with a counselor or clinician at your student health center. These professionals can tell you whether you should cut down or abstain. If you have a severe drinking problem, alcoholism in your family, or other medical problems, you should stop drinking completely. Your counselor or clinician will advise you about what is right for you.

If you need to cut down on your drinking, these steps can help you:

- **Write your reasons for cutting down or stopping.** There are many reasons you may want to cut down or stop drinking. You might want to improve your health, sleep better, or get along better with your family or friends.
- **Set a drinking goal.** Determine a limit for how much you will drink. You may choose to cut down, or to not drink at all. If you aren't sure what goal is right for you, talk with your counselor. Once you determine your goal, write it down on a piece of paper. Put it someplace you can see it, such as on your refrigerator or bathroom mirror.
- **Keep a journal of your drinking.** Write down every time you have a drink. Try to keep your journal for 3 or 4 weeks. This will show you how much you drink and when. You may be surprised. How different is your goal from the amount you drink now?
- **Keep little or no alcohol at home.** You don't need the temptation.
- **Drink slowly.** When you drink, sip slowly. Take a break of 1 hour between drinks. Drink a nonalcoholic beverage, such as soda, water, or juice, after every alcoholic drink you consume. Do not drink alcohol on an empty stomach. Eat food when you are drinking.

- **Take a break from alcohol.** Pick a day or two each week when you will not drink at all. Then try to stop drinking for 1 week. Think about how you feel physically and emotionally on these days. When you succeed and feel better, you may find it easier to cut down for good.
- **Learn how to say no.** You do not have to drink when other people are drinking or take a drink when offered one. Practice ways to say no politely. Stay away from people who give you a hard time about not drinking.
- **Stay active.** Use the time and money you once spent on drinking to do something fun with your family or friends. Go out to eat, see a movie, or play sports or a game.
- **Get support.** Cutting down on your drinking may be difficult at times. Ask your family and friends for support to help you reach your goal. Talk to your counselor if you are having trouble cutting down. Get the help you need to reach your goal.

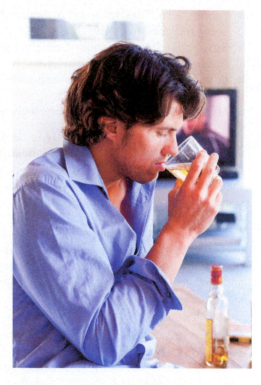

- **Avoid temptations.** Watch out for people, places, or times that lead you to drink even if you did not want to. Plan ahead of time what you will do to avoid drinking when you are tempted. Do not drink when you are angry, upset, or having a bad day.
- **Remember, don't give up!** Most people don't cut down or give up drinking all at once. As with a diet, it is not easy to change. That's okay. If you don't reach your goal the first time, try again. Remember, get support from people who care about you and want to help.

- What are some practical steps you can take to cut down on your drinking?

- Have you ever decided to reduce the amount of alcohol you consume? If so, what were the steps that you took?

7.8 Explain treatment options available to alcoholics.

Only a very small percentage of alcoholics ever receive care in special treatment facilities. Numerous factors contribute to this low rate of treatment utilization, including an inability or unwillingness to admit to an alcohol problem, the social stigma, the abstinence that seeking treatment would require, and desire to deal with alcohol problems on one's own.[70] Importantly, high costs of many programs keep people from enrolling. Most problem drinkers who seek help have experienced a turning point when the person recognizes that alcohol controls his or her life.

Alcoholics who decide to quit drinking will experience *detoxification*, the process by which addicts end their dependence on a drug. Withdrawal symptoms include hyperexcitability, confusion, agitation, sleep disorders, convulsions, tremors, depression, headache, and seizures. For a small percentage of people, alcohol withdrawal results in a severe syndrome known as **delirium tremens (DTs)**, characterized by confusion, delusions, agitated behavior, and hallucinations.

The alcoholic who is ready for help has several avenues of treatment: psychologists and psychiatrists specializing in treatment, private treatment centers, hospitals specifically designed to treat alcoholics, community mental health facilities, and support groups such as **Alcoholics Anonymous (AA)**.

Private Treatment Facilities

On admission to a private treatment facility, the patient receives a complete physical examination to determine whether any underlying medical problems will interfere with treatment. Shortly after detoxification, alcoholics begin their treatment for psychological addiction. Most treatment facilities keep their patients from 3 to 6 weeks. Treatment at private centers can cost several thousand dollars, but some insurance programs or employers will assume most of this expense.

Therapy

Several types of therapy are commonly used in alcoholism recovery programs. In family therapy, the person and family members examine the psychological reasons underlying the addiction and environmental factors enabling it. In individual and group therapy, alcoholics learn positive coping skills for situations that have regularly caused them to turn to alcohol. Typically, the alcoholic will participate in some or all of these types of therapy as part of the recovery process.

While there are many recovery management strategies for adults, understanding an appropriate recovery support system for college students has received less attention. In particular, there has been a lack of campus-based services for recovering students. The high prevalence of alcohol use and other drug use on college campuses makes attending college a threat to sobriety. However, many campuses recognize the need to create recovery-friendly space and supportive environments for students engaged in recovery. Common features of such programs include a designated campus meeting space, drug-free housing options, individual or group counseling, relapse prevention, and sober leisure activities. In addition, such programs emphasize peer support and incorporate Alcoholics Anonymous' twelve-step approach.[71]

Relapse

Success in recovery varies with the individual. Treating an addiction requires more than getting the addict to stop using a substance; it also requires getting the person to break a pattern of behavior that has dominated his or her life. Many alcoholics refer to themselves as "recovering" throughout their lifetime rather than "cured." In fact, only about a third of people who are abstinent less than a year will remain abstinent.[72]

People seeking to regain a healthy lifestyle must not only confront their addiction, but also guard against the tendency to relapse. For alcoholics, it is important to identify situations that could trigger a relapse, such as becoming angry or frustrated and being around other people who drink.

During the initial recovery period, it can help to join a support group, maintain stability (resisting the urge to move, travel, assume a new job, or make other drastic life changes), set aside time each day for reflection, and maintain a pattern of assuming responsibility for one's own actions. To be effective, recovery programs must be able to help an alcoholic improve his or her self-esteem and resume personal growth.

Additional points to remember:

1. In alcohol use disorder, you typically can't control your drinking or your emotions and both need "fixing."
2. Counseling or therapy for you and your family should be a priority. Learning new skills, learning to control stress, anxiety, anger, and frustration should be a focus for the alcoholic and their loved ones.
3. Rebuilding trust and support should be a goal within the alcoholic's close relationships.
4. Setting short and long term goals is important.
5. Learning to recognize your unique triggers is a first step on your path to recovery.
6. You didn't become an alcoholic overnight, and you won't get better overnight. Be self-compassionate, work toward your goals, and remember that you have the strength to break the addiction cycle.

- Why do so few alcoholics receive treatment?
- What treatment options are available for alcoholics?
- Why is family therapy a component of alcohol treatment programs?

7.9 Examine reasons that people start smoking and factors that contribute to tobacco use by college students.

Approximately 36 million Americans age 18 and older report using tobacco products (cigarettes, cigars, smokeless tobacco, and pipe tobacco) at least once in the past month.[73] In 2015, 16.7 percent of men and 13.6 percent of women were current cigarette smokers. Nearly 13 percent of adults age 18 to 24 are cigarette smokers, yet adults age 25 to 44 had the highest percentage of current cigarette smoking (18 percent). The percentage of smokers then decreases with age, with 17 percent of adults age 45 to 64 and 8 percent of adults age 65 years and older reported to be current smokers.[74]

Why Do People Use Tobacco?

Nicotine Addiction Beginning smokers usually feel the effects of nicotine with their first puff. These symptoms, called **nicotine poisoning**, can include dizziness, lightheadedness, rapid and erratic pulse, clammy skin, nausea, vomiting, and diarrhea. Symptoms cease as tolerance develops, which happens as quickly as the second or third cigarette. Many regular smokers experience no "buzz" but continue to smoke because stopping is too difficult.

Behavioral Dependence People who smoke are not just physically but also psychologically dependent. Nicotine tricks the brain into creating pleasurable associations with sensory stimuli or environmental cues that may trigger the urge for a cigarette.[75] Some former smokers remain vulnerable to sensory and environmental cues for many years after they quit.

Weight Control Nicotine is an appetite suppressant and slightly increases the basal metabolic rate. After smoking a cigarette, one's metabolism quickly increases, then returns to normal; heavy smokers have such surges throughout the day. When a smoker quits, the metabolic rate slows down, and appetite returns. People tend to eat more, particularly sweets. Fear of gaining weight is one of the biggest reasons smokers are reluctant to quit. To avoid weight gain after quitting smoking, avoid crash diets, keep low-calorie treats handy, and drink plenty of water.

Advertising The tobacco industry spends an estimated $26 million per day on advertising and promotional material.[76] With the number of smokers declining by about 1 million each year, the industry must actively recruit new smokers.[77] Studies have found that children are three times more susceptible to advertising run by tobacco companies than are adults, that children are more likely to smoke as a result of cigarette marketing than because of peer pressure, and that tobacco company advertising and promotion can be cited as the culprit for a third of underage experimentation with smoking.[78]

Tobacco products are heavily advertised to specific populations. In women's magazines, ads imply that smoking is the key to financial success, desirability, beauty, weight control, independence, social acceptance, and being "cool." These ads have apparently been working; from the mid-1970s through the early 2000s, cigarette sales to women increased dramatically. Not coincidentally, cigarette-induced lung cancer had surpassed breast cancer as the leading cancer killer among women by 1987 and has remained the leading cancer killer in every year since.[79]

Women are not the only targets of gender-based cigarette advertisements. Ads depict men in locker rooms, charging over

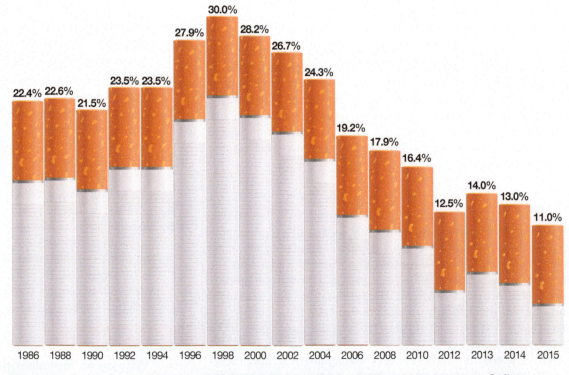

Figure 7.8 **Trends in the Prevalence of Cigarette Smoking in the Past Month among College Students**

Source: Data from L.D. Johnston et al., *Monitoring the Future National Survey Results on Drug Use, 1975–2015, Volume II, College Students and Adults Ages 19–50* (Ann Arbor: Institute for Social Research, University of Michigan, 2016).

rugged terrain in off-road vehicles, or riding stallions into the sunset in blatant appeals to a need to feel and appear masculine. Minorities are also often the targets of heavy marketing. Tobacco advertising, particularly menthol cigarettes, is much more common in magazines aimed at African Americans, such as *Jet* and *Ebony*, than in similar magazines aimed at broader audiences, such as *Time* and *People*. Billboards and posters spreading the cigarette message have dotted the landscape in Hispanic communities for many years, especially in low-income areas. Tobacco companies also sponsor community-based events such as festivals and annual fairs.

Financial Costs to Society

In the United States, tobacco use is the single most preventable cause of death. Close to a half a million Americans die each year of tobacco-related diseases.[80] Another 16 million people suffer from health disorders caused by tobacco.[81] Estimates show annual costs attributed to smoking in the United States are between $289 billion and $333 billion.[82] The economic burden of tobacco use totals more than $170 billion in direct medical expenditures and more than $150 billion in lost productivity.[83] It is estimated that the costs of smoking-related health problems and productivity losses are $19.16 per pack of cigarettes sold.[84]

College Students and Tobacco Use

Although college students are the targets of heavy tobacco advertising campaigns, cigarette smoking among U.S. college students has decreased in recent years. In a 2016 survey, just over 10 percent of college students reported having smoked cigarettes in the past 30 days (**Figure 7.8**).[85] College men have slightly higher rates of smoking (13 percent) compared to women (8 percent); however, when students are asked how many students they think have smoked in the last thirty days, they perceive that rates are

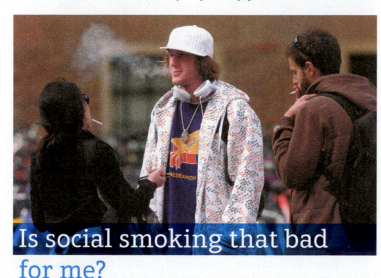

Is social smoking that bad for me?

An occasional puff once in a while when you are out with friends can't hurt, right? Wrong! There is no "safe" amount of tobacco use. Any smoking or exposure to smoke increases your risks for negative health effects such as heart disease and lung cancer.

as high as 75 percent![86] Men also use more cigars and smokeless tobacco than women.[87]

Why Do College Students Smoke?

Some college students smoke to relax or reduce stress. Other key reasons students smoke are to fit in or because they are addicted. For some students, weight control is an important motivator, and fear of weight gain is a common reason for smoking relapse. Students diagnosed or treated for depression are much more likely to use tobacco compared to students who are not.

Many college student smokers identify themselves as "social smokers," that is, they smoke only when they are with people, not when they are alone. Social smokers typically smoke on weekends, at night, at social events, or just hanging out with friends. Often, social smokers smoke to fit in with groups and to help ease social interactions.[88]

However, even occasional smoking carries the risks of damaging health effects. Smoking less than a pack of cigarettes a week has been shown to damage blood vessels and to increase the risk of heart disease and cancer.[89] Pregnant women who smoke only occasionally still run a risk of giving birth to babies with health problems.

Unlike social smokers, most students who smoke regularly and are nicotine dependent do want to stop smoking, but in spite of their efforts or desire to quit, they continue to smoke throughout college. To reduce the incidence of smoking among students, colleges and universities need to engage in antismoking efforts, control tobacco advertising, provide smoke-free residence halls, and offer greater access to smoking-cessation programs.

As policies designed to reduce cigarette smoking increase, the use of electronic cigarettes poses an additional challenge. Electronic cigarette use is banned on many campuses, airlines, and in many other public settings. Because e-cigarettes are not yet regulated by the FDA and their effects on health remain in question, many campuses are being proactive in reducing potential health threats.

67% of regular current smokers may eventually die of smoking-related diseases, according to a large Australian Study.

Check Yourself

- The tobacco industry has been accused of targeting college students in its marketing campaigns. Do you agree? If so, give examples of tobacco marketing that target young adults.

- What factors make college students more likely to use tobacco?

- What is your campus doing to reduce tobacco use by students?

7.10 Tobacco: Its Components and Effects

Learning Outcome

7.10 Compare and contrast tobacco products on the market.

Smoking, the most common form of tobacco use, delivers a strong dose of nicotine as well as 7,000 other chemical substances, including arsenic, formaldehyde, and ammonia, directly to the lungs. Among these chemicals are more than 69 known or suspected carcinogens (cancer-causing agents).[90] Inhaling hot toxic gases exposes sensitive mucous membranes to irritating chemicals that weaken the tissues and contribute to cancers of the mouth, larynx, and throat. The heat from tobacco smoke is also harmful to tissues.

Nicotine

The highly addictive chemical stimulant **nicotine** is the major psychoactive substance in all tobacco products. When tobacco leaves are burned in a cigarette, pipe, or cigar, the smoker inhales nicotine into the lungs. Sucking or chewing tobacco releases nicotine into the saliva; it is then absorbed through the mucous membranes in the mouth.

Nicotine is a powerful central nervous system stimulant that produces a variety of physiological effects. In the cerebral cortex, it produces an aroused, alert mental state. It stimulates production of adrenaline, increases heart and respiratory rates, constricts blood vessels, and thus increases blood pressure because the heart must work harder to pump blood through narrowed vessels.

Tar and Carbon Monoxide

Cigarette smoke is a complex mixture of chemicals and gases produced by the burning of tobacco and its additives. When inhaled, particulate matter condenses in the lungs to form a sludge called **tar**, which contains carcinogenic agents, such as benzopyrene, and chemical irritants, such as phenol. Phenol has the potential to combine with other chemicals that contribute to developing lung cancer.

In healthy lungs, millions of tiny hairlike projections (*cilia*) in the lining of the upper respiratory passages sweep away foreign matter, which is then expelled from the lungs by coughing. However, nicotine paralyzes the cilia for up to 1 hour following a single cigarette, allowing tars and other solids in tobacco smoke to accumulate and irritate lung tissue.

Cigarette smoke also contains poisonous gases, the most dangerous of which is **carbon monoxide**. In the human body, carbon monoxide enters the lungs and combines with hemoglobin, reducing or blocking the blood's ability to carry oxygen to cells. The more a person smokes, the greater the oxygen deprivation, eventually leading to flu-like symptoms, tiredness, headache, nausea, dizziness, and increased heart rate. Women who smoke during pregnancy can harm the fetus, particularly in the early trimesters. Over time there may be life-threatening CVD risks to the smoker and those who are exposed to secondary smoke.

Tobacco Products

Cigarettes *Filtered cigarettes* are the most common form of tobacco available today. Almost all manufactured cigarettes have filters designed to reduce levels of gases such as hydrogen cyanide and carbon monoxide, but these products may actually deliver more hazardous gases to the user than nonfiltered brands. Some smokers use low-tar and low-nicotine products as an excuse to smoke more cigarettes, but they wind up exposing themselves to more harmful substances than they would with a smaller number of regular-strength cigarettes.

Clove cigarettes contain about 40 percent ground cloves and 60 percent tobacco. Many users mistakenly believe that these products are made entirely of ground cloves and that smoking them eliminates the risks associated with tobacco. In fact, clove cigarettes contain higher levels of tar, nicotine, and carbon monoxide than do regular cigarettes. In addition, the numbing effect of eugenol, an ingredient in cloves, allows smokers to inhale more deeply. The same effect is true of *menthol cigarettes*: The throat-numbing effect of the menthol allows for deeper inhalation. Menthol cigarettes also have higher carbon monoxide concentrations than do regular cigarettes.

Cigars As cigarette use has declined, sales of large cigars have more than tripled.[91] Many people believe that cigars are safer than cigarettes when, in fact, the opposite is true. Cigars have higher levels of cancer-causing substances, more tar per gram of tobacco smoked, and higher levels of toxins than do cigarettes.[92] In addition,

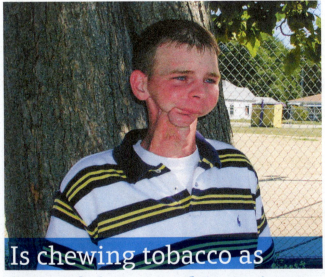

Is chewing tobacco as harmful as smoking cigarettes?

Dental problems are common among users of smokeless tobacco Contact with tobacco juice causes receding gums, tooth decay, bad breath, and discolored teeth. Damage to both the teeth and jawbone can contribute to loss of teeth. This young cancer survivor began using smokeless tobacco at age 13; by age 17, he was diagnosed with squamous cell carcinoma. He has undergone surgery to remove neck muscles, lymph nodes, and his tongue, and he now educates others about the dangers of chewing tobacco.

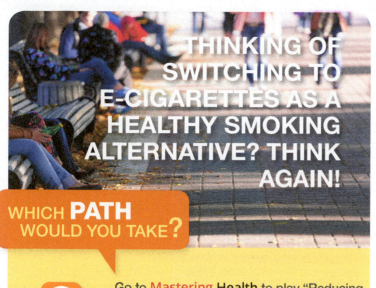

THINKING OF SWITCHING TO E-CIGARETTES AS A HEALTHY SMOKING ALTERNATIVE? THINK AGAIN!

WHICH PATH WOULD YOU TAKE?

Go to Mastering Health to play "Reducing Tobacco Use" and see how your actions today affect your future health.

cigar smoking causes many of the same diseases as cigarette smoking and using smokeless tobacco do. Regular cigar smokers are at risk for developing cancers of the lung, oral cavity, larynx, esophagus, and possibly pancreas. Cigar smokers have 4 to 10 times the risk of dying from lung, laryngeal, oral, or esophageal cancer compared to people who have never smoked.[93] Most cigars contain as much nicotine as several cigarettes, and when cigar smokers inhale, nicotine is absorbed as rapidly as it is with cigarettes. Those who don't inhale still expose the lips, tongue, throat, and larynx to toxic chemicals in tobacco smoke, and high levels of nicotine are still absorbed through the mouth's mucous membranes. A single cigar can provide as much nicotine as a pack of cigarettes.[94]

Pipes and Hookahs Pipes have had a long history of use throughout the world, including ritualistic and ceremonial usage for many cultures. Often thought to be safer than cigarettes or cigars, pipes are not risk-free. According to research by the National Cancer Institute and the American Cancer Society, pipe smoking carries risks similar to those of cigar smoking. Of concern is the increasing prevalence, particularly among college students, of the use of hookahs, or water pipes. Hookah smoking involves burning flavored tobacco in a water pipe and inhaling the smoke through a hose. Hookahs are marketed as reducing risks from hazardous chemicals by filtering the smoke through water before you inhale. However, many of the same harmful toxins and chemicals found in cigarettes—those associated with lung cancer, respiratory disease, low birth weight babies, and periodontal disease—are also found in hookah smoke.[95] Health risks associated with hookah use also include the possibility of infectious disease transmission by sharing a pipe.

Bidis Bidis are small, hand-rolled cigarettes in flavors such as vanilla, chocolate, and cherry. They have become increasingly popular with college students. Bidis are actually far more toxic than cigarettes and those that do not list ingredients should be avoided. Smoke from a bidi contains three to five times more nicotine than cigarettes do.[96] The leaf wrappers of bidis are nonporous, which

means that smokers must suck harder to inhale and inhale more to keep the bidi lit. This results in much more exposure to higher amounts of tar, nicotine, carbon monoxide, and other chemicals.

Smokeless Tobacco Smokeless tobacco is just as addictive as cigarettes and actually contains more nicotine; holding an average-sized dip or chew in the mouth for 30 minutes delivers as much nicotine as smoking four cigarettes. A 2-can-a-week snuff user gets as much nicotine as a 10-pack-a-week smoker.

Chewing tobacco comes in three forms—loose leaf, plug, or pouch—and contains tobacco leaves treated with molasses and other flavorings. The user "dips" the tobacco by placing a small amount between the lower lip and teeth to stimulate the flow of saliva and release the nicotine. **Dipping** rapidly releases nicotine into the bloodstream. While cigarette smoking has been on the decline in the United States among youth, use of smokeless tobacco by youth has held steady since 1999.[97]

Snuff is a finely ground form of tobacco that can be inhaled, chewed, or placed against the gums. It comes in dry or moist powdered form or sachets (tea bag–like pouches). "Snus" is the latest form of smokeless tobacco to hit the market in the United States. Popular for more than 100 years in Sweden, these small sachets of tobacco are placed inside the cheek and sucked.

See It! Videos

What are the dangers of e-cigarettes for children? Watch **GMA Investigates Liquid Nicotine** in the Study Area of Mastering Health.

Electronic Cigarettes and Vaping Electronic cigarettes (also called *e-cigarettes*, *electronic nicotine delivery systems*, *vape pens*, or simply *vapes*) typically deliver nicotine, flavorings (e.g., mint, chocolate) and other additives as vapor instead of smoke. When a user draws air through one of these devices, an airflow sensor activates the battery and heats the atomizer to vaporize propylene glycol and nicotine. Newer forms of devices offer flavored vaping devices that do not have batteries or produce heat; rather the user just simply inhales. On inhalation, the aerosol vapor delivers a dose of nicotine into the lungs, after which residual aerosol is exhaled into the environment. Beyond exposing users to chemicals such as nicotine, carbonyl compounds, and volatile organic compounds, the health effects of e-cigarette fluids, including solvents, flavorings, and toxicants, are not fully understood.[98]

In a recent survey of college students, about 11 percent of college students reported using e-cigarettes in the past, with 5 percent reporting usage in the past 30 days.[99] Students who use e-cigarettes are more likely to be heavy drinkers. While many campuses and many student apartments and rental houses have become tobacco or smoke free, the availability of e-cigarettes—and their barely detectable odor—may have allowed students to get around those bans and be able to more easily co-use alcohol and nicotine.[100]

Check Yourself

- How does nicotine affect the body?
- Why do some people mistakenly believe that some tobacco products are less harmful than others?

Health Hazards of Tobacco Products

Learning Outcome

7.11 **Summarize the health risks of tobacco products.**

Cigarette smoking adversely affects the health of every person who smokes, as well as the health of everyone nearby. Each day, tobacco contributes to approximately 1,200 deaths from cancer, cardiovascular disease, and respiratory disorders.[101] In addition, tobacco use can negatively affect the health of almost every system in your body (**Figure 7.9**).

Cancer

Lung cancer is the leading cause of cancer deaths in the United States. The American Cancer Society estimates that tobacco smoking causes 90 percent of all cases of lung cancer in men and 78 percent of cases in women.[102] There were an estimated 222,500 *new* cases of lung cancer in the United States in 2017 alone, and an estimated 155,870 Americans died from the disease in 2017.[103]

Smokers' risk of developing lung cancer depends on several factors. Someone who smokes two packs a day is 15 to 25 times more likely to develop lung cancer than a nonsmoker. A second factor is when you started smoking; an earlier start greatly increases risk. The combination of the number of smoking years multiplied by the dose smoked (number of cigarettes smoked/day) equals the number of *pack years*: a number often associated with a person's smoking-attributable health risks. A third factor associated with increased risk is whether you inhale deeply when you smoke.

A major risk of chewing tobacco is **leukoplakia**, leathery white patches inside the mouth produced by contact with irritants in tobacco juice (**Figure 7.10**). While leukoplakia does not develop into cancer in most cases, it may be precancerous and can eventually progress to cancer without proper treatment or may already be cancerous on initial sighting.[104]

Over 49,670 cases of oral cancer were diagnosed in 2017, the vast majority of which were caused by smokeless tobacco or

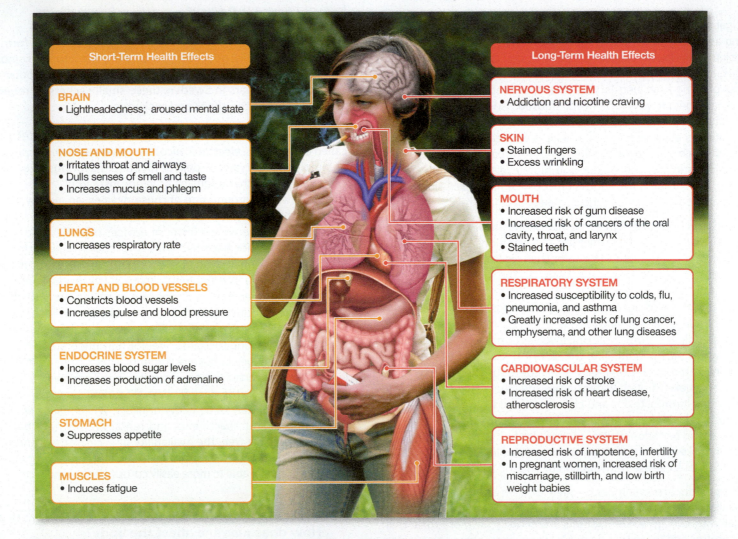

Short-Term Health Effects

BRAIN
• Lightheadedness; aroused mental state

NOSE AND MOUTH
• Irritates throat and airways
• Dulls senses of smell and taste
• Increases mucus and phlegm

LUNGS
• Increases respiratory rate

HEART AND BLOOD VESSELS
• Constricts blood vessels
• Increases pulse and blood pressure

ENDOCRINE SYSTEM
• Increases blood sugar levels
• Increases production of adrenaline

STOMACH
• Suppresses appetite

MUSCLES
• Induces fatigue

Long-Term Health Effects

NERVOUS SYSTEM
• Addiction and nicotine craving

SKIN
• Stained fingers
• Excess wrinkling

MOUTH
• Increased risk of gum disease
• Increased risk of cancers of the oral cavity, throat, and larynx
• Stained teeth

RESPIRATORY SYSTEM
• Increased susceptibility to colds, flu, pneumonia, and asthma
• Greatly increased risk of lung cancer, emphysema, and other lung diseases

CARDIOVASCULAR SYSTEM
• Increased risk of stroke
• Increased risk of heart disease, atherosclerosis

REPRODUCTIVE SYSTEM
• Increased risk of impotence, infertility
• In pregnant women, increased risk of miscarriage, stillbirth, and low birth weight babies

Figure 7.9 **Effects of Smoking on the Body and Health**

Mastering **Health & Nutrition** Long- and Short-Term Effects of Tobacco

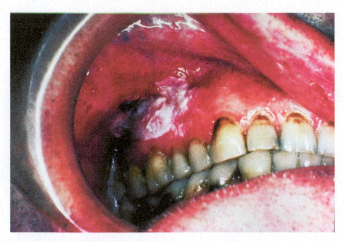

Figure 7.10 Leukoplakia
Leukoplakia, which can appear on the tongue or in the mouth as shown here, can be a precursor to oral cancer.

cigarettes.[105] Smokeless tobacco users have significantly higher rates of oral cancer than do nonusers. Warning signs include lumps in the jaw, neck, or lips; white, smooth, or scaly patches in the mouth or on the neck, lips, or tongue; mouth sores or bleeding that doesn't heal in 2 weeks; and difficulty speaking or swallowing. The time between first use and contracting cancer is shorter for smokeless tobacco users than for smokers.

Tobacco is linked to other cancers as well. The rate of pancreatic cancer is more than twice as high for smokers as for nonsmokers. Smokers are at increased risk to develop cancers of the lip, tongue, salivary glands, and esophagus. Long-term use of smokeless tobacco increases the risk of cancers of the larynx, esophagus, nasal cavity, pancreas, colon, kidney, and bladder.

Cardiovascular Disease

Smoking tobacco is a major risk factor for cardiovascular disease and stroke.[106] Smoking contributes to heart disease by aging the arteries.[107] This occurs because smoking and exposure to environmental tobacco smoke encourage and accelerate the buildup of fatty deposits (*plaque*) in the heart and major blood vessels (*atherosclerosis*). Smokers can experience a 50 percent increase in plaque accumulation in the arteries compared with ex-smokers. Nonsmokers regularly exposed to environmental tobacco smoke can have a 20 to 25 percent increase in plaque buildup.[108] For unknown reasons, smoking decreases blood levels of HDLs, the "good cholesterol" that helps to protect against heart attacks.

Smoking also contributes to **platelet adhesiveness**, the sticking together of red blood cells associated with blood clots. Smoking decreases oxygen supplied to the heart and contributes to irregular heart rhythms, which can trigger a heart attack. Smokers are two to four times as likely to suffer strokes as nonsmokers.[109] A stroke occurs when a small blood vessel in the brain bursts or is blocked by a blood clot, denying the brain oxygen and nourishment. Depending on the brain area affected, stroke can result in paralysis, loss of mental functioning, or death. Smoking contributes to strokes by raising blood pressure, which increases stress on vessel walls. Platelet adhesiveness contributes to blood clot formation.

Respiratory Disorders

Smokers are more prone to breathlessness, chronic cough, and excess phlegm production than are nonsmokers their age. Ultimately, smokers are up to 25 times more likely to die of lung disease than are nonsmokers.[110]

Chronic bronchitis may develop in smokers because their inflamed lungs produce more mucus, which they constantly try to expel along with foreign particles. This results in the persistent cough known as "smoker's hack." Smokers are also more prone to respiratory ailments such as influenza, pneumonia, and colds, and smoking exacerbates asthma symptoms.

Emphysema is a chronic disease in which the alveoli (the tiny air sacs in the lungs) are destroyed, impairing the lungs' ability to obtain oxygen and remove carbon dioxide and making breathing very difficult. Because the heart has to work harder to do even the simplest tasks, it may become enlarged and death from heart damage may result. There is no known cure, and the damage is irreversible. Approximately 80 to 90 percent of all cases of emphysema are related to cigarette smoking.[111]

Sexual Dysfunction and Fertility Problems

Despite attempts by tobacco advertisers to make smoking appear sexy, research shows that smoking can actually cause impotence in men. Studies have found that male smokers are much more likely to experience erectile dysfunction than are nonsmokers.[112] Women who smoke increase their risk for infertility, ectopic pregnancy, spontaneous abortion, and stillbirth. Smoking also increases the risk of sudden infant death syndrome and the chances of a baby being born with a cleft lip or cleft palate.[113] Smoking during pregnancy increases the chance of premature birth and the risk of low birth weight (less than 5.5 pounds), which in turn increases the likelihood of illness or death of an infant.[114]

Other Health Effects

Studies have shown tobacco use to be a serious risk factor in the development of gum disease.[115] In addition, smoking increases the risk of macular degeneration, one of the most common causes of blindness in older adults. It also causes premature skin wrinkling, staining of the teeth, yellowing of the fingernails, and bad breath. Nicotine speeds up the process by which the body uses and eliminates drugs, making medications less effective. In addition, recent research suggests smoking significantly increases the risk for Alzheimer's disease.[116]

Check Yourself

- **What are the major health risks from smoking tobacco? Which health risks are likely to affect people during their college years?**

- **Explain how the use of tobacco products affects the lungs and heart and who might be at particular risk.**

- **Name at least four types of cancer that are linked to the use of tobacco and what factors increase or decrease individual risks.**

7.12 Environmental Tobacco Smoke

Learning Outcome

7.12 Describe the risks of environmental tobacco smoke.

Environmental tobacco smoke (ETS), also known as *second-hand smoke*, is divided into two categories: **mainstream smoke** (smoke exhaled by a smoker) and **sidestream smoke** (smoke from the burning end of a cigarette). People who breathe smoke from someone else's smoking product are said to be *involuntary smokers* or *passive smokers*. Between 1988 and 2008, detectable levels of nicotine exposure in nonsmoking Americans decreased from 87.9 percent to 25.3 percent.[117]

Risks from Environmental Tobacco Smoke

Although involuntary smokers breathe less tobacco than active smokers do, they still face risks from exposure. ETS contains hundreds of chemicals known to be toxic or carcinogenic, including formaldehyde, benzene, vinyl chloride, arsenic ammonia, and hydrogen cyanide.[118] Every year, ETS is estimated to be responsible for approximately 3,400 lung cancer deaths in nonsmoking adults, 46,000 coronary and heart disease deaths in nonsmoking adults who live with smokers, and higher risk of death in newborns from sudden infant death syndrome.[119]

The Environmental Protection Agency (EPA) has designated secondhand smoke as a known (group A) carcinogen. More than 70 cancer-causing agents are found in secondhand smoke.[120] There is also strong evidence that secondhand smoke interferes with normal functioning of the heart, blood, and vascular systems, significantly increasing the risk for heart disease. Studies indicate that nonsmokers exposed to secondhand smoke were far more likely to have coronary heart disease and stroke than were non-smokers who had not been exposed to smoke.[121]

Children and Environmental Tobacco Smoke

More than 53 percent of U.S. children age 3 to 11 are exposed to ETS.[122] Disparities in ETS also occur along racial and class lines. African Americans have been found to have higher levels of exposure to ETS than whites and Hispanics; exposure is also higher for low-income people.[123]

Exposure to ETS increases children's risk of lower respiratory tract infections, leading to an estimated 150,000 to 300,000 lower respiratory tract infections in children under 18 months of age and lung infections resulting in 7,500 to 15,000 hospitalizations each year.[124] In addition, children exposed to secondhand smoke have a greater chance of coughing, wheezing, asthma, and chest colds, along with a decrease in lung function. Children exposed to secondhand smoke daily in the home miss more school days and have more colds and acute respiratory infections than do those not exposed.

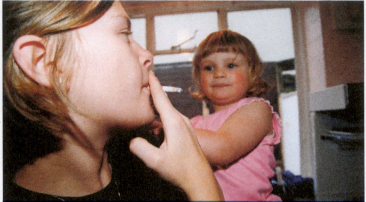

What are the health risks of secondhand smoke?

Environmental tobacco smoke is linked to deaths from cancer and heart disease in adults and sudden infant death syndrome in infants. Because their bodies and brains are still developing, babies and children are particularly vulnerable to the toxins in secondhand smoke.

Secondhand smoke also affects children's cognitive abilities. One study found that children exposed to high levels of secondhand smoke were twice as likely to develop learning disabilities, conduct disorders, and other behavioral disorders.[125] Boys were more likely to be at risk of developing learning disabilities than girls.[126]

Environmental Tobacco Smoke and Additional Health Problems

ETS can cause allergic reactions such as itchy eyes, difficulty breathing, headaches, nausea, and dizziness. It may also increase risk of breast cancer in women; cancers of the nasal sinus cavity and pharynx in adults; and leukemia, lymphoma, and brain tumors in children.[127] The level of carbon monoxide in cigarette smoke contained in enclosed places is 4,000 times higher than that allowed in the clean air standard recommended by the EPA.

Check Yourself

- What are the health risks of exposure to ETS? Which populations are particularly susceptible? What can be done to reduce risks?

- Considering the risks of ETS to children, do you think parents should be prohibited from using tobacco? Would you favor smoking bans in all public Places? Homes with children? Why or why not?

7.13

Alcohol and Tobacco

7.13 Describe policy efforts to discourage tobacco use.

It has been more than 40 years since the U.S. government began warning that tobacco use was hazardous to the nation's health. Despite all the education on the health hazards of tobacco use, health care spending and lost productivity associated with smoking costs between $289 billion and $333 billion each year.[128]

In 1998, the tobacco industry reached the Master Settlement Agreement with 46 states. The agreement requires tobacco companies to pay out more than $206 billion over 25 years. The agreement includes a variety of measures to support antismoking education and advertising and to fund research to determine effective smoking-cessation strategies. The agreement also curbs certain advertising and promotions directed at youth.

Unfortunately, most of the money designated for tobacco control and prevention at the state level has not been used for this purpose. Facing budget woes, many states have drastically cut spending on antismoking programs. In the few states that have spent the settlement money on smoking-cessation programs, there has been some reported success in decreasing cigarette use.[129]

The Family Smoking Prevention and Tobacco Control Act of 2009 allows the FDA to forbid tobacco advertising geared toward children, to lower the amount of nicotine in tobacco products, to ban sweetened cigarettes that appeal to young people, and to require ingredient information and ban products that lack this information.

Recently, the FDA announced plans to target tobacco's addictive properties and effects on health. Because almost 90% of adult smokers started smoking before the age of 18, and nearly 2,500 youth smoke their first cigarette every day in the U.S., the FDA's new comprehensive plan will develop policies that lower nicotine levels in cigarettes to non-addictive levels, thereby decreasing addiction of new smokers and helping current smokers to quit.[130] They also plan to prohibit labels such as "light" and "low tar."[131]

Major efforts are underway to assess the effects of such policy and promote a plan reflecting these goals. One of the most significant impacts of the law is that it requires more prominent health warnings on advertising of tobacco products. Ads for smokeless tobacco now must contain a warning that fills 20 percent of the advertising space. The FDA attempted to require cigarette packages and advertising to have larger, graphical warnings depicting the negative consequences of smoking, but a federal judge declared the requirement unconstitutional.

Many universities, hospitals, public buildings, and businesses have taken a proactive stance by banning the use of tobacco products on their property.

Recently, questions about the safety of e-cigarettes have prompted the FDA to issue a warning about potential health risks. There is no quality control in the manufacturing of the product, with many e-cigarettes manufactured in China under uncontrolled conditions.

As cities in the past took action to ban cigarette smoking in public places, some cities are following suit with e-cigarettes as well, including New York City, Chicago, and Los Angeles. Additionally, many employers are struggling with employees wanting to "vape" indoors on break, and some employers are charging employees who use e-cigarettes and tobacco a higher price for their insurance premiums.[132]

SMOKE FREE INSIDE & OUT
SMOKING IS NOT PERMITTED
- ALL BUILDINGS ON CAMPUS
- ALL OUTDOOR AREAS
- ALL PARKING LOTS

- Which policies do you think have been most successful in discouraging tobacco use?

- What would you recommend as further steps?

7.14 Mindfulness: Breaking the Tobacco Habit

7.14 Discuss strategies for quitting tobacco use.

Approximately 70 percent of U.S. adult smokers want to quit smoking, and up to 55 percent make a serious attempt to quit each year.[133] Quitting is often a lengthy process involving several unsuccessful attempts before success is finally achieved. Even successful quitters suffer occasional slips. Smokers who are unable to quit can expect to lose at least one decade of life compared to people who do not smoke.

Benefits of Quitting

Many tissues damaged by smoking repair themselves (see Figure 7.11). Within 12 hours, carbon monoxide levels return to normal, and "smoker's breath" disappears.[134] Within weeks, the mucus that clogs airways is eliminated, and circulation and sense of taste and smell improve. Many ex-smokers have more energy, sleep better, and feel more alert.

After 1 year of no smoking, the risk for heart disease decreases.[135] Women are less likely to bear low birth weight babies.[136] After 10 smoke-free years, the risk of developing cancer of the lung, larynx, pancreas, kidney, bladder, or cervix is considerably reduced.[137]

Another benefit is money saved. The cost of a single pack of cigarettes ranges from about $5.19 (including tax) to as much as $12.60 in the most expensive state, so a pack-a-day smoker who lives in an area where cigarettes cost $8.00 per pack spends $56.00 per week, or $2,912 per year.[138]

How Can You Quit?

Many people quit "cold turkey"—they simply decide not to smoke again. Others choose programs based on behavior modification and self-reward, attend treatment centers, or work privately with a physician. Plans that combine several approaches have shown the most promise.

Nicotine addiction may be one of the toughest addictions to overcome. Symptoms of **nicotine withdrawal** include irritability, restlessness, nausea, vomiting, and intense cravings. The evidence is strong that consistent pharmacological treatments can double a smoker's chances of quitting.

Nicotine Replacement Products Nontobacco products that replace depleted levels of nicotine in the bloodstream have helped some people stop using tobacco; the dose of nicotine is gradually reduced until the smoker is fully weaned from the drug. Nicotine gum delivers about as much nicotine as a cigarette but doesn't produce the same rush. Users experience no withdrawal symptoms and fewer cravings. Nicotine lozenges, like the gum, are available over the counter. The nicotine patch is a small, thin patch that, when placed on the smoker's upper body, delivers a continuous flow of nicotine through the skin, helping to relieve cravings. It is recommended that people who use the patch as a part of their smoking-cessation program use it for 9 to 10 weeks.[139] During this time, the dose of nicotine is gradually reduced until the smoker is fully weaned from the drug. The patch costs less than a pack of cigarettes—about $4—and some insurance plans will pay for it.[140]

Nicotine nasal spray, which requires a prescription, is much more powerful. Patients must be careful not to overdose; as little as 40 milligrams of nicotine at once could be lethal. The spray should be used for no more than 3 months and never for more than 6 months so that smokers don't find themselves dependent on it; also, people with nasal or sinus problems, allergies, or asthma shouldn't use the spray.

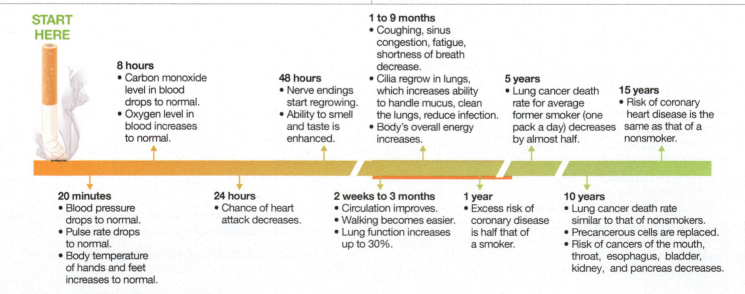

START HERE

20 minutes
- Blood pressure drops to normal.
- Pulse rate drops to normal.
- Body temperature of hands and feet increases to normal.

8 hours
- Carbon monoxide level in blood drops to normal.
- Oxygen level in blood increases to normal.

24 hours
- Chance of heart attack decreases.

48 hours
- Nerve endings start regrowing.
- Ability to smell and taste is enhanced.

2 weeks to 3 months
- Circulation improves.
- Walking becomes easier.
- Lung function increases up to 30%.

1 to 9 months
- Coughing, sinus congestion, fatigue, shortness of breath decrease.
- Cilia regrow in lungs, which increases ability to handle mucus, clean the lungs, reduce infection.
- Body's overall energy increases.

1 year
- Excess risk of coronary disease is half that of a smoker.

5 years
- Lung cancer death rate for average former smoker (one pack a day) decreases by almost half.

10 years
- Lung cancer death rate similar to that of nonsmokers.
- Precancerous cells are replaced.
- Risk of cancers of the mouth, throat, esophagus, bladder, kidney, and pancreas decreases.

15 years
- Risk of coronary heart disease is the same as that of a nonsmoker.

Figure 7.11 When Smokers Quit

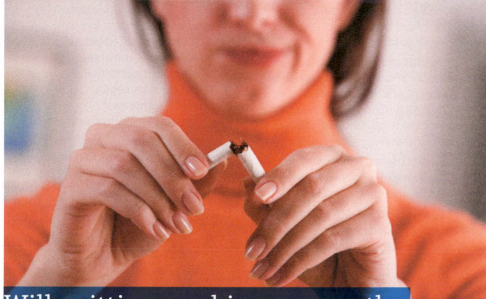

Will quitting smoking reverse the damage that's already been done?

When you quit using tobacco, your body immediately starts to repair the damage. Over time, the body's repair processes reduce the former smoker's risks of heart disease and cancer; after 10 years, heart disease and lung cancer risks are comparable to those of nonsmokers.

The nicotine inhaler also requires a prescription. The smoker inhales air saturated with nicotine, which is absorbed through the lining of the mouth, entering the body much more slowly than the nicotine in cigarettes does.

Smoking-Cessation Medications Bupropion (brand name Zyban), an antidepressant, is FDA approved as a smoking-cessation aid. Varinicline (brand name Chantix) reduces nicotine cravings and the urge to smoke and blocks the effects of nicotine at nicotine receptor sites in the brain. Both drugs may cause changes in behavior such as agitation, depression, hostility, and suicidal thoughts or actions. People taking one of these drugs who experience any unusual changes in mood are advised to stop taking the drug immediately and contact their health care professional.[141]

Mindfulness for Smoking Cessation

Recently, mindfulness-based therapies have been found to offer greater chances of success for people who are trying to quit smoking. Mindfulness interventions have also been shown to decrease negative effects and craving in smokers. Researchers have found that people who use mindfulness training may have better outcomes than those who use standard methods of quitting. In their mindfulness strategies, researchers used the acronym RAIN to help people manage their nicotine cravings[142]:

- Recognize the craving that is occurring, and relax with it.
- Accept the moment. Pay attention to how your body is feeling.
- Investigate the experience. Ask yourself what is happening to your body in this moment.
- Note what is happening. As you acknowledge anxiousness, irritability, and other feelings, realize that they are nothing more than body sensations that will pass.

Using mindfulness techniques in this way will help the body become familiar with the cravings and learn that it can adapt. Cravings usually last from 90 seconds to 3 minutes. Simply using the acronym above helps many smokers acknowledge and get through the craving—cravings that should then become weaker over time.[143]

Skills for Behavior Change

Tips For Quitting Smoking

If you're a smoker and you're ready to quit, try these tips:

- Use the four Ds: Delay (put off smoking for 10 minutes, then another 10 after that, etc.), Deep breathing, Drink water, Do something else.
- Keep "mouth toys" such as hard candy, gum, toothpicks, straws, and carrot sticks handy.
- If you've had trouble stopping before, ask your doctor about nicotine gum, patches, nasal sprays, inhalers, or lozenges.
- Have your teeth cleaned.
- Examine associations that trigger your urge to smoke.
- Tell family and friends that you've stopped so they won't offer you cigarettes.
- Spend time in places that prohibit smoking.
- To shake up your routine and distract you from smoking, take up a new sport, hobby, or organizational commitment.
- Throw out your cigarettes or keep them in a place that makes smoking inconvenient, such as in the freezer or at a friend's house.

Check Yourself

- What are the benefits of stopping the use of tobacco products right now?

- What are some products that are marketed as helping people quit smoking? How effective are they?

- Discuss behavioral strategies that can help smokers break the habit of smoking. What type of mindfulness strategies would you suggest to friends or family members who are trying to quit smoking?

Summary

LO 7.1 Although consumption trends are creeping downward, students are under extreme pressure to consume alcohol. Negative consequences associated with alcohol use among college students include academic problems, traffic accidents, dropping out of school, unplanned sex, alcohol poisoning, and injury.

LO 7.2 Alcohol's effect on the body is measured by blood alcohol concentration (BAC), the ratio of alcohol to total blood volume.

LO 7.3 Alcohol depresses the central nervous system (CNS); short-term effects include decreased respiratory rate, pulse rate, and blood pressure. Alcohol use is a contributing factor to injuries, poor sexual decision-making, rape, and weight gain. Drinking large amounts quickly can lead to alcohol poisoning.

LO 7.4 Long-term alcohol overuse can cause nervous system damage, cardiovascular damage, liver disease, and increased cancer risk. Drinking during pregnancy can cause fetal alcohol spectrum disorders (FASDs).

LO 7.5 Drinking impairs driving abilities. Alcohol-impaired drivers are involved in 1 out of 3 crash deaths in the United States.

LO 7.6 Alcohol use becomes alcohol use disorder when it interferes with school, work, or relationships or entails legal violations. Causes are biological, social, and cultural.

LO 7.7 Being worried about one's alcohol consumption is a cause for concern. A counselor or clinician can advise on steps to take to cut down on drinking.

LO 7.8 Most alcoholics deny having a problem until they reach a major crisis. Treatment options include detoxification at private facilities, therapy, and self-help programs such as Alcoholics Anonymous. Most alcoholics relapse; alcoholism is a behavioral and chemical addiction.

LO 7.9 Tobacco use is widespread in the United States and costs the nation $289 to $333 billion per year. Tobacco companies target college students in their marketing campaigns.

LO 7.10 Tobacco is available in smoking and smokeless forms, both of which contain nicotine, an addictive psychoactive substance. Little is known about the health risks of electronic cigarettes, which are growing in popularity.

LO 7.11 Hazards of smoking include increased rates of cancer, heart and circulatory disorders, and respiratory and gum diseases. Smoking during pregnancy presents risks for the fetus. Smokeless tobacco dramatically increases oral cancer risk.

LO 7.12 Environmental tobacco smoke (secondhand smoke) puts nonsmokers at risk for cancer and heart disease.

LO 7.13 The U.S. Food and Drug Administration (FDA) regulates the sale and advertising of tobacco products.

LO 7.14 To quit, smokers must kick a chemical addiction *and* a behavioral habit. Nicotine replacement products or drugs can help wean smokers off nicotine. Mindfulness strategies can also help.

Pop Quiz

*Visit **Mastering Health** to personalize your study plan with Chapter Review Quizzes and Dynamic Study Modules.*

LO 7.1 1. When Amanda goes out with her friends, she usually has four or five beers in a row within a couple of hours. This type of high-risk drinking is called
 a. tolerance.
 b. alcoholic addiction.
 c. alcohol overconsumption.
 d. binge drinking.

LO 7.2 2. BAC is the
 a. concentration of plant sugars in the bloodstream.
 b. percentage of alcohol in a beverage.
 c. ratio of alcohol to body weight.
 d. ratio of alcohol to total blood volume.

LO 7.3 3. Drinking large amounts of alcohol in a short period of time that leads to passing out is known as
 a. learned behavioral tolerance.
 b. alcoholic unconsciousness.
 c. alcohol poisoning.
 d. acute metabolism syndrome.

LO 7.6 4. To adapt to his father's alcoholic behavior, Jake played the obedient son. What role did he assume?
 a. Family hero   c. Scapegoat
 b. Mascot   d. Lost child

LO 7.8. 5. The alcohol withdrawal syndrome that results in confusion, delusion, agitated behavior, and hallucination is known as
 a. automatic detoxification.
 b. delirium tremens.
 c. acute withdrawal.
 d. transient hyperirritability.

LO 7.10 6. You are out in a very smoky club and the air is hazy—you suddenly notice that you don't feel well, have a headache, feel dizzy, and your heart is racing. What might be the most likely cause of your symptoms?
 a. That you are really out of shape and should stop dancing
 b. that you should have eaten dinner before clubbing and need some food
 c. That you are experiencing the start of carbon monoxide poisoning and should leave
 d. that you are coming down with a sudden case of the flu and should go home and rest.

LO 7.10. 7. What is the major psychoactive ingredient in tobacco products?
 a. Carbon monoxide
 b. Tar
 c. Formaldehyde
 d. Nicotine

LO 7.10 8. What does nicotine do to cilia?
 a. Instantly destroys them
 b. Thickens them
 c. Paralyzes them
 d. Accumulates on them

LO 7.11 9. A major health risk of chewing tobacco is
 a. lung cancer.
 b. leukoplakia.
 c. heart disease.
 d. emphysema.

LO 7.14 10. Quitting smoking
 a. usually results in minor withdrawal symptoms.
 b. does little to reverse damage to the lungs.
 c. can be aided by nicotine replacement.
 d. is best done by transitioning to "light" cigarettes.

Answers to these questions can be found on page A-1. If you answered a question incorrectly, review the module identified by the Learning Outcome. For even more study tools, visit Mastering Health.

Think About It!

LO 7.1 **1.** When it comes to drinking alcohol, how much is too much? How can you avoid drinking amounts that will affect your judgment? If you see a friend having too many drinks at a party, what actions could you take?

LO 7.2 **2.** Would a person be more intoxicated after having four one-shot gin and tonics instead of four 12-oz. cans of regular (non-craft) beers? Why or why not? What factors would you need to know to judge a particular beer?

LO 7.3–7.4 **3.** At what point in your life should you start worrying about the long-term effects of alcohol abuse?

LO 7.6 **4.** Is there a difference between a problem drinker and an alcoholic? What factors can cause someone to develop alcohol use disorder?

LO 7.9 **5.** What are some of the main reasons college students choose to use tobacco?

LO 7.10 **6.** Discuss the various ways in which tobacco is used. Is any method less addictive or less hazardous to health than another?

LO 7.11 **7.** Discuss health hazards associated with tobacco. Who should be responsible for the medical expenses of smokers? Insurance companies? Smokers themselves?

LO 7.14 **8.** Describe the various ways to stop using tobacco. Which would be most effective for you? Why?

Nutrition

ASSESS YOURSELF: How Healthy Are Your Eating Habits? Find out in the Study Area at Mastering Health.

Advice about food comes at us from all directions. Knowing what to eat, how much to eat, and how to choose can be a mind-boggling conundrum. Why does something so good ultimately end up being a problem for so many? Why does what we eat now, affect us now and in the future? What influences our eating habits, and how can we learn to eat more healthfully?

True **hunger** occurs when there is a lack of basic foods. When we're hungry, our brains initiate a physiological response that prompts us to seek food for the energy and **nutrients** our bodies need for proper functioning. Most people in the United States have never known true hunger. Most of us eat because of our **appetite**, a learned psychological desire to consume food and learned behaviors related to time of day. Other reasons for eating include cultural and social meanings attached to food, convenience and advertising, habit or custom, emotional eating, perceived nutritional value, social interaction, and financial means.

Nutrition is the science that investigates the relationship between physiological function and the essential elements of the foods we eat. Your health depends largely on what and how much you eat.

Understanding Nutrition: Digestion and Caloric Needs

8.1 **Describe the digestive process, and identify daily calorie needs.**

Food provides the chemicals we need for activity and body maintenance. Our bodies cannot synthesize certain *essential nutrients* (or cannot synthesize them in adequate amounts); we must obtain them from the foods we eat. Of the six groups of essential nutrients, the four we need in the largest amounts—water, proteins, carbohydrates, and fats—are called *macronutrients*. The other two groups—vitamins and minerals—are needed in smaller amounts, so they are called *micronutrients*.

Before the body can use foods, the digestive system must break down larger food particles into smaller, more usable forms. The sequence of functions by which the body breaks down foods

and either absorbs or excretes them is the *digestive process* (**Figure 8.1**).

Recommended Intakes for Nutrients

The recommended amounts of each nutrient group are known as the *Dietary Reference Intakes (DRIs)*. The DRIs, which are published by the Food and Nutrition Board of the Institute of Medicine, establish the amount of each nutrient needed to prevent deficiencies or reduce the risk of chronic disease and identify maximum safe intake levels for healthy people.[1] The DRIs are umbrella guidelines and include the following categories:

■ **Recommended Dietary Allowances (RDAs)** are daily nutrient intake levels that meet the nutritional needs of 97 to 98 percent of healthy individuals.

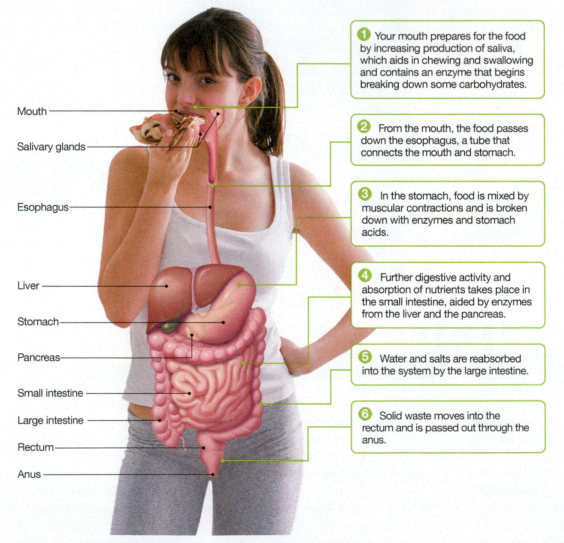

Mouth

Salivary glands

Esophagus

Liver

Stomach

Pancreas

Small intestine

Large intestine

Rectum

Anus

❶ Your mouth prepares for the food by increasing production of saliva, which aids in chewing and swallowing and contains an enzyme that begins breaking down some carbohydrates.

❷ From the mouth, the food passes down the esophagus, a tube that connects the mouth and stomach.

❸ In the stomach, food is mixed by muscular contractions and is broken down with enzymes and stomach acids.

❹ Further digestive activity and absorption of nutrients takes place in the small intestine, aided by enzymes from the liver and the pancreas.

❺ Water and salts are reabsorbed into the system by the large intestine.

❻ Solid waste moves into the rectum and is passed out through the anus.

Figure 8.1 The Digestive Process
The entire digestive process takes approximately 24 hours.

- **Adequate Intakes (AIs)** are daily intake levels that are assumed to be adequate for most healthy people. AIs are used when there isn't enough research to support establishing an RDA.
- **Tolerable Upper Intake Levels (ULs)** are the highest amounts of a nutrient that an individual can consume daily without risking adverse health effects.
- **Acceptable Macronutrient Distribution Ranges (AMDRs)** are ranges of protein, carbohydrate, and fat intake that provide adequate nutrition and are associated with a reduced risk for chronic disease.

Whereas the RDAs, AIs, and ULs are expressed as amounts—usually milligrams (mg) or micrograms (μg)—AMDRs are expressed as percentages. The AMDR for protein, for example, is 10 to 35 percent, meaning that no less than 10 percent and no more than 35 percent of the calories you consume should come from proteins. But that raises a new question: What are calories?

Calories

A *kilocalorie* is a unit of measure used to quantify the amount of energy in food. On nutrition labels and in consumer publications, the term is shortened to **calorie**. *Energy* is defined as the capacity to do work. We derive energy from the energy-containing nutrients in the foods we eat. These nutrients—proteins, carbohydrates, and fats—provide calories. Vitamins, minerals, and water do not. It's important to know your approximate caloric needs, based on your age, gender, and activity level. **Table 8.1** shows the caloric needs for various individuals.

Americans consume about 900 more calories per day than they did 50 years ago (see **Figure 8.2**).[2] In general, it isn't the actual amount of food, but the number of calories in the foods we choose to eat that has increased. When these trends are combined with our increasingly sedentary lifestyle, it is not surprising that we have seen a dramatic rise in obesity. With an understanding of nutrition, you will be able to make more informed choices about your diet and lifestyle.

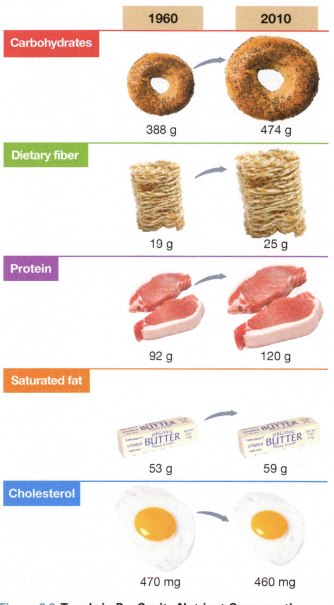

Figure 8.2 Trends in Per Capita Nutrient Consumption
Since 1960, Americans have increased their daily caloric intake from 3,100 to 4,000 and their daily consumption of carbohydrates, protein, and saturated fat.

Source: Data are from the USDA Center for Nutrition Policy and Promotion, February 1, 2015, www.ers.usda.gov/data-products/food-availability-(per-capita)-data-system/.aspx#26715.

TABLE 8.1	Estimates of Daily Calorie Needs		
	Calorie Range		
	Sedentary[a]		**Active**[b]
Children			
2–3 years old	1,000	→	1,400
Females			
4–13 years old	1,200–1,600	→	1,400–2,200
14–18	1,800	→	2,400
19–25	2,000	→	2,400
26–50	1,800	→	2,200–2,400
51+	1,600	→	2,000–2,200
Males			
4–12 years old	1,200–1,800	→	1,600–2,400
13–18	2,000–2,400	→	2,600–3,200
19–20	2,600	→	3,000
21–40	2,400	→	2,800–3,000
41–60	2,200	→	2,800
61+	2,000	→	2,400–2,600

[a] A lifestyle that includes only the light physical activity associated with typical day-to-day life.
[b] A lifestyle that includes physical activity equivalent to walking more than 3 miles per day at 3 to 4 miles per hour in addition to the light physical activity associated with typical day-to-day life.

Source: U.S. Department of Agriculture and U.S. Department of Health and Human Services, *2015–2020 Dietary Guidelines for Americans*, 8th ed., Appendix 2, Table A2-1. (Washington, DC: U.S. Government Printing Office).

Check Yourself

- Describe the digestive process, from mouth to excretion.
- What are your estimated daily calorie needs?
- What factors influence your calorie needs?

8.2 Essential Nutrients: Water and Protein

Learning Outcome

8.2 Explain the functions of water and protein in the body.

Water

Humans can survive for several weeks without food but for only about 1 week without water. The human body consists of 50 to 70 percent water by weight. The water in our system bathes cells, aids in fluid and electrolyte balance, maintains pH balance, and transports molecules and cells throughout the body. Water is the major component of blood, which carries oxygen and nutrients to the tissues, removes metabolic wastes, and keeps cells in working order.

Individual needs for water vary according to dietary factors, age, size, overall health, environmental temperature and humidity, and exercise. The latest DRIs suggest that most people can meet their hydration needs simply by eating a healthy diet and drinking in response to thirst. The general recommendations for women has been approximately 9 cups of total water from all beverages and foods each day; for men, the recommendation is an average of 13 cups.[3] Critics have questioned whether we really need to consume this much additional water, as the average healthy person gets considerable water in the foods they eat and through other beverages.[4] In fact, fruits and vegetables are 80 to 95 percent water, meats are more than 50 percent water, and even dry bread and cheese are about 35 percent water!

Contrary to popular opinion, caffeinated drinks, including coffee, tea, and soda, also count toward total fluid intake. Consumed in moderation, caffeinated beverages have not been found to dehydrate people whose bodies are used to caffeine, as many people believe.[5]

There are situations in which a person needs additional fluids to avoid **dehydration**, a state of abnormal depletion of body fluids. Dehydration can develop within a single day, especially when you engage in strenuous physical activity in a hot climate. Dehydration is also a risk when you have a fever or an illness involving vomiting or diarrhea and in people with kidney disease, diabetes, or cystic fibrosis. Older adults and the very young are also at increased risk for dehydration.

Excessive water intake can also pose a serious health risk if it prompts *hyponatremia*, a condition characterized by low blood levels of the mineral sodium. If you are an athlete and wonder about water consumption, visit the American College of Sports Medicine's website (www.acsm.org) to download its brochure "Selecting and Effectively Using Hydration for Fitness."[6]

Protein

Next to water, **proteins** are the most abundant substances in the human body. Proteins are major components of nearly every cell; they've been called the "body builders" because of their role in developing and repairing bone, muscle, skin, and blood cells. Proteins are the key elements of antibodies that protect us from disease, of enzymes that control chemical activities in the body, and of hormones that regulate body functions. Proteins help transport iron, oxygen, and nutrients to all body cells and supply

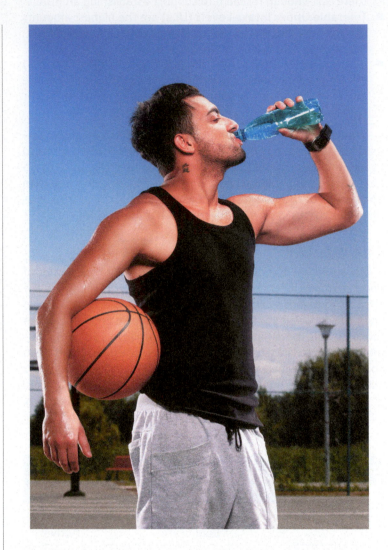

Drinking water is important to maintain normal body functioning. If you're exercising in hot weather or sweating profusely, it's crucial to stay adequately hydrated.

another source of energy to cells when fats and carbohydrates are not available. Every gram of protein you eat provides 4 calories. Adequate amounts of protein in the diet are vital to many body functions and, ultimately, to survival.

Your body breaks down proteins into smaller nitrogen-containing **amino acids**. Nine of the 20 amino acids are **essential amino acids**, which the body must obtain from the diet; the other 11 can be produced by the body. Dietary protein that supplies all the essential amino acids is called **complete protein**. Typically, protein from animal products is complete.

Nearly all proteins from plant sources are **incomplete proteins**, lacking one or more of the essential amino acids. However, it is easy to combine plant foods to produce a complete protein meal (**Figure 8.3**). Plant sources of protein fall into three general categories: *legumes* (e.g., beans, peas, peanuts, and soy products), *grains* (e.g., wheat, corn, rice, and oats), and *nuts and seeds*.

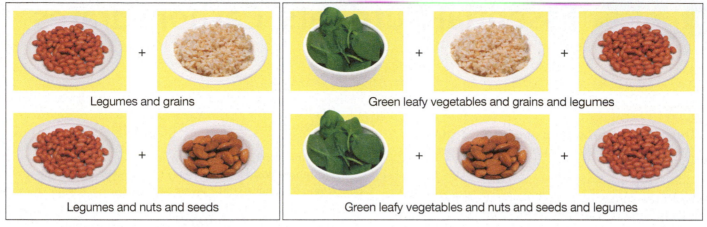

Figure 8.3 Complementary Proteins
Eaten in the right combinations, plant-based foods can provide complementary proteins and all essential amino acids.

| Legumes and grains | Green leafy vegetables and grains and legumes |
| Legumes and nuts and seeds | Green leafy vegetables and nuts and seeds and legumes |

Certain vegetables, such as leafy green vegetables and broccoli, also contribute valuable plant proteins. Consuming a variety of foods from these categories will provide all the essential amino acids.

Although protein deficiency poses a threat to the global population, few Americans suffer from protein deficiencies. In fact, the average American age 20 and over consumes 83 grams of protein daily, much of it from high-fat animal flesh and dairy products.[7] The AMDR for protein is 10 to 35 percent of calories. The RDA is 0.8 gram (g) per kilogram (kg) of body weight. Some experts indicate that the AMDR range may be appropriate; however, typical consumers may need more situation-specific clarification.[8]

To calculate your recommended protein intake per day, divide your body weight in pounds by 2.2 to get your weight in kilograms, then multiply by 0.8. For example, a woman who weighs 130 pounds should consume about 47 grams of protein each day. A 6-ounce steak provides 53 grams of protein—more than she needs!

People who need to eat extra protein include pregnant women and patients who are fighting a serious infection, recovering from surgery or blood loss, or recovering from burns. In these instances, proteins that are lost to cellular repair and development need to be replaced. Athletes also require more protein to build and repair muscle fibers.[9] In addition, a sedentary person may find it easier to stay in energy balance when consuming a high-protein, low-carbohydrate diet because protein takes longer to digest than carbohydrates. Protein also releases certain satiety hormones that contribute to feeling full longer.

Toward Sustainable Seafood The U.S. Department of Agriculture (USDA) recommends consuming fish twice a week to reduce saturated fat and cholesterol levels and increase omega-3 fatty acid levels. However, environmental concerns call into question the sustainability and safety of such consumption. Overfishing and human activities have reduced the populations of many species. Large portions of the world's oceans are *dead zones* that do not have enough oxygen to support marine life. These dead zones are primarily caused by agricultural and chemical runoff, sewage, ocean warming, and other factors.

Farming fish can counteract the loss of wild fish populations, but these farms pose additional health risks and environmental concerns. Some farmed fish are laden with antibiotics, some are nourished by human and animal wastes, and highly concentrated levels of parasites and bacteria from fish farm runoff may reach wild fish populations through adjacent waterways. Some farmed fish are fed wild fish, resulting in a net loss of fish from the sea.

Not surprisingly, high levels of chemicals, parasites, bacteria, waste products, and toxins are found in many of the fish available on the market. Mercury, a waste product of many industries, binds to proteins and stays in an animal's body, accumulating as the mercury moves up the food chain. In humans, mercury can damage the nervous system and kidneys and cause birth defects and developmental problems. Polychlorinated biphenyls (PCBs) can build up in the fatty tissue of fish. Other chemical and environmental assaults cause diseases and mutations in fish that make it difficult for them to navigate and hunt for foods. Taking time to investigate where your fish are coming from and the standards followed in harvesting, producing, and selling seafood should be an important part of your nutritional plan.

Purchasing seafood from regularly inspected, environmentally responsible sources will support fisheries and fish farms that are healthy for you and the environment. Several major environmental groups have developed guides to inform consumers of safe and sustainable seafood choices, including the Monterey Bay Aquarium in California (http://mobile.seafoodwatch.org) and the Environmental Protection Agency (https://www.epa.gov/choose-fish-and-shellfish-wisely/fish-and-shellfish-advisories-and-safe-eating-guidelines).

Check Yourself

- Why is water considered an essential nutrient? Are you getting enough water each day?

- What are the functions of protein in the body?

- Why is it important that we get enough protein in our diets?

8.2

Nutrition

Carbohydrates supply us with the energy we need to sustain normal daily activity. The human body metabolizes carbohydrates more quickly and efficiently than it does proteins, so carbohydrates can be a quick source of energy for the body. Carbohydrates are easily converted to glucose, the fuel for the body's cells. Carbohydrates also play an important role in the functioning of internal organs, the nervous system, and muscles. They are the best fuel for moderate to intense exercise because they can be readily broken down to glucose even when you're breathing hard and your muscle cells are getting less oxygen.

Like proteins, carbohydrates provide 4 calories per gram. The RDA for adults is 130 grams of carbohydrate per day.[10] There are two major types of carbohydrates: simple carbohydrates and complex carbohydrates.

Simple Carbohydrates

Simple carbohydrates, or *simple sugars*, are found naturally in fruits, many vegetables, and dairy foods. The most common form of simple carbohydrates is *glucose*. Fruits and berries contain *fructose* (commonly called *fruit sugar*). Glucose and fructose are **monosaccharides**. Eventually, the human body converts all types of simple sugars to glucose to provide energy to cells.

Disaccharides are combinations of two monosaccharides. Perhaps the best-known example is *sucrose* (granulated table sugar). *Lactose* (milk sugar), found in milk and milk products, and *maltose* (malt sugar) are other common disaccharides. Disaccharides must be broken down into monosaccharides before the body can use them.

Americans typically consume far too many refined carbohydrates (i.e., carbohydrates containing only sugars and starches, discussed below), which have few health benefits and are a major factor in our growing epidemic of overweight and obesity. Many of the simple sugars in these foods come from *added sugars*, sweeteners that are put in during processing to flavor foods, make sodas taste good, and ease our craving for sweets. A classic example is the amount of added sugar in one can of soda: more than 10 teaspoons per can! All that refined sugar can cause tooth decay and put on pounds.

Sugar is found in high amounts in a wide range of food products. Such diverse items as ketchup, barbecue sauce, and flavored coffee creamers derive 30 to 65 percent of their calories from sugar. Knowing what foods contain these sugars, considering the amounts you consume each day that are hidden in foods, and then trying to reduce these levels can be a great way to reduce excess weight. Read food labels carefully before purchasing. If sugar or one of its aliases (including *high fructose corn syrup* and *cornstarch*) appears near the top of the ingredients list, then that product contains a lot of sugar and is probably not your best nutritional bet. Also, most labels list the amount of sugar as a percentage of total calories.

Complex Carbohydrates

Complex carbohydrates are found in grains, cereals, legumes, and other vegetables. Also called *polysaccharides*, they are

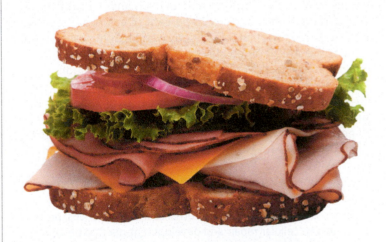

Why are whole grains better than refined grains?

A recent study that followed more than 367,000 participants over 14 years found that the higher the consumption of whole grains, the lower the risk for death from cardiovascular disease, diabetes, and cancer. The risk of death was reduced by an average of 17 percent. Unfortunately, nearly 100 percent of Americans fail to meet their recommended intakes for whole grains.

Sources: T. Huang et al., "Consumption of Whole Grains and Cereal Fiber and Total and Cause-Specific Mortality: Prospective Analysis of 367,442 Individuals," *BMC Medicine* 13, no. 1 (2015): 59; Scientific Report of the 2015 Dietary Guidelines Advisory Committee, "Advisory Report to the Secretary of Health and Human Services and the Secretary of Agriculture," 2015, Available at: http://health.gov/dietaryguidelines/2015-scientific-report.

formed by long chains of monosaccharides. Like disaccharides, they must be broken down into simple sugars before the body can use them. Starches, glycogen, and fiber are the main types of complex carbohydrates.

Starches and Glycogen **Starches**, which make up the majority of the complex carbohydrate group, come from flours, breads, pasta, rice, corn, oats, barley, potatoes, and related foods. The body breaks down these complex carbohydrates into the monosaccharide glucose, which can be easily absorbed by cells and used as energy. Polysaccharides can also be stored in body muscles and the liver as **glycogen**. When the body requires a sudden burst of energy, it breaks down glycogen into glucose.

Fiber **Fiber**, sometimes referred to as "bulk" or "roughage," is the indigestible portion of plant foods that helps move foods through the digestive system, delays absorption of cholesterol and other nutrients, and softens stools by absorbing water. Dietary fiber is found only in plant foods such as fruits, vegetables, nuts, and grains.

Fiber is either *soluble* or *insoluble*. Soluble fibers, such as pectins, gums, and mucilages, dissolve in water, form gel-like substances, and can be digested easily by bacteria in the colon. Major food sources of soluble fiber include citrus fruits, berries, oat bran, beans (e.g., kidney, garbanzo, pinto, and navy beans), and some vegetables. Insoluble fibers, such as lignins and cellulose, typically do not dissolve in water and cannot be fermented by bacteria in the colon. They are found in most fruits and vegetables and in **whole grains** such as brown rice, wheat, bran, and whole-grain breads and cereals (see **Figure 8.4**).

Despite growing evidence supporting the benefits of whole grains and high-fiber diets, fiber intake among the general public remains low. Most experts believe that Americans should double their current consumption of dietary fiber. The AMDR for carbohydrates is 45 to 65 percent of total calories, and health experts recommend that the majority of this intake be fiber-rich carbohydrates.

A diet that is high in fiber is associated with a reduced risk for obesity, heart disease, constipation, and possibly even type 2 diabetes and colon and rectal cancers. The DRI for dietary fiber is 25 grams per day for women and 38 grams per day for men.[11] The best way to increase your fiber intake is to eat fewer refined carbohydrates and more fiber-rich carbohydrates, including whole-grain breads and cereals, fresh fruits, legumes and other vegetables, nuts, and seeds.

As with most nutritional advice, however, too much of a good thing can pose problems. A sudden increase in dietary fiber may cause flatulence (intestinal gas), cramping, or bloating. Consume plenty of water or other sugar-free liquids to reduce such side effects.

Find out more about the benefits of fiber in the **Skills for Behavior Change**.

8.3

Nutrition

Skills for **Behavior Change**

Bulk Up Your Fiber Intake!

To increase your intake of dietary fiber:

- Whenever possible, select 100 percent whole-grain breads that are low in fat and sugars, with 3 or more grams of fiber per serving. Read labels. Just because bread is brown doesn't mean that it's better for you.
- Eat whole, unpeeled fruits and vegetables rather than drinking their juices. The fiber in whole fruit tends to slow blood sugar increases and helps you feel full longer.
- Substitute whole-grain pastas, bagels, and pizza crust for the refined, white flour versions.
- Add wheat crumbs or grains to meat loaf and burgers to increase fiber intake.
- Toast grains to bring out their nutty flavor and make foods more appealing.
- Sprinkle ground flaxseed on cereals, yogurt, and salads. You can also add flaxseed to casseroles, burgers, and baked goods. Flaxseeds have a mild flavor and are also high in beneficial fatty acids.

Check Yourself

- **What are the functions of carbohydrates in the body?**
- **What are the preferred sources of carbohydrates?**
- **Why is fiber important in the diet?**

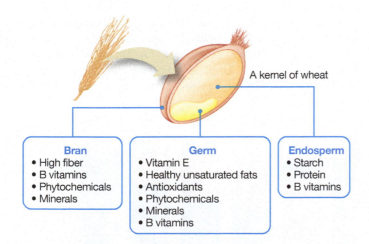

A kernel of wheat

Bran
- High fiber
- B vitamins
- Phytochemicals
- Minerals

Germ
- Vitamin E
- Healthy unsaturated fats
- Antioxidants
- Phytochemicals
- Minerals
- B vitamins

Endosperm
- Starch
- Protein
- B vitamins

Figure 8.4 Anatomy of a Whole Grain
Whole grains are more nutritious than refined grains because whole grains contain the bran, germ, and endosperm of the seed—sources of fiber, vitamins, minerals, and beneficial phytochemicals (chemical compounds that occur naturally in plants).

Source: Adapted from Joan Salge Blake, Kathy D. Munoz, and Stella Volpe, *Nutrition: From Science to You*, 3rd ed. © 2015, page 132. Printed and electronically reproduced by permission of Pearson Education, Inc., Upper Saddle River, New Jersey.

Essential Nutrients: Fats

8.4 **Describe the functions of fats in the body.**

Fats, perhaps the most misunderstood nutrient, are the most energy dense, providing 9 calories per gram. Fats are a significant source of our body's fuel. The body can store only a limited amount of carbohydrate, so the longer you exercise, the more fat your body burns. Fats also play a vital role in maintaining healthy skin and hair, insulating body organs against shock, maintaining body temperature, and promoting healthy cell function. Fats make foods taste better and carry vitamins A, D, E, and K to cells. They also make you feel full after eating. So why are we constantly urged to cut back on fats? It's because some fats are less healthy than others and because excessive consumption of fats can lead to weight gain and other problems.

Triglycerides, which make up about 95 percent of total body fat, are the most common form of fat circulating in the blood. When we consume too many calories from any source, the liver converts the excess into triglycerides, which are stored throughout our bodies.

Another oily substance in foods derived from animals is **cholesterol**. We don't need to consume any dietary cholesterol because our liver can make all that we need. In the *2015–2020 Dietary Guidelines for Americans*, experts essentially removed previous recommendations to consume less than 300 mg of cholesterol per day and said not to worry so much about cholesterol. Instead, you should focus on reducing saturated fat in your diet. Eggs, which have 215 mg of cholesterol, have very little saturated fat and therefore are not the culprits we used to think they were. This doesn't mean that you should chow down on all the high-cholesterol foods you can, but rather consider calories, amount of fat, and other nutrients first, and use moderation when it comes to cholesterol.[12]

Neither triglycerides nor cholesterol can travel independently in the bloodstream. Instead, they are "packaged" inside protein coats to form compounds called lipoproteins. **High-density lipoproteins (HDLs)** are relatively high in protein and low in cholesterol and triglycerides. A high level of HDLs in the blood is healthful because HDLs remove cholesterol from dying cells and from plaque within blood vessels, eventually transporting cholesterol to the liver and eliminating it from the body. **Low-density lipoproteins (LDLs)** are much higher in both cholesterol and triglycerides than HDLs. They travel in the bloodstream delivering cholesterol to body cells; however, LDLs that are not taken up by cells degrade and release their cholesterol into the bloodstream. This cholesterol can then stick to the lining of blood vessels, contributing to the plaque that causes heart disease.

Types of Dietary Fats

Fat molecules include *fatty acid* chains of oxygen, carbon, and hydrogen atoms. Fatty acid chains that cannot hold any more hydrogen in their chemical structure are called **saturated fats**. These generally come from animal sources such as meat, dairy, and poultry and are solid at room temperature. **Unsaturated fats** have room for additional hydrogen atoms in their chemical structure and are liquid at room temperature. They come from plants and include most vegetable oils.

The terms *monounsaturated fatty acids (MUFAs)* and *polyunsaturated fatty acids (PUFAs)* refer to the relative number of hydrogen atoms missing in a fatty acid chain. Peanut and olive oils are high in monounsaturated fats. Corn, sunflower, and safflower oils are high in polyunsaturated fats.

There is controversy about which unsaturated fats are most beneficial. MUFAs, such as olive oil, which seem to lower LDL levels and increase HDL levels, are currently preferred. **Figure 8.5** shows fats in common vegetable oils.

PUFAs come in two forms: *omega-3 fatty acids* (in many fatty fish) and *omega-6 fatty acids* (in corn, soybean, and cottonseed oils). Both are classified as *essential fatty acids*—we must receive them from our diets. *Linoleic acid*, an omega-6 fatty acid, and alpha-linolenic acid, an omega-3 fatty acid, are needed to make

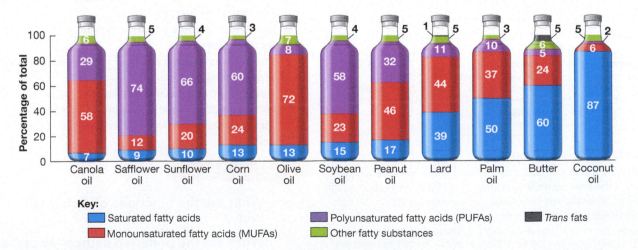

Figure 8.5 Percentages of Saturated, Polyunsaturated, Monounsaturated, and *Trans* Fats in Common Vegetable Oils

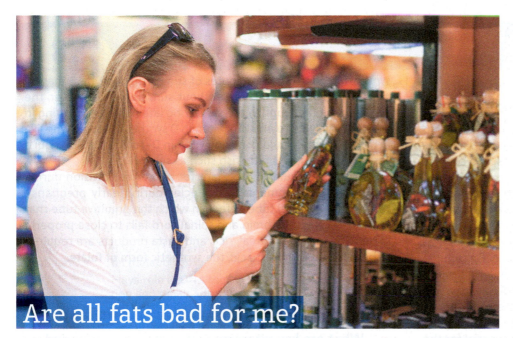

Are all fats bad for me?

Not all fats are the same, and your body needs some fat to function healthily. Try to reduce saturated fats, those that come in meat, dairy, and poultry products; avoid *trans* fats, those that can come in stick margarine, commercially baked goods, and deep-fried foods; and replace these with monounsaturated fats, such as those in peanut and olive oils.

hormone-like compounds that control immune function, pain perception, and inflammation and reduce risks for cardiovascular disease. EPA and DHA, derivatives of alpha-linolenic acid that are found abundantly in oily fish such as salmon and tuna, are associated with a reduced risk for heart disease.[13]

The AMDR for fats is 20 to 35 percent of calories, with 5 to 10 percent coming from essential fatty acids. Within this range, we should minimize our intake of saturated fats.

Avoiding *Trans* Fatty Acids

For decades, Americans shunned butter, red meat, and other foods because of their saturated fats. What they didn't know was that foods low in saturated fat, such as margarine, can be just as harmful because they contain **trans fatty acids**. Research shows that consuming *trans* fats decreases levels of HDL cholesterol and increases levels of LDL cholesterol as well as increasing risks of cardiovascular disease and type 2 diabetes.[14]

Although small amounts of *trans* fatty acids do occur in some animal products, most are in processed foods made with partially hydrogenated oils (PHOs).[15, 16] PHOs are produced when food manufacturers add hydrogen to a plant oil, solidifying it, helping it resist rancidity, and giving the food in which it is used a longer shelf life. This process straightens out the fatty acid chain so that it is more like a saturated fatty acid, and it has similar harmful effects, lowering HDLs and raising LDLs. *Trans* fats have been used in margarines, many commercial baked goods, and restaurant deep-fried foods.

In 2015, the U.S. Food and Drug Administration (FDA) ruled that PHOs are no longer "generally recognized as safe" for consumption. Food companies have until July 2018 to remove all PHOs

from their products.[17] In the meantime, *trans* fats have been removed from most foods. The FDA allows foods with less than 1 gram of *trans* fat per serving to be labeled as *trans*-fat free. However, if you see the words *partially hydrogenated oils, fractionated oils, shortening, lard,* or *hydrogenation* on a food label, then *trans* fats are present, even if the amount listed on the label is zero.

A Healthy Approach to Fats

The AMDR for fats is 20 to 35 percent of total calories. Saturated fat should make up less than 10 percent of your total calories, and you should keep *trans*-fat intake to an absolute minimum.[18] Instead of trying to eat a low-fat diet, replace the saturated and *trans* fats you eat with healthful unsaturated fats from plants and fish. Many studies have shown that balanced higher-fat diets such as the Mediterranean diet, which is rich in plant oils and fish, produce significant improvements in body weight and cardiovascular risk factors.[19]

Follow these dietary guidelines to add more healthy fats to your diet:

- Eat sustainable fatty seafood (bluefish, herring, mackerel, salmon, sardines, or tuna) at least twice weekly.
- Use olive, peanut, soy, and canola oils instead of butter or lard.
- Add leafy green vegetables, walnuts, walnut oil, and ground flaxseed to your diet.
- Read the Nutrition Facts panel on food labels to find out how much fat is in your food.
- Chill meat-based soups and stews, remove any fat that hardens on top, then reheat to serve.
- Fill up on fruits and vegetables.
- Avoid all products with *trans* fatty acids. For healthy toppings on your bread, try vegetable spreads, bean spreads, nut butters, sugar-free jams, or fat-free cheese.
- Choose lean meats, fish, or skinless poultry. Broil, steam, poach, or bake whenever possible. Drain off fat after cooking.
- Choose fewer cold cuts, bacon, sausages, hot dogs, and organ meats that are high in fat and sodium.
- Select nonfat and low-fat dairy products, but remember that many nonfat and low-fat foods have higher amounts of carbohydrates and sugars. Choose wisely.

Check Yourself

- **What role do fats play in the body and why should you make sure you have some fat in your diet?**

- **What are more and less healthful sources of fats?**

- **Consider the types of fat that you typically eat— How might you best cut down on your fat Intake?**

Increasingly, nutrition research is focusing on components of foods that are not nutrients themselves, but interact with nutrients to promote human health.[24] Foods that may confer health benefits beyond the nutrients they contribute to the diet—whole foods, fortified foods, enriched foods, or enhanced foods—are called **functional foods**. When functional foods are included as part of a varied diet, they have the potential to affect health in positive ways.[25]

Some of the most popular functional foods contain **antioxidants**. These substances appear to protect against oxidative stress, a complex process in which *free radicals* (atoms with unpaired electrons) destabilize other atoms and molecules, prompting a chain reaction that can damage cells, cell proteins, or genetic material in the cells. Free radical formation is a natural process that cannot be avoided, but antioxidants combat it by donating their electrons to stabilize free radicals, activating enzymes that convert free radicals to less damaging substances, or reducing or repairing the damage they cause.

Among the more commonly cited antioxidants are vitamins C and E, as well as the minerals copper, iron, manganese, selenium, and zinc. Other potent antioxidants are **phytochemicals**, compounds that occur naturally in plants and are thought to protect them against ultraviolet radiation, pests, and other threats. Common examples include the *carotenoids*, pigments found in red, orange, and dark green fruits and vegetables. Beta-carotene, the most researched carotenoid, is a precursor of vitamin A, meaning that vitamin A can be produced in the body from beta-carotene. Both vitamin A and beta-carotene have antioxidant properties.

Polyphenols, which include a group known as *flavonoids*, are the largest class of phytochemicals. They are found in an array of fruits and vegetables as well as soy products, tea, and chocolate. Like carotenoids, they are thought to have potent antioxidant properties.[26]

Although research supporting the health benefits of antioxidant nutrients and phytochemicals is not conclusive, studies do show that individuals who are deficient in antioxidant vitamins and minerals have an increased risk for age-related diseases and that antioxidants consumed in whole foods, mostly fruits and vegetables, may reduce these individuals' risks.[27] In contrast, antioxidants that are consumed as supplements do not necessarily confer such a benefit, and some studies suggest that they may be harmful, acting as "pro-oxidants" and increasing the risk of certain cancers and overall mortality in some populations, such as smokers.[28]

Health Claims of Superfoods

In food advertisements, in fitness and food magazines, and even among health care organizations, functional foods are increasingly

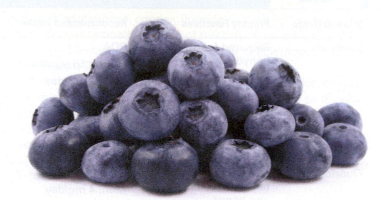

Blueberries are a great source of antioxidants.

being referred to as "superfoods." Do superfoods live up to their new name? Let's look at a few.

Salmon is a rich source of the omega-3 fatty acids EPA and DHA, which combat inflammation, improve HDL/LDL blood profiles, and reduce the risk for cardiovascular disease. These essential fatty acids may also promote a healthy nervous system, reducing the risk for mood disorders and age-related dementia.[29]

Yogurt makes it onto most superfood lists because it contains living, beneficial bacteria called probiotics. You will see their genus name—for example, *Lactobacillus* or *Bifidobacterium*—in the list of ingredients on the product's label. Probiotics colonize the large intestine, where they help to complete digestion and produce certain vitamins and may reduce the risk of diarrhea and other bowel disorders, boost immunity, and help regulate body weight.[30]

Cocoa is particularly rich in phytochemicals called flavonols that have been shown in many studies to reduce the risk for cardiovascular disease, diabetes, and even arthritis. Dark chocolate has a higher level of flavonols than milk chocolate.[31]

Given such claims, it's easy to get carried away by the idea that superfoods have superpowers. But eating a square of dark chocolate won't rescue you from the ill effects of a fast-food burger and fries. What matters is your whole diet. Focus on including superfoods as components of a varied diet that is rich in fresh fruits, legumes and other vegetables, whole grains, lean sources of protein, and nuts and seeds.

- How do functional foods benefit health?

- How can you incorporate more functional foods into your diet?

8.8 Planning a Healthy Diet: Using the Food Label

8.8 Understand each component of the food label.

To help consumers evaluate the nutritional values of packaged foods, the FDA and the USDA developed the Nutrition Facts panel that is typically displayed on the side or back of packaged foods. One of the most helpful items on the panel is the **% daily values (%DVs)** list, which tells you how much of an average adult's allowance for a particular substance (fat, fiber, calcium, etc.) is provided by a serving of the food. The %DV is calculated on the basis of a diet of 2,000 calories per day, so your values may be different from those listed on a label. The panel also includes information on the serving size and calories.

In 2016, the FDA published a new label that is more helpful for consumers. It identifies the calories per serving in much larger type and uses a serving size that better reflects the amount of the food that people typically eat. **Figure 8.6** walks you through a typical Nutrition Facts panel.

See It! Videos

Learn how the new FDA mandate will affect packaging labels. Watch **Changes Coming to Nutrition Labels** in the Study Area of Mastering Health.

Sample Label for Macaroni and Cheese

Original Label

Start here. Serving sizes are standardized to make shopping easier.

Calories per serving and the number of servings are listed on the label.

% Daily Values tell you if the food is high or low in a nutrient based on a 2,000 calorie diet.

Vitamin A, vitamin C, calcium, and iron are required on the label. Other vitamins and minerals are voluntary.

Nutrition Facts

Serving size 2/3 cup (55g)
Servings Per Container About 8

Amount Per Serving

Calories 230   Calories from Fat 40

	% Daily Value*
Total Fat 8g	12%
Saturated Fat 1g	5%
Trans Fat 0g	
Cholesterol 0mg	0%
Sodium 160mg	7%
Total Carbohydrate 37g	12%
Dietary Fiber 4g	16%
Sugars 1g	
Protein 3g	
Vitamin A	10%
Vitamin C	8%
Calcium	20%
Iron	45%

* Percent Daily Values are based on a 2,000 calorie diet. Your Daily Values may be higher or lower depending on your calorie needs:

	Calories:	2,000	2,500
Total Fat	Less than	65g	80g
Sat Fat	Less than	20g	25g
Cholesterol	Less than	300mg	300mg
Sodium	Less than	2,400mg	2,400mg
Total Carbohydrate		300g	375g
Dietary Fiber		25g	30g

New Label

Nutrition Facts

8 servings per container
Serving size   2/3 cup (55g)

Amount Per serving

Calories   230

	% Daily Value*
Total Fat 8g	10%
Saturated Fat 1g	5%
Trans Fat 0g	
Cholesterol 0mg	0%
Sodium 160mg	7%
Total Carbohydrate 37g	13%
Dietary Fiber 4g	14%
Sugars 12g	
Includes 10g Added Sugars	20%
Protein 3g	
Vitamin D 2mcg	10%
Calcium 260mg	20%
Iron 8mg	45%
Potassium 235mg	6%

* The % Daily Value (DV) tells you how much a nutrient in a serving of food contributes to a daily diet. 2,000 calories a day is used for general nutrition advice.

New labels have bolder and larger type for serving sizes.

Calories from fat is removed.

% Daily Values are listed first and explained in a new detailed footnote.

Added Sugars are listed separately.

Vitamin D, calcium, iron, and potassium are required. Other vitamins and minerals are voluntary.

Figure 8.6 Reading a Food Label

Source: U.S. Food and Drug Administration, "How to Understand and Use the Nutrition Facts Panel," April 2015, www.fda.gov/Food/IngredientsPackagingLabeling/LabelingNutrition/ucm274593.htm; U.S. Food and Drug Administration, "Changes to the Nutrition Facts Label," August 2016, http://www.fda.gov/Food/GuidanceRegulation/GuidanceDocumentsRegulatoryInformation/LabelingNutrition/ucm385663.htm.

▶ Mastering Health & Nutrition Understanding Food Lables

■ **What are the key components of a food label? How can they help you make better food choices?**

Planning a Healthy Diet: Dietary Guidelines and MyPlate

8.9 Explain the principles for a healthy diet contained in the MyPlate food guidance system.

Now that you have some idea of your nutritional needs, let's discuss what a healthy diet looks like, how you can begin to fill your needs, and how you can meet the challenge of getting the foods you need on campus.

Dietary Guidelines for Americans

The Dietary Guidelines for Americans are a set of recommendations for healthy eating; they are revised every 5 years. The *2015–2020 Dietary Guidelines for Americans* provide advice about consuming fewer calories, making informed food choices, and being physically active to attain and maintain a healthy weight, reduce your risk for chronic disease, and improve your overall health. To help consumers understand and implement the Dietary Guidelines, the USDA has developed an easy-to-follow graphic and guidance system called MyPlate, which can be found at www.choosemyplate.gov and is illustrated in **Figure 8.7**.

The MyPlate Food Guidance System

The MyPlate food guidance system takes into consideration the dietary and caloric needs for a wide variety of individuals, such as pregnant or breast-feeding women, people who are trying to lose weight, and adults with different activity levels. When you visit the interactive website, you can create personalized dietary and exercise recommendations based on the information you enter.

MyPlate's key messages, which support the Dietary Guidelines, include the following.

Balance Calories Find out how many calories you need for a day. This is important for managing your weight. Go to www.choosemyplate.gov to find your calorie level. Being physically active also helps you balance calories.

- Enjoy your food, but eat less. Take time to fully enjoy your food as you eat it. Eating too fast or when your attention is elsewhere can lead to consuming too many calories. Pay attention to hunger cues before, during, and after meals. Use them to recognize when to eat and when you've had enough.
- Avoid large portions. Use a smaller plate, bowl, and glass. Portion out food before you eat. When eating out, choose a smaller size option, share a dish, or take home part of your meal.

Increase Some Foods Eat more vegetables, fruits, whole grains, and fat-free or 1 percent milk and dairy products. These foods have the nutrients you need for health, including potassium, calcium, vitamin D, and fiber. Make them the basis for meals and snacks.

- Make half your plate fruits and vegetables. Choose red, orange, and dark-green vegetables such as tomatoes, sweet potatoes, and broccoli. Add fruit to meals as part of main or side dishes or as dessert.
- Make at least half your grains whole grains. Substitute whole-wheat bread for white bread or brown rice for white rice.
- Switch to fat-free or 1 percent milk. They have the same amount of calcium and other essential nutrients as whole milk but fewer calories and less saturated fat.
- Experiment with spices and herbs. They have interesting flavors that can add zest to food without the extra hit of sodium. Remember to replace them when they get old or lose flavor.

Reduce Some Foods Cut back on foods that are high in solid fats, added sugars, and salt. Enjoy these foods as occasional treats, not everyday foods.

- Compare the amounts of sodium in foods such as soup, bread, and frozen meals, and choose the foods with lower numbers.

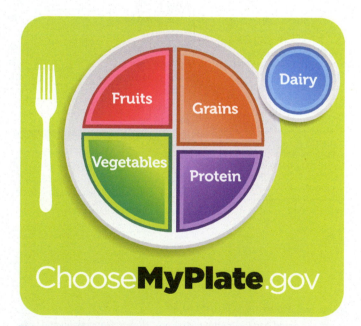

Figure 8.7 The MyPlate Food Guidance System
The USDA MyPlate food guidance system takes a new approach to dietary and exercise recommendations. Each colored section of the plate represents a food group. An interactive tool on www.choosemyplate.gov can provide individualized recommendations for users.
Source: U.S. Department of Agriculture, 2013, www.choosemyplate.gov.

Look for "low sodium," "reduced sodium," or "no salt added" on the food label.

- Drink water instead of sugary drinks. Cut calories by drinking water or unsweetened beverages. Soda, energy drinks, and sports drinks are a major source of added sugar and calories in American diets.

Understand Serving Sizes MyPlate presents personalized dietary recommendations in terms of numbers of servings of particular nutrients. But how much is one serving? Is it different from a portion? Although these two terms are often used interchangeably, they actually mean very different things. A *serving* is the recommended amount you should consume, whereas a *portion* is the amount you choose to eat at any one time. Many people select portions that are much bigger than recommended servings. See **Figure 8.8** for an easy way to recognize serving sizes.

Unfortunately, we don't always get a clear idea from food producers and advertisers about what a serving really is. Consider a bottle of chocolate milk: The food label may list one serving size as 8 fluid ounces and 150 calories. However, note the size of the entire bottle. If it holds 16 ounces, drinking the whole thing means consuming two servings, which serve up 300 calories.

Eat Nutrient-Dense Foods Although eating the proper number of servings from MyPlate is important, it is also important to recognize that there are large caloric, fat, and energy differences among foods within a given food group. For example, salmon and hot dogs provide vastly different nutrient levels per ounce. Salmon is rich in essential fatty acids and is considered nutrient dense. Hot dogs are loaded with saturated fats, cholesterol, and sodium—all substances that we should limit. It is important to eat foods that have a high nutritional value for their caloric content.

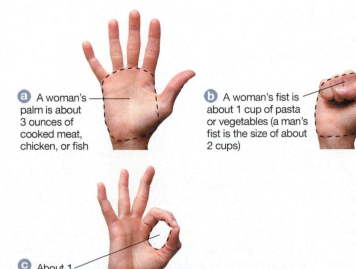

a A woman's palm is about 3 ounces of cooked meat, chicken, or fish

b A woman's fist is about 1 cup of pasta or vegetables (a man's fist is the size of about 2 cups)

c About 1 tablespoon of vegetable oil

Figure 8.8 What's a Serving?
Your hands can guide you in estimating portion sizes.

Reduce Empty Calorie Foods Avoid *empty calories*, that is, calories that have little or no nutritional value. Sugar is sugar, but when you eat it in a piece of fruit, you're getting dietary fiber, lots of vitamins and minerals, and phytochemicals. In contrast, when you drink a 12-ounce soft drink, you're getting nearly 200 empty calories. Don't be fooled by fruit drinks. Unless the label states that they're 100 percent juice, they may also be loaded with added sugar. Even 100 percent fresh-squeezed orange juice has 20 grams (5 teaspoons!) of naturally occurring sugar in an 8-ounce serving. Bottled coffees, teas, and energy drinks are usually even higher in sugar and empty calories. Ice cream, alcoholic beverages and sodas, most bakery sweets, sausages, and pizza are other examples of empty-calorie foods.[32]

Physical Activity Strive to be physically active for at least 30 minutes per day, preferably with moderate to vigorous activity levels on most days. Physical activity does not mean that you have to go to the gym, jog 3 miles a day, or hire a personal trainer. Any activity that gets your heart pumping (e.g., gardening, playing basketball, heavy yard work, brisk walks, swimming, or dancing) is a good way to get moving. In addition to personalized recommendations on diet, MyPlate personalized plans will also offer recommendations for weekly physical activity.

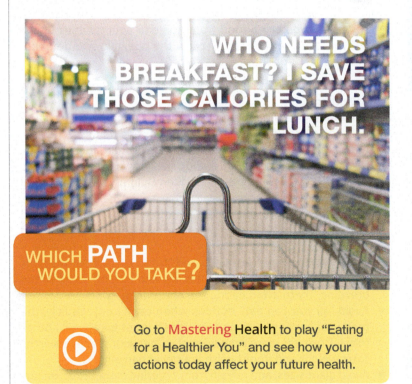

WHO NEEDS BREAKFAST? I SAVE THOSE CALORIES FOR LUNCH.

WHICH PATH WOULD YOU TAKE?

Go to Mastering Health to play "Eating for a Healthier You" and see how your actions today affect your future health.

Check Yourself

- What are the main guidelines of the MyPlate food guidance system?

- Which parts of MyPlate can you most easily adopt in your diet? Which are the most challenging? Why?

8.10 Toward Healthy, Mindful Eating in College

8.10 Provide examples of what college students can do to eat more healthfully and mindfully.

Many college students find it hard to fit a well-balanced meal into their day, even though healthy eating is important if you are to keep energy levels up and get the most out of your classes. Starting with a healthy breakfast that includes fiber-rich carbohydrates, protein, and healthy unsaturated fat (such as a banana, peanut butter, and whole-grain bread sandwich or a bowl of oatmeal topped with fruit and nuts) is important. Equally important is selecting healthy foods for regular meals and snacks that include high-fiber carbohydrates, low-fat proteins, and minimal sugars. Don't skip meals—just look at an overall daily balance in intake while keeping calories within a healthy range for you.

If your campus is like many others, you've probably noticed a distinct move toward fast-food restaurants in your student unions. Generally speaking, you can eat more healthfully and for less money if you bring food from home or your campus dining hall. If you must eat fast food, follow the tips below to get more nutritional bang for your buck:

- Ask for nutritional analyses of items. Most fast-food chains now have them.
- Remember that not all salads are healthy. Choose salads carefully, and avoid heavy dressings, croutons and noodles, cheeses, bacon (as in Cobb salads or taco salads), sugar-laden cranberries, and other Items that end up making your salad equal to the highest-calorie items on the menu. Lightly dip your forkful in the dressing rather than slathering it over the entire surface. Remember that "no-fat" dressings often are high in sugar and sodium. Load up on leafy greens, grilled chicken or tofu, and vegetables.
- If you crave french fries, try baked "fries," or order onion rings instead as a slightly healthier option, and pick off some of the breading. Try to avoid eating the entire serving.
- Avoid "all you can eat" options when eating out. Usually, the food is of lower quality and includes a lot of breads and other fillers. Don't eat more than normal to "get your money's worth." Extra weight and poor health are never bargains.
- Avoid giant sizes, and refrain from ordering extra sauce, bacon, cheese, dressings, and other extras that add additional calories, sodium, carbohydrates, and fat.
- Limit your consumption of sodas and other beverages that are high in added sugars.
- At least once a week, substitute a vegetable-based meat substitute into your fast-food choices. Most places now offer veggie burgers or similar products, which provide excellent sources of protein and often have considerably less fat and fewer calories. Ditch the top part of the bun to save calories.

In the dining hall, try these ideas:

- Choose lean meats, grilled chicken, fish, or vegetable dishes. Avoid fried chicken, fatty cuts of red meat, and meat dishes smothered in creamy or oily sauce.
- When choosing items from a made-to-order food station, ask the preparer to hold the butter, oil, mayonnaise, sour cream, or cheese- or cream-based sauces.
- If there is something you would like but don't see in your dining hall, speak to your food services manager and provide suggestions.

Between classes, avoid vending machines. Reach into your backpack for an apple, a banana, small portions of dried fruit and nuts, or whole-grain crackers or celery spread with peanut butter. Energy bars can be a nutritious option, but not always. Check the Nutrition Facts panel for bars that are below 200 calories and provide at least 3 grams of dietary fiber and low sugar. Cereal bars usually provide less protein than energy bars; however, cereal bars also tend to be much lower in calories and sugar and high in fiber.

Choose fruits and veggies in season—they'll cost less. Remember that frozen options are generally just as nutritious as fresh and are likely to be cheaper when fresh items are not in your budget.

Maintaining a nutritious diet within the confines of student life can be challenging. However, if you take the time to plan healthy meals, you will find that you are eating better, enjoying it more, and saving money.

Mindful Eating

A slower, more thoughtful and focused way of consuming food, known as **mindful eating**, can help you to avoid processed foods and unhealthy food and beverage choices.

Have you ever eaten your meal standing at the kitchen counter, sitting in front of your computer, or while on the way somewhere in the car? Some research has suggested that a slower, more thoughtful way of eating may reduce body weight and lead to healthier food choices. Eating on autopilot or using food as a reward interferes with the body's ability to feel hunger, stop when full, or enjoy food. It's easy to overeat and gain weight. The key is to slow down, focus on what you are putting in your mouth, and enjoy food, free of distractions. Mindful eating is eating intentionally—eating with the understanding and awareness that what you're putting in your mouth has an effect on your body. That eating isn't just filling up the gas tank—something to do as quickly as possible. It's an opportunity to get to know yourself, what you enjoy, and what your body is telling you.

Once you develop a healthy relationship with food, you're less likely to use food as a coping mechanism to deal with stress, social rejection, anxiety, depression, or even anger. This is the goal of

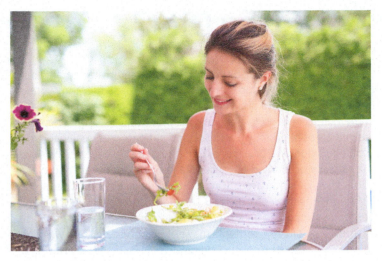

Mindful eating gives you the opportunity to slow down, savor your food, and enjoy the process of eating healthfully.

mindful eating. Mindfulness applied to eating may be achieved with these simple steps[33]:

- **Eat at the table.** Food eaten at the table is often eaten more slowly. When you eat in the car or between classes, you tend to eat in haste, choosing foods for convenience. Foods eaten at the table tend to be healthier options.
- **Make food the main focus.** Notice the colors, smells, flavors, and textures of your food. Get rid of distractions such as smart-phones, tablets, or television while eating.
- **Slow down. Savor the flavor.** Take small bites and focus on the taste and texture of your food. Rather than just wolfing down your food and washing it down with a beverage, try to distin-guish individual tastes and textures. As a young adult, you have over 10,000 taste buds that are replaced every few weeks. Use them as you will have fewer with age and may miss out on the best tastes of your life!
- **Choose foods you enjoy.** Plan meals that are colorful, satisfy-ing, and also nourishing to the body, and make sure different food groups are included. Make sure you have some greens and reds/oranges on every plate.
- **Eating should nourish your soul.** Learn to use all your senses to eat foods that are both satisfying to your soul and nourish your body.
- **Eat until you are satisfied and then stop.** Become aware of your own cues for when to begin eating and when to stop. Focus on when you get full and how that feels rather than pushing through it and feeling bloated.
- **Start slowly to begin the practice of mindful eating.** Because old eating habits may be hard to change, begin by eating just one meal a day or per week in a more attentive manner.

What's Healthy on the Menu?

No matter what type of cuisine you enjoy, there will always be healthier and less healthy options on the menu. To help you order

wisely, here are some lighter options and high-fat pitfalls. "Best" choices contain fewer than 30 grams of fat, a generous meal's worth for an active, medium-sized woman. "Worst" choices have up to 100 grams of fat.

Breakfast
- *Best:* Hot or cold high-fiber, low-sugar cereal with low-fat milk; 2-egg omelet with fresh vegetables, savory cheese such as low-fat feta or blue cheese, tofu, a side of fresh fruit, and whole-grain toast.
- *Worst:* Belgian waffle; biscuits and gravy, cheesy eggs, and hash browns; meat lover's omelets with extra cheese, loaded with bacon and hollandaise sauce.
- *Tips:* Ask for spinach, tomatoes, low-fat cream cheese, zucchini, mushrooms, and onions in a scramble. Forgo the bacon or sau-sage unless you can get turkey sausage or veggie or soy-based sausage from vendors of established products. Read labels to ensure low fat, high fiber, and low sodium.

Sandwiches
- *Best:* Grilled chicken breast; turkey; hummus and red pepper.
- *Worst:* Reuben; triple cheeseburger with bacon or other mon-ster burgers.
- *Tips:* Ask for mustard; hold the mayonnaise and high-fat cheese. Load up sandwiches with veggies such as tomatoes, lettuce, cucumbers, sprouts, and bell peppers.

Seafood
- *Best:* Halibut or snapper; salmon; grilled scallops; steamed crab or lobster.
- *Worst:* Fried seafood platter; blackened catfish.
- *Tips:* Order fish broiled, baked, grilled, or steamed—not panfried or sautéed. Ask for lemon instead of tartar sauce. Avoid creamy and buttery sauces.

Italian
- *Best:* Pasta with ripe or sun-dried tomato and low-fat feta; spa-ghetti with marinara or tomato-and-meat sauce.
- *Worst:* Fettuccine Alfredo; fried calamari; lasagna.
- *Tips:* Stick with plain bread instead of garlic bread made with butter or oil. Avoid cream- or egg-based sauces. Try vegetarian pizza, and don't ask for extra cheese.

Mexican
- *Best:* Bean burrito (no cheese); chicken fajitas.
- *Worst:* Beef chimichanga; quesadilla; chile relleno; refried beans.
- *Tips:* Choose soft tortillas (not fried) with fresh salsa, not guaca-mole. Ask for beans made without lard or fat, and have cheeses and sour cream provided on the side or left out altogether.

Check Yourself

- **What challenges do you face when trying to eat more healthfully?**

- **What are some steps that you can take to eat more mindfully?**

8.10

Nutrition

8.11 **Describe the benefits and drawbacks of a vegetarian diet.**

The word **vegetarian** can mean different things to different people. *Vegans* eat no animal products at all, while many vegetarians eat dairy or other animal products but not animal flesh, and some eat seafood but not beef, pork, or poultry. Approximately 8 million Americans are either vegetarian or vegan and 37 percent of Americans have tried vegetarian eating out in the last year.[34] Women are most likely to be vegans, and young adults (ages 18 to 34), make up the largest group of vegetarians overall.[35]

Common reasons for pursuing a vegetarian lifestyle include concern for animal welfare, the environmental costs of meat production, food safety, personal health, weight loss, and weight maintenance. Generally, people who follow a balanced vegetarian diet weigh less and have better cholesterol levels, fewer problems with constipation and diarrhea, and a lower risk of heart disease than do nonvegetarians. A recent analysis of 29 studies involving a total of more than 20,000 participants found that vegetarians have an average blood pressure several points lower than that of nonvegetarians.[36] Another recent study indicated significant reductions in body mass index, total and LDL cholesterol levels, and glucose levels among vegans in comparison to meat eaters and overall reductions in ischemic heart disease and cancer.[37]

With proper meal planning and eating a variety of healthful foods throughout the day, vegetarianism provides a healthful alternative to a high-fat, high-calorie, meat-based diet. Purely vegan diets may be deficient in some important vitamins and minerals, though many foods are fortified with these nutrients, or vegans can obtain them from supplements. Pregnant women, children, older adults, and sick people who are vegans or vegetarians need to take special care to ensure that their diets are adequate. Seek advice from a health care professional if you have questions.

Do Vegetarians Need to Take Supplements?

Dietary supplements are products that are intended to supplement existing diets. Ingredients range from vitamins, minerals, and herbs to enzymes, amino acids, fatty acids, and organ tissues. A majority of Americans—68 percent—take at least one dietary supplement.[38] Among supplements users, 98 percent take vitamin and mineral supplements.[39] The FDA does not evaluate the safety and efficacy of supplements before they are marketed; it can take action to remove a supplement from the market only after the supplement has been proved harmful.

Whether you need dietary supplements is a matter of debate. The Office of Dietary Supplements, part of the National Institutes of Health, and other national groups indicate that the best source of nutrients is a varied, healthful diet. For the average person with a balanced and healthy diet, supplements may help ensure that you get adequate amounts of essential nutrients, but are not intended to prevent or treat diseases. In fact, a task force recently concluded that there is insufficient evidence to recommend taking multivitamin and mineral supplements to prevent cardiovascular disease or cancer.[40]

The people who may benefit from using multivitamin and mineral supplements include pregnant and breast-feeding women, older adults who are ill or who are not getting essential nutrients in their diets, vegans, people on a very low-calorie weight-loss diet, individuals dependent on alcohol, and patients with malabsorption problems/digestive or other significant health problems. However, the efficacy of many dietary supplements is unproven, and claims about their benefits are often not backed by science. For example, although ingestion of omega-3 through fish consumption continues to be supported as a means of reducing the risk of heart disease, omega-3 in supplements may not be as beneficial as was once thought, with several conflicting reports surfacing in recent years.[41]

Taking high-dose supplements of the fat-soluble vitamins A, D, and E can be harmful or even fatal. Moreover, supplements often do not contain the ingredients listed on the label.

If you do decide to take dietary supplements, choose brands that have the U.S. Pharmacopeia (USP) or Consumer Lab seal. This ensures that the supplement is free of toxic ingredients and contains the ingredients stated on the label. Store your supplements in a dark, dry place (not the bathroom or other damp spots); make sure they are out of reach of small children; and check the expiration date, throwing them away once that date has been reached.

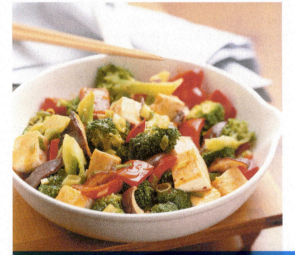

Are vegetarian diets healthy?

Adopting a vegan or vegetarian diet can be a very healthy way to eat. Take care to prepare your food healthfully by limiting the use of oils and avoiding added sugars and sodium. Make sure you get all the essential amino acids by eating meals like this tofu and vegetable stir fry. To further enhance it, add a whole grain such as brown rice.

Check Yourself

- What are some of the benefits and drawbacks of a vegetarian diet?

- What would be your biggest reasons for becoming a vegetarian? For not opting for vegetarianism?

8.12 Is Organic for You?

Learning Outcome

8.12 **Explain the nature of organic foods.**

Concerns about food safety, genetically modified foods, and the health impacts of chemicals used in the growth and production of food have led many people to turn to foods that are **organic**—foods and beverages developed, grown, or raised without the use of synthetic pesticides, chemicals, or hormones. Any food sold in the United States as organic has to meet criteria set by the USDA under the National Organic Rule and can carry a USDA seal verifying products as "certified organic."

Under the National Organic Rule, a product that is certified may carry one of the following terms: "100 percent Organic" (100 percent compliance with organic criteria), "Organic" (must contain at least 95 percent organic materials), "Made with Organic Ingredients" (must contain at least 70 percent organic ingredients), or "Some Organic Ingredients" (contains less than 70 percent organic ingredients—usually listed individually). To be labeled with any of these terms, the foods must be produced without the use of hormones, antibiotics, herbicides, insecticides, chemical fertilizers, genetic modification, or germ-killing radiation. However, reliable monitoring systems to ensure credibility are still under development and enforcement is lacking.

Products that are labeled "all natural," "free-range," or "hormone free" are not necessarily organic. Free range may mean that hundreds of chickens are let out of their cages and are walking in wastes and intermingling with diseased birds in a very crowded unsanitary building. Distinguishing those free range chickens from those raised in your local community and who have the luxury of acres of pasture, may difficult to determine. Ask questions and don't pay more for misleading labels.The term *natural* on food labels is not currently regulated; it is a marketing term that has no real meaning except to imply healthiness. What is "natural" chicken compared to "unnatural" chicken, for example? The FDA is currently investigating concerns related to the use of the term "natural" and may shortly develop regulations on its use.[43]

The market for organic foods has been increasing faster than food sales in general for many years. Whereas only a small subset of the population once bought organic foods, 82 to 84 percent of U.S. families now buy them at least occasionally,

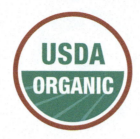

USDA label for certified organic foods.

and sales of organic foods represent nearly 5 percent of total food sales.[44] In the third quarter of 2016, sales of organic vegetables were up nearly 8 percent and sales of organic fruits were up 17.5 percent compared to the third quarter of 2015.[45]

Common reasons why people choose to buy organic foods include preferring the taste and wanting to limit exposure to pesticides and food additives. Some people purchase organic products because of environmental concerns, since organic farming limits pesticide use and takes other measures to reduce pollution. The U.S. Environmental Protection Agency regulates pesticide use and, while ensuring Americans that only low levels of pesticide residue remain on conventionally grown foods, advises consumers to scrub produce under running water and, if possible, peel it.[46]

Is buying organic better for you? That depends on what aspect of the food is being studied and how the studies are conducted. Research provides a controversial picture of the benefits of organic meats, dairy products, and eggs compared to conventional products. While organic meats provide higher fatty acid levels, consumer brand preferences, appearance of packaging, and texture appear to influence consumer perceptions more than actual nutritional benefits do.[47] Other research indicates that in terms of food safety, we don't have sufficient knowledge to say whether organic foods' higher prices are justified for safety reasons alone.[48].

The word **locavore** has been coined to describe people who eat only food grown or produced locally, usually within close proximity to their homes. Foods sold at farmers markets, homegrown foods, or those grown by independent farmers are thought to be fresher and to require far fewer resources to get them to market and keep them fresh for longer periods of time. Unfortunately,, because organic, locally grown foods at farmers markets and in local stores usually come at a hefty price, many people can't afford them or can't justify paying that much.

Consumers should not assume that locally grown foods are always organic or less likely to be contaminated with microorganisms. Pesticide residues and harmful bacteria can be found in foods purchased from local farms as well as in foods shipped from distant countries.[49] Additionally, issues about the raising, harvesting, transport and refrigeration of locally or regionally grown foods have been raised, as regulations and enforcement policies are often not in place. To reduce risk, wash your produce before eating, be cautious about home grown and preserved products, and cook meats and seafood to temperature.

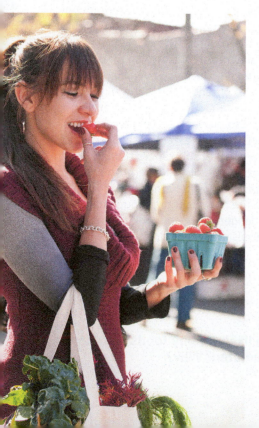

Check Yourself

- Which organic foods are you currently buying? Why did you choose these?

- To make the best use of your finances, which foods carry the greatest risks and which foods should you substitute for them?

8.13 Food Technology

Learning Outcome

8.13 Identify technologies being used in food production today.

Food Irradiation

Food irradiation involves exposing foods to low doses of radiation, or ionizing energy, which breaks chemical bonds in the DNA of harmful bacteria, destroying them or keeping them from reproducing. Essentially, the radiation passes through the food without leaving any radioactive residue.[50] It also kills harmful insects that might enter the United States, delays sprouting and ripening in transit, and keeps foods from spoiling.

Irradiation lengthens food products' shelf life and impedes the spread of deadly microorganisms, particularly in high-risk foods such as ground beef, pork, chicken, shellfish, lettuce, spinach, and eggs. Use of food irradiation is limited because of consumers' concerns about its safety and because irradiation facilities are expensive to build. Still, food irradiation is now common in over 40 countries. Irradiated foods are marked with the "radura" logo.

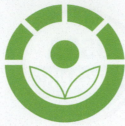

U.S. FDA label for irradiated foods.

Genetically Modified Food Crops

Genetic modification involves the insertion or deletion of genes into the DNA of an organism. In the case of **genetically modified (GM) foods**, this is usually done to enhance production by making disease- or insect-resistant plants, improving yield, or controlling weeds. There continues to be considerable controversy about the use of GM foods in the food chain. Many countries ban them. Many researchers are concerned that GM foods carry serious risks to humans and ecosystems, disrupting the delicate balance between insects, birds, and other species and foods. Others worry about seeds being controlled by large corporations. Organic farmers are concerned about pesticide- and chemical-infused GM seeds drifting into their fields. Proponents argue that GM crops grow faster and have average yields that are 22 percent higher than those of traditional crops and can be credited with helping to feed millions of people who would otherwise face starvation or malnutrition.[51] In addition, GM foods are sometimes created to boost the level of specific nutrients. For example, currently under development is a GM variety of rice that is high in vitamin A and iron. Another use that is under development is the production and delivery of vaccines through GM foods.

Soybeans and cotton are the most common GM crops, followed by corn. An estimated 75 percent of processed foods on supermarket shelves are genetically modified.[52]

Although the genetic engineering of insect-resistant crops has reduced the use of insecticides, it has simultaneously increased the use of herbicides (which kill weeds). This has not only led to the evolution of so-called "superweeds," but has also killed off beneficial weeds such as milkweed.[53] As a result, butterfly populations that depend on these weeds, particularly the monarch butterfly, have been decimated.[54]

The long-term safety of GM foods—for humans, other species, and the environment—is still in question. The American Association for the Advancement of Science reports that foods containing GM ingredients pose no more risk than the same foods composed of crops modified over time by conventional plant-breeding techniques. The World Health Organization states that no adverse effects on human health have been shown from consumption of GM foods in countries that have approved their use.[55] The debate surrounding the risks and benefits of GM foods is not likely to end soon.

Arguments for the Development of Genetically Modified Foods

- People have been manipulating food crops—primarily through selective breeding and hybridization—since the beginning of agriculture. Genetic modification is fundamentally the same thing, just more precise.
- Modified fruits and vegetables produce higher levels of antioxidants, which reduce the risk of heart disease and cancer, and vitamin A to prevent blindness.
- Genetically modified seeds and products are tested for safety, and there has never been a substantiated claim for a human illness resulting from consumption of a GM food.
- Genetically modified crops have the potential to reduce world hunger. They can be created to grow more quickly than conventional crops, increasing productivity and allowing for faster cycling of crops, which means a higher food yield. In addition, nutrient-enhanced crops can address malnutrition, and crops engineered to resist spoiling or damage can allow for transportation to areas affected by drought or natural disaster.

Arguments against the Development of Genetically Modified Foods

- Genetic modification could cause an allergic reaction. Allergic reactions occur in humans when their immune system recognizes a protein as a foreign invader. Research suggests that some GM foods may cause allergic reactions.
- GM foods have the potential to reduce absorption of essential nutrients. For example, if the gene inserted to make the new GM food increases the phytate content of the food, this reduces the absorption of certain minerals, such as calcium and iron. Modified soy products may also produce less phytoestrogens, which are known to reduce the risk of heart disease and cancer.
- Plants naturally produce low levels of substances that are toxic to humans. While these toxins do not produce problems for humans, there is a concern that adding a new gene to produce a GM plant may cause the new plant to produce toxins at higher levels that could be dangerous if eaten. For instance, GM potatoes produce higher levels of glycoalkaloids.

Check Yourself

- **What are two technologies that are being used in production of our food?**

- **Are you more or less likely to buy foods that have been modified or irradiated? Why?**

Food Allergies and Intolerances

8.14 Define food allergies and intolerances.

Although many people today *think* they have a food allergy, it is estimated that only 5 percent of children and 4 percent of adults actually do.[56]

Food Allergies

A **food allergy**, or hypersensitivity, is an abnormal response to a food that is triggered by the immune system. Symptoms of an allergic reaction vary in severity and may include a tingling sensation in the mouth; swelling of the lips, tongue, and throat; difficulty breathing; skin hives; vomiting; abdominal cramps; and diarrhea. A severe reaction called *anaphylaxis* can cause widespread inflammation, difficulty breathing, and cardiovascular problems such as a sudden drop in blood pressure that can be life threatening.[57] Anaphylaxis may occur within seconds to hours after eating the foods to which one is seriously allergic.

The Food Allergen Labeling and Consumer Protection Act requires food manufacturers to label foods clearly to indicate the presence of (or possible contamination by) any of the eight major food allergens: milk, eggs, peanuts, wheat, soy, tree nuts (walnuts, pecans, cashews, pistachios, etc.), fish, and shellfish. Although over 160 foods have been identified as allergy triggers, these eight foods account for 90 percent of all food allergies in the United States.[58]

If you suspect that you have had an allergic reaction to food, see an allergist to be tested to determine the source of the problem. Because there are several diseases that share symptoms with food allergies (for instance, ulcers and cancers of the gastrointestinal tract can cause vomiting, bloating, diarrhea, nausea, and pain), you should have any persistent symptoms checked out as soon as possible. If particular foods seem to bother you consistently, look for alternatives or modify your diet. If you have a true food allergy, you might not be able to consume even the smallest amount of a substance safely.

Food Intolerance

In contrast to allergies, **food intolerance** can cause symptoms of gastric upset, but the upset is not the result of an immune system response. Probably the best example of a food intolerance is *lactose intolerance*, which is common, although the number of Americans with the condition is unknown.[59] Lactase is an enzyme produced by the small intestine that helps to break the bonds in the lactose molecule. If a person doesn't produce enough lactase, undigested lactose remains in the small intestine, drawing water by osmosis. This dilates the small intestine and speeds the transit of the food mass, resulting in diarrhea. When the undigested lactose reaches the large intestine, gut bacteria ferment it. Gas is formed, and the person experiences bloating and abdominal pain.

Food intolerance also occurs in response to some food additives, such as the flavor enhancer MSG, certain dyes, sulfites, gluten, and other substances. In some cases, the food intolerance may have psychological triggers.

Celiac Disease

Celiac disease is an immune disorder that causes malabsorption of nutrients from the small intestine in genetically susceptible people. It is thought to affect as many as 1 in every 141 Americans, most of whom are undiagnosed.[60] When a person with celiac disease consumes gluten—a protein found in wheat, rye, and barley—the person's immune system attacks the small intestine and stops nutrient absorption. Pain, cramping, and other symptoms often follow in the short term. Untreated, celiac disease can lead to other health problems, such as osteoporosis, nutritional deficiencies, and cancer. Individuals diagnosed with celiac disease are encouraged to consult a dietitian for help in designing a gluten-free diet. If you suspect that you have celiac disease, see a doctor. Blood tests looking for specific antibodies or a small intestine biopsy can help to determine whether you have celiac disease or other GI issues.

Increasing numbers of products are available for people who need to follow a gluten-free diet. Specially formulated gluten-free breads, pasta, and cereal products can allow people with celiac disease to enjoy meals similar to those without the disease. Reading food labels is particularly important because many foods that seem safe may have hidden sources of gluten. Bouillon cubes, cold cuts, and soups are three examples of processed foods that may contain wheat, barley, or rye.

Peanuts are among the eight most common food allergens.

- What causes food allergies and intolerances?

- What is the difference between a food allergy and an intolerance?

8.15 Provide examples of food safety concerns and tips for reducing exposure to unsafe food.

Eating unhealthy food is one thing. Eating food that has been contaminated with a pathogen, toxin, or other harmful substance is quite another. As outbreaks of foodborne illness (commonly called *food poisoning*) make the news, the food industry has come under fire. The Food Safety Modernization Act, passed into law in 2011, included new requirements for food processors to take actions to prevent contamination of foods. The act gave the FDA greater authority to inspect food-manufacturing facilities and to recall contaminated foods.[61]

Are you concerned that the chicken you are buying doesn't look pleasingly pink or that your "fresh" fish smells a little *too* fishy? You may have good reason to be worried. The Centers for Disease Control and Prevention (CDC) estimates that foodborne illnesses from 31 pathogens cause 9.4 million illnesses, 55,961 hospitalizations, and 1,351 deaths in the United States annually.[62] Although the incidence of infection with certain microbes has declined, the incidence of infection with other microbes has risen or stayed essentially unchanged; therefore, the CDC reports that foodborne infections are an ongoing public health concern requiring improved prevention.[63]

Most foodborne infections and illnesses are caused by several common types of bacteria and viruses. The following are some of the most common[64]:

- **Norovirus.** Transmitted through contact with the vomit or stool of infected people, norovirus is the most common cause of foodborne illness in the United States annually. Washing hands and all kitchen surfaces can help to prevent transmission.
- **Salmonella.** Commonly found in the intestines of birds, reptiles, and mammals, the species *Salmonella* can spread to humans through foods of animal origin. Infection is more likely in people with poor underlying health or weakened immune systems.
- **Clostridium perfringens.** This is a bacterial species found in the intestinal tracts of humans and animals.
- **Campylobacter.** Most raw poultry has *Campylobacter* in it; bacterial infection most often results from eating undercooked chicken, raw eggs, or foods contaminated with juices from raw chicken. Shellfish and unpasteurized milk are also sources.
- **Staphylococcus aureus.** *Staph* lives on human skin, in infected cuts, and in the nose and throat.

Foodborne illnesses can also be caused by a toxin in food originally produced by a bacterium or other microbe in the food. These toxins can produce illness even if the microbes that produced them are no longer there. For example, botulism is caused by a deadly neurotoxin produced by the bacterium *Clostridium botulinum*. This bacterium is widespread in soil, water, plants, and intestinal tracts, but it can grow only in environments with limited or no oxygen. Potential food sources include improperly canned food and vacuum-packed or tightly wrapped foods. Botulism is rare, and most cases occur as a result of eating home-canned vegetables; however, store-bought foods from cans that are dented, pierced, leaking, or bulging may also harbor the botulism toxin.[65]

Signs of foodborne illnesses vary tremendously and usually include one or several symptoms: diarrhea, nausea, cramping, and vomiting. Depending on the amount and virulence of the pathogen, symptoms may appear as early as 30 minutes after eating contaminated food or as long as several days or weeks later. Most of the time, symptoms occur 5 to 8 hours after eating and last only a day or two. Foodborne diseases can be fatal for certain populations, such as the very young; older adults; or people with severe illnesses such as cancer, diabetes, kidney disease, or AIDS.

Several factors contribute to foodborne illnesses, including inadequate oversight of both foreign and domestic suppliers by uncoordinated and underfunded federal agencies. Moreover, federal agencies can be slow to identify and respond to outbreaks.[66] The task is enormous. Food can become contaminated in the field by contaminated irrigation water or runoff from nearby animal feedlots, or during harvesting if farm laborers have not washed their hands properly after using the toilet. Food-processing equipment, facilities, or workers may contaminate food, or it can become contaminated if not kept clean and cool during transport or on store shelves.

In addition, the actual location where food is grown might not be known because mass distribution centers take in foods from many growers, repackage it, and send it to different companies for labeling. Good luck if you want to know whether your milk came from Wisconsin or California. Most food labels say, "Distributed by" rather than listing the actual location of production. This is a major area of concern.

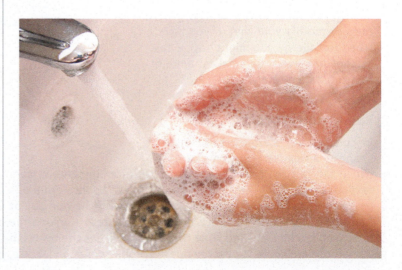

95%

is the percentage of people who fail to wash their hands with soap long enough to kill harmful bacteria that can spread diseases. Ten percent skip the sink entirely, and 62 percent of men and 40 percent of women don't wash their hands after using the toilet.

The bacterium *Escherichia coli*, species of which produce a dangerous toxin, is present in unprocessed cow manure, which is commonly used as a fertilizer on both organic and conventional farms. Although the level of the bacteria drops significantly within 60 days, it can survive on fields for up to 120 days and can even be resuscitated after heavy rains.[67] No regulations prohibit farmers from using animal manure to fertilize crops. In addition, *E. coli* quickly reproduces in the summer months as cattle await slaughter in crowded, overheated pens. This increases the chances of meat coming to market already contaminated.

Other key factors associated with the increasing spread of foodborne diseases include the inadvertent introduction of pathogens into new geographic regions and insufficient education about food safety. Globalization of the food supply, climate change, and global warming are also factors that may influence the increasing spread.

Avoiding Risks in the Home

Part of the responsibility for preventing foodborne illness lies with consumers. Although 75 percent of cases of foodborne illness are caused by foods consumed in restaurants, delis, or banquet facilities, about 9 percent result from unsafe handling of food at home.[68] Fortunately, consumers can take several steps to reduce the likelihood of contaminating their food (see Figure 8.9). Among the most basic precautions are washing your hands frequently while preparing food and washing all produce before eating it.

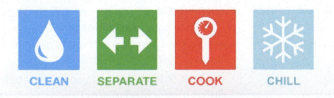

Figure 8.9 The Four Core Practices for Food Safety
This logo reminds consumers how to prevent foodborne illness.
Source: Partnership for Food Safety Education, 2017, www.fightbac.org/safe-food-handling

Also, avoid cross-contamination in the kitchen by using separate cutting boards and utensils for meats and produce.

Temperature control is also important. Refrigerators must be set at 40 degrees or less. Be sure to cook meats to the recommended temperature to kill contaminants before eating. Hot foods must be kept hot and cold foods must be kept cold to avoid unchecked bacterial growth. Eat leftovers within 3 days. If you're unsure how long something has been sitting in the fridge, don't take chances. When in doubt, throw it out. See Skills for Behavior Change for more tips about reducing risk of foodborne illness when shopping for and preparing food.

Skills for Behavior Change

Reduce Your Risk For Foodborne Illness

- **When shopping, put perishable foods in your cart last. Check for cleanliness throughout the store, especially at the salad bar and at the meat and fish counters. Never buy dented cans of food, particularly those where the lid or seam shows signs of denting. Check the "sell by" or "use by" date on foods and find out what those terms really mean. Not all sell by or use by labels mean the food is no longer edible.**
- **Once you get home, put dairy products, eggs, meat, fish, and poultry in the refrigerator immediately. If you don't plan to eat meats within 2 days, freeze them. You can keep an unopened package of hot dogs or luncheon meats for about 2 weeks.**
- **When refrigerating or freezing raw meats, make sure their juices can't spill onto other foods.**
- **Never thaw frozen foods at room temperature. Put them in the refrigerator to thaw, or thaw them in the microwave, following manufacturer's instructions.**
- **Wash your hands with soap and warm water before preparing food. Wash fruits and vegetables before peeling, slicing, cooking, or eating them—but do not wash meat, poultry, or eggs. Wash cutting boards, countertops, and other utensils and surfaces with detergent and hot water after food preparation.**
- **Use a meat thermometer to ensure that meats are completely cooked. To find out proper cooking temperatures for different types of meat, visit http://foodsafety.gov.**
- **Refrigeration slows the secretion of bacterial toxins into foods. Never leave leftovers out for more than 2 hours. On hot days, don't leave foods out for longer than 1 hour.**
- **In an era of reusable bags, wash bags regularly and keep meats in bags separate from fresh produce and other foods.**

Check Yourself

- What are some of the greatest food safety issues in America today? Which ones are most likely to affect you right now?

- Have you ever experienced a foodborne illness? If so, what were possible causes, and how could you have avoided the illness?

Summary

LO 8.1 Recognizing that we eat for more reasons than just survival is the first step toward improving our nutritional habits.

LO 8.1–8.7 The essential nutrients include water, proteins, carbohydrates, fats, vitamins, and minerals. Water makes up 50 to 60 percent of our body weight and is necessary for nearly all life processes. Proteins are major components of our cells and are key elements of antibodies, enzymes, and hormones. Carbohydrates are our primary sources of energy. Fats play important roles in maintaining body temperature and cushioning and protecting organs. Vitamins are organic compounds, and minerals are inorganic compounds. We need both in relatively small amounts to maintain healthy body function. Functional foods may provide health benefits in addition to the nutrients they contribute to the diet.

LO 8.8 Food labels provide information on serving size and number of calories in a food, as well as the amounts of various nutrients and the percentage of recommended daily values those amounts represent.

LO 8.9 A healthful diet is adequate, moderate, balanced, varied, and nutrient dense. The *Dietary Guidelines for Americans* and the MyPlate food guidance system provide guidelines for healthy eating. These recommendations, developed by the USDA, place emphasis on balancing calories and making appropriate food choices.

LO 8.10 College students face unique challenges in eating healthfully. Learning to make better choices at restaurants, to eat healthfully on a budget, and to eat nutritiously at home or in the dorm are all possible when you use the information in this chapter. Mindful eating can help you make healthier choices and enjoy the process of eating more.

LO 8.11 Vegetarianism can provide a healthy alternative for people who want to eat less or no meat.

LO 8.12 Organic foods are grown and produced without the use of synthetic pesticides, chemicals, or hormones. The USDA offers certification of organics. These foods have become increasingly available and popular as people take more interest in eating healthfully and sustainably.

LO 8.11–8.15 Foodborne illnesses, food irradiation, allergies, food intolerances, GM foods, and other food safety and health concerns are becoming increasingly important to health-wise consumers. Recognizing potential risks and taking steps to prevent problems are part of a sound nutritional plan.

Pop Quiz

Visit **Mastering Health** *to personalize your study plan with Chapter Review Quizzes and Dynamic Study Modules.*

LO 8.2 1. What is the most crucial nutrient for life?
a. Water
c. Minerals
b. Fiber
d. Protein

LO 8.2 2. Which of the following nutrients is required for the repair and growth of body tissue?
a. Carbohydrates
c. Vitamins
b. Proteins
d. Fats

LO 8.3 3. Which of the following nutrients moves food through the digestive tract?
a. Water
c. Minerals
b. Fiber
d. Starch

LO 8.4 4. What substance plays a vital role in maintaining healthy skin and hair, insulating body organs against shock, maintaining body temperature, and promoting healthy cell function?
a. Fats
c. Proteins
b. Fibers
d. Carbohydrates

LO 8.4 5. Triglycerides make up about ___ percent of total body fat.
a. 5
c. 55
b. 35
d. 95

LO 8.4 6. Which of the following is a healthier fat to include in the diet?
a. *Trans* fat
b. Saturated fat
c. Unsaturated fat
d. Hydrogenated fat

LO 8.5 7. Which vitamin helps to maintain bone health?
a. B_{12}
c. B_6
b. D
d. Niacin

LO 8.6 8. Which of the following is a trace mineral?
a. Calcium
c. Potassium
b. Sodium
d. Iron

LO 8.9 9. Which of the following foods would be considered a healthy, nutrient-dense food?
a. Nonfat milk
c. Soft drink
b. Celery
d. Potato chips

LO 8.14 10. Lucas's doctor diagnoses him with celiac disease. Which of the following foods should Lucas cut out of his diet to eat gluten-free?
a. Shellfish
c. Peanuts
b. Eggs
d. Wheat

Answers to these questions can be found on page A-1. If you answered a question incorrectly, review the module identified by the Learning Outcome. For even more study tools, visit Mastering Health.

Think About It!

LO 8.2–8.6 1. What are the major types of nutrients that you need to obtain from the foods you eat? What happens if you fail to get enough of some of them? In what ways do women's nutrient needs differ from men's?

LO 8.9 2. What are the major food groups in the MyPlate plan? From which groups do you eat too few servings? Too many? What can you do to increase or decrease your intake of selected food groups?

LO 8.10 3. What are the major problems that you face when trying to eat healthy foods? List five actions that you and others like you could take immediately to improve your eating.

LO 8.11 4. Distinguish among varieties of vegetarianism. Which types are most likely to lead to nutrient deficiencies? What can be done to ensure that even people who follow the strictest vegetarian diet receive enough of the major nutrients? If vegetarianism isn't for you, what can you do to increase your vegetable consumption and eat more alternative sources of protein?

LO 8.14 5. How does a food intolerance differ from a food allergy?

LO 8.15 6. What are the major risks for foodborne illnesses, and what can you do to protect yourself? What can be done to protect food safety in the larger community?

Weight Management and Body Image

9

The keys to weight management seem simple enough: Eat too many calories without exercising, and you will gain weight; reduce calories and increase exercise, and the pounds will slide right off. But if all it took were eating less and exercising more, Americans would merely reevaluate their diets, cut calories, and exercise. Unfortunately, it's not that easy. And the problem goes beyond body weight to increasingly common issues of self-perception and disordered eating among both men and women.

What factors predispose people to problems with weight? Although diet and exercise are clearly major contributors, genetics and physiology are also important. Learned behaviors in the home and influences at school, in social environments, in the media, and in the environments where we live, work, and play are all important to our weight profiles.[1] Experts realize that a complex web of interactive factors influences what we eat, how much we eat, and when we eat as well as how we expend energy. Figuring out what these factors are and developing key strategies to reduce risk are key.

203

Obesity in the United States and Worldwide

Learning Outcome

9.1 Examine obesity trends in the United States.

The United States has the dubious distinction of having the highest proportion of obesity in the world at 13 percent, followed by China and India, whose populations together make up 15 percent of the obese population.[2] Young and old, rich and poor, rural and urban, educated and uneducated Americans have one thing in common: They are fatter than virtually all previous generations.[3]

The word **obesogenic** means something that is characterized by environments that promote increased food intake, nonhealthful foods, and physical inactivity. It has increasingly become an apt descriptor of our society. The map in **Figure 9.1** illustrates the rapidly increasing levels of obesity in the United States over the last two decades.

Obesity has become steadily more prevalent in recent decades, with disproportionate risks among certain populations.[4] Obesity rates for children age 2 to 5 have shown slight decreases or appear to have stabilized in recent years; however, the rates remain high, with over 9.4 percent of our youngest children already obese. Obesity rates have risen in almost all other groups. Nearly 17.5 percent of children age 6 to 11 and 20.6 percent of adolescents age 12 to 19 are obese today, and rates of extreme obesity are increasing.[5] Children and adolescents living in low-income, low-education, and higher-unemployment homes are at significantly greater risk of developing obesity, while those from higher-income homes with more educated parents have decreasing risk.[6]

A Youthful Start on Obesity However, today's youth have easy access to a vast array of high-fat, high-calorie foods; have fewer physical education requirements in schools; are more restricted in terms of playing outdoors, particularly in high-crime areas; and are more obese than ever before. Nearly 55 percent of obese children are still obese in adolescence, and 80 percent of obese adolescents will be obese adults—with 70 percent of those continuing to be obese after age 30.[23]

Research also points to higher rates of overweight and obesity among some adult populations in the United States. Hispanic men (79.6 percent) and non-Hispanic white men (73 percent) are more likely to be overweight or obese than are non-Hispanic black men (69 percent).[7] Non-Hispanic black women (82.2 percent) and Hispanic women (77.1 percent) are more likely to be overweight or obese than are non-Hispanic white women (63.7 percent).[8] In sharp contrast, 46.6 percent of Asian men and 34.6 percent of Asian women in the United States are overweight or obese.[9]

The United States is not alone in the obesity epidemic. In fact, obesity has more than doubled globally since 1980, with over 1.9 billion overweight and 600 million obese adults.[10] Obesity was once predominantly a problem in high-income countries; today, increasing numbers of low- and middle-income countries have overweight and obesity problems.[11] The global epidemic of high rates of overweight and obesity in multiple regions of the world has come to be known as **globesity**. Increases in sedentary occupations, mass marketing of high-fat, high-carbohydrate foods, and an increase in the food energy supply to the world's population through international distribution have contributed to the rise in obesity.[12]

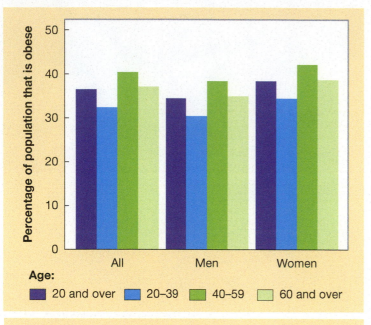

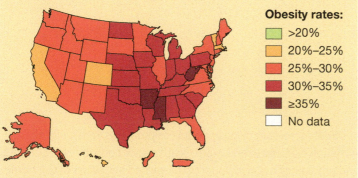

Figure 9.1 Prevalence of Obesity in Adults Age 20 Years or Older by Age and Sex

Source: E.J. Benjamin, et al. "Heart Disease and Stroke Statistics—2017 Update: A Report from the American Heart Association," *Circulation* 135, no. 10 (2017): e146–e603; Centers for Disease Control and Prevention/National Center for Health Statistics, NHANES, 2011 TO 2014; Centers for Disease Control and Prevention, OBESITY PREVALENCE Map, 2012–2014.

Check Yourself

- How have levels of obesity changed in the United States over the last two decades?

- Why do you think disparities in obesity levels exist among certain populations in the United States?

9.2 Health Effects of Overweight and Obesity

Learning Outcome

9.2 **List health effects associated with overweight and obesity.**

Although smoking is still the leading cause of preventable death in the United States, obesity is rapidly gaining on it. Obesity is linked to cardiovascular disease (CVD), stroke, cancer, hypertension, diabetes, depression, digestive problems, gallstones, sleep apnea, osteoarthritis, decreased mobility, restrictions on activities of daily living, and loss of independence.[13] **Figure 9.2** summarizes these and other potential health consequences of obesity.

Short- and long-term health consequences of obesity are not our only concern. Obese populations have a 42 percent higher annual health care cost than healthy-weight populations. Severely obese adults have health care costs that are 81 percent higher per capita than those of healthy adults. Lifetime medical costs for major diseases increase by over 50 percent for obese individuals—twice that amount for severely obese people. Longer hospital stays, longer recovery times, and increased medications are all part of these costs.[14]

Other effects of overweight and obesity can be more subtle. Consequences can include depression, anxiety, low self-esteem, poor body image, and suicidal acts and thoughts; binge eating and unhealthy weight-control practices; lack of adequate health care because doctors spend less time with and do fewer interventions on overweight patients and are reluctant to perform preventive health screenings; and reluctance to visit the doctor and get necessary preventive health care services.

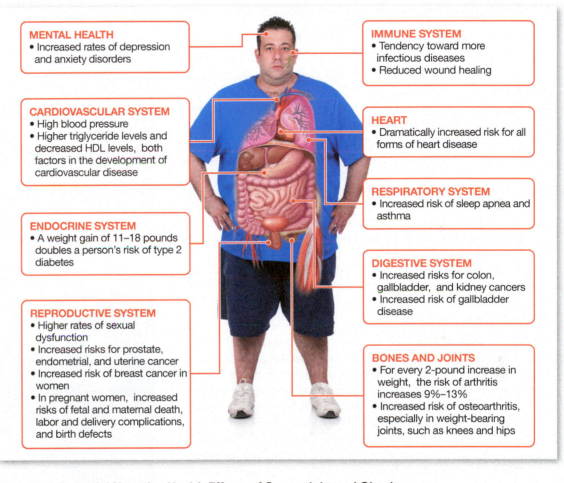

MENTAL HEALTH
• Increased rates of depression and anxiety disorders

IMMUNE SYSTEM
• Tendency toward more infectious diseases
• Reduced wound healing

CARDIOVASCULAR SYSTEM
• High blood pressure
• Higher triglyceride levels and decreased HDL levels, both factors in the development of cardiovascular disease

HEART
• Dramatically increased risk for all forms of heart disease

RESPIRATORY SYSTEM
• Increased risk of sleep apnea and asthma

ENDOCRINE SYSTEM
• A weight gain of 11–18 pounds doubles a person's risk of type 2 diabetes

DIGESTIVE SYSTEM
• Increased risks for colon, gallbladder, and kidney cancers
• Increased risk of gallbladder disease

REPRODUCTIVE SYSTEM
• Higher rates of sexual dysfunction
• Increased risks for prostate, endometrial, and uterine cancer
• Increased risk of breast cancer in women
• In pregnant women, increased risks of fetal and maternal death, labor and delivery complications, and birth defects

BONES AND JOINTS
• For every 2-pound increase in weight, the risk of arthritis increases 9%–13%
• Increased risk of osteoarthritis, especially in weight-bearing joints, such as knees and hips

Figure 9.2 **Potential Negative Health Effects of Overweight and Obesity**

▶ Mastering **Health & Nutrition** Obesity Health Effects

Check Yourself

■ **What are some potential effects on the body of overweight and obesity?**

■ **Do you consider the most significant consequences of overweight and obesity to be physical, financial, emotional, or other?**

9.3 Factors Contributing to Overweight and Obesity: Genetics, Physiology, and the Environment

9.3 Explain the impact of genetics, physiology, and environment on body weight.

Several factors appear to influence why one person becomes obese and another remains thin.

Body Type and Genes

New research suggests that there is a genetic basis for our appetite and that some people inherit a lower sensitivity to **satiety**—the feeling of fullness when nutritional needs are satisfied and the stomach signals "no more."[15] Thus, some people may be more prone to grazing and food cravings than others. The *fat mass and obesity-associated (FTO)* gene may be among the most important.[16]

If your genes play a key role in obesity tendencies, are you doomed to a lifelong battle with your weight? Probably not. A healthy lifestyle may be able to override "obesity" genes. Results of a recent study of 5,079 adult twin pairs indicates that physical activity suppresses genetic variability in body weight, indicating that exercise may override genetic influences on risk of obesity.[17]

Physiological Factors

Metabolic Rates Although number of calories consumed is important, metabolism also helps determine weight. The **basal metabolic rate (BMR)** is the minimum rate at which the body uses energy when working to maintain basic vital functions. The BMR for the average healthy adult is 1,200 to 1,800 calories per day.

The **resting metabolic rate (RMR)** includes the BMR plus any energy expended through daily sedentary activities such as food digestion, sitting, studying, or standing. The **exercise metabolic rate (EMR)** accounts for all remaining daily calorie expenditures. For most of us, these calorie expenditures come from activities such as walking, climbing stairs, and mowing the lawn.

In general, the younger you are, the higher is your BMR. Growth consumes a good deal of energy, and the BMR is highest during infancy, puberty, and pregnancy. After age 30, a person's BMR slows down by 1 to 2 percent a year. Less activity, shifting priorities from fitness to family and career, and loss in muscle mass also contribute to weight gain in many middle-aged people.

Theories abound concerning mechanisms regulating metabolism and food intake. Some sources indicate that the hypothalamus (the part of the brain that regulates appetite) closely monitors levels of certain nutrients in the blood; when they fall, the brain signals us to eat. According to one theory, the monitoring system in obese people makes cues to eat more frequent and intense than in other people. Another theory, **adaptive thermogenesis**, suggests that the brain slows metabolic activity and

energy expenditure as a form of defensive protection against possible starvation, which makes weight loss difficult.

On the other side of the BMR equation is the **set point theory**, which suggests that our bodies fight to maintain our weight around a narrow range or at a set point. If we go on a drastic diet, our bodies slow our BMR to conserve energy. The good news is that set points can be changed, slowly and steadily, via a healthy diet, steady weight loss, and exercise.

Yo-yo diets, in which people repeatedly lose weight then gain it back, are doomed to fail. When such dieters resume eating, their BMR is set lower, making them almost certain to regain the lost pounds. After repeated losses and gains, it becomes increasingly hard to lose weight and easy to regain it.

Hormonal Influences: Ghrelin and Leptin Much research has centered on the role of genes such as FTO on regulating *ghrelin*—a hormone that has been shown to play a key role in metabolism—specifically in determining appetite and food intake control (particularly

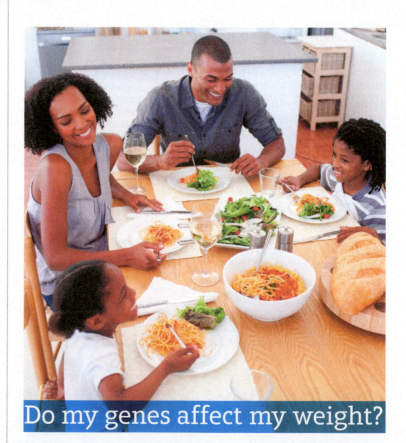

Do my genes affect my weight?

Many factors help to determine weight and body type, including heredity and genetic makeup, environment, and learned eating patterns, which are often connected to family habits.

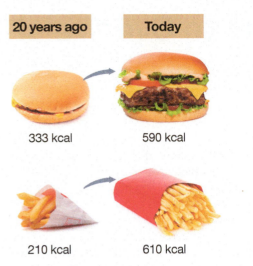

20 years ago	Today
333 kcal	590 kcal
210 kcal	610 kcal

Figure 9.3 Today's Bloated Portions
The increase in average portion sizes has made it tougher than ever to manage your weight.
Source: Data are from National Heart, Lung, and Blood Institute, "Portion Distortion," March 2017, www.nhlbi.nih.gov/health/educational/wecan/eat-right/portion-distortion.htm.

in controlling satiety), gastrointestinal motility, gastric acid secretion, endocrine and exocrine pancreatic secretions, glucose and lipid metabolism, *and* cardiovascular and immunological processes.[18]

Another hormone, *leptin*, is produced by fat cells; its levels in the blood increase as fat tissue increases. When blood levels of leptin rise, appetite drops. Scientists believe that leptin signals that you are getting full, slows food intake, and promotes energy. Researchers believe that when leptin levels are low, people are more prone to overeating and weight gain. More research on leptin's role is necessary. Obese people seem to have excess ghrelin production and faulty leptin receptors, although the exact reasons why these hormones function improperly is not clear. It may be that environmental and psychological cues are stronger than biological signals in some individuals.[19] Also, different genes may influence weight gain at certain periods of life, particularly during adolescence and young adulthood.[20]

Fat Cells and Predisposition to Fatness Some obese people may have excessive numbers of fat cells. Where an average-weight adult has approximately 25 to 35 billion fat cells and a moderately obese adult has 60 to 100 billion, an extremely obese adult has as many as 200 billion.[21] This condition, **hyperplastic obesity**, usually appears in early childhood and perhaps, because of the mother's dietary habits, even before birth. Critical periods for the development of hyperplasia are the last 2 to 3 months of fetal development, the first year of life, and the period between ages 9 and 13. Central to this theory is the belief that the number of fat cells in a body does not increase appreciably during adulthood. However, the ability of each of these cells to swell (**hypertrophy**) and shrink does carry over into adulthood. People with large numbers of fat cells may be able to lose weight by decreasing the size of each fat cell in adulthood, but with the next calorie binge, the cells swell and sabotage weight-loss efforts. Weight gain may be tied to both the number of fat cells in the body and the capacity of individual fat cells to enlarge.

Thrifty Gene Metabolism In a carefully controlled laboratory study, 12 obese men and women were asked to fast for 1 day and remain as inpatients for 6 weeks, consuming 50 percent of their normal calories each day. Those who lost the least weight were those whose metabolism slowed down significantly in response to caloric restriction.[22] Individuals in these studies have what researchers refer to as *thrifty metabolism*. In contrast, those with a *spendthrift metabolism* had metabolisms that kept chugging along when caloric intake decreased, losing significantly more weight than the thrifty group. Researchers are unsure whether these responses to dieting have a genetic basis or develop over time.

Environmental Factors

Automobiles, remote controls, and desk jobs lead us to sit more and move less. Our culture also urges us to eat more. Combined, these environmental influences are a clear recipe for weight gain.

- We are bombarded with media messages and advertising for low-price, high-calorie foods and super-sized portions. Standard portions have increased dramatically in the past 20 years (Figure 9.3).
- Because of our fast-paced lives, we eat out more and consume too many prepackaged, high-fat meals, fast food, sugar-laden soft drinks, and high-calorie coffee drinks.
- Bottle-feeding infants may increase their energy intake compared to breast-feeding.
- Misleading food labels confuse consumers about portion and serving sizes.

Skills for **Behavior Change**

Beware of Portion Distortion

To avoid overeating when you dine out, follow these strategies:

- Order the smallest size available. Focus on taste, not quantity.
- Take your time, and give your fullness indicator a chance to kick in while there is still time to stop eating before you overeat.
- Dip your food in dressings, gravies, and sauces on the side rather than pouring extra calories over the top.
- Order a healthy appetizer as your main course along with a small side salad or veggie side.
- Split an entrée with a friend or put half of your meal in a take-out box, and eat only what's left at the restaurant.
- Avoid buffets and all-you-can-eat establishments. If you go to them, use small plates, and fill them with salads, vegetables, and other high-protein, low-calorie, low-fat options. Look for high-quality, reasonably priced foods, and emphasize flavor. Practice mindful eating, and savor the flavor, noticing texture, smell, and taste. Put your fork down between bites.

Check Yourself

- **What are the influences of genetics, physiology, and the environment on body weight? Which do you consider most important?**

Factors Contributing to Overweight and Obesity: Lifestyle

9.4 Explain the impact of psychosocial, economic, and lifestyle factors on body weight.

Psychosocial and Economic Factors

Our friends and loved ones are often key influences in our eating behaviors. In fact, according to recent research, young adults who are overweight and obese tend to befriend and date overweight and obese people in much the same way that smokers or exercisers tend to hang out with other smokers or exercisers. People may gain or lose weight on the basis of social undermining of weight-loss attempts ("Let's order pizza!") or support for weight loss.[24]

Socioeconomic status can have a significant effect on obesity risk. People in poverty may have less access to fresh, nutrient-dense foods and opt for less expensive, high-calorie processed food. Those who work multiple jobs, work odd hours, and have long commutes might not have the time or energy to cook nutritious food. Personal trainers and gym memberships may be too expensive or inconveniently located. Lack of lighting, sidewalks, trails, and other places to walk or bike can make it unsafe and difficult to exercise.[25]

Lifestyle Factors

Although heredity, metabolism, and environment all have an impact on weight management, the way we live our lives is also responsible. In general, Americans are eating more and moving less than ever before, becoming overweight as a result. According to data from the 2016 *National Health Interview Survey*, slightly more than 52.8 percent of adults age 18 and over in the United States met the guidelines for aerobic activity through involvement in leisure-time activity.[26] Just over 22 percent met the minimum guidelines for both aerobic exercise and muscle strengthening.[27] Think about how well you have managed to meet these guidelines in the last month.

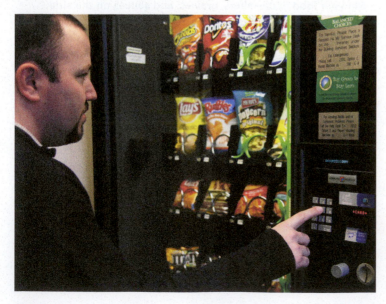

Do you know people who seemingly can eat whatever they want without gaining weight? With few exceptions, if you were to monitor the level and intensity of their activity, you would discover why. Even if their schedule does not include intense exercise, it probably includes a high level of activity.

Rather than focusing only on how much formal exercise we get in each day, health and fitness experts have begun to focus on how much time we spend sitting. If the body isn't moving, it's not burning many calories. Research indicates a dose-response association between sitting time and mortality from all causes and from cardiovascular disease, independent of leisure-time activity; that is, the more time you spend sitting, the worse your health is likely to be, whether you exercise or not. Because muscle activity burns energy, passive sitting is one of the worst things you can do if you are trying to burn calories. If you stood up while reading this chapter, the large and small muscle groups in your legs would be constantly working to keep you from falling over—and would thus be burning more calories. These little extra bouts of movement may make a big difference in daily calories burned, weight management, and overall health.

Other lifestyle factors that may increase your obesity risks are:

- **Pathogens and toxins.** Could the bacteria in your gastrointestinal tract increase your obesity risks? Is it possible that something in the environment may make you more or less susceptible to pathogens that affect weight gain or loss? Obese and nonobese individuals have different intestinal flora, and research is examining possible mechanisms for increased risk as well as environmental factors.[28]
- **Drugs.** Several studies have examined the role of prescription drugs such as antidepressants, allergy medications, antibiotics, heart and high blood pressure pills, diabetes drugs, and cancer medications in increased weight gain and weight fluctuation.[29]
- **Sleep deprivation.** Sleep-deprived people tend to have significant drops in leptin levels. How might that effect weight?[30]

Skills for Behavior Change

Finding the Fun in Healthy Eating And Exercise

With a little creativity, you can make weight management a fun, positive part of your life. Try these tips:

- **Cook and eat with friends.** Share the responsibility for making the meal while you spend time with people you like.
- **Experiment with new foods** to add variety to your meals.
- **Vary your exercise routine.** Change the exercise or your location, join a team for the social aspects in addition to exercise, or run a race just for the challenge.

- **What lifestyle changes can contribute positively or negatively to weight management?**

9.5 Assessing Body Weight and Body Composition

Learning Outcome

9.5 Distinguish among overweight, overfatness, obesity, and underweight.

Everyone has his or her own ideal weight, based on individual variables such as body structure, height, and fat distribution. Traditionally, experts used measurement techniques such as height–weight charts to determine whether an individual fell into the ideal weight, overweight, or obese category. However, these charts can be misleading because they don't take body composition (a person's ratio of fat to lean muscle) or fat distribution into account.

People who are extremely muscular may fall into the overweight category on weight charts, as we will discuss later in this chapter. More accurate measures of evaluating healthy weight and health risks might be by assessing "overfatness" and how fat is distributed in a person's body.

Many people worry about becoming fat, but some fat is essential for healthy body functioning. Fat regulates body temperature, cushions and insulates organs and tissues, and is the body's main source of stored energy. Body fat is composed of two types of fat: essential and storage. *Essential fat* is the fat necessary for maintenance of life and reproductive functions. *Storage fat*, the nonessential fat that many of us try to shed, makes up the remainder of our fat reserves.

Overweight and Obesity

In general, **overweight** is a body weight more than 10 percent above healthy levels, whereas **obesity** refers to a body weight that is more than 20 percent above recommended levels for health.

Experts usually define overweight and obesity in terms of BMI, a measure to be discussed later, or percentage of body fat, as determined by some of the methods we'll discuss shortly. Although opinion varies somewhat, most experts agree that men's bodies should contain between 8 and 20 percent total body fat, and women's total body fat should be within the range of 20 to 30 percent. These ranges vary at various ages and stages of life, but generally, men who exceed 22 percent body fat and women who exceed 35 percent are considered overweight (see Table 9.1).

Underweight

Men with only 3 to 7 percent body fat and women with approximately 8 to 15 percent are considered **underweight**, which can seriously compromise health. Extremely low body fat can cause hair loss, visual disturbances, skin problems, a tendency for bones to fracture easily, digestive system disturbances, heart irregularities, gastrointestinal problems, difficulties in maintaining body temperature, and **amenorrhea** (loss of menstrual periods) in women. Rates of underweight individuals have declined in recent decades as overweight and obesity rates have increased.

TABLE 9.1 Body Fat Percentage Norms for Men and Women*

Men's Age (years)	Very Lean	Excellent	Good	Fair	Poor	Very Poor
20–29	<7%	7%–10%	11%–15%	16%–19%	20%–23%	>23%
30–39	<11%	11%–14%	15%–18%	19%–21%	22%–25%	>25%
40–49	<14%	14%–17%	18%–20%	21%–23%	24%–27%	>27%
50–59	<15%	15%–19%	20%–22%	23%–24%	25%–28%	>28%
60–69	<16%	16%–20%	21%–22%	23%–25%	26%–28%	>28%
70–79	<16%	16%–20%	21%–23%	24%–25%	26%–28%	>28%
Women's Age (years)	**Very Lean**	**Excellent**	**Good**	**Fair**	**Poor**	**Very Poor**
20–29	<14%	14%–16%	17%–19%	20%–23%	24%–27%	>27%
30–39	<15%	15%–17%	18%–21%	22%–25%	26%–29%	>29%
40–49	<17%	17%–20%	21%–24%	25%–28%	29%–32%	>32%
50–59	<18%	18%–22%	23%–27%	28%–30%	31%–34%	>34%
60–69	<18%	18%–23%	24%–28%	29%–31%	32%–35%	>35%
70–79	<18%	18%–24%	25%–29%	30%–32%	33%–36%	>36%

* Assumes nonathletes. For athletes, recommended body fat is 5 to 15 percent for men and 12 to 22 percent for women. Please note that there are no agreed-upon national standards for recommended body fat percentage.

Source: Based on data from The Cooper Institute, Dallas Texas, www.cooperinstitute.org.

Check Yourself

- **What are the differences between overweight and obesity?**

- **Why is percentage of body fat a better way to evaluate someone's health than looking at weight alone?**

Assessing Body Weight and Body Composition: BMI and Other Methods

9.6 Compare and contrast different methods of body composition assessment.

Body mass index (BMI) is a description of body weight relative to height, numbers highly correlated with total body fat. Find your BMI in inches and pounds in **Figure 9.4**, or you can calculate your BMI by dividing your weight in kilograms by height in meters squared:

$$BMI = weight\ (kg)/height\ squared\ (m^2)$$

A BMI calculator is also available at www.nhlbi.nih.gov.

Desirable BMI levels (classes) vary with age and by sex; however, most BMI tables for adults do not account for such variables. **Healthy weight** is defined as having a BMI of 18.5 to 24.9, the range of lowest statistical health risk.[31] A BMI of 25 to 29.9 indicates *overweight* and the potential for health risks.[32] A BMI of 30 to 39.9 is classified as **obese** with a significant low risk of health problems.[33] A BMI of 40 to 49.9 is **morbidly obese**, and a new category of BMI of 50 or higher—one increasing in numbers—has been labeled as **super obese**.[34] Nearly 5 percent of obese men and almost 10 percent of obese women are morbidly obese.[35]

Although useful measures, BMI levels don't include water, muscle, and bone mass or account for the fact that muscle weighs more than fat. BMI levels can be inaccurate for people who are under 5 feet tall, are highly muscled, or are older and have little muscle mass. More precise methods of determining body fat, described below, should be used for these individuals.

Youth and BMI

The labels *obese* and *morbidly obese* have been used for years for adults, though there is growing concern about the consequences of pinning these potentially stigmatizing labels on children. When subjected to bias and discrimination, people are actually likely to eat more rather than to curtail eating behavior.[36] BMI ranges above normal weight for children and teens are often labeled as "at risk of overweight" and "overweight." These ranges take into account normal differences in body fat between boys and girls and the differences in body fat that occur at various ages. Specific guidelines for calculating youth BMI are available at the Centers for Disease Control and Prevention website, www.cdc.gov.

Waist Circumference and Ratio Measurements

Knowing where you carry your fat may be more important than knowing how much you carry. Men and postmenopausal women tend to store fat in the

Height (feet and inches)	100	120	140	160	180	200	220	240	260
4'6"	24 27	29 31	34 36	39 41	43 46	48 51	53 55	58 60	63
4'8"	22 25	27 29	31 34	36 38	40 43	45 47	49 52	54 56	58
4'10"	21 23	25 27	29 31	33 36	38 40	42 44	46 48	50 52	54
5'0"	20 22	23 25	27 29	31 33	35 37	39 41	43 45	47 49	51
5'2"	18 20	22 24	26 27	29 31	33 35	37 38	40 42	44 46	48
5'4"	17 19	21 22	24 26	28 29	31 33	34 36	38 40	41 43	45
5'6"	16 18	19 21	23 24	26 27	29 31	32 34	36 37	39 40	42
5'8"	15 17	18 20	21 23	24 26	27 29	30 32	33 35	37 38	40
5'10"	14 16	17 19	20 22	23 24	26 27	29 30	32 33	34 36	37
6'0"	14 15	16 18	19 20	22 23	24 26	27 29	30 31	33 34	35
6'2"	13 14	15 17	18 19	21 22	23 24	26 27	28 30	31 32	33
6'4"	12 13	15 16	17 18	20 21	22 23	24 26	27 28	29 30	32
6'6"	12 13	14 15	16 17	19 20	21 22	23 24	25 27	28 29	30
6'8"	11 12	13 14	15 17	18 19	20 21	22 23	24 25	26 28	29
6'10"	11 12	13 14	15 16	17 18	19 20	21 22	23 24	25 26	27
7'0"	10 11	12 13	14 15	16 17	18 19	20 21	22 23	24 25	26

Weight (pounds)

Key:

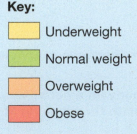

- Underweight
- Normal weight
- Overweight
- Obese

Figure 9.4 Body Mass Index
Locate the intersection of your weight and height to determine BMI. (BMI values have been rounded off to the nearest whole number.)

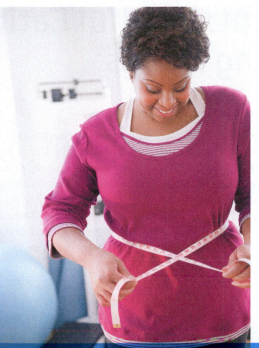

How can I tell if I am overweight?

Observing the way you look and how your clothes fit can give you a general idea of whether you weigh more or less than in the past. But for evaluating your weight and body fat levels in terms of potential health risks, it's best to use more scientific measures, such as BMI, waist circumference, waist-to-hip ratio, or a technician-administered body composition test.

abdominal area. Premenopausal women usually store fat in the hips, buttocks, and thighs. Waist circumference measurement is increasingly recognized as a useful tool in assessing abdominal fat, which is considered more threatening to health than fat in other regions.

A waistline greater than 40 inches (102 centimeters) in men and 35 inches (88 centimeters) in women may be particularly indicative of greater health risk.[37] This may be important for determining the risk of diabetes, cardiovascular disease, hypertension, or stroke.[38] If a person is less than 5 feet tall or has a BMI of 35 or above, waist circumference standards used for the general population might not apply.

The waist-to-hip ratio measures regional fat distribution. The higher your waist-to-hip ratio, the greater is your chance of having increased health risks.[39] Newer research has pointed to waist-to-hip ratio being more effective than waist circumference alone or BMI use for measuring body fat in children and adolescents.[40]

Measures of Body Fat

There are many other ways to assess body fat levels. One low-tech way is simply to look in the mirror or consider how your clothes fit now compared with how they fit in the past. If you want to take a more precise measurement of your percentage of body fat, more accurate techniques are available, including caliper measurement, underwater weighing, and various body scans (Figure 9.5). These

methods usually involve the help of a professional and typically must be done in a lab or clinical setting. Before undergoing any procedure, make sure you understand the expense, the potential for inaccuracy, the risks, and the tester's training. Also consider why you are seeking this assessment and what you plan to do with the results.

Underwater (hydrostatic) weighing:
Measures the amount of water a person displaces when completely submerged. Fat tissue is less dense than muscle or bone, so body fat can be computed within a 2%–3% margin of error by comparing weight underwater and out of water.

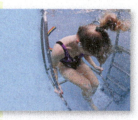

Skinfolds:
Involves "pinching" a person's fold of skin (with its underlying layer of fat) at various locations of the body. The fold is measured using a specially designed caliper. When performed by a skilled technician, it can estimate body fat with an error of 3%–4%.

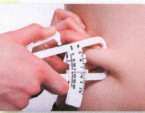

Bioelectrical impedance analysis (BIA):
Involves sending a very low level of electrical current through a person's body. As lean body mass is made up of mostly water, the rate at which the electricity is conducted gives an indication of a person's lean body mass and body fat. Under the best circumstances, BIA can estimate body fat with an error of 3%–4%.

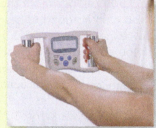

Dual-energy X-ray absorptiometry (DXA):
The technology is based on using very-low-level X ray to differentiate between bone tissue, soft (or lean) tissue, and fat (or adipose) tissue. The margin of error for predicting body fat is 2%–4%.

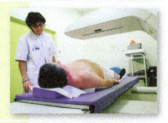

Bod Pod:
Uses air displacement to measure body composition. This machine is a large, egg-shaped chamber made from fiberglass. The person being measured sits in the machine wearing a swimsuit. The door is closed and the machine measures how much air is displaced. That value is used to calculate body fat, with a 2%–3% margin of error.

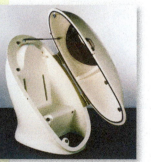

Figure 9.5 Overview of Various Body Composition Methods
Source: Adapted from J. Thompson and M. Manore, *Nutrition: An Applied Approach*, 4th ed., © 2015. Printed and electronically reproduced by permission of Pearson Education, Inc., Upper Saddle River, New Jersey.

Check Yourself

- **Which of the various assessment methods do you consider the most accurate? Which is the most accessible to the average person?**

9.7 Weight Management: Mindful Eating and Improving Eating Habits

9.7 Explain how energy expenditure and energy intake affect weight management and ways to successfully manage your weight.

At some point in our lives, almost all of us will decide to lose weight or modify our diet. Many will have mixed success. Success often involves adjusting long-term eating behaviors, such as developing the habits of mindfulness and healthy snacking.

Understanding Calories and Energy Balance

A *calorie* is a unit of measure that indicates the amount of energy gained from food or expended through activity. Each time you consume 3,500 calories more than your body needs to maintain weight, you gain a pound of storage fat. Conversely, each time your body expends an extra 3,500 calories, you lose a pound of fat. If you consume 140 calories (the amount in one can of regular soda) more than you need every single day and make no other changes in diet or activity, you would gain 1 pound in 25 days (3,500 calories ÷ 140 calories per day = 25 days). Conversely, if you walk for 30 minutes each day at a pace of 15 minutes per mile (172 calories burned) in addition to your regular activities, you would lose 1 pound in 20 days (3,500 calories ÷ 172 calories per day = 20.3 days) as a result of the negative caloric balance. This is an example of the concept of energy balance described in **Figure 9.6**.

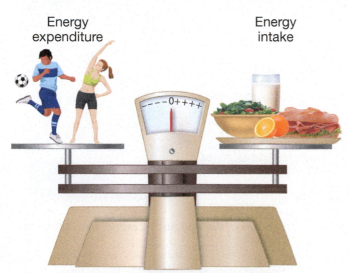

Energy expenditure

Energy intake

Energy expenditure = Energy intake

Figure 9.6 The Concept of Energy Balance
According to this concept, if you consume more calories than you burn, you will gain weight. If you burn more than you consume, you will lose weight. If both are equal, your weight will not change.

The Importance of Exercise

Any increase in the intensity, frequency, and duration of daily exercise can have a significant impact on total calorie expenditure because lean (muscle) tissue is more metabolically active than fat tissue. Exact estimates vary, but experts currently think that 2 to 50 more calories per day are burned per pound of muscle than for each pound of fat tissue. Thus, the base level of calories needed to maintain a healthy weight varies greatly from person to person.

The number of calories spent depends on three factors:

1. The number and proportion of muscles used
2. The amount of weight moved
3. The length of time the activity takes.

An activity involving both the arms and legs burns more calories than the same activity involving only the legs. An activity performed by a heavy person burns more calories than the same activity performed by a lighter person, and an activity performed for 40 minutes requires twice as much energy as the same activity performed for only 20 minutes.

Becoming Mindful of your Eating Triggers

If you are like the 66 percent of American adults who eat in front of the TV or computer, it should be no surprise that you are eating faster and more, with more awareness of the screen than your food.[41] *Mindless eating*—putting food in your mouth that you don't really taste or notice while consuming more than you should—may be a key contributor to excess calorie consumption and weight gain. When we eat mindlessly, we may miss feelings of satiety and ignore tendencies to use restraint. *Mindful eating* means eating with awareness—awareness of *why* we are eating (was it a trigger, or are we really hungry?), *what* we are eating (should we really be eating this?), and *how much* we are eating. Slowing down and experiencing the smell, taste and textures of foods rather than just shoving food in your mouth and washing it down with a beverage are part of mindful eating. Also, consider the speed with which you consume food, whether you are truly hungry when you eat that huge plate of food, or whether you are eating because it's a habit to eat at three times per day.

Once you have assessed your eating behavior, think about what triggered that "eat" urge. Before you can change an unhealthy eating habit, you must first determine what triggers you to eat. Keeping a log of eating triggers—*when, what, where,* and *how much* you eat—for 2 to 3 days can help you identify what is pushing those "eat everything in sight" buttons for you.

Typically, dietary triggers involve patterns and problems in everyday living rather than real hunger pangs. Ask yourself: Are you really hungry? Or are you eating for comfort or distraction? Focus on why you have your hand on the chips or find yourself grazing in the refrigerator. If you eat while working or watching TV, limit what you put on your plate and put the rest away.

Eat slowly. Chew more, taste your food rather than swilling it down in a rush of soda or other beverages. Try new flavors, and focus on when you have had enough and should stop eating. Order smaller portions when eating out. Eat on a smaller plate. Put down the cell phone or shut off the TV while eating, and give eating priority status. Pay attention to what is going into your mouth.

Improving Your Eating Habits

Once you have evaluated your behaviors and determined your triggers, you can begin to devise a plan for improved eating. If you are unsure where to start, seek assistance from reputable sources such as MyPlate (www.choosemyplate.gov). Registered dietitians, some physicians (not all doctors have a strong background in nutrition), health educators and exercise physiologists with nutritional training, and other health professionals can provide reliable information. Be wary of people who call themselves nutritionists or nutritional life coaches; there are no such official designations. Avoid weight-loss programs that promise quick "miracle" results or those run by "trainees," who are often people who have taken short courses on nutrition and exercise that are designed to sell products or services.

Before engaging in any weight-loss program, ask about the credentials of the adviser; assess the nutrient value of the prescribed diet; verify that the dietary guidelines are consistent with reliable nutrition research; and analyze the suitability of the diet to your tastes, budget, and lifestyle. Any diet that requires radical behavior changes or sets up artificial dietary programs through prepackaged products that don't teach you how to eat healthfully is likely to fail. Supplements and fad diets that claim fast weight loss will invariably mean fast weight regain. The most successful plans allow you to make food choices in real-world settings and do not ask you to sacrifice everything you enjoy.

You will also need to address triggers that you may have for eating that are unrelated to hunger. For example, if you tend to eat in stressful situations, try to acknowledge the feelings of stress and anxiety, and develop stress management techniques to practice daily. If you find yourself eating when you are bored or tired, identify the times when your energy is low, and fill them with activities other than eating, such as exercise breaks, or cultivate a new interest or hobby that keeps your mind and hands busy. If your trigger for eating is feeling angry or upset, analyze your emotions, and look for a noneating activity to deal with them, such as taking a quick walk or calling a friend. If it is the sight and smell of food that triggers you to eat, stop buying high-calorie foods that tempt you, or store them in an inconvenient place, out of sight. Avoid walking past or sitting or standing near the table of tempting treats at a meeting, party, or other gathering.

See It! Videos

How can you control your urge to go overboard with meal portions? Watch **Experiment Shows Portion Control Is the Key to Healthy Eating** in Mastering Health.

Millions of people drink diet soda to help maintain or control their weight. According to a growing body of research, this weight-loss strategy may actually contribute to weight gain. According to new research, overweight or obese individuals who opt for diet beverages actually consume more calories from food at meals and from snacks than people who choose sugared beverages. Why is this? Although the exact mechanism remains in question, researchers speculate that artificial sweeteners may change the way we perceive fullness and may increase appetite. Others suggest a form of "cognitive distortion" whereby we justify a few more snacks or dessert because our drinks have fewer calories.[42]

Skills for Behavior Change

Tips for Sensible Snacking

- **Keep healthy munchies around.** Buy 100 percent whole-wheat breads. If you need to spice up your snack, use low-fat or soy cheese, low-fat cream cheese, peanut butter, hummus, or other healthy favorites. Some baked or popped crackers are low in fat and calories and high in fiber. Look for these on your grocery shelves or in campus vending machines.
- **Keep "crunchies" on hand.** Apples, pears, red or green pepper strips, carrots, and celery all are good choices. Wash the fruits and vegetables, and cut them up to carry with you to eat them when a snack attack comes on.
- **Quench your thirst with hot drinks.** Hot tea, heated milk, plain or decaffeinated coffee, hot chocolate made with nonfat milk or water, or soup broths will help keep you satisfied.
- **Choose natural beverages.** Drink plain water, 100 percent juice in small quantities, or other low-sugar choices to satisfy your thirst. Avoid certain juices, energy drinks, and soft drinks that have added sugars, low fiber, and no protein. Usually, they are high in calories and low in longer-term satisfaction.
- **Eat nuts instead of candy.** Although nuts are relatively high in calories, they are also loaded with healthy fats and make a healthy snack when consumed in moderation.
- **If you must have a piece of chocolate, keep it small.** Note that because of its antioxidant content, dark chocolate is better than milk chocolate or white chocolate.
- **Avoid high-calorie energy bars.** Eat energy bars only if you are exercising hard and don't have an opportunity to eat a regular meal. If you buy energy bars, look for ones with a good mixture of fiber and protein and that are low in fat and calories.

Check Yourself

- What are three potential triggers for overeating, and how can they be overcome?
- What steps should you take before engaging in any weight-loss program?

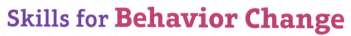

9.8 Weight Management: Assessing Diet Programs

Learning Outcome

9.8 Identify strengths and weaknesses of popular diet programs.

People looking to lose weight and improve eating habits often turn to diet programs for advice and guidance.

Table 9.2 analyzes several diets that are currently popular. For information on other plans, check out the regularly updated list of reviews on the website of the Academy of Nutrition and Dietetics at www.eatright.org.

TABLE 9.2 Analyzing Popular Diet Programs

Diet Name	Basic Principles	Good for Diabetes and Heart Health?	Weight Loss Effectiveness	Pros, Cons, and Other Things to Consider
DASH (Dietary Approaches to Stop Hypertension)	A balanced plan developed to fight high blood pressure and reduce risks of cardiovascular disease and diabetes. Eat fruits, vegetables, whole grains, lean protein, and low-fat dairy. Avoid sweets, fats, red meat, and sodium.	Yes	Not specifically designed for weight loss but a balanced approach that does lead to loss	A balanced, safe, and healthy diet, rated the number one best diet overall by *U.S. News & World Report* in 2016 and 2017. Very effective in improving cholesterol levels and other biomarkers long term.
TLC (Therapeutic Lifestyle Change)	Developed by NIH. Focused on cardiovascular disease risk reduction with fruits and vegetables, lean protein, low fat, etc. Balanced and effective.	Yes	Weight loss likely; cholesterol key	Safe, balanced, and healthy diet, tied for number four best diet overall with the Mayo Clinic diet and the Weight Watchers diet by *U.S. News & World Report* in 2017. Particularly good for heart health and cholesterol reduction.
Mediterranean	A plan that emphasizes fruits, vegetables, fish, whole grains, beans, nuts, legumes, olive oil, and herbs and spices. Poultry, eggs, cheese, yogurt, and red wine can be enjoyed in moderation. Sweets and red meat are saved for special occasions.	Yes	Very effective, safe, and easy to follow	Widely considered to be one of the most healthy, safe, and balanced diets. Weight loss may not be as dramatic, but long-term health benefits have been demonstrated. Rated the number two best diet overall by *U.S. News & World Report* in 2017.
Weight Watchers	New "Beyond the Scale" program, which emphasizes three components: eating healthier, fitness that fits your life, and "developing skills and supportive connections to help you stay on track." Involves tracking food, nutritional values, and exercise. In-person group meetings and online membership are options.	Yes (depending on individual choices)	Very effective, safe	Consistently rated by experts as one of the top three or four most effective weight loss programs. Flexible programs that don't deny foods but rather teach about healthy choices. Works for both short- and long-term weight loss. Support groups are available, but the program can be done online in the privacy of the home with coaches. Check your campus or community for meetings and watch for specials, as some plans require membership fees. Rated number one weight-loss diet by *U.S. News & World Report* in 2016.
MIND Diet	Combines the best elements of DASH and Mediterranean diets in a healthy dietary regimen.	Yes	Effective, focus on real food	Number three best overall diet rating by *U.S. News and World Report* in 2017. Noteworthy for the potential to boost brain power and reduce risk of cognitive decline.
Flexitarian Diet	High scores for nutritional completeness and easy-to-follow approach for long-term success for all members the of family	Yes	Very effective	Ranked among the top five diets in 2017 as safe, effective, and sustainable.

Sources: Opinions on diet pros and cons are based on *U.S. News & World Report*, "Best Diets Overall," 2017, http://health.usnews.com/best-diet/best-overall-diets?int=9c2508. Dietary reviews, particularly of fad diets, are available online from registered dieticians at the Academy of Nutrition and Dietetics, 2016; B. Johnson et al., "Comparisons of Weight Loss among Diet Programs in Overweight and Obese Adults: A Meta-analysis," *Journal of the American Medical Association* 312, no. 9 (2014): 923–33.

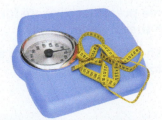

Check Yourself

■ **What are important factors to consider when evaluating current diet programs?**

9.9 Weight Management: In Perspective

Learning Outcome

9.9 **List steps to successful weight management.**

Supportive friends, relatives, community resources, and policies that support healthy food choices and exercise options all increase the likelihood of successful weight loss. People of the same age, sex, height, and weight can have resting metabolic rates that differ by as much as 1,000 calories a day. This may explain why extra food intake may lead to weight gain in one person and weight loss and hunger in another person. Depression, stress, cultural influences, and the availability of high-fat, high-calorie foods can also make weight loss harder.

To reach and maintain the weight at which you will be healthy and feel your best, develop a program of exercise and healthy

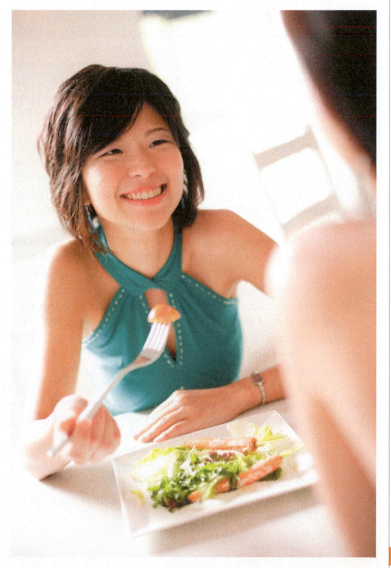

It's important to enjoy your meals, but stay aware of your weight management goals. Be adventurous, and enliven your meals and snacks with a wide variety of healthy options.

eating that you can maintain. It is unrealistic and potentially dangerous to try to lose weight in a short period of time. Instead, try to lose a healthy 1 to 2 pounds during the first week, and stay with this slow-and-easy regimen. Adding exercise and cutting back on calories to expend about 500 calories more than you consume each day will help you lose weight at a rate of 1 pound per week.

Skills for Behavior Change

Keys to Successful Weight Management

The key to successful weight management is finding a sustainable way to control what you eat and to make exercise a priority.

- To get started, ask yourself some key questions. Why do you want to make this change right now? What are your goals?
- Write down the things you find positive about your diet and exercise behaviors. Then write down things that need to be changed. For each change you need to make, list three or four small things you can change right now.
- What resources on campus or in your community could help? Who among your friends and family members will help you?
- Keep a food and exercise log for 2 or 3 days. Note the good things you are doing, the things that need improvement, and the triggers you need to address.

Make a Plan

- Set realistic short- and long-term goals.
- Establish a plan. What diet and exercise changes can you make this week? Once you have made the changes for 1 week, plot a course for 2 weeks, and so on.
- Look for balance. Remember that it is calories taken in and burned over time that make the difference.

Change Your Habits

- Notice whether you're hungry before starting a meal. Eat slowly, noting when you start to feel full. Stop before you are full.
- Eat a substantial breakfast. This will prevent you from being too hungry and overeating at lunch.
- Keep healthful snacks on hand for when you get hungry.
- Don't constantly deprive yourself or set unrealistic guidelines.

Incorporate Exercise

- Be active; slowly increase your time, speed, distance, or resistance levels.
- Vary your physical activity. Find activities you love. Try things you haven't tried before.
- Find an exercise partner to help you stay motivated.
- Make exercise a fun break. Go for a walk in a place that interests you.

Check Yourself

- **What are the key components of a successful weight management plan?**

9.10 Explain measures that may be taken when body weight poses an extreme threat to health.

In cases of extreme health risk, dramatic weight loss may be recommended. Severely obese patients may be given powdered formulas with daily values of 400 to 700 calories plus vitamin and mineral supplements. Such **very-low-calorie diets (VLCDs)** should never be undertaken without strict medical supervision.

One dangerous potential complication of VLCDs or starvation diets is *ketoacidosis*, in which a patient's blood becomes more acidic, causing severe damage to body tissues. Risk is greatest for those with untreated type 1 diabetes, anorexia nervosa, or bulimia nervosa. If fasting continues, the body turns to its last resort—protein—for energy, breaking down essential muscle and organ tissue to stay alive. Within about 10 days after the typical adult begins a complete fast, the body will have depleted its energy stores, and death may occur.

Dieters often turn to commercially marketed weight-loss supplements. U.S. Food and Drug Administration (FDA) approval is not required for over-the-counter "diet aids" or supplements, whose effectiveness is largely untested and unproven. Virtually all people who use supplements and diet pills to lose weight eventually regain it.[43]

Today, nearly 65 prescription, over-the-counter, alternative, and off-label drugs are available for weight loss. Alli causes about 30 percent of fats consumed to pass through the digestive system. Qsymia is an appetite suppressant and antiseizure drug that reduces the desire for food. Belviq affects serotonin levels, helping patients feel full. Newer drugs, such as Contrave, combine antidepressants with other approved drugs and carry warnings specific to both. When used as part of a long-term, comprehensive weight-loss program, weight-loss drugs have the potential to help the severely obese lose weight and keep it off; however, few of these drugs are without side effects. Investigate side effects and check with your doctor before using any of these drugs.[44]

Don't assume that herbal supplements are any safer. For instance, *Hoodia gordonii*, a plant native to Africa, is a purported appetite suppressant. Many supplements contain this substance, including some that contain additional unproven ingredients such as bitter orange and other stimulants. To date, it is not FDA approved. Products containing ephedra can cause rapid heart rate, seizures, insomnia, and elevated blood pressure, all without significant effects on weight. St. John's wort and other herbs reported to suppress appetite have not been shown to be effective.

People who are severely overweight and have diabetes or hypertension may be candidates for surgical options. In *gastric banding*, an inflatable band partitions off the stomach, leaving only a small opening between its two parts so that the stomach is smaller and the person feels full more quickly. In *sleeve gastrectomy*, about 75 percent of the stomach is removed, leaving only a tube (about the size of a banana) that is connected directly to the intestines.

In *gastric bypass*, up to 70 percent of the stomach is sutured off, drastically reducing how much food a person can eat and absorb. Results are fast and dramatic, but there are many risks, including blood clots in the legs, a leak in a staple line in the stomach, pneumonia, infection, and death. Undigested foods may rush through the small intestine, causing cramping and uncontrollable diarrhea.[45] The stomach pouch that remains after surgery is small (about the size of a lime), so the person can eat or drink only a tiny amount at a time. Possible side effects include nausea and vomiting, vitamin and mineral deficiencies, and dehydration.

A *biliopancreatic diversion* or *duodenal switch procedure* reduces the size of the stomach less than a gastric bypass while bypassing less of the small intestine. This surgery has a greater risk of complications and death than other options.[46]

Research has shown unexpected results from gastric surgeries: complete remission of type 2 diabetes in the majority of cases, with drastic reductions in blood glucose levels in others.[47] However, about one-third of these patients will relapse and begin to show diabetic symptoms within 5 years after surgery.

Liposuction is a cosmetic (not weight loss) surgical procedure in which fat cells are removed from specific areas of the body. Risks include severe scarring, and even death has resulted. In many cases, people who have liposuction regain fat or require multiple surgeries to repair lumpy, irregular surfaces.

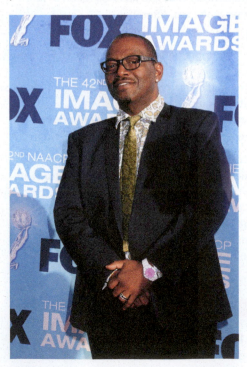

Former *American Idol* judge and record producer Randy Jackson, shown here, and NBC weatherman Al Roker have undergone gastric bypass surgery to shed well over 100 pounds each and to reduce the risks of serious chronic diseases such as type 2 diabetes.

- **What measures can be taken when body weight poses a risk to health? What are their risks?**

9.11 Trying to Gain Weight

9.11 Describe healthy strategies for trying to gain weight.

For some people, trying to gain weight is a challenge for a variety of metabolic, hereditary, psychological, and other reasons. If you are one of these individuals, the first priority is to determine why you cannot gain weight.

Perhaps you're an athlete and you burn more calories than you manage to eat. Perhaps you're stressed out and skipping meals to increase study time. Or stress, depression, or other emotional issues may make it difficult to focus on food and take good care of your body. Among older adults, the senses of taste and smell may decline, which makes food less tasty and therefore less pleasurable to eat. Visual problems and other disabilities may make meals more difficult to prepare, and dental problems may make eating more difficult.

People who engage in extreme energy-burning sports and exercise routines may be at risk for caloric and nutritional deficiencies, which can lead not only to weight loss, but also to immune system problems and organ dysfunction; weakness, which leads to falls and fractures; slower recovery from diseases; and a host of other problems.

People who are too thin need to take the same kind of steps as those who are overweight or obese to find out what their healthy weight is and attain that weight.

The Skills for Behavior Change feature gives ideas and tips for gaining weight. Depending on your situation, you may aim to gain as much as a pound per week, which would mean adding up to 500 calories a day to your diet. It is important that these calories be added in the form of energy-dense, nutritious choices from a variety of foods. For example, you could choose to eat a thick slice of whole-grain toast topped with peanut butter and a banana for breakfast or garnish a salad with olive oil, avocado, nuts, and sunflower seeds for lunch. One cup of whole-wheat flakes provides 128 calories, while a cup of granola provides 464 calories. Similarly, plain low-fat yogurt contains 154 calories per cup, while strawberry low-fat yogurt offers 238 calories per cup. Just be sure that the calories you add are coming from high-quality sources, not high-fat junk food.

Skills for Behavior Change

Tips for Gaining Weight

- Eat at regularly scheduled times.
- Eat more frequently, spend more time eating, eat high-calorie foods first if you fill up fast, and always start with the main course.
- Take time to shop, cook, and eat slowly.
- Put extra spreads such as peanut butter, cream cheese, or cheese on your foods. Make your sandwiches with extra-thick slices of bread, and add more filling. Take seconds whenever possible, and eat high-calorie, nutrient-dense snacks such as nuts and cheese during the day.
- Supplement your diet. Add high-calorie drinks that have a healthy balance of nutrients, such as whole milk.
- Try to eat with people you are comfortable with. Avoid people who you feel are analyzing what you eat or who make you feel that you should eat less.
- If you are sedentary, be aware that moderate exercise can increase appetite. If you are exercising to extremes, moderate your activities until you've gained some weight.
- Avoid diuretics, laxatives, and other medications that cause you to lose body fluids and nutrients.
- Relax. Many people who are underweight operate in high gear most of the time. Slow down, get more rest, and take steps to control stress and anxiety.

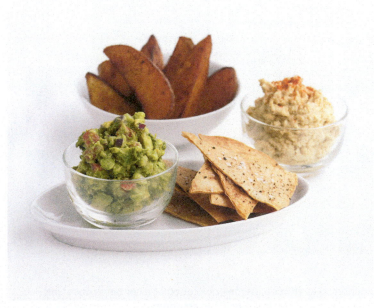

A snack of guacamole and whole-grain tortilla chips or hummus and baked potatoes is a healthy, nutrient-dense way to increase calorie intake.

- What are some steps to be taken when weight needs to be gained? Do you think this is as difficult a task as trying to lose weight?

9.12 Understanding and Improving Body Image

9.12 Identify the elements of the body image continuum, and list steps that can be taken to build a more positive body image.

When you look in the mirror, do you like what you see? If you feel disappointed, frustrated, or even angry, you're not alone. In a recent national poll, 67 percent of women and 53 percent of men reported worrying about their appearance regularly—women, more than every other issue in their lives, and men, more than every issue but finances.[48] Negative feelings about one's body can contribute to behaviors that can threaten your health—and your life. In contrast, a healthy body image can help reduce stress and lead to personal empowerment and joyful living.

Body image includes several components:

- How you see yourself in your mind
- What you believe about your appearance
- How you feel about your body
- How you sense and control your body as you move
- How you act on your thoughts and feelings about your body.

A *negative body image* is either a distorted perception of your shape or feelings of discomfort, shame, or anxiety about your body. A *positive body image* is a true perception of your appearance. You understand that everyone is different, and you celebrate

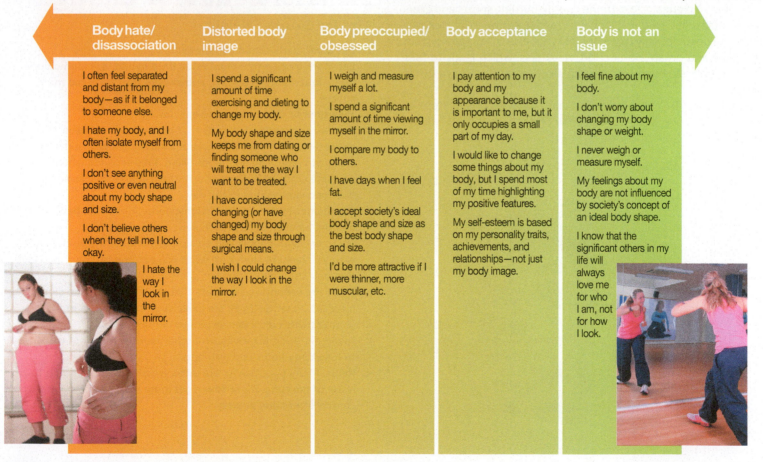

Body hate/ disassociation	Distorted body image	Body preoccupied/ obsessed	Body acceptance	Body is not an issue
I often feel separated and distant from my body—as if it belonged to someone else.	I spend a significant amount of time exercising and dieting to change my body.	I weigh and measure myself a lot.	I pay attention to my body and my appearance because it is important to me, but it only occupies a small part of my day.	I feel fine about my body.
I hate my body, and I often isolate myself from others.	My body shape and size keeps me from dating or finding someone who will treat me the way I want to be treated.	I spend a significant amount of time viewing myself in the mirror.	I would like to change some things about my body, but I spend most of my time highlighting my positive features.	I don't worry about changing my body shape or weight.
I don't see anything positive or even neutral about my body shape and size.	I have considered changing (or have changed) my body shape and size through surgical means.	I compare my body to others.	My self-esteem is based on my personality traits, achievements, and relationships—not just my body image.	I never weigh or measure myself.
I don't believe others when they tell me I look okay.	I wish I could change the way I look in the mirror.	I have days when I feel fat.		My feelings about my body are not influenced by society's concept of an ideal body shape.
I hate the way I look in the mirror.		I accept society's ideal body shape and size as the best body shape and size.		I know that the significant others in my life will always love me for who I am, not for how I look.
		I'd be more attractive if I were thinner, more muscular, etc.		

Figure 9.7 Body Image Continuum

This continuum shows a range of attitudes and behaviors toward body image. Functioning at either extreme—not caring at all or being obsessed—leads to problems. When you are functioning in the "body acceptance" area, you are taking care of your body and emotions.

Source: Adapted from Smiley/King/Avery, "Eating Issues and Body Image Continuum," Campus Health Service 1996. Copyright © 1997 Arizona Board of Regents for University of Arizona.

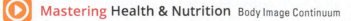 **Mastering** Health & Nutrition Body Image Continuum

your uniqueness. **Figure 9.7** will help you identify whether your body image is positive, negative, or somewhere in between.

Factors Influencing Body Image

Images of celebrities in the media set the standard for what we find attractive, leading some people to go to dangerous extremes to have the biggest biceps or fit into size zero jeans.

Social media images of unrealistically thin bodies—coupled with catch phrases telling young people to "get thin" or "be fit"—can be hard to avoid.[49, 50] With more than two-thirds of American adults 20 years and older overweight or obese, a significant disconnect exists between the media's idealized images and the typical American body.[51] At the same time, the media bombards us with messages telling us that we just don't measure up.

Parents are especially influential. For instance, fathers who validate the acceptability of their daughters' appearance throughout puberty and mothers who model body acceptance can help their daughters maintain a positive body image.[52]

Interactions with people outside the family can contribute to negative body image. Being overweight is now the most commonly reported reason children are bullied at school,[53] and teasing and bullying contribute to a negative body image. Moreover, associations within one's cultural group appear to influence body image. For example, studies have found that white females experience the highest rates of body dissatisfaction but that the body dissatisfaction levels of minority women increase the more they are exposed to mainstream media.[54]

People diagnosed with a body image disorder show differences in the brain's ability to regulate *neurotransmitters* linked to mood[55] in a way similar to that of depression and anxiety disorders, including obsessive-compulsive disorder. One study linked distortions in body image to a malfunction in the brain's visual processing region.[56]

Building a Positive Body Image

To develop a more positive body image, start by challenging some commonly held myths and attitudes in contemporary society[57]:

- **Myth 1: How you look is more important than who you are.** Is your weight important in defining who you are? How much does it matter to you to have friends who are thin? How important do you think being thin is in attracting a partner?
- **Myth 2: Anyone can look like the celebrities if they work hard enough.** While exercise and healthy eating can improve anyone's health status, not everyone has the genes to be muscular, tall, or curvy. We can exercise and eat our way to health but not to a particular shape.
- **Myth 3: Extreme dieting is an effective weight-loss strategy.** Are you attracted to fad diets or quick-weight-loss products? How far would you go to attain the "perfect" body?
- **Myth 4: Things will go better for me after I achieve the perfect body.** A certain shape or weight is not the key to a happy, wonderful life. Investing in healthy relationships and working toward life goals can bring lasting happiness.

Body Dysmorphic Disorder

Approximately 2 percent of people in the United States suffer from **body dysmorphic disorder (BDD)**.[58] Persons with BDD are obsessively concerned with their appearance and have a distorted view of their own body. Although the precise cause of BDD isn't known, an anxiety disorder such as obsessive-compulsive disorder is often present. Contributing factors may include genetic susceptibility, childhood teasing, physical or sexual abuse, low self-esteem, and rigid sociocultural expectations of attractiveness.[59]

People with BDD may try to fix their perceived flaws through abuse of steroids, excessive bodybuilding, cosmetic surgeries, extreme tattooing, or other appearance-altering behaviors.[60] Not only do such actions fail to address the underlying problem, but they also are actually considered diagnostic signs of BDD. Psychiatric treatment, including psychotherapy and/or antidepressant medications, can help.

Skills for **Behavior Change**

Ten Steps to a Positive Body Image

One way to turn negative thoughts positive is to think about how to look more healthfully and happily at yourself and your body. The more you try, the better you will feel about the body you have.

- **Step 1. Appreciate all of the amazing things your body does for you**—running, dancing, breathing, laughing, dreaming.
- **Step 2. Make a list of things you like about yourself that aren't related to how much you weigh or how you look.**
- **Step 3. Remind yourself that true beauty is *not* skin deep.** When you feel good about yourself and who you are, you carry yourself with a sense of confidence, self-acceptance, and openness that is attractive.
- **Step 4. Look at yourself as a whole person instead of focusing on specific body parts.**
- **Step 5. Surround yourself with positive people.** It is easier to feel good about yourself when you are around people who are supportive.
- **Step 6. Shut down those voices in your head that tell you your body is not "right" or that you are a "bad" person.**
- **Step 7. Wear comfortable clothes that make you feel good about your body.** Work with your body, not against it.
- **Step 8. Become a critical viewer of social and media messages.** Pay attention to images, slogans, and attitudes that make you feel bad about your appearance.
- **Step 9. Show appreciation for your body.** Take a bubble bath, make time for a nap, or find a peaceful place outside to relax.
- **Step 10. Use the time and energy you might have spent worrying about food, calories, and your weight to do something to help others.** Reaching out to other people can help you feel better about yourself and make a positive change in our world.

Source: "10 Steps to Positive Body Image," from National Eating Disorders Association website, Accessed February 13, 2016. National Eating Disorders Association. Reprinted with permission. For more information, visit www.NationalEatingDisorders.org or call NEDA's helpline at 1-800-931-2237.

Check Yourself

- Where do you place yourself on the body image continuum? What steps can you take to improve your body image?

What Is Disordered Eating?

9.13 Identify the elements of the eating issues continuum.

The eating issues continuum in **Figure 9.8** identifies thoughts and behaviors associated with disordered eating.

Some people who exhibit disordered eating patterns progress to a clinical **eating disorder**—a diagnosis that can be applied only by a physician to a patient who exhibits severe disturbances in thoughts, behavior, and body functioning. The American Psychiatric Association (APA) has defined several eating disorders: *anorexia nervosa*, *bulimia nervosa*, *binge-eating disorder*, and a cluster of less-distinct conditions collectively referred to as **Other Specified Feeding or Eating Disorder (OSFED)**.[61]

Twenty million women and 10 million men in the United States will suffer from some sort of eating disorder over their lifetime.[62]

Although anorexia nervosa and bulimia nervosa primarily affect people in their teens and twenties, other age groups can be affected, from children to older adults. In 2016, 2.7 percent of college students reported having been diagnosed with anorexia or bulimia and 1.5 perent of them reported that an eating disorder had had a negative effect on their academic performance[63] Eating disorders are on the rise among men, who make up nearly 25 percent of all anorexia and bulimia patients.[64]

Many people with eating disorders feel controlled in other aspects of their lives and try to gain a sense of power through food. Many are clinically depressed, suffer from obsessive-compulsive disorder, anxiety, or have other psychiatric problems. In addition, individuals with low self-esteem, negative body image, and a high tendency for perfectionism are at risk.[65]

Eating disordered	Disruptive eating patterns	Food preoccupied/ obsessed	Concerned in a healthy way	Food is not an issue
I worry about what I will eat or when I will exercise all the time.	My food and exercise concerns are starting to interfere with my school and social life.	I think about food a lot.	I pay attention to what I eat in order to maintain a healthy body.	I am not concerned about what or how much I eat.
I follow a very rigid eating plan and know precisely how many calories, fat grams, or carbohydrates I eat every day.	I use food to comfort myself.	I'm obsessed with reading books and magazines about dieting, fitness, and weight control.	Food and exercise are important parts of my life, but they only occupy a small part of my time.	I feel no guilt or shame no matter what I eat or how much I eat.
I feel incredible guilt, shame, and anxiety when I break my diet.	I have tried diet pills, laxatives, vomiting, or extra time exercising in order to lose or maintain my weight.	I sometimes miss school, work, and social events because of my diet or exercise schedule.	I enjoy eating, and I balance my pleasure with my concern for a healthy body.	Exercise is not really important to me. I choose foods based on cost, taste, and convenience, with little regard to health.
I regularly stuff myself and then exercise, vomit, or use laxatives to get rid of the food.	I have fasted or avoided eating for long periods of time in order to lose or maintain my weight.	I divide food into "good" and "bad" categories.	I usually eat three balanced meals daily, plus snacks, to fuel my body with adequate energy.	My eating is very sporadic and irregular.
My friends and family tell me I am too thin, but I feel fat.	If I cannot exercise to burn off calories, I panic.	I feel guilty when I eat "bad" foods or when I eat more than what I feel I should be eating.	I am moderate and flexible in my goals for eating well and being physically active.	I don't worry about meals; I just eat whatever I can, whenever I can.
I am out of control when I eat.	I feel strong when I can restrict how much I eat.	I am afraid of getting fat.	Sometimes I eat more (or less) than I really need, but most of the time I listen to my body.	I enjoy stuffing myself with lots of tasty food at restaurants, holiday meals, and social events.
I am afraid to eat in front of others.	I feel out of control when I eat more than I wanted to.	I wish I could change how much I want to eat and what I am hungry for.		
I prefer to eat alone.				

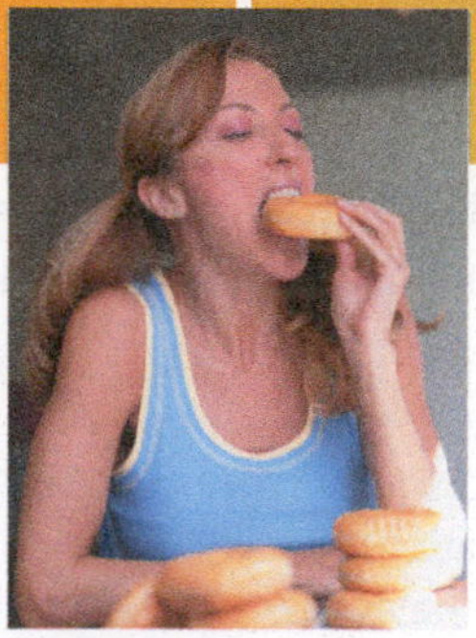

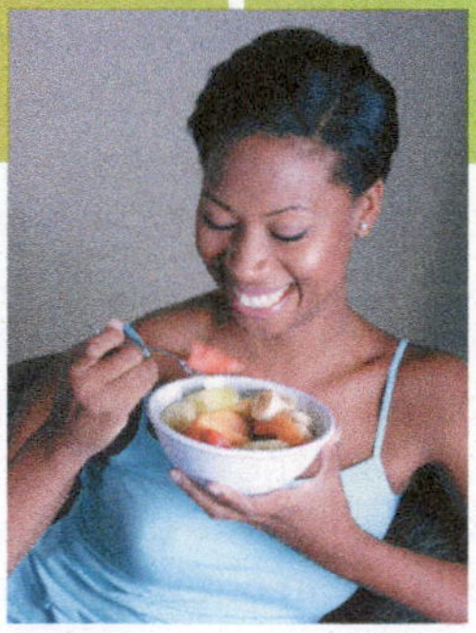

Figure 9.8 Eating Issues Continuum
This continuum shows progression from eating disorders to normal eating. The goal is to be concerned in a healthy way.

Source: Adapted from Smiley/King/Avery, "Eating Issues and Body Image Continuum," Campus Health Service 1996. Copyright © 1997 Arizona Board of Regents for University of Arizona.

- **Where do you place yourself on the eating issues continuum?**

Learning Outcome

9.14 List the criteria, effects, and treatment of anorexia nervosa.

Anorexia nervosa is a persistent, chronic eating disorder characterized by deliberate food restriction and severe, life-threatening weight loss. It involves self-starvation motivated by an intense fear of gaining weight along with an extremely distorted body image.

Initially, most people with anorexia nervosa lose weight by reducing total food intake, particularly of high-calorie foods. Eventually, they progress to restricting their intake of almost all foods. The little they do eat, they may purge through vomiting, use of laxatives, or excessive exercise. Although they lose weight, people with anorexia nervosa never seem to feel thin enough.

An estimated 0.9 to 2.0 percent of females suffer from anorexia nervosa in their lifetime.[66]

The APA criteria for anorexia nervosa are as follows[67]:

- Refusal to maintain body weight at or above a minimally normal weight for age and height
- Intense fear of gaining weight or becoming fat, even though considered underweight by all medical criteria
- Disturbance in the way in which one's body weight or shape is experienced, undue influence of body weight or shape on self-evaluation, or denial of the seriousness of the current low body weight.

Figure 9.9 illustrates the physical symptoms and negative health consequences associated with anorexia nervosa. Because it involves starvation and can lead to heart attacks and seizures, anorexia nervosa has the highest death rate (20 percent) of any psychological illness.[68]

Causes of anorexia nervosa are complex and variable. Many people with anorexia have coexisting psychiatric problems, including low self-esteem, depression, an anxiety disorder such as obsessive-compulsive disorder, and substance abuse. Some people with anorexia nervosa have a history of being physically or sexually abused, and others have troubled interpersonal relationships. Cultural norms that value appearance and glorify thinness as beauty are factors, as are weight-based shame, peer comparisons, and weight bias.[69] Physical factors are thought to include an imbalance of neurotransmitters and genetic susceptibility.[70]

Once the patient's condition has been stabilized, treatment involves long-term therapy that focuses on the psychological, social, environmental, and physiological factors that have led to the problem. Through therapy, the patient works on adopting new eating behaviors, building self-confidence, and finding other ways to deal with life's problems. Support groups can also help. With treatment, long-term full recovery rates range from 44 to 76 percent.[71]

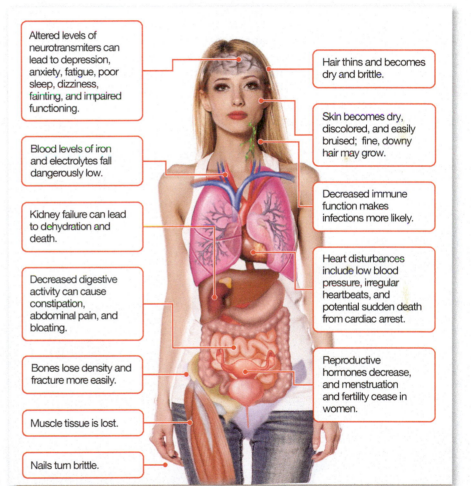

Altered levels of neurotransmiters can lead to depression, anxiety, fatigue, poor sleep, dizziness, fainting, and impaired functioning.

Hair thins and becomes dry and brittle.

Skin becomes dry, discolored, and easily bruised; fine, downy hair may grow.

Blood levels of iron and electrolytes fall dangerously low.

Decreased immune function makes infections more likely.

Kidney failure can lead to dehydration and death.

Heart disturbances include low blood pressure, irregular heartbeats, and potential sudden death from cardiac arrest.

Decreased digestive activity can cause constipation, abdominal pain, and bloating.

Reproductive hormones decrease, and menstruation and fertility cease in women.

Bones lose density and fracture more easily.

Muscle tissue is lost.

Nails turn brittle.

Figure 9.9 What Anorexia Nervosa Can Do to the Body

Check Yourself

- What factors might put a person at risk for anorexia nervosa?

- How is anorexia nervosa treated?

9.15 Eating Disorders: Bulimia Nervosa and Binge Eating Disorder

Learning Outcome

9.15 List the criteria, effects, and treatments for bulimia nervosa and binge eating.

Individuals with **bulimia nervosa** often binge on huge amounts of food and then engage in some kind of purging or compensatory behavior, such as vomiting, taking laxatives, or exercising excessively, to rid themselves of the calories they have just consumed. People with bulimia are obsessed with their bodies, weight gain, and appearance, although their problem is often hidden from the public eye because their weight may fall within a normal range or they may be overweight. Up to 3 percent of adolescents and young women are bulimic; rates among men are about 10 percent of the rate among women.[72] The APA criteria include recurrent episodes of binge eating and recurrent inappropriate compensatory behavior such as self-induced vomiting, use of laxatives or diuretics, fasting, or excessive exercise. The behavior must occur at least once a week for 3 months.[73]

Figure 9.10 shows the physical symptoms and negative health consequences associated with bulimia nervosa.

A combination of genetic and environmental factors is thought to cause bulimia nervosa.[74] A family history of obesity, an underlying anxiety disorder, and an imbalance in neurotransmitters are all possible contributing factors. One study showed that brain circuitry involved in regulating impulsive behavior seems to be less active in women with bulimia than in healthy women.[75] However, it is unknown whether such differences exist before bulimia develops or arise as a consequence of the disorder.

Individuals with **binge-eating disorder** gorge but do not take excessive measures to lose the weight they gain; they are often clinically obese. As in bulimia, binge-eating episodes are typically characterized by eating large amounts of food rapidly, even when not feeling hungry, and feeling guilty or depressed after overeating.[76]

The prevalence of binge-eating disorder is thought to be 1.4 percent.[77] The APA criteria for binge-eating disorder are similar to those for bulimia nervosa but without compensatory behavior.[78] Individuals diagnosed with the condition also show three or more of the following behaviors: eating much more rapidly than normal; eating until uncomfortably full; eating large amounts when not physically hungry; eating alone because of embarrassment over how much one is eating; and feeling disgusted, depressed, or very guilty after overeating.

Because eating disorders are caused by a combination of factors, there are no simple solutions. Without treatment, approximately 20 percent of people with a serious eating disorder will die as a result. With treatment, long-term full recovery rates range from 50 to 70 percent for bulimia nervosa.[79]

Treatment often focuses first on reducing the threat to life. Once the patient's condition has been stabilized, long-term therapy focuses on the psychological, social, environmental, and physiological factors that led to the problem. Through therapy, the patient works on adopting new eating behaviors, building self-confidence, and finding healthy ways to deal with life's problems. Support groups can help the family and the individual learn positive actions and interactions. Treatment of an underlying anxiety disorder or depression may also be a focus.

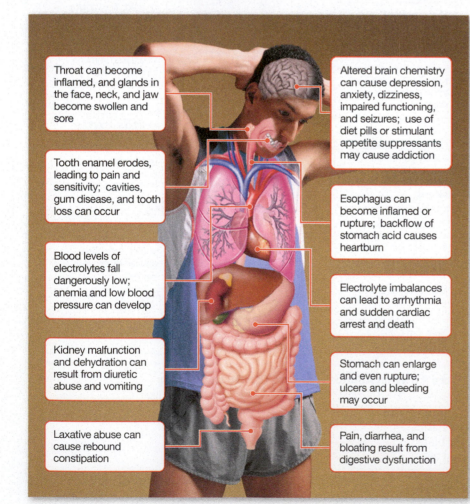

- Throat can become inflamed, and glands in the face, neck, and jaw become swollen and sore
- Tooth enamel erodes, leading to pain and sensitivity; cavities, gum disease, and tooth loss can occur
- Blood levels of electrolytes fall dangerously low; anemia and low blood pressure can develop
- Kidney malfunction and dehydration can result from diuretic abuse and vomiting
- Laxative abuse can cause rebound constipation
- Altered brain chemistry can cause depression, anxiety, dizziness, impaired functioning, and seizures; use of diet pills or stimulant appetite suppressants may cause addiction
- Esophagus can become inflamed or rupture; backflow of stomach acid causes heartburn
- Electrolyte imbalances can lead to arrhythmia and sudden cardiac arrest and death
- Stomach can enlarge and even rupture; ulcers and bleeding may occur
- Pain, diarrhea, and bloating result from digestive dysfunction

Figure 9.10 What Bulimia Nervosa Can Do to the Body

Check Yourself

- What factors might put a person at risk for bulimia nervosa and binge-eating disorder?

- How are bulimia nervosa and binge-eating disorder treated?

9.16 Exercise Disorders

Learning Outcome

9.16 List the criteria, effects, and treatment for exercise disorders.

Although exercise is generally beneficial to health, in excess it can be a problem. In addition to being a common compensatory behavior used by people with anorexia or bulimia, exercise can become a compulsion or contribute to muscle dysmorphia and the female athlete triad.

In a recent study, researchers showed that participants used excessive exercise or **compulsive exercise** as a way to regulate their emotions.[80] **Compulsive exercise**, or *anorexia athletica*, is characterized not by a *desire* to exercise but by a *compulsion* to do so, with guilt and anxiety if the person doesn't work out.

Compulsive exercise can contribute to injuries to joints and bones. It can also put significant stress on the heart, especially if combined with disordered eating. Psychologically, people who engage in compulsive exercise are often plagued by anxiety and/or depression.

Muscle Dysmorphia

Muscle dysmorphia is a form of body image disturbance and exercise disorder in which a person (usually male) believes that his body is insufficiently lean or muscular.[81] Men with muscle dysmorphia believe that they look "puny" when in reality they look normal or may even be unusually muscular. Behaviors characteristic of muscle dysmorphia include comparing oneself unfavorably to others, checking one's appearance in the mirror, and camouflaging one's appearance. Men with muscle dysmorphia also are likely to abuse anabolic steroids and dietary supplements.[82]

The Female Athlete Triad

Female athletes in competitive sports often strive for perfection. In an effort to be the best, they may put themselves at risk for a

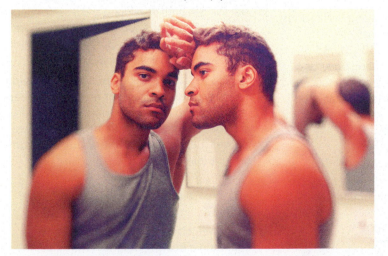

Men with muscle dysmorphia may have unusually muscular bodies but suffer from very low self-esteem.

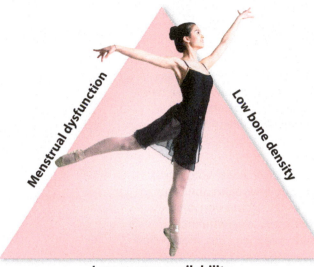

Figure 9.11 The Female Athlete Triad
The female athlete triad is a cluster of three interrelated health problems.

(Triangle labels: Menstrual dysfunction; Low bone density; Low energy availability)

syndrome called the **female athlete triad**, which consists of three interrelated problems (**Figure 9.11**): low energy (food) intake, typically prompted by disordered eating; menstrual dysfunction such as amenorrhea; and poor bone density.[83]

How does the female athlete triad develop? First, a chronic pattern of low food intake and intensive exercise depletes nutrients that are essential to health. The body begins to burn stores of fat tissue for energy, reducing levels of the female reproductive hormone *estrogen* and thus stopping menstruation. Depletion of fat-soluble vitamins, calcium, and estrogen weakens the athlete's bones, leaving her at high risk for fracture.

The triad is particularly prevalent in athletes in highly competitive individual sports that emphasize leanness, such as gymnasts, figure skaters, cross-country runners, and ballet dancers.

Warning signs include dry skin; light-headedness or fainting; fine, downy hair covering the body; multiple injuries; and changes in endurance, strength, or speed. Associated behaviors include preoccupation with food and weight, compulsive exercising, use of weight-loss products or laxatives, self-criticism, anxiety, and depression. Treatment requires a multidisciplinary approach involving the athlete's coach or trainer, a psychologist, and family members and friends.

See It! Videos
Can you go too far with extreme exercise? Watch **Young Boys, Exercising to Extremes** in the Study Area of Mastering Health.

Check Yourself

- **What are the criteria, effects, and treatment for exercise disorders? How might these differ for men and women?**

Summary

LO 9.1 Overweight, obesity, and weight-related health problems have reached epidemic levels in the United States, largely because of obesogenic behaviors in an obesogenic environment.

LO 9.2 Societal costs from obesity include increased health care costs, lowered worker productivity, low self-esteem, and obesity-related stigma. Individual health risks from overweight and obesity include a variety of chronic diseases.

LO 9.3–9.4 Many factors contribute to risk for obesity, including environmental factors, poverty, education level, genetics, developmental factors, endocrine influences, psychosocial factors, eating cues, metabolic changes, and lifestyle.

LO 9.5–9.6 Percentage of body fat is a reliable indicator for levels of overweight and obesity. *Overweight* is most commonly defined as a BMI of 25 to 29, and *obesity* is defined as a BMI of 30 or greater. Waist circumference is believed to be related to risk for several chronic diseases, particularly type 2 diabetes. Body mass index is one of the most commonly used body fat assessments, however, it is not the most accurate.

LO 9.7–9.9 Sensible, mindful eating and exercise offer the best options for weight loss and maintenance. The best diet programs allow you to make healthy choices in real-world settings without sacrificing everything enjoyable. Successful weight management includes making a plan and changing habits.

LO 9.10 Diet pills, surgery, and very-low-calorie diets are drastic measures for weight loss and may carry significant risks.

LO 9.11 To gain weight, a person should increase intake of energy-dense, nutritious foods.

LO 9.12 Negative feelings about one's body can contribute to behaviors that can threaten health. In contrast, a healthy body image can contribute to reduced stress and personal empowerment. Body image disorders affect men and women of all ages. Body image can be affected by culture, media, and individual physiological and psychological factors.

LO 9.13–9.15 Disordered eating and eating disorders such as anorexia nervosa, bulimia nervosa, and binge-eating disorder can lead to serious health problems and even death.

LO 9.16 Although exercise is healthy in moderation, if it becomes a compulsion it can lead to disorders such as muscle dysmorphia and the female athlete triad.

Pop Quiz

Visit Mastering Health to personalize your study plan with Chapter Review Quizzes and Dynamic Study Modules.

LO 9.3 1. The rate at which your body consumes food energy to sustain basic functions is your
a. basal metabolic rate.
b. resting metabolic rate.
c. body mass index.
d. set point.

LO 9.5 2. Which of the following statements is *false*?
a. A slowing basal metabolic rate may lead to weight gain after age 30.
b. Hormones are implicated in hunger impulses and eating behavior.
c. The more muscles you have, the fewer calories you'll burn.
d. Overweight and obesity can have serious health consequences, even before middle age.

LO 9.6 3. Which of the following statements about BMI is *false*?
a. BMI is based on height and weight measurements.
b. BMI is accurate for everyone, including people with high muscle mass.
c. Children's BMIs are used to determine a percentile ranking among their age peers.
d. BMI stands for "body mass index."

LO 9.6 4. Which of the following BMI ratings is considered overweight?
a. 20   b. 25   c. 30   d. 35

LO 9.6 5. Which of the following body circumferences is most strongly associated with risk of heart disease and diabetes?
a. Hip circumference
b. Chest circumference
c. Waist circumference
d. Thigh circumference

LO 9.7 6. One pound of additional body fat is created through consuming how many extra calories?
a. 1,500   b. 3,500
c. 5,000   d. 7,000

LO 9.7 7. To lose weight, you must establish a(n)
a. negative caloric balance.
b. energy balance.
c. positive caloric balance.
d. set point.

LO 9.9 8. Successful, healthy weight loss is characterized by
a. a lifelong pattern of healthful eating and exercise.
b. cutting out fats and carbohydrates.
c. never eating foods that are considered bad for you.
d. a pattern of repeatedly losing and regaining weight.

LO 9.12 9. Which of the following is *not* a contributor to negative body image?
a. Idealized media images of celebrities
b. Increases in portion sizes
c. Cultural attitudes about body ideals
d. Neurotransmitter regulation in the brain

LO 9.15 10. Which of the following eating disorders includes compensatory behavior in its definition?
a. Anorexia nervosa
b. Bulimia nervosa
c. Binge-eating disorder
d. Muscle dysmorphia

Answers to these questions can be found on page A-1. If you answered a question incorrectly, review the module identified by the Learning Outcome. For even more study tools, visit Mastering Health.

Think About It!

LO 9.1 1. Why do you think that obesity rates are rising in both developed and less-developed regions of the world? What strategies can we take collectively and individually to reduce risks of obesity nationally? Internationally?

LO 9.3 2. List the risk factors for your being overweight or obese right now. Which seem most likely to determine whether you will be obese in middle age? If newer theories prove true, how might they influence future weight loss efforts?

LO 9.5–9.6 3. Which measurement would you choose to assess your fat levels? Why?

LO 9.7–9.11 4. Are you satisfied with your body weight? If so, what do you do to maintain a healthy weight? What lifestyle changes could you make to improve your weight and overall health?

Fitness

Most Americans are aware of the wide range of physical, social, and mental health benefits of physical activity and that they should be more physically active. Physiological changes resulting from regular physical activity reduce the likelihood of coronary artery disease, high blood pressure, type 2 diabetes, obesity, and other chronic diseases. Engaging regularly in physical activity also helps to control stress and increase self-esteem.

Despite these benefits, 25.9 percent of American adults engage in no leisure-time physical activity,[1] a situation that is linked to the current high rates of obesity, type 2 diabetes, and other chronic and mental health diseases.[2]

In general, college students are more physically active than older adults, but a recent survey indicated that 41.6 percent of college women and 49 percent of college men do not do the recommended amount of moderate to vigorous physical activity per week.[3]

College is a great time to develop attitudes and behaviors that can increase the quality and quantity of your life. This chapter offers knowledge and strategies to help you get moving.

10.1 Distinguish among physical activity for health, for fitness, and for performance.

Physical activity is any body movement that works your muscles, uses more energy than is used when resting, and enhances health.[4] Physical activities can vary by intensity. For example, walking to class on flat ground typically requires little effort, while walking to class uphill is more intense and harder to do. The three general categories of physical activity are defined by their purpose: physical activity for health, physical activity for physical fitness, and physical activity for performance.

Exercise is defined as planned, structured, and repetitive bodily movement done to improve or maintain one or more components of physical fitness, such as cardiorespiratory endurance, muscular strength or endurance, or flexibility. Although all exercise is physical activity, not all physical activity is considered exercise. For example, walking from your car to class is physical activity, whereas going for a brisk 30-minute walk is considered exercise.

Physical Activity for Health

Adding more physical activity to your day can benefit your health.[5] We know that physical activity is good for health, and we know that physical inactivity contributes to increased risk of negative health outcomes. We can define **sedentary** as any activity that expends no more than 1.5 times the resting energy level while seated or reclined. Typically, we describe physical activity in terms of **METS**, the metabolic equivalent used to estimate the amount of energy (oxygen) the body uses during physical activity. Typically, 1 MET equals the energy used when sitting or resting quietly (couch potato time); a MET of 2 equals twice the energy level used at MET level 1 (a casual walk, or doing housework); a MET level 3 equals three times the at rest energy used; and so on. Jogging or aerobic exercise might be at 5 to 6 METS. There are three primary levels of physical activity: (1) *light/lifestyle/physical activities* (<3 METS), (2) *moderate physical activities* (3 to 6 METS), and (3) *vigorous activities* (>6 METS). If you've spent much time on treadmills and elliptical machines, you have seen the MET levels go up with the intensity of your workout. Generally, as fitness improves, you are able to exercise at a higher MET level.

Although regular exercise and high levels of physical activity can protect against disease and premature death, sedentary time has an independent effect on disease and mortality.[6] Research shows that risk for cardiovascular disease, cancers, and type 2 diabetes increases with high amounts of sitting time.[7] Indeed, it is estimated that physical inactivity is responsible for 30 percent of the cases of ischemic heart disease, 27 percent of cases of type 2 diabetes, and 21 to 25 percent of cases of breast and colon cancer worldwide.[8] Table 10.1 summarizes physical activity guidelines.

Physical Activity for Fitness

Physical fitness refers to a set of health- and performance-related attributes. These attributes—cardiorespiratory fitness, muscular strength and endurance, flexibility, and body composition—allow us to perform moderate- to vigorous-intensity physical activities on a regular basis without getting too tired and with energy left over to handle physical or mental emergencies. Figure 10.1 identifies the major health-related components of physical fitness.

TABLE 10.1 Physical Activity Guidelines for Americans

Key Guidelines for Health*	For Additional Fitness or Weight Loss Benefits*	PLUS
150 min/week moderate intensity OR 75 min/week of vigorous intensity OR Equivalent combination of moderate and vigorous intensity (i.e., 100 min moderate intensity = 25 min vigorous intensity)	300 min/week moderate intensity OR 150 min/week of vigorous intensity OR Equivalent combination of moderate and vigorous intensity (i.e., 200 min moderate intensity = 50 min vigorous intensity) OR More than the previously described amounts	Muscle strengthening activities for *all* the major muscle groups at least 2 days/week

* Accumulate this physical activity in sessions of 10 minutes or more at one time.

Source: Office of Disease Prevention and Health Promotion, U.S. Department of Health and Human Services, *2008 Physical Activity Guidelines for Americans: Be Active, Healthy, and Happy!* ODPHP Publication no. U0036 (Washington, DC: U.S. Department of Health and Human Services, 2008), available at www.health.gov.

Note: An advisory committee has been established to review research related to the current guidelines and health and to discuss the guidelines with the public. The goal is to have the second edition of the Physical Activity Guidelines for Health available for the public in 2018. Check out the website for more information! https://health.gov/paguidelines/second-edition

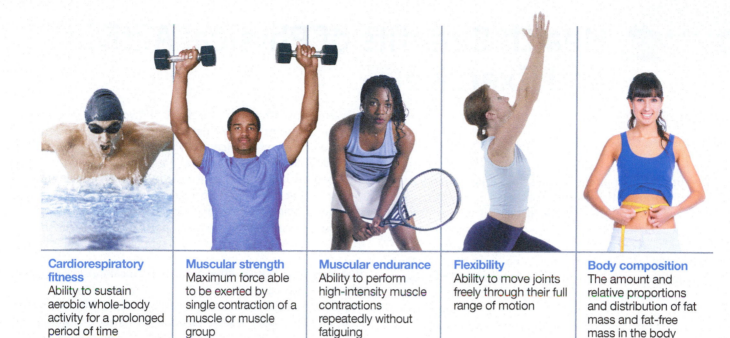

Cardiorespiratory fitness
Ability to sustain aerobic whole-body activity for a prolonged period of time

Muscular strength
Maximum force able to be exerted by single contraction of a muscle or muscle group

Muscular endurance
Ability to perform high-intensity muscle contractions repeatedly without fatiguing

Flexibility
Ability to move joints freely through their full range of motion

Body composition
The amount and relative proportions and distribution of fat mass and fat-free mass in the body

Figure 10.1 Components of Physical Fitness

Cardiorespiratory Fitness **Cardiorespiratory fitness** is the ability of the heart, lungs, and blood vessels to supply the body with oxygen efficiently. The primary category of physical activity known to improve cardiorespiratory fitness is **aerobic exercise**. The word *aerobic* means "with oxygen" and describes any exercise that requires oxygen to make energy for prolonged activity. Aerobic activities such as swimming, cycling, and jogging are among the best exercises for improving or maintaining cardiorespiratory fitness.

Cardiorespiratory fitness is measured by determining **aerobic capacity** (or **power**), the volume of oxygen the muscles consume during exercise. Maximal aerobic power ($VO_{2\ max}$) is defined as the maximal volume of oxygen that the muscles consume during exercise. The most common measure of maximal aerobic capacity is a walk or run test on a treadmill. For greatest accuracy, this is done in a lab and requires special equipment and technicians to measure the precise amount of oxygen entering and exiting the body during the exercise session. Submaximal tests can be used to get a more general sense of cardiorespiratory fitness; one such test is the 1-mile walk test.

Muscular Strength **Muscular strength** refers to the amount of force a muscle or group of muscles is capable of exerting in one contraction. A common way to assess the strength of a particular muscle group is to measure the maximum amount of weight you can move one time (and no more), or your one repetition maximum (1 RM).

Muscular Endurance **Muscular endurance** is the ability of a muscle or group of muscles to exert force repeatedly without fatigue or the ability to sustain a muscular contraction. The more repetitions of an endurance activity (e.g., push-ups) you can perform successfully, or the longer you can hold a certain position (e.g., wall sit), the greater is your muscular endurance. General muscular endurance is often measured by using the number of curl-ups an individual can do; this test is described in the Assess Yourself module in Mastering Health.

Flexibility **Flexibility** refers to the range of motion, or the amount of movement possible, at a particular joint or series of joints: the greater the range of motion, the greater the flexibility. One of the most common measures of general flexibility is the sit-and-reach test, described in the Assess Yourself module in Mastering Health.

Body Composition **Body composition**, the fifth and final component of a comprehensive fitness program, describes the relative proportions and distribution of fat and lean (muscle, bone, water, organs) tissues in the body.

Physical Activity for Performance

Physical fitness for athletes involves attributes that improve their ability to perform athletic tasks. These attributes can also help nonathletes increase their fitness levels and their ability to perform daily tasks. These skill-related components of physical fitness (also called sports skills) are *agility*, *balance*, *coordination*, *power*, *speed*, and *reaction time*. Participating regularly in any sport or activity can improve your sports skills, as can performing drills that mimic a sport-specific skill.

Check Yourself

- **What are the differences between physical activity for health, for fitness, and for performance?**

- **What is the difference between Physical Activity, Exercise, and Physical Fitness?**

- **What are the core components of physical fitness and why are each of these important?**

10.1

Fitness

Health Benefits of Physical Activity and Exercise

10.2 List the health benefits of physical activity and exercise.

The first step in starting a physical fitness program is identifying where you are in terms of fitness levels and coming up with goals that are best for you, your current health status and what you would like to accomplish overall. A person who wants to run a marathon might have different goals than someone who is unfit and wants to be able to lose weight, take long walks and be active without gasping for breath! Once you have a clear set of goals, you should next consider anything that might get in the way of your achieving those goals. Once you have contemplated these factors, you are ready to create an individual physical activity or exercise program to meet your physical fitness goals. Before we start, and to help you get motivated, let's take a look at the many physical and psychological benefits of physical activity.

What Are the Health Benefits of Regular Physical Activity?

Regular physical activity improves more than 50 different physiological, metabolic, and psychological aspects of life. **Figure 10.2** summarizes some of the major health-related benefits.

Reduced Risk of Cardiovascular Diseases Aerobic exercise is good for the heart and lungs and reduces the risk for cardiovascular diseases. It improves blood flow and eases performance of everyday tasks. Regular exercise makes the cardiovascular and respiratory systems more efficient by strengthening the heart muscle, thus enabling more blood to be pumped with each stroke, and increasing the number of *capillaries* (small blood vessels that allow gas exchange between blood and surrounding tissues) in trained skeletal muscles, thus supplying more blood to working muscles. Exercise also improves the respiratory system by increasing the amount of oxygen inhaled and distributed to body tissues.[9]

Regular physical activity of moderate intensity can reduce hypertension (chronic high blood pressure), a cardiovascular disease itself and a significant risk factor for other cardiovascular diseases and stroke.[10] Regular aerobic activity also improves the blood lipid profile. It typically increases high-density lipoproteins (HDLs, or "good" cholesterol), which are associated with lower risk for coronary artery disease because of their role in removing plaque built up in the arteries.[11] Triglycerides (a blood fat) typically decrease with aerobic activity. Low-density lipoproteins (LDLs, or "bad" cholesterol) and total cholesterol are also often improved with exercise.[12]

Reduced Risk of Metabolic Syndrome and Type 2 Diabetes Regular physical activity reduces the risk of *metabolic syndrome*, a combination of risk factors that produces a synergistic increase in risk heart disease and diabetes.[13] Specifically, metabolic syndrome includes high blood pressure, abdominal obesity, low levels of HDLs, high levels of triglycerides, and impaired glucose tolerance.[14] Regular participation in moderate- to vigorous-intensity physical activities reduces the risk for each factor individually and collectively.[15]

Research indicates that a healthy dietary intake combined with sufficient physical activity could prevent many cases of type 2 diabetes.[16] Doing the recommended 150 minutes of moderate- to vigorous-intensity aerobic activity per week has been shown to improve glucose tolerance and insulin sensitivity to manage diabetes.[17]

Reduced Cancer Risk After decades of research, most cancer epidemiologists believe that 25 to 37 percent of cancers can be avoided by healthier lifestyle and environmental choices.[18] Recent research assessing the impact of sedentary time on cancer indicates that the risk for several types of cancer is associated with high levels of sedentary time.[19] The American Cancer Society reports that approximately 20 percent of cancers are linked to physical inactivity and dietary choices, and other research shows that up to 30 percent of some cancers could be prevented with regular physical activity and healthy diet choices.[20]

Improved Bone Mass and Reduced Risk of Osteoporosis A common affliction for older people is *osteoporosis*, a disease characterized by low bone mass and deterioration of bone tissue, which increases the risk of fracture. Regular weight-bearing and strength-building physical activities are recommended throughout life to maintain bone health and prevent osteoporotic fractures However, it appears that the full bone-related benefits of physical activity are best achieved when sufficient hormone levels (estrogen in women, testosterone in men) and adequate calcium, vitamin D, and total caloric intakes are also considered.[21]

Improved Weight Control For many people, the desire to lose weight or maintain a healthy weight is the main reason for physical activity. On the most basic level, physical activity requires your body to generate energy through calorie expenditure; if calories expended exceed calories consumed over a span of time, the net result will be weight loss.

Physical activity also has a direct positive effect on metabolic rate, keeping it elevated for several hours following vigorous physical activities.[22] This increase in metabolic rate can lead to body composition changes as well as increased muscle mass. Over time, that can lead to improved weight control. After weight loss, increased physical activity and increased strength can improve your chances of maintaining the weight loss. If you are currently at a healthy body weight, regular physical activity can prevent significant weight gain.

Improved Immunity Research shows that regular moderate-intensity physical activity reduces an individual's susceptibility to disease through improving the body's ability to fight infections.[23] Regular exercise has also been shown to reduce inflammation that is associated with higher risk of chronic conditions such as cardiovascular

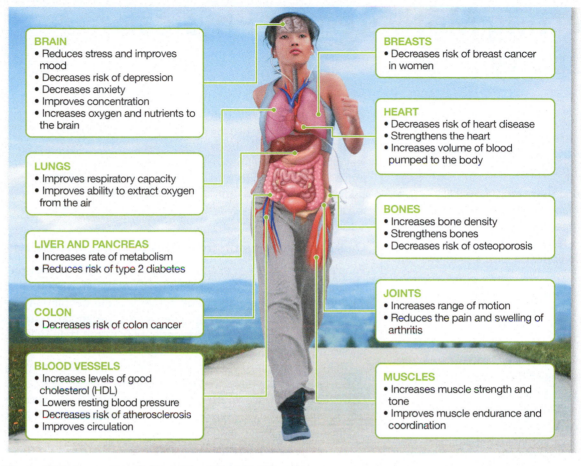

BRAIN
• Reduces stress and improves mood
• Decreases risk of depression
• Decreases anxiety
• Improves concentration
• Increases oxygen and nutrients to the brain

LUNGS
• Improves respiratory capacity
• Improves ability to extract oxygen from the air

LIVER AND PANCREAS
• Increases rate of metabolism
• Reduces risk of type 2 diabetes

COLON
• Decreases risk of colon cancer

BLOOD VESSELS
• Increases levels of good cholesterol (HDL)
• Lowers resting blood pressure
• Decreases risk of atherosclerosis
• Improves circulation

BREASTS
• Decreases risk of breast cancer in women

HEART
• Decreases risk of heart disease
• Strengthens the heart
• Increases volume of blood pumped to the body

BONES
• Increases bone density
• Strengthens bones
• Decreases risk of osteoporosis

JOINTS
• Increases range of motion
• Reduces the pain and swelling of arthritis

MUSCLES
• Increases muscle strength and tone
• Improves muscle endurance and coordination

Figure 10.2 Some Health Benefits of Regular Exercise

Mastering Health & Nutrition Health Benefits of Regular Exercise

disease or cancer.[24] Often, the relationship between physical activity and improved immunity has been attributed in part to the increases in natural killer cells (NKCs) that have been shown to occur in response to acute exercise. NKCs work by recognizing and eliminating virus-infected and neoplastic cells and thus serve a vital role in body defenses. Through exercise, the effects of NKCs may be enhanced, along with other cellular changes in disease-fighting neutrophils, lymphocytes, anti-inflammatory cytokines, and others. Moderate levels of exercise seem to be most important in improved immune response.[25] People who routinely engage in higher levels of exercise (e.g., extreme athletes, iron-man, marathon, or other intense physical training programs) have been shown to be at greater risk for upper respiratory tract infections in the first 8 hours after an intense exercise session.[26]

Improved Back Strength Regular whole-body exercise and exercises that target the specific muscles of the back (and the rest of the core) create a strong platform for the entire body. A strong, healthy back helps you maintain proper posture and avoid posture-related stress in the neck, shoulders, hips, knees, and ankles. It also gives you a good foundation for a range of exercise and reduces the likelihood of injury.

Improved Mental Health and Stress Management People who engage in regular physical activity are likely to notice psychological

benefits, such as feeling better about themselves and an overall sense of well-being.[27] Although these mental health benefits are difficult to quantify, they are frequently mentioned as reasons for continuing to be physically active. Learning new skills, developing increased ability and capacity in recreational activities, and sticking with a physical activity plan also improve self-esteem.[28] In addition, regular physical activity can improve a person's physical appearance, further increasing self-esteem.[29]

There is increasing evidence that regular physical activity positively affects cognitive function across the lifespan. Research has associated regular activity and fitness (aerobic and muscular) levels with improved academic performance in school, and higher levels of sedentary time has been associated with poorer performance on some measures.[30] Study-related fatigue and performance on laboratory tasks to assess executive cognitive functions improved with regular aerobic exercise, and these effects were seen both immediately after the intervention and during follow-ups 1 and 3 months later.[31] Furthermore, first-year medical students who reported using the recreation center frequently in the 3 weeks before an exam had higher scores on exams than did those who used it less frequently.[32] The most frequent use was associated with the highest exam scores.[33] Regular aerobic activity, even when initiated as an adult, has also been associated with reduced risk for and improvement in dementia and Alzheimer's disease in adults.[34]

Longer Lifespan Experts have long debated the relationship between physical activity and longevity. Several studies indicate significant decreases in long-term health risk and increases in years lived, particularly among those who have several risk factors and use physical activity as a means of risk reduction.[35] The largest benefits from physical activity occur in sedentary individuals who add a little physical activity to their lives, with additional benefits as physical activity levels increase.[36] Additionally, data show that the more sedentary time adults report, the greater is the reduction in the ability to perform activities of daily living.[37] It is not just structured exercise that is important, but moving as much as possible and sitting as little as possible.

Check Yourself

■ **What are five health benefits of physical activity?**

10.3 Getting Motivated for Physical Activity

There are many reasons for wanting to be more physically active and physically fit, including the many health benefits discussed earlier in this text. Taking some time to reflect on your personal circumstances, goals, and desires regarding physical fitness will probably make it easier for you to come up with a plan you can stick to.

What If I Have Been Inactive for a While?

If you have been physically inactive for the past few months or longer, first make sure that your physician clears you for exercise. Consider consulting a personal trainer or fitness instructor to help you get started. In this phase of your fitness program, the *initial conditioning stage*, you may begin at levels lower than those recommended for physical fitness. Starting slowly will ease you into a workout regime with a minimum of soreness. For example, you might start your cardiorespiratory program by simply moving more and reducing your sedentary time each day. Take the stairs instead of the elevator, walk farther from your car to the store, and plan for organized movement each day, such as a 10- to 15-minute walk. In addition, you can start your muscle fitness program with simple body weight exercises, emphasizing proper technique and body alignment before adding any resistance.

Overcoming Common Obstacles to Physical Activity

People offer a variety of excuses to explain why they do not exercise, ranging from personal ("I don't have time") to environmental ("I don't have a safe place to be active"). Some people may be reluctant to exercise if they are overweight, are embarrassed to work out with their more "fit" friends, or feel that they lack the knowledge and skills required.

Think about your obstacles to physical activity and write them down. Consider anything that gets in the way of your exercising, however minor. Once you have honestly evaluated why you are not as physically active as you want to be, review **Table 10.2** for suggestions on overcoming your hurdles.

Incorporating Fitness into Your Life

When designing your program, you should consider several factors to boost your chances of achieving your physical fitness goals.

Some activities are more intense or vigorous than others and result in more calories used; **Figure 10.3** shows the caloric cost of various activities when done for 30 minutes. Choose activities that are appropriate for you, that you genuinely like doing, and that are convenient. For example, you might choose jogging over swimming because you like to run and there are beautiful trails nearby, while you don't really like the water and the pool is difficult to get to. Likewise, choose activities that are suitable for your current fitness level. If you are overweight or obese and haven't exercised in months, don't sign up for the advanced aerobics classes. Start slow, plan fun activities, and progress to

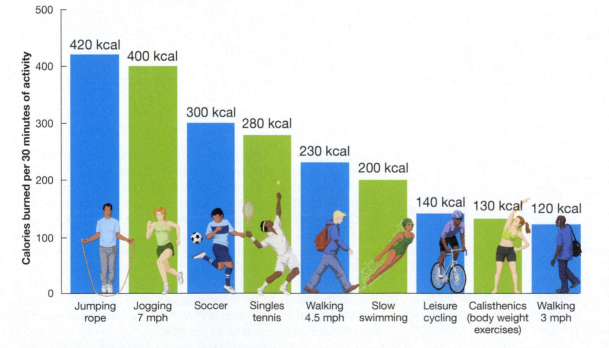

Figure 10.3 Calories Burned by Different Activities
The harder you exercise, the more energy you expend. Estimated calories burned for various moderate and vigorous activities are listed for a 30-minute bout of activity.

10.2 Overcoming Obstacles to Physical Activity

Obstacle	Possible Solution
Lack of time	• Look at your schedule. Where can you find 30-minute time slots? Perhaps you need to focus on shorter times (10 minutes or more) throughout the day. • Multitask. Read while riding an exercise bike, or listen to lectures or podcasts while walking. • Be physically active during your lunch and study breaks as well as between classes. Skip rope or throw a Frisbee with a friend. • Select activities that require less time, such as brisk walking or jogging. • Ride your bike to class, or park your car (or get off the bus) farther from your destination.
Social influence	• Invite family and friends to be active with you. • Join a class to meet new people. • Explain the importance of exercise and your commitment to physical activity to people who may not support your efforts. • Find a role model to support your efforts. • Plan for physically active dates—go dancing or bowling.
Lack of motivation, willpower, or energy	• Schedule your workout time just as you would any other important commitment. • Enlist the help of an exercise partner to make you accountable for working out. • Give yourself an incentive. • Schedule your workouts for times when you feel most energetic. • Remind yourself that exercise gives you more energy. • Get things ready for your workout. For example, if you choose to walk in the morning, set out your walking clothes the night before, or pack your gym bag before going to bed.
Lack of resources	• Select an activity that requires minimal equipment, such as walking, jogging, jumping rope, or calisthenics. • Identify inexpensive resources on campus or in the community. • Use active forms of transportation. • Take advantage of no-cost opportunities, such as playing catch in the park or in a green space on campus.

Source: Adapted from National Center for Chronic Disease Prevention and Health Promotion, "How Can I Overcome Barriers to Physical Activity?," Updated February 2011, www.cdc.gov.

more challenging activities as your physical fitness improves. You might choose simply to walk more in an attempt to achieve the recommended goal of 10,000 steps per day; keep track with a pedometer or step counter; see **Table 10.3** for more on this handy gadget and other fitness equipment you may consider purchasing or using at a health club. Try to make exercise a part of your

How can I motivate myself to be more physically active?

One great way to motivate yourself is to sign up for an exercise class. Find something that interests you—dance, yoga, aerobics, martial arts, acrobatics—and get yourself involved. The structure, schedule, social interaction, and challenge of learning a new skill can be terrific motivators that make exercising and being physically active exciting and fun.

routine by incorporating it into something you already have to do, such as getting to class or work.

Take a *mindfulness* break. Making time for some outdoor exercise ("green exercise") is a great way to get mental health benefits in addition to the physical ones.[38] Take a walk through your campus, purposefully focusing on the outdoor setting. Listen to the sounds, and take note of the smells. Breathe, and allow yourself to only think about the moment you are living in, free from external stressors. Open green space is a great place for a yoga mat and taking a time-out. Stadium stairs and benches can be incorporated into an exercise routine, and even trees can become exercise equipment.

Check Yourself

- **What are some common obstacles people face when they decide to be more physically active? How can these obstacles be overcome?**

- **What factors should you consider when choosing an exercise activity?**

10.4 Some Popular Fitness Gadgets and Equipment

Learning Outcome

10.4 Identify common types of fitness equipment and their uses.

TABLE 10.3 Some Popular Fitness Gadgets and Equipment

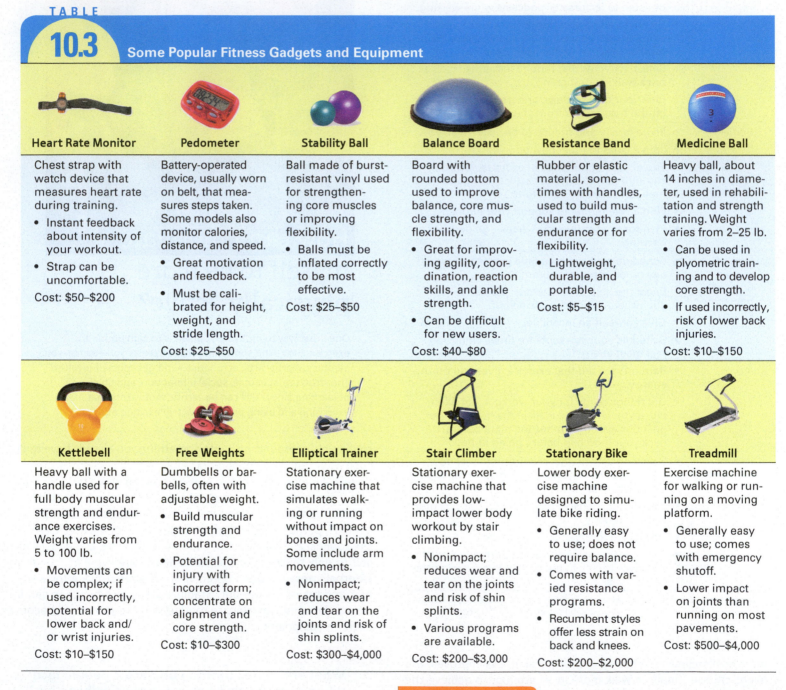

Heart Rate Monitor	Pedometer	Stability Ball	Balance Board	Resistance Band	Medicine Ball
Chest strap with watch device that measures heart rate during training. • Instant feedback about intensity of your workout. • Strap can be uncomfortable. Cost: $50–$200	Battery-operated device, usually worn on belt, that measures steps taken. Some models also monitor calories, distance, and speed. • Great motivation and feedback. • Must be calibrated for height, weight, and stride length. Cost: $25–$50	Ball made of burst-resistant vinyl used for strengthening core muscles or improving flexibility. • Balls must be inflated correctly to be most effective. Cost: $25–$50	Board with rounded bottom used to improve balance, core muscle strength, and flexibility. • Great for improving agility, coordination, reaction skills, and ankle strength. • Can be difficult for new users. Cost: $40–$80	Rubber or elastic material, sometimes with handles, used to build muscular strength and endurance or for flexibility. • Lightweight, durable, and portable. Cost: $5–$15	Heavy ball, about 14 inches in diameter, used in rehabilitation and strength training. Weight varies from 2–25 lb. • Can be used in plyometric training and to develop core strength. • If used incorrectly, risk of lower back injuries. Cost: $10–$150
Kettlebell	**Free Weights**	**Elliptical Trainer**	**Stair Climber**	**Stationary Bike**	**Treadmill**
Heavy ball with a handle used for full body muscular strength and endurance exercises. Weight varies from 5 to 100 lb. • Movements can be complex; if used incorrectly, potential for lower back and/or wrist injuries. Cost: $10–$150	Dumbbells or barbells, often with adjustable weight. • Build muscular strength and endurance. • Potential for injury with incorrect form; concentrate on alignment and core strength. Cost: $10–$300	Stationary exercise machine that simulates walking or running without impact on bones and joints. Some include arm movements. • Nonimpact; reduces wear and tear on the joints and risk of shin splints. Cost: $300–$4,000	Stationary exercise machine that provides low-impact lower body workout by stair climbing. • Nonimpact; reduces wear and tear on the joints and risk of shin splints. • Various programs are available. Cost: $200–$3,000	Lower body exercise machine designed to simulate bike riding. • Generally easy to use; does not require balance. • Comes with varied resistance programs. • Recumbent styles offer less strain on back and knees. Cost: $200–$2,000	Exercise machine for walking or running on a moving platform. • Generally easy to use; comes with emergency shutoff. • Lower impact on joints than running on most pavements. Cost: $500–$4,000

Check Yourself

■ What are five types of fitness equipment? Which would you be likely to use and why?

10.5 Fitness Program Components

10.5 Describe how to set SMART goals and list the parts of the FITT principle.

Set SMART Goals

Your physical fitness goals and objectives should be both achievable and in line with what you truly want. To set successful goals, try using the *SMART system*. SMART goals are *s*pecific, *m*easurable, *a*ction-oriented, *r*ealistic, and *t*ime-oriented. A vague goal would be "Improve fitness by exercising more." Following are SMART goals:

- **Specific.** "I'll participate in a resistance training program that targets all of the major muscle groups 3 to 5 days per week."
- **Measurable.** "I'll improve my fitness classification to average."
- **Action-oriented.** "I'll meet with a personal trainer to learn how to safely do resistance exercises and to plan a workout."
- **Realistic.** "I'll increase the weight I can lift by 20 percent."
- **Time-oriented.** "I'll try my new weight program for 8 weeks, then reassess."

Use the FITT Principle

The **FITT (frequency, intensity, time, and type)** principle shown in **Figure 10.4** can be used to devise a workout plan. To achieve the desired level of fitness, consider the following elements:

- **Frequency** refers to how often you must exercise.
- **Intensity** refers to how hard your workout must be.
- **Time**, or *duration*, refers to how many minutes or repetitions of an exercise are required per session.
- **Type** refers to the kind of exercises performed.

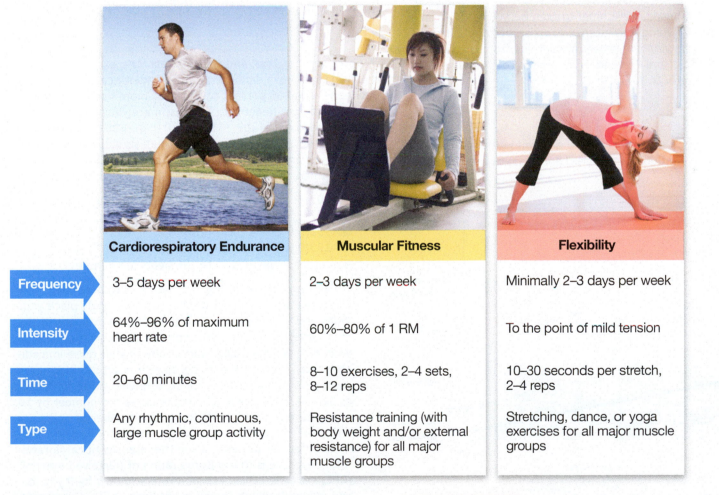

	Cardiorespiratory Endurance	Muscular Fitness	Flexibility
Frequency	3–5 days per week	2–3 days per week	Minimally 2–3 days per week
Intensity	64%–96% of maximum heart rate	60%–80% of 1 RM	To the point of mild tension
Time	20–60 minutes	8–10 exercises, 2–4 sets, 8–12 reps	10–30 seconds per stretch, 2–4 reps
Type	Any rhythmic, continuous, large muscle group activity	Resistance training (with body weight and/or external resistance) for all major muscle groups	Stretching, dance, or yoga exercises for all major muscle groups

Figure 10.4 The FITT Principle Applied to Cardiorespiratory Fitness, Muscular Strength and Endurance, and Flexibility

- What is an example of a SMART goal for fitness?
- What are the four parts of the FITT principle?

10.6 The FITT Principle for Cardiorespiratory Fitness

10.6 List the FITT requirements for cardiorespiratory fitness.

The most effective aerobic exercises for building cardiorespiratory fitness are total-body activities involving the large muscle groups. The FITT prescription for cardiorespiratory fitness includes 3 to 5 days per week of vigorous, rhythmic, continuous activity at 64 to 96 percent of your estimated maximal heart rate for 20 to 60 minutes.[39]

Frequency

To improve your cardiorespiratory fitness, you must exercise vigorously at least three times a week or moderately at least five times a week. If you are a newcomer to exercise, you can still make improvements by doing less intense exercise but doing it more days a week, following the recommendations from the Centers for Disease Control and Prevention for moderate physical activity 5 days a week (refer to Table 10.1).

Intensity

The most common methods used to determine the intensity of cardiorespiratory endurance exercises are target heart rate, rating

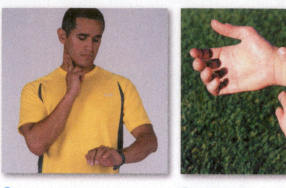

ⓐ Carotid pulse   ⓑ Radial pulse

Figure 10.6 Taking a Pulse
Palpation of the carotid (neck) or radial (wrist) artery is a simple way of determining heart rate.

of perceived exertion, and the talk test. The exercise intensity required to improve cardiorespiratory endurance is a heart rate between 64 and 96 percent of your maximum heart rate. To calculate this target **heart rate**, first estimate your maximal heart rate with the formula [$207 - 0.7$(age)] (Figure 10.5). The example below is based on a 20-year-old. Substitute your age to determine your own maximal heart rate, then multiply by 0.64 and 0.94 to determine the lower and upper limits of your target range.

1. $207 - 0.7(20) =$ maximal heart rate for a 20-year old
2. $207 - 14 = 193$ (maximal heart rate)
3. $193(0.64) = 123.52$ (lower target limit)
4. $193(0.94) = 185.28$ (upper target limit)
5. Target range $=$ 124 to 186 beats per minute

Take your pulse during your workout to determine how close you are to your target heart rate. Lightly place your index and middle fingers (not your thumb) over one of the major arteries in your neck or on the artery on the inside of your wrist (Figure 10.6). Start counting your pulse immediately after you stop exercising, as your heart rate decreases rapidly. Using a watch or a clock, take your pulse for 6 seconds (the first pulse is "0") and multiply this number by 10 (add a zero to your count) to get the number of beats per minute.

Another way of determining the intensity of cardiorespiratory exercise is to use Borg's rating of perceived exertion (RPE) scale. Perceived exertion refers to how hard you feel you are working, which you might base on your heart rate, respiration rate, sweating, and level of fatigue. This scale uses a rating from 6 (no exertion at all) to 20 (maximal exertion). An RPE of 12 to 16 is generally recommended for training the cardiorespiratory system.

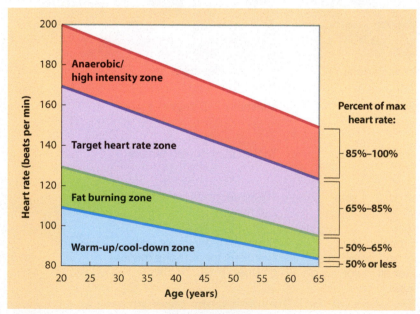

Figure 10.5 Target Heart Rate Ranges
These ranges are based on calculating the maximum heart rate as $207 - 0.7$(age) and the training zone as 64 to 96 percent of maximum heart rate. Individuals with low fitness levels should start below or at the low end of these ranges. Based on data from the American Heart Association.

The easiest method of measuring cardiorespiratory exercise intensity is the "talk test." A "moderate" level of exercise (heart rate at 64 to 76 percent of maximum) is a conversational level of exercise. At this level, you are able to talk with a partner while exercising. If you can talk but only in short fragments and not sentences, you may be at a "vigorous" level of exercise (heart rate at 76 to 96 percent of maximum). If you are breathing so hard that talking is difficult, the intensity of your exercise may be too high. Conversely, if you are able to sing or laugh heartily while exercising, the intensity of your exercise is not sufficient for maintaining and/or improving cardiorespiratory fitness.

Time

For cardiorespiratory fitness benefits, the American College of Sports Medicine (ACSM) recommends that vigorous activities be performed for at least 20 minutes at a time, and moderate activities should be performed for at least 30 minutes.[40] You can also set a time goal for the entire week as long as your sessions last at least 10 minutes (150 minutes per week for moderate intensity and 75 minutes per week for vigorous intensity).

Type

Any sort of rhythmic, continuous, and vigorous physical activity that can be done for 20 or more minutes will improve cardiorespiratory fitness. Examples include walking briskly, cycling, jogging, fitness classes, and swimming.

Incorporating Cardiorespiratory Fitness into Daily Life

Before we became a car culture, much of our transportation was human powered. Bicycling and walking were important means of transportation and recreation in the United States. These modes not only helped keep people in good physical shape, but also had little or no impact on the environment. Even in the first few decades after the automobile started to be popularized, people continued to get around under their own power. Since World War II, however, the development of automobile-oriented communities has led to a steady decline in bicycling and walking.

The more we use our cars to get around, the more congested our roads, the more polluted our air, and the more sedentary our lives become. That is why many people are embracing a movement toward more active transportation. *Active transportation* means getting out of your car and using your own power to get from place to place—whether walking, riding a bike, skateboarding, or roller skating. Each of these activities can also be incorporated into your life as a form of exercise that contributes to cardiorespiratory fitness.

The following are just a few of the many reasons to make active transportation a bigger part of your life[41]:

- **You will be adding more exercise into your daily routine.** People who walk, bike, or use other active forms of transportation to complete errands are physically active.

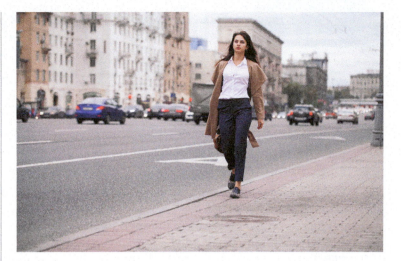

Put on your walking shoes, and join the green revolution! Active transportation is an excellent way to protect the environment and add physical activity to your day, especially on nonexercise days.

- **Walking or biking can save you money.** With rising gas prices and parking fees in addition to increasing car maintenance and insurance costs, fewer automobile trips could add up to considerable savings. During the course of a year, regular bicycle commuters who ride 5 miles to work can save about $500 on fuel and more than $1,000 on other expenses related to driving.
- **Walking or biking may save you time!** Cycling is usually the fastest mode of travel door to door for distances up to 6 miles in city centers. Walking is simpler and faster for distances of about a mile.
- **You will enjoy being outdoors.** Research is emerging on the physical and mental health benefits of nature and being outdoors. So much of what we do is inside, with recirculated air and artificial lighting, that our bodies don't get enough fresh air and sunlight.
- **You will be making a significant contribution to the reduction of air pollution.** Driving less means fewer pollutants being emitted into the air. Annually, personal transportation accounts for the consumption of approximately 136 billion gallons of gasoline, or the production of 1.2 billion tons of carbon dioxide. Leaving your car at home just 2 days a week will reduce greenhouse gas emissions by an average of 1,600 pounds per year.

10.6

Fitness

Check Yourself

- What are the FITT requirements for cardiorespiratory fitness?

- How can you incorporate cardiorespiratory fitness into your daily life?

The FITT Principle for Muscular Strength and Endurance

10.7 **List the FITT requirements for muscular strength and endurance.**

The FITT prescription for muscular strength and endurance includes 2 to 3 days per week of exercises that train the major muscle groups, using enough sets and repetitions and enough resistance to maintain or improve muscular strength and endurance.[42]

Frequency

For frequency, the FITT principle recommends performing 8 to 10 exercises that train the major muscle groups 2 to 3 days a week. Overloading the muscles, a normal part of resistance training (described below), Is believed to cause microscopic tears in muscle fibers. The rebuilding process that increases the muscle's size and capacity takes about 24 to 48 hours. Thus, resistance-training exercise programs should include at least 1 day of rest between workouts before the same muscles are overloaded again. But don't wait too long between workouts—one of the important principles of strength training is the idea of *reversibility*. Reversibility means that if you stop exercising, the body responds by deconditioning. Within 2 weeks, muscles begin to revert to their untrained state.[43] The saying "use it or lose it" applies here!

Intensity

To determine the intensity of exercise needed to improve muscular strength and endurance, you need to know the maximum amount of weight you can lift (or move) in one contraction. This value is called your **one repetition maximum (1 RM)** and can be individually determined or predicted from a 10 RM test. Once your 1 RM has been determined, it is used as the basis for intensity recommendations for improving muscular strength and endurance. Muscular strength is improved when resistance loads are greater than 60 percent of your 1 RM, whereas muscular endurance is improved using loads of less than 60 percent of your 1 RM.

Everyone begins a resistance-training program at an initial level of strength. To become stronger, you must *overload* your muscles, that is, regularly create a degree of tension in your muscles greater than that to which you are accustomed. Overloading your muscles forces them to adapt by getting larger, stronger, and capable of producing more tension. If you underload your muscles, you will not increase strength. If you create too great an overload, you may experience muscle injury, muscle fatigue, and potentially a loss in strength. Once you have reached your strength goal, no further overload is necessary; your challenge at that point is to maintain your level of strength by engaging in a regular (once or twice per week) total-body resistance exercise program.

Time

The time recommended for muscular strength and endurance exercises is measured not in minutes of exercise, but rather in repetitions and sets. The types of demands that you put on your body will result in the kind of adaptation that will follow.

Repetitions and Sets. To increase muscular strength, you need higher intensity and fewer repetitions and sets. Use a resistance of at least 60 percent of your 1 RM, performing 8 to 12 repetitions per set, with two to four sets performed overall. If improving muscular endurance is your goal, use less resistance and more repetitions and sets. The recommendations for improving muscular endurance are to perform one or two sets of 15 to 25 repetitions using a resistance that is less than 50 percent of your 1 RM.

Resistance training to improve muscular strength and endurance can be done with free weights, machines, or even your own body weight.

10.4 Methods of Providing Exercise Resistance

Calisthenics (Body Weight Resistance)	Free Weights (Fixed Resistance)	Weight Machines (Variable Resistance)
• Using your own body weight to develop muscular strength, endurance. • Improves overall muscular fitness—in particular core strength and overall muscle tone.	• Provides constant resistance throughout full range of movement. • Requires balance and coordination; promotes development of core strength.	• Resistance is altered so the muscle's effort is consistent throughout full range of motion. • Provides more controlled motion and isolates certain muscle groups.
Examples: Push-ups, pull-ups, curl-ups, dips, leg raises, and chair sits. For an extra challenge, you can do these exercises on a stability ball or balance board.	**Examples:** Barbells, dumbbells, medicine balls, and kettlebells. Resistance bands can be used for resistance instead of weights.	**Examples:** Weight machines in gyms, homes (Nautilus or Bowflex), and rehabilitation centers.

Rest Periods. The amount of rest between exercises is key to an effective strength-training workout. Resting between exercises can reduce fatigue and help with performance and safety in subsequent sets. A rest period of 2 to 3 minutes is recommended according to the guidelines for general health benefits. However, the rest period in working to develop strength or endurance will vary. Note that the rest period refers specifically to the muscle group being exercised, and it is possible to alternate muscle groups. For example, you can alternate a set of push-ups with a set of curl-ups; the muscle groups that are worked in one set can rest while you are working the other muscle groups.

Type

To improve muscular strength or endurance, resistance training is most often recommended using either your own body weight or devices that provide a fixed or variable resistance (see Table 10.4). Some cardiorespiratory training activities also enhance muscular endurance: Thousands of repetitions are performed during a 20-minute (or longer) workout using relatively low resistance when jogging or when training on an exercise device such as a stationary bicycle, rowing machine, or stair-climbing machine.

When selecting the type of strength-training exercises to do, keep several important principles in mind. The first of these is *specificity*. According to the specificity principle, the effects of resistance-exercise training are specific to the muscles exercised; only the muscle or muscle group that is overloaded responds to the demands placed on it. For example, if you regularly do curls,

the muscles involved—your biceps—will become larger and stronger, but the other muscles in your body will not. This sort of training may put opposing muscle groups—in this case the triceps—at increased risk for injury. To improve total body strength, you must include exercises for all the major muscle groups. You must also ensure that your overload is sufficient to increase strength and not only endurance.

Another important concept to consider is *exercise selection*. Exercises that work a single joint (e.g., chest presses) are effective for building specific muscle strength, whereas multiple-joint exercises (e.g., a squat coupled with an overhead press) are more effective for increasing overall muscle strength. Selecting 8 to 10 exercises targeting all major muscle groups is generally recommend and will ensure that exercises are balanced for opposing muscle groups.

Finally, for optimal training effects, it is important to pay attention to *exercise order*. When training all major muscle groups in a single workout, complete large-muscle group exercises (e.g., the bench press or leg press) before small-muscle group exercises, multiple-joint exercises before single-joint exercises (e.g., biceps curls, triceps extension), and high-intensity exercises before lower-intensity exercises.

Check Yourself

■ **What are the FITT requirements for muscular strength and endurance?**

10.8 The FITT Principle for Flexibility

10.8 List the FITT requirements for flexibility.

Improving your flexibility enhances the efficiency of your movements, increases well-being, and reduces stress. Furthermore, inflexible muscles are susceptible to injury; flexibility training helps to reduce the incidence and severity of lower back problems and muscle or tendon injuries and reduces joint pain and deterioration.[44]

Frequency

The FITT principle calls for doing flexibility training a minimum of 2 to 3 days per week. Daily training is even better.

Intensity

Hold static (still) stretching positions at an individually determined point of tension. You should feel tension or mild discomfort in the muscle(s) stretched, but not pain.[45]

Time

Hold each stretch at the point of tension for 10 to 30 seconds for each stretch; repeat two or three times in close succession.[46]

Type

The most effective exercises for building flexibility involve stretching of major muscle groups when the body is already warm, such as after cardiorespiratory activities. The safest such exercises involve **static stretching**, which slowly and gradually lengthens a muscle or group of muscles and their attached tendons. The primary strategy is to decrease the resistance to stretch (tension) within a tight muscle targeted for increased range of motion.[47] With each repetition, your range of motion improves temporarily as a result of the slightly lessened sensitivity of tension receptors in the stretched muscles; when these exercises are done regularly, range of motion increases. **Figure 10.7** shows some basic stretching exercises.

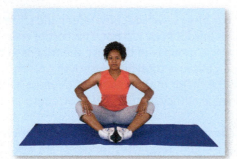

a Stretching the inside of the thighs

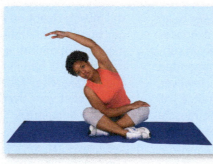

b Stretching the upper arm and the side of the trunk

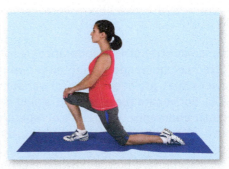

c Stretching the triceps

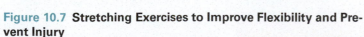

d Stretching the trunk and the hip

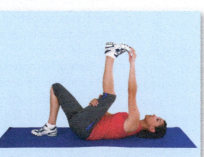

e Stretching the hip, back of the thigh, and the calf

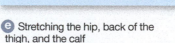

f Stretching the front of the thigh and the hip flexor

Figure 10.7 Stretching Exercises to Improve Flexibility and Prevent Injury
Use these stretches as part of your warm-up and cool-down. Hold each stretch for 10 to 30 seconds, and repeat each of them two or three times for each limb.

- What are the FITT requirements for flexibility?

10.9 Developing and Staying Motivated with a Mindful Fitness Plan

Learning Outcome

10.9 Describe how to stay with and adjust your fitness program over time.

Develop a Progressive Plan

Begin an exercise regimen by picking an exercise and gradually increasing your workout frequency. For example, in week 1, you might exercise 3 days for 20 minutes per day and then move to 4 days in week 3 or 4. Then consider increasing your duration to 30 minutes per session over the next couple of weeks. In general, most people can tolerate an increase of 5 to 10 minutes a session every 1 to 2 weeks during the first month.

Vary your exercise. Variety is a fundamental strength training principle that is also relevant to cardiorespiratory fitness and flexibility training. Changes in one or more parts of your workout not only produce a higher level of physical fitness and reduce the risk of overuse injuries (because different muscle groups are used), but also keep you motivated and interested.

Reevaluate your overall goals and plans every month or so. To keep yourself motivated, review your progress, make changes when necessary, and continue to reevaluate regularly.

Design Your Exercise Session

A comprehensive workout includes a warm-up, cardiorespiratory and/or resistance training, and then a cool-down.

Warm-ups involve large body movements, generally using light cardiorespiratory activities, followed by range-of-motion exercises of the muscle groups to be used during the exercise session. Usually 5 to 15 minutes long, a warm-up can be shorter when you are geared up and ready to go and longer when you are struggling to get moving or your muscles are cold or tight. Warm-ups slowly increase heart rate, blood pressure, breathing rate, and body temperature; improve joint lubrication; and increase muscles' and tendons' elasticity and flexibility.

The next stage of your workout may involve cardiorespiratory training, resistance training, or a little of each. If you are doing aerobic and resistance exercise in the same session, you should perform your aerobic exercise first. This order will provide additional warm-up for the resistance session, and your muscles will not be fatigued for the aerobic workout.

Cool-downs include 5 to 10 minutes of low-intensity activity and 5 to 10 minutes of stretching. Because of the body's increased temperature, the cool-down is an excellent time to stretch to improve flexibility. The cool-down gradually reduces heart rate, blood pressure, and body temperature; reduces the risk of blood pooling in the extremities; and helps speed recovery between exercise sessions.

Motivate Yourself with Mindfulness

Some goals take several weeks to achieve. In the meantime, to keep yourself motivated, be mindful of the benefits you are getting. Focus on how you feel after a brisk walk or run. Is your breathing fast and is your face flushed? Do you feel warm and can you feel your heart beating? Focus on the warmth of your skin and how your muscles feel. Inhale deeply. Exhale. Repeat several times. Notice how your body is relaxing, yet you feel more alive, more energized, less stressed. Focus on those feelings and nothing else. Allow yourself to bask in the moment.

Journal about how exercise made you feel and the changes you noticed in your body. Do you sleep better after exercise? Do you feel more relaxed after a stressful day? Journaling these simple benefits can keep you on track as you work toward bigger goals.

Skills for Behavior Change

Plan It, Start It, Stick With It!

The most successful physical activity program is one that is realistic and appropriate for your skill level and needs.

- **Make it enjoyable.** Pick activities you like to do so you will make the effort and find the time to do it.
- **Start slowly.** If you have been physically inactive for a while or are a first-time exerciser, any type and amount of physical activity is a step in the right direction. Keep in mind that it is an achievement to get to the fitness center or to put your sneakers on for a walk! Start slowly and let your body adapt to avoid excess pain the next day (a real reaction to using muscles you have not used much or as intensely before). Do not be discouraged; you will be able to increase your activity each week, and soon you will be on your way to meeting the physical activity recommendations and your personal goals.
- **Make only one lifestyle change at a time.** It is not realistic to change everything at once. Success with one behavioral change will increase your belief in yourself and encourage you to make other positive changes.
- **Set reasonable expectations for yourself and your physical fitness program.** It takes several months to really feel the benefits of physical activity. Be patient.
- **Choose a time to exercise and stick with it.** Set priorities, and keep to a schedule. Try exercising at different times of the day to learn what works best for you. Be flexible so that if something comes up, you will be able to find time later that day for some physical activity. Avoid an all-or-nothing attitude.
- **Keep a record of your progress.** Include the intensity, time, and type of physical activities and your emotions and personal achievements.
- **Take lapses in stride.** Sometimes life gets in the way. Start again, and do not despair; your commitment to physical fitness will have ebbs and flows like everything else in life.

Check Yourself

- What are strategies for staying with and adjusting your fitness program over time?

10.10 **Explain the benefits of a strong core.**

Yoga, tai chi, and Pilates have become increasingly popular in the United States. All three of these forms of exercise have the potential to improve **core strength**, flexibility, balance, coordination, and agility. They also develop the mind–body connection through concentration on breathing and body position.

Core Strength Training

The body's core muscles, including the deep back and abdominal muscles that attach to the spine and pelvis, are the foundation for all movement.[48] Contraction of these muscles provides the basis of support for movements of the upper and lower body and powerful movements of the extremities. A weak core generally results in poor posture, low back pain, and muscle injuries. A strong core provides a stable center of gravity and so a more stable platform for movements, thus reducing the chance of injury.

You can develop core strength using exercises such as calisthenics, yoga, and Pilates. Core strength does not happen from one single exercise but rather is the result of a structured regime of postures and exercises.[49] Holding yourself in a front or reverse plank ("up" and reverse of a push-up position) and holding or doing abdominal curl-ups are examples of exercises that increase core strength. The use of instability devices (stability ball, wobble boards, etc.) and exercises to train the core have also become popular.[50]

Yoga

Yoga, based on ancient Indian practices, blends the mental and physical aspects of exercise—a union of mind and body that participants often find relaxing and satisfying. If done regularly, yoga improves flexibility, vitality, posture, agility, balance, coordination, and muscular strength and endurance. Many people report an improved sense of general well-being, too.

The practice of yoga focuses attention on controlled breathing as well as physical exercise and incorporates a complex array of static stretching exercises expressed as postures (*asanas*). During a session, participants move to different asanas and may hold them for 30 seconds or longer.

Some forms of yoga are more meditative in their practice; others are more athletic. *Ashtanga yoga*, also called "power yoga," focuses on a series of poses done in a continuous, repeated flow, with controlled breathing. *Bikram yoga*, also known as *hot yoga*, is unique in that classes are held in rooms heated to 105°F, which practitioners claim helps the potential for increasing flexibility.

Tai Chi

Tai chi is an ancient Chinese form of exercise that combines stretching, balance, muscular endurance, coordination, and meditation. It increases range of motion and flexibility while reducing muscular tension. Tai chi involves a series of positions called *forms* that are performed continuously. Tai chi is often described as "meditation in motion" because it promotes serenity through gentle movements, connecting the mind and body.

Pilates

Pilates was developed by Joseph Pilates in 1926 as an exercise style that combines stretching with movement against resistance, frequently aided by devices such as tension springs or heavy rubber bands. It teaches body awareness, good posture, and easy, graceful body movements while improving flexibility, coordination, core strength, muscle tone, and economy of motion.

Pilates differs from yoga and tai chi in that it includes sequences of movements specifically designed to increase strength. Some Pilates exercises are done on specially designed equipment; others can be performed on mats.

Strengthening core body muscles can enhance flexibility and help lower stress levels.

10.10

Fitness

Check Yourself

- What are some benefits of having a strong core?

- What types of exercise increase core strength?

10.11 Activity and Exercise for Special Populations

10.11 Explain challenges and considerations related to physical activity for older people and those with common health conditions.

All individuals can benefit from a physically active lifestyle. People with the considerations mentioned here should consult a physician before beginning an exercise program.

Asthma

For individuals with asthma, regular physical activity strengthens respiratory muscles, improves immune system functioning, and helps in weight maintenance.

Before engaging in exercise, ensure that your asthma is under control. Ask about adjusting medications (for example, your doctor may recommend you use your inhaler 15 minutes before exercising). When exercising, keep your inhaler nearby. Warm up and cool down properly; it is particularly important that you allow your lungs and breathing rate to adjust slowly. Protect yourself from asthma triggers when exercising. Finally, if you have symptoms while exercising, stop and use your inhaler; if an asthma attack persists, call 9-1-1.[51]

Obesity

Limitations such as heat intolerance, shortness of breath during physical activity, lack of flexibility, frequent musculoskeletal injuries, and difficulty with balance in weight-bearing activities need to be addressed. Programs for individuals who are obese should emphasize physical activities that can be sustained for 30 minutes or more, such as walking, swimming, or bicycling, with caution recommended in heat or humidity. Start slow (5 to 10 minutes of activity at 55 to 65 percent of maximal heart rate), then work up to at least 30 to 60 minutes of exercise per day—150 to 300 minutes per week. Obese individuals can improve health with cardiorespiratory and resistance-training activities.[52]

Coronary Heart Disease and Hypertension

Although regular physical activity reduces the risk of coronary heart disease, vigorous activity acutely increases risk of sudden cardiac death and heart attack. Individuals with coronary heart disease must consult their physicians and might need to participate in a supervised exercise program for individuals with heart disease.[53]

Physical activity is an integral component for the prevention and treatment of hypertension. Using the FITT prescription, individuals who are hypertensive should engage in physical activity on most, if not all, days at moderate intensity for 30 minutes or more.[54]

Diabetes

Physical activity benefits individuals with diabetes by controlling blood glucose (for type 2 diabetics) by improving insulin transport into cells, controlling body weight, and reducing risk of heart disease.

Before individuals with type 1 diabetes engage in physical activity, they must learn how to manage their resting blood glucose levels. Individuals with type 1 diabetes should have an exercise partner; eat 1 to 3 hours before exercise; eat complex carbohydrates after exercise; avoid late-evening physical activities; and monitor blood glucose before, during, and after exercise.

One of the most important factors for individuals with type 2 diabetes is the time or length of their physical activity. Because a critical objective of the management of type 2 diabetes is to reduce body fat (obesity), the longer exercise periods are recommended—at least 30 minutes, working up to 60 minutes per session or 300 minutes per week. Multiple 10-minute sessions can be used to accumulate these totals. It is prudent to reduce the intensity of the activity to a target heart rate range of 40 to 60 percent of maximal heart rate.

Older Adults

A physically active lifestyle increases life expectancy by limiting development and progression of chronic diseases and disabling conditions, reducing the risk for age-related cognitive decline, enhancing mental acuity, and improving quality of life. The general recommendation for older adults is to engage in regular physical activity. For individuals with arthritis, osteoarthritis, and other musculoskeletal problems, non-weight-bearing activities, such as cycling and swimming or other water exercises, are recommended. Movement is important, even if physical activity levels must be modified.[55]

Athletes like Jay Cutler, an NFL quarterback and a type 1 diabetic, are living proof that chronic conditions need not prevent you from achieving your physical activity goals.

- What should older people and those with health conditions be aware of when choosing a program of physical exercise?
- Have you had to make any accommodations in your fitness program because of an existing health condition?

10.12 Explain nutritional habits that support healthy exercise.

To make the most of your workouts, follow the recommendations of the MyPlate plan and make sure that you eat sufficient carbohydrates, the body's main source of fuel. Your body stores carbohydrates as glycogen primarily in the muscles and liver and then uses this stored glycogen for energy when you are physically active. Fats are also an important source of energy, packing more than double the energy per gram of carbohydrates. Protein plays a role in muscle repair and growth but is not normally a source of energy. Another important nutrient to consider is water (or fluids containing water).

Timing Your Food Intake

When you eat is almost as important as *what* you eat. Eating a large meal before exercising can cause upset stomach, cramping, and diarrhea because your muscles have to compete with your digestive system for energy. After a large meal, wait 3 to 4 hours before you begin exercising. A smaller meals or snack can be eaten about an hour before activity. Not eating at all before a workout can cause low blood sugar levels that, in turn, cause weakness and slower reaction times.

It is also important to refuel after your workout. Help your muscles recover and prepare for the next bout of activity by eating a snack or meal that contains plenty of carbohydrates plus a bit of protein.

Staying Hydrated

In addition to eating well, staying hydrated is crucial for active individuals who want to maintain a healthy, fully functional body.

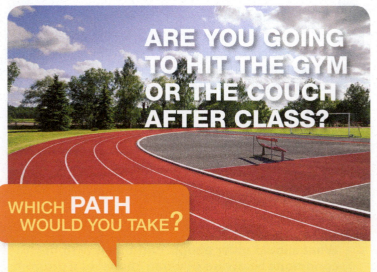

ARE YOU GOING TO HIT THE GYM OR THE COUCH AFTER CLASS?

WHICH PATH WOULD YOU TAKE?

Go to Mastering Health to play "Improving Your Personal Fitness" and see how your actions today affect your future health.

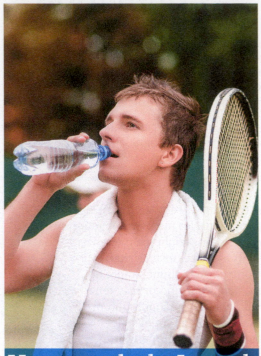

How much do I need to drink before, during, and after physical activity?

The American College of Sports Medicine and the National Athletic Trainers' Association recommend consuming 14 to 22 ounces of fluid several hours before exercise and about 6 to 12 ounces per 15 to 20 minutes during exercise—assuming that you are sweating.

How much fluid do you need to stay well hydrated? Keep in mind that the goal of fluid replacement is to prevent excessive dehydration (greater than 2 percent loss of body weight). The ACSM and the National Athletic Trainers Association recommend consuming 5 to 7 milliliters of fluid per kilogram of body weight (approximately 0.7 to 1.07 ounce per 10 pounds of body weight), 4 hours before exercising.[56] Drinking fluids during exercise is also important, though it is difficult to provide guidelines for how much or when because intake should be based on time, intensity, and type of activity performed. A good way to monitor how much fluid you need to replace is to weigh yourself before and after your workout. The difference in weight is how much you should drink. For example, if you lost 2 pounds during a training session, you should drink 32 ounces of fluid.[57]

What are the best fluids to drink? For exercise sessions lasting less than 1 hour, plain water is sufficient for rehydration. If your exercise session exceeds 1 hour and you sweat profusely, consider a sports drink containing electrolytes. The electrolytes in these

10.5 Performance-Enhancing Dietary Supplements and Drugs: Their Uses and Effects

Substance	Primary Uses	Side Effects
Creatine Naturally occurring compound that helps supply energy to muscle	• Improve postworkout recovery • Increase muscle mass • Increase strength • Increase power	• Weight gain, nausea, muscle cramps • Large doses have a negative effect on the kidneys
Ephedra and ephedrine Stimulant that constricts blood vessels and increases blood pressure and heart rate Illegal; banned by FDA in 2006; banned by sports organizations	• Lose weight • Increase performance	• Nausea, vomiting • Anxiety and mood changes • Hyperactivity • In rare cases, seizures, heart attack, stroke, psychotic episodes
Anabolic steroids Synthetic versions of the hormone testosterone Nonmedical use is illegal; banned by major sports organizations	• Improve strength, power, and speed • Increase muscle mass	• In adolescents, stops bone growth; therefore, reduces adult height • Masculinization of females; feminization of males • Mood swings • Severe acne, particularly on the back • Sexual dysfunction • Aggressive behavior • Potential heart and liver damage
Steroid precursors Substances that the body converts into anabolic steroids, e.g., androstenedione (andro), dehydroepiandrosterone (DHEA) Nonmedical use is illegal; banned by major sports organizations	• Converted in the body to anabolic steroids to increase muscle mass	• In addition to side effects noted with anabolic steroids: body hair growth, increased risk of pancreatic cancer
Human growth hormone Naturally occurring hormone secreted by the pituitary gland that is essential for body growth Nonmedical use is illegal; banned by major sports organizations	• Antiaging agent • Improve performance • Increase muscle mass	• Structural changes to the face • Increased risk of high blood pressure • Potential for congestive heart failure

Sources: Mayo Clinic Staff, "Tween and Teen Health: Hazards of Performance Enhancing Drugs." MayoClinic.com, July 2017, www.mayoclinic.com.

products are minerals and ions such as sodium and potassium needed for proper functioning of your nervous and muscular systems. Replacing electrolytes is particularly important for endurance athletes engaging in long bouts of exercise or competition. In endurance events lasting more than 4 hours, an athlete's overconsumption of plain water can dilute the sodium concentration in the blood with potentially fatal results, an effect called **hyponatremia** or **water intoxication**.

What about mixing alcohol and exercise? Drinking alcohol can contribute to weight gain, derailing efforts to stay fit. Additionally, a hangover from drinking the night before leads to dehydration and other negative symptoms that can inhibit exercise performance. Consuming alcohol immediately before or during exercise also impairs judgment and motor coordination. After the workout, it's important to rehydrate with water (or other recovery fluids) and refuel first before drinking any alcohol. (See Chapter 7 for more on the effects of alcohol.)

Dietary Supplements

There is a burgeoning market for dietary supplements that claim to deliver the nutrients needed for muscle recovery, as well as some that include additional "performance-enhancing" ingredients. Supplements do not require FDA approval, and ingredients may cause side effects and interact with prescription medicines. See Table 10.5 for a list of some of the most popular performance-enhancing drugs and supplements, their purported benefits, and associated risks.

Check Yourself

- What are some of the most important nutritional aspects of fitness?

- How does hydration affect exercise?

Fitness-Related Injuries: Prevention and Treatment

10.13 **Distinguish between traumatic injuries and overuse injuries, and discuss how to prevent common fitness-related injuries.**

The two basic types of fitness-related injuries are traumatic injuries and overuse injuries. **Traumatic injuries** occur suddenly and violently, most often by accident. Typical traumatic injuries are broken bones, torn ligaments and muscles, contusions, and lacerations.

Some traumatic injuries are unavoidable—for example, spraining your ankle by landing on another person's foot after jumping up for a rebound in basketball. Others are preventable through proper training, appropriate equipment and clothing, and common sense. If your traumatic injury causes a noticeable loss of function and immediate pain or pain that does not go away after 30 minutes, consult a physician.

Overtraining is the most frequent cause of injuries related to physical fitness training. Doing too much intense exercise, doing too much exercise without variation, or not allowing for sufficient rest and recovery time can increase the likelihood of **overuse injuries**. Overuse injuries occur because of the cumulative, day-after-day stresses placed on tendons, muscles, and joints.

Common Overuse Injuries

Common sites of overuse injuries are the hip, knee, shoulder, and elbow joints. Three of the most common overuse injuries are plantar fasciitis, shin splints, and runner's knee.

Plantar Fasciitis *Plantar fasciitis* is an inflammation of the plantar fascia, a broad band of dense, inelastic tissue (fascia) that runs from the heel to the toes on the bottom of your foot. The main function of the plantar fascia is to protect the nerves, blood vessels, and muscles of the foot from injury. In repetitive weight-bearing physical activities such as walking and running, the plantar fascia may become inflamed. Common symptoms are pain and tenderness under the ball of the foot, at the heel, or at both locations.[58] The pain of plantar fasciitis is particularly noticeable during your first steps in the morning. If not treated properly, this injury may progress to the point that weight-bearing activities are too painful to endure.

Shin Splints *Shin splints*, a general term for any pain that occurs on the front part of the lower legs, is used to describe more than 20 different medical conditions. The most common type of shin splints occurs along the inner side of the tibia and is usually a combination of muscle irritation and irritation of the tissues attaching the muscles to the bone.

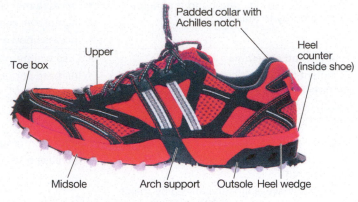

Figure 10.8 **Anatomy of a Running Shoe**
A good running shoe should fit comfortably, allow room for your toes to move, have a firm but flexible midsole, and have a firm grip on your heel to prevent slipping.

Specific pain on the tibia or on the fibula (the adjacent smaller bone) should prompt examination for a possible stress fracture.

Runner's Knee *Runner's knee* describes a series of problems involving the muscles, tendons, and ligaments of the knee. The most common cause is abnormal movements of the patella (kneecap). Women are more commonly affected because their wider pelvis results in a lateral pull on the patella by the muscles that act on the knee. In women (and some men), this causes irritation to cartilage on the back of the patella and to nearby tendons and ligaments. The main symptom is pain experienced when downward pressure is applied to the kneecap after the knee is straightened fully. Additional symptoms include pain, swelling, redness, and tenderness around the patella and a dull aching pain in the center of the knee.[59]

Falls and Other Injuries

Older people and those who have been sedentary for prolonged periods of time and/or who are starting a new weight-bearing physical activity program are at the greatest risk for injuries, particularly strains, sprains, and falls. Because bone density and muscle mass diminish over time, the risk of broken bones and torn muscles, tendons, and ligaments is greater in older adults than at other stages of life. However, research suggests that exercise may keep older adults on their feet and injury free. Strength training is particularly important for older and disabled individuals. In a

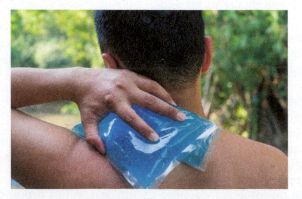

Applying ice to an injury such as a sprain can help to relieve pain and reduce swelling, but never apply the ice directly to the skin, as that could lead to frostbite.

recent 15-year study, seniors who engaged in strength training at least twice a week Increased their overall muscle mass and strength and reduced their risk of premature disability and death.[60]

Treatment of Fitness-Training Related Injuries

First-aid treatment for virtually all fitness-training related injuries involves **RICE**: rest, ice, compression, and elevation. *Rest* is required to avoid further irritation of the injured body part. *Ice* is applied to relieve pain and constrict the blood vessels to reduce internal or external bleeding. To prevent frostbite, wrap the ice or cold pack in a layer of wet toweling or elastic bandage before applying to your skin. A new injury should be iced for approximately 20 minutes every hour for the first 24 to 72 hours. *Compression* of the injured body part can be accomplished with a 4- or 6-inch-wide elastic bandage; this applies indirect pressure to damaged blood vessels to help stop bleeding. Be careful, though, that the compression wrap does not interfere with normal blood flow. Throbbing or pain indicates that a compression wrap should be loosened. *Elevation* of an injured extremity above heart level also helps to control internal or external bleeding by forcing the blood to flow upward to reach the injured area.

Preventing Injuries

Using common sense and identifying and using proper gear and equipment can help you avoid an injury. Varying your physical activities and setting appropriate and realistic short- and long-term goals will also help. It is important to listen to your body when working out. Warning signs include muscle stiffness and soreness, bone and joint pains, and whole-body fatigue that does not go away.

Appropriate Footwear Proper footwear, replaced in a timely manner, can decrease the likelihood of foot, knee, hip, or back injuries. Running, jumping, and other high-impact activities have significant effects on your joints. Consider the impact for a runner who has poor mechanics or an overweight individual who participates in weight-bearing activities. The force not absorbed by the running shoe is transmitted upward into the foot, leg, thigh, and back. Our bodies can absorb forces such as these but may be injured by the cumulative effect of repetitive impact (such as running 40 miles per week). Thus, the shoes' ability to absorb shock is critical—not just for people who run, but for anyone who engages in weight-bearing activities.

In addition to providing shock absorption, an athletic shoe should provide a good fit for maximum comfort and performance (see **Figure 10.8**). To get the best fit, shop at a sports or fitness specialty store where there is a large selection to choose from and salespeople are available who are trained in properly fitting athletic shoes. Because different activities place different stresses on your feet and joints, you should choose shoes specifically designed for your sport or activity. Shoes of any type should be replaced once they lose their cushioning.

Protective Equipment It is essential to use well-fitted, appropriate protective equipment that is best for you and your body. For example, using the correct racquet with the proper tension helps prevent the general inflammatory condition known as tennis elbow. Likewise, eye injuries can occur in virtually all physical activities,

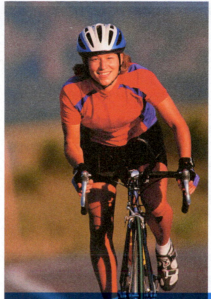

How can I avoid injury when I am physically active?

Reducing your risk for exercise-related injuries requires common sense and some preventative measures. Wear protective gear, such as helmets, knee pads, elbow pads, eyewear, and supportive footwear, that is appropriate for your activity. Vary your activities to avoid overuse injuries. Dress for the weather, try to avoid exercising in extreme conditions, and always stay well hydrated. Finally, respect your personal physical limitations, listen to your body, and respond effectively to it.

although some activities (such as baseball, basketball, and racquet sports) are riskier than others.[61] As many as 90 percent could be prevented by wearing appropriate eye protection, such as goggles with polycarbonate lenses.[62]

An estimated 66 to 88 percent of head injuries among cyclists can be prevented by wearing a helmet.[63] In a recent study of college students, 36 percent of students who rode a bike in the past 12 months reported never wearing a helmet, and 24.5 percent said they wore one only sometimes or rarely.[64] The direct medical cost of cyclists' failure to wear helmets is an estimated $81 million a year.[65]

Cyclists aren't the only ones who should be wearing helmets—so should people who skateboard, use kick-scooters, ski, in-line skate, play contact sports, and snowboard. Look for helmets that meet standards established by the American National Standards Institute or the Snell Memorial Foundation.

Check Yourself

- **What is the difference between traumatic injuries and overuse injuries?**

- **How can you prevent and treat fitness-related injuries?**

10.14 Describe signs and prevention of heat-related injuries and hypothermia.

Exercising in the Heat

Exercising in hot or humid weather increases the risk of a heat-related injury, in which the body's rate of heat production can exceed its ability to cool. The three heat stress illnesses, in order of increasing severity, are heat cramps, heat exhaustion, and heatstroke.

Heat cramps, heat-related involuntary and forcible muscle contractions that cannot be relaxed, can usually be prevented by intake of fluid and electrolytes lost during sweating. **Heat exhaustion** is a mild form of shock, in which blood pools in the arms and legs away from the brain and major organs, caused by excessive water loss because of intense or prolonged exercise or work in a hot and/or humid environment. Symptoms include nausea, headache, fatigue, dizziness and faintness, and, paradoxically, "goose bumps" and chills. In sufferers from heat exhaustion, the skin is cool and moist. **Heatstroke**, or *sunstroke*, is a life-threatening emergency condition with high morbidity and mortality rates.[66] Heatstroke occurs when the body's heat production significantly exceeds its cooling capacities. Core body temperature can rise from normal (98.6°F) to 105°F to 110°F; this rapid increase can cause brain damage, permanent disability, or death. Common signs of heatstroke are dry, hot, and usually red skin; very high body temperature; and rapid heart rate. If you experience any of these symptoms, stop exercising immediately. Move to the shade or a cool spot to rest, and drink plenty of cool fluids. If heatstroke is suspected, seek medical attention immediately.

Heat stress illnesses may also occur when the danger is not so obvious. Serious or fatal heat stroke may result from prolonged immersion in a sauna, hot tub, or steam bath or from exercising in a "sauna suit." Similarly, exercising in the heat with heavy clothing and equipment, such as a football uniform, puts one at risk.

To prevent heat stress, follow certain precautions. If possible, acclimatize yourself to hot or humid climates through 10 to 14 days of gradually increased activity in the hot environment. Replace fluids before, during, and after exercise. Wear light, breathable clothing that is appropriate for the activity and environment. Use common sense; for example, when the temperature is 85°F and the humidity is 80 percent, postpone a lunchtime run until evening when it is cooler.

Pay particular attention to your pets if you take them running or walking with you. Pets can quickly succumb to heatstroke and rely on you for hydration. They can also quickly burn their pads on hot pavement. Be responsible, and take care of yourself and your pets.

Exercising in the Cold

When you exercise in cool weather, especially in windy conditions, your body's rate of heat loss is frequently greater than its rate of heat production. This may lead to **hypothermia**, a condition in which the body's core temperature drops below 95°F.[67] Hypothermia doesn't require frigid temperatures; it can result from prolonged, vigorous exercise in 40°F to 50°F temperatures, particularly if there is rain, snow, or strong wind.

As the body's core temperature drops from the normal 98.6°F to about 93.2°F, shivering begins, which increases body temperature using the heat given off by muscle activity. You may also experience cold hands and feet, poor judgment, apathy, and amnesia. Shivering ceases as core temperatures drop to between 87°F and 90°F, a sign that the body has lost its ability to generate heat. Death usually occurs at body core temperatures between 75°F and 80°F.[68]

To prevent hypothermia, analyze weather conditions, including wind and humidity, before engaging in outdoor activity. Have a friend join you for cold weather outdoor activities, and wear layers of appropriate clothing to prevent excessive heat loss and frostbite. Keep your head, hands, and feet warm. Do not allow yourself to become dehydrated.

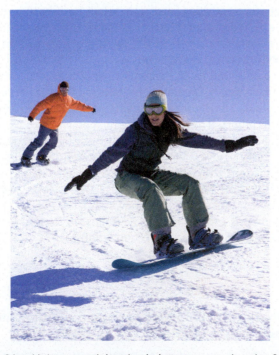

Having a friend join you and dressing in layers are two key tips for making cold weather exercise both safe and fun.

- What are the signs and treatment of heat cramps, heat exhaustion, and heatstroke?

- How can you prevent hypothermia?

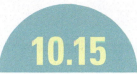

10.15 Smart Shopping for Fitness

Learning Outcome

10.15 List important factors to keep in mind when choosing fitness equipment, facilities, and clothing.

You can achieve your personal physical fitness goals without becoming a member of a fitness or wellness center, without buying equipment, and without spending lots of money on the latest fitness fashions. All you need is a good pair of shoes, comfortable clothing to suit the environment in which you will be physically active, your own body to use as resistance, and a safe place for activity. However, you may enjoy the outing or experience created by going to a fitness or wellness center, or you may prefer to have some exercise equipment in your home. The following will help to guide your selections.

Choosing Facilities

- Visit several facilities before making a decision—and if possible during the time of day when you intend to use them (so you can see how busy or crowded they are at that time).
- Determine the hours of operation. Are they convenient for you?
- Consider the exercise classes offered. What is the schedule? Can you try one for free? Are classes included in the price of membership, or do they cost extra?
- Consider the equipment. Is it sufficient for your training needs (e.g., aerobic exercise machines; resistance-training equipment, including both free weights and machines; mats; and other items to assist with stretching)? Is it kept clean and in good condition? Does the facility offer instruction in how to use the equipment?
- Consider the locker room. Is it kept clean? Are there lockers free for your use if you need them?
- Consider the location. How convenient is it (e.g., on your way to or from work or school, close to your home)?
- Consider the personnel (including their training in first aid and CPR), options for working with a personal trainer, and how friendly and approachable staff members are.
- Consider the financial implications. What membership benefits, student rates, or other discounts are available? Will they hold your membership for the summer, so you do not have to continue paying if you are not attending school in the area? Steer clear of clubs that pressure you for a long-term commitment and do not offer trial memberships or grace periods that allow you to get a refund.

Buying Equipment

- Ignore claims that an exercise device provides lasting "no-sweat" results in a short time.
- Question claims that an exercise device can target or burn fat or lead to miracle cures for "cellulite."

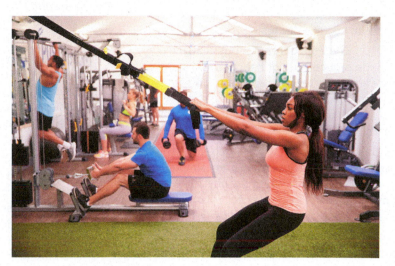

Before you sign on the dotted line, check out the classes, equipment, and personnel a fitness center offers.

- Be skeptical of testimonials and before-and-after pictures of satisfied customers.
- Calculate the cost, including shipping and handling fees, sales tax, delivery and setup charges, or long-term commitments.
- Obtain details on warranties, guarantees, and return policies.
- Consider how this piece of equipment will fit in your home. Where will you store it? Will you be able to get to it easily?
- Check out consumer reports or online resources for the best product ratings and reviews.

Buying Exercise Clothing

- Choose your exercise clothing on the basis of comfort, not looks. It should be neither too loose nor too tight.
- Invest in a good pair of sneakers.
- Consider the environment (temperature, humidity, ventilation) when making your selection.
- Choose clothing that helps you to feel good about yourself and the activity you are undertaking.

Check Yourself

- **What should you keep in mind when choosing fitness equipment, facilities, and clothing?**
- **Which of these factors are most important to you?**

Summary

LO 10.1 Physical fitness involves achieving minimal levels in the health-related components of fitness: cardiorespiratory, muscular strength, muscular endurance, flexibility, and body composition.

LO 10.2 Benefits of regular physical activity include reduced risk of heart attack, some cancers, hypertension, and type 2 diabetes and improved blood profile, weight control, stress management, and more healthy years.

LO 10.3 If you are new to exercise, start slowly, keep your fitness program simple, and consider consulting your physician and/or a fitness instructor for recommendations. Identify and plan for barriers.

LO 10.4 Fitness gadgets and equipment can motivate and keep you interested.

LO 10.5 Planning to improve fitness involves setting SMART goals and FITT principles to achieve them.

LO 10.6 For health benefits, moderate-intensity activities for 30 minutes at least 5 days a week. For cardiorespiratory fitness, vigorous, continuous activities 3 to 5 days per week are best.

LO 10.7 Three key principles for developing muscular strength and endurance are overload, specificity of training, and variation.

LO 10.8 Improve flexibility by engaging in two or three repetitions of static stretching exercises at least 2 to 3 days a week.

LO 10.9 A regular workout should include a warm-up with stretching, strength-development exercises, aerobic activities, and a cool-down with stretching. Mindfulness techniques can help motivate you to stay with your fitness plan.

LO 10.10 Core strength training is important for maintaining full mobility and stability and for preventing injury.

LO 10.11 Individuals with special conditions, such as asthma, heart disease, and diabetes, should consult with a physician before beginning an exercise program.

LO 10.12 Fueling properly for exercise involves eating a balance of healthy foods 3 to 4 hours before exercise and proper hydration.

LO 10.13–10.15 Fitness training injuries are generally caused by overuse or trauma. Proper footwear and equipment can help prevent injuries. Exercise in the heat or cold requires special precautions.

Pop Quiz

Visit Mastering Health to personalize your study plan with Chapter Review Quizzes and Dynamic Study Modules.

LO 10.1 1. The maximum volume of oxygen consumed by the muscles during exercise defines
  a. target heart rate.
  b. muscular strength.
  c. aerobic capacity.
  d. muscular endurance.

LO 10.1 2. Flexibility is the range of motion around
  a. specific bones.
  b. a joint or series of joints.
  c. the tendons.
  d. the muscles.

LO 10.1 3. Theresa wants to lower her ratio of fat to total body weight. She wants to work on her
  a. flexibility.
  b. muscular endurance.
  c. muscular strength.
  d. body composition.

LO 10.1 4. Miguel is a runner who can sustain moderate-intensity, whole-body activity for an extended time. This ability relates to what component of physical fitness?
  a. Flexibility
  b. Body composition
  c. Cardiorespiratory fitness
  d. Muscular strength and endurance

LO 10.6 5. The "talk test" measures
  a. exercise intensity.   b. exercise time.
  c. exercise frequency. d. exercise duration.

LO 10.6 6. Aerobic exercise includes:
  a. brisk walking.
  b. bench-pressing weights.
  c. stretching exercises.
  d. holding yoga poses.

LO 10.7 7. Isabella has been lifting 95 pounds while doing leg curls. To become stronger, she began lifting 105 pounds while doing leg curls. What principle of strength development does this represent?
  a. Reversibility
  b. Overload
  c. Strain increase
  d. Specificity of training

LO 10.10 8. Which of the following includes sequences of movements designed to increase strength?
  a. Pilates
  b. Ashtanga yoga
  c. Tai chi
  d. Bikram yoga

LO 10.11 9. People with type 2 diabetes
  a. should not engage in physical activity.
  b. should avoid weight-bearing activities.
  c. should limit physical activity to 30 minutes a day or less.
  d. can improve blood glucose levels through physical activity.

LO 10.13 10. Overuse injuries can be prevented by
  a. monitoring quantity and quality of workouts.
  b. engaging in only one type of aerobic training.
  c. working out daily.
  d. working out with a friend.

Answers to these questions can be found on page A-1. If you answered a question incorrectly, review the module identified by the Learning Outcome. For even more study tools, visit Mastering Health.

Think About It!

LO 10.1 1. How are muscle strength and muscle endurance different? How might you increase muscle strength and muscle endurance?

LO 10.1–10.2 2. How do you define *physical fitness*? Identify at least four physiological and psychological benefits of physical activity.

LO 10.3 3. How do you motivate yourself to exercise? What and who helps you to be physically active?

LO 10.5–10.8 4. Describe the FITT prescription for cardiorespiratory fitness, muscular strength and endurance, and flexibility training.

LO 10.10 5. Why is core strength important? What are some ways to increase your core strength every day?

LO 10.12 6. Why is when you eat as important as what you eat?

LO 10.14 7. What precautions do you need to take when exercising outdoors in the heat and in the cold?

Cardiovascular Disease, Cancer, and Diabetes

11

An overwhelming percentage of deaths in the United States are due to three major causes: cardiovascular disease, diabetes, and cancer. Over 92 million Americans—1 of every 3 adults—suffer from one or more types of **cardiovascular disease (CVD)**, diseases of the heart and blood vessels.[1] CVD has been the leading killer of U.S. adults every year since 1900 with the exception of the flu pandemic of 1918. Growing rates of obesity, hypertension, and diabetes are key contributors to the increasing numbers of CVD cases in the United States and worldwide.

Diabetes is one of the fastest-growing health threats in the world today, with over 422 million people classified as diabetic.[2] Diabetes is the primary cause of death each year for over 76,000 Americans and is a contributing factor in hundreds of thousands more deaths from CVD, kidney disease, and other diseases.[3]

As recently as 50 years ago, a cancer diagnosis was typically a death sentence. Cancer remains the second leading cause of death in the United States.[4] In 2017, there were nearly 1.7 million *new* cancer diagnoses, and nearly 601,000 deaths.[5] The good news is that cancer death rates have been declining in the last decades. Early detection and better treatments have dramatically improved the prognosis for many people with higher survival rates for most cancers.

The cardiovascular system is the network of organs and vessels through which blood flows, carrying oxygen and nutrients to all parts of the body. It includes the heart, arteries, arterioles (small arteries), veins, venules (small veins), and capillaries (minute blood vessels).

The Heart: A Mighty Machine

The heart is a muscular, four-chambered pump, roughly the size of your fist. It is a highly efficient, extremely flexible organ that contracts over 100,000 times each day, -pumping the equivalent of 2,000 gallons of blood to all areas of the body. In a 70-year lifetime, an average human heart beats 2.5 billion times.

The human body contains approximately 6 quarts of blood, which transports nutrients, oxygen, waste products, hormones, and enzymes throughout the body. Blood aids in regulating body temperature, cellular water levels, and acidity levels of body components and helps defend the body against toxins and harmful microorganisms. Adequate blood supply is essential to health.

The heart's four chambers work together to circulate blood constantly throughout the body. The two large upper chambers, the **atria**, receive blood from the rest of the body; the two lower chambers, the **ventricles**, pump the blood out again. Small valves regulate a steady, rhythmic flow of blood and prevent leakage or backflow between chambers.

Blood Flow through Heart and Vessels

Heart activity depends on a complex interaction of biochemical, physical, and neurological signals. To understand blood flow through the heart, follow the steps in **Figure 11.1**, from deoxygenated blood entering the heart to oxygenated blood being pumped into the blood vessels. Different types of blood vessels are required for different parts of this process. **Arteries** carry blood away from the heart. All arteries carry oxygenated blood except the pulmonary arteries, which carry deoxygenated blood to the lungs, where the blood picks up oxygen and releases carbon dioxide. The arteries branch off from the heart, then divide into smaller vessels called **arterioles**, then into even smaller **capillaries**. Capillaries have thin walls that permit the exchange of oxygen, carbon dioxide, nutrients, and waste products between the blood and body cells. Carbon dioxide and other waste products are transported to the lungs and kidneys through **veins** and **venules** (small veins).

Your heartbeat is governed by an electrical impulse that directs the heart muscle to move, resulting in sequential contraction of the chambers. This signal starts in a small bundle of highly specialized cells in the right atrium, called the **sinoatrial node (SA node)**, which serves as a natural pacemaker. The average adult heart at rest beats 70 to 80 times per minute.

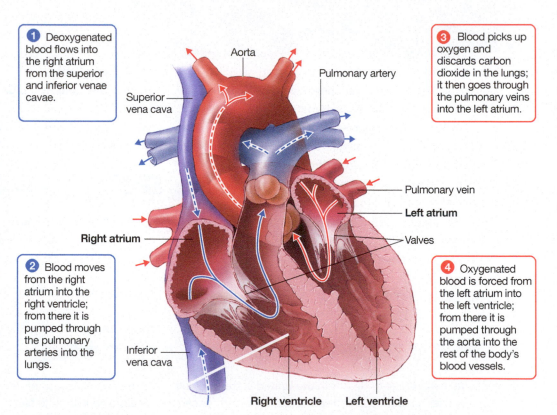

1 Deoxygenated blood flows into the right atrium from the superior and inferior venae cavae.

2 Blood moves from the right atrium into the right ventricle; from there it is pumped through the pulmonary arteries into the lungs.

3 Blood picks up oxygen and discards carbon dioxide in the lungs; it then goes through the pulmonary veins into the left atrium.

4 Oxygenated blood is forced from the left atrium into the left ventricle; from there it is pumped through the aorta into the rest of the body's blood vessels.

Aorta · Pulmonary artery · Superior vena cava · Pulmonary vein · **Left atrium** · Valves · **Right atrium** · Inferior vena cava · Right ventricle · Left ventricle

Figure 11.1 Blood Flow within the Heart

Cardiovascular Disease: An Epidemiological Overview

Learning Outcome

11.2 Describe patterns in the prevalence of cardiovascular disease relative to gender and ethnicity.

The good news is that U.S. death rates from CVD have declined over the past decade by about 33 percent.[6] However, CVD still claims more than 17 million lives around the globe each year—more lives than the next two leading causes of death combined (all forms of cancer and chronic lower respiratory diseases). By 2030, CVD deaths are expected to increase to nearly 24 million per year. (Even in the United States, CVD remains the leading cause of death).[7] Consider the following:

- Many CVD-related fatalities are *sudden cardiac deaths*, an abrupt, profound loss of heart function (cardiac arrest) that causes death either instantly or shortly after symptoms occur. Fifty percent of men and 64 percent of women who die suddenly have had no previous symptoms.[8]
- CVD has claimed the lives of more women than men every year since 1984. (**Figure 11.2**).[9, 10]
- Among women, African Americans and Asian/Pacific Islanders (particularly South Asians) have the highest percentages of CVD deaths. Forty-seven percent of all non-Hispanic black women have some form of CVD.[11]
- Among men, Asian/Pacific Islanders and African Americans have the highest percentages of CVD deaths, at 32.8 percent and 31.7 percent, respectively.[12]
- American Indian and Alaska Natives have the lowest percentages of deaths from CVD.[13]
- Among individuals age 20 to 39, 20.3 percent have metabolic syndrome (MetS), a dangerous grouping of key risk factors for CVD. Among individuals age 40 to 59, rates jump to 40.8 percent; and for those 60 and over, rates are nearly 52 percent.[14]
- 25 percent of men and 38 percent of women will die within 1 year of having an initial heart attack.[15]

Much of the improvement in death rates is due to better diagnosis, early intervention, and steadily improving treatments, including new drugs. We've also improved our understanding about diet, activity, and other behaviors that affect the risk of CVD and created policies and programs designed to reduce risks. Unfortunately, soaring costs for medicines, hospitalization, home health care, rehabilitation services, and outpatient tests make recovery challenging.

The economic burden of CVD on our society is huge—more than $316 billion in direct and indirect costs.[16] Of this amount, nearly $194 billion is direct costs, including physicians and other professionals, hospital services, prescribed medication, and home health care.[17] Indirect costs, attributed to projected losses in future productivity, make up the remainder of the roughly $122 billion in costs.[18] According to some sources,

by 2035, nearly 45 percent of the U.S. population will have CVD, at an estimated cost of over 1.1 trillion dollars per year. Medical costs for coronary heart disease alone will increase by more than 100 percent.[19] While economic concerns are huge, the effects of CVD on patients, families, communities, and society may be even greater.

With an international trend toward obesity, more and more countries face epidemic CVD rates. The World Health Organization (WHO) estimates CVD accounts for 31 percent of all deaths globally.[20] Unfortunately, over 75 percent of the world's deaths from CVD occur in low- and middle-income countries, places where people have more risks and fewer options for prevention and treatment.[21] As health care options dwindle for vulnerable populations in the United States, increasing numbers of people will access health care later in their disease course, be unable to afford expensive treatments, and face poorer outcomes than those with means.

Although death rates are relatively easy to calculate the fear and depression that can accompany CVD are harder to measure. Imagine the anxiety caused by wondering whether your heart will fail each time you exercise or during sexual activity. Knowing more about your specific CVD risks, your limitations, and what you can do about them is key to taking healthy action.

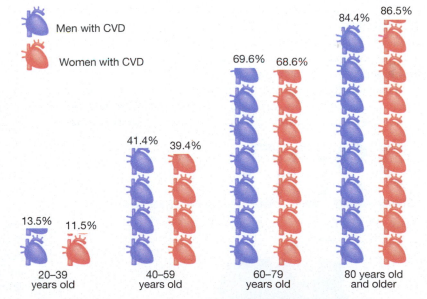

Figure 11.2 Prevalence of Cardiovascular Disease in U.S. Adults Age 20 and Older by Age and Sex

Source: Data from E. Benjamin et al., "Heart Disease and Stroke Statistics—2017 Update: A Report from the American Heart Association," *Circulation* 135, no. 10 (2017): e146–3603.

Check Yourself

- **What are some patterns in cardiovascular disease incidence, relative to gender and/or ethnicity?**

11.3 Key Cardiovascular Diseases: Hypertension

Learning Outcome

11.3 Define hypertension and explain how it is measured.

The major cardiovascular diseases are hypertension, atherosclerosis, coronary heart disease, and stroke. Each of these diseases causes deaths and disabilities; their causes and treatments are discussed in the following modules.

Force exerted on artery walls as the heart pumps is referred to as **blood pressure**. Blood pressure is measured by two numbers—for example, 110/80 mmHg, stated as "110 over 80 millimeters of mercury." The top number refers to **systolic pressure**, the pressure applied to the walls of the arteries when the heart contracts, pumping blood to the rest of the body. The bottom number is **diastolic pressure**, the pressure applied to the walls of the arteries during the heart's relaxation phase, when blood reenters the chambers of the heart in preparation for the next heartbeat.

Normal blood pressure varies depending on weight, age, and physical condition. High blood pressure, or **hypertension**, refers to sustained high blood pressure. Historically, hypertension has referred to a blood pressure of 140 or above. However, in November, 2017, new guidelines for diagnosis and treatment of hypertension were developed, effectively lowering the definition of high blood pressure to 130/80 millimeters of mercury. When only systolic pressure is high, the condition is known as *isolated systolic hypertension (ISH)*, the most common form of high blood pressure in older Americans. See **Table 11.1** for a summary of the new blood pressure guidelines.

In general, the higher your blood pressure, the greater is your risk for CVD. This is because blood pressure that remains in a higher-than-optimal range can lead to heart or vessel damage

2200 Americans die every day of CVD.

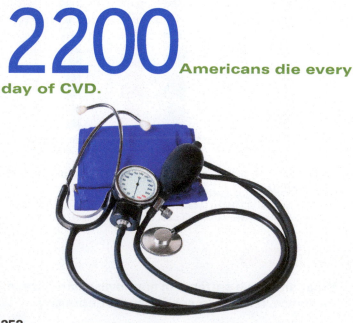

TABLE 11.1 Blood Pressure Classifications

Classification	Systolic Reading (mmHg)		Diastolic Reading (mmHg)
Normal	<120	And	<80
Elevated	120–129	Or	<80
Hypertension			
Stage 1	130–139	Or	80–89
Stage 2	140>	Or	90>

Note: If systolic and diastolic readings fall into different categories, treatment is determined by the highest category. Readings are based on the average of two or more properly measured, seated readings on each of two or more health care provider visits.

ACC/AHA/AAPA/ABC/ACPM/AGS/APhA/ASH/ASPC/NMA/PCNA Guideline for the Prevention, Detection, Evaluation, and Management of High Blood Pressure in Adults. Journal of the American College of Cardiology 2017, doi: 10.1016/j.jacc.2017.11.006.

over time, increasing the chance of heart attack, stroke, heart failure, kidney damage, and a host of other issues. Hypertension is known as the silent killer; it typically has few overt symptoms, so people often don't know they have it.

The prevalence of hypertension in the United States continues to increase in spite of significant efforts aimed at treatment and control. At 45 percent, African Americans are the ethnic group with the highest rate of high blood pressure in the United States.[22] Rates are also much higher among older adults, men, and people who don't have a high school education. Systolic blood pressure tends to increase with age, whereas diastolic blood pressure increases until age 55 and then declines. Prevalence rates in men under the age of 45 are expected to triple under the new definition, with rates among women doubling.[23] Women tend to have higher rates of hypertension after age 65.[24]

Treatment of hypertension can involve dietary changes such as reducing sodium intake, weight loss (when appropriate), regular exercise, reducing alcohol consumption, treatment of sleep disorders such as sleep apnea, and the practice of relaxation techniques and effective coping and communication skills. Use of diuretics and other medications such beta-blockers, alpha-blockers, or ACE inhibitors may also be part of treatment, as directed by a physician. Drugs alone do not seem to be the complete answer for most people with hypertension; the majority of individuals who are being treated with drugs still do not have their blood pressure under control.[25]

Check Yourself

- What is hypertension, and what are its causes and treatments?

11.4 Key Cardiovascular Diseases: Atherosclerosis

11.4 List the major factors contributing to atherosclerosis.

The term **atherosclerosis** is based on the Greek words *athero* (meaning gruel or paste) and *sclerosis* (hardness). In this condition, fatty substances, cholesterol, cellular waste products, calcium, and fibrin (a clotting material in the blood) build up in the inner lining of an artery. *Hyperlipidemia* (an abnormally high blood lipid level) is a key factor in this process, and the resulting buildup is called **plaque**.

As plaque accumulates, vessel walls become narrow and may eventually block blood flow or cause vessels to rupture (**Figure 11.3**). The pressure buildup is similar to that achieved when you put your thumb over the end of a hose while water is on. Pressure builds within arteries just as pressure builds in the hose. If vessels are weakened and pressure persists, the vessels may burst or the plaque itself may break away from the walls of

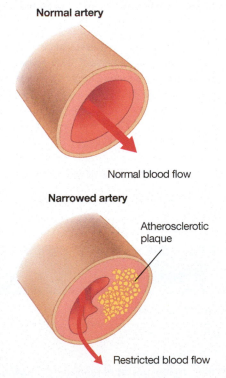

Normal artery

Normal blood flow

Narrowed artery

Atherosclerotic plaque

Restricted blood flow

Figure 11.3 Atherosclerosis and Coronary Artery Disease In atherosclerosis, arteries become clogged by a buildup of plaque. When atherosclerosis occurs in coronary arteries, blood flow to the heart muscle is restricted and a heart attack may occur.

Source: Adapted from Joan Salge Blake, *Nutrition and You*, 2nd ed. © 2014. Reprinted by permission of Pearson Education, Inc., Upper Saddle River, New Jersey.

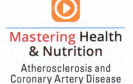

Mastering Health & Nutrition

Atherosclerosis and Coronary Artery Disease

the vessels and obstruct blood flow. In addition, fluctuation in the blood pressure levels within arteries can damage internal arterial walls, making it even more likely that plaque will stick to injured wall surfaces and accumulate.

Atherosclerosis is often called **coronary artery disease (CAD)** because of the damage to the body's main coronary arteries on the outer surface of the heart. These are the arteries that provide blood to the heart muscle itself. Most heart attacks result from blockage of these arteries. Atherosclerosis and other circulatory impairments also often reduce blood flow and limit the heart's blood and oxygen supply, a condition known as **ischemia**.

When atherosclerosis occurs in the lower extremities, such as in the feet, calves, or legs, or in the arms, it is called **peripheral artery disease (PAD)**. Over 8.5 million people—particularly non-Hispanic blacks, women under the age of 60, and men over the age of 60 in the United States—have PAD, and many are not receiving treatment because they are asymptomatic or don't recognize subtle symptoms.[26] Most often characterized by pain and aching in the legs, calves, or feet on walking or exercise (known as *intermittent claudication*), PAD is a leading cause of disability in people over the age of 50 for both men and women. Smokers, and diabetics tend to develop it more frequently.[27] In recent years, increased attention has been drawn to the role of PAD in subsequent blood clots and resultant heart attacks, particularly among people who sit in cramped airplanes for long distances without getting up and moving. Sometimes PAD in the arms can be caused by trauma, certain diseases, radiation therapy, surgery, repetitive motion syndrome, or a combination of factors. Damage to vessels and threats to health can be severe, with a two to three times greater risk of stroke and heart attack among people who have PAD.[28] Risk for PAD increases with age in both men and women.

Atherosclerosis treatment focuses on lifestyle changes, drugs that reduce the risk of plaque, medical procedures to open vessels, or surgery to open clogged vessels. Millions of Americans take drugs designed to reduce triglycerides and low-density lipoprotein (sometimes called "bad cholesterol" because of its association with CVD) and increase high-density lipoprotein (sometimes called "good cholesterol" because it can help to protect against CVD). *Statins* are the most commonly prescribed medications for atherosclerosis; however, they are not without risk. The most common risk is muscle pain that ranges from mild to severe. Other potential side effects are digestive issues, liver damage, increased risk of diabetes, and memory loss. People who are considering taking statins should discuss the risks and benefits with their health care providers.

- **What is atherosclerosis, and what are its causes?**

- **What are the symptoms of peripheral artery disease? Who is most at risk for this disease?**

11.5 Key Cardiovascular Diseases: Coronary Heart Disease

Learning Outcome

11.5 List the major factors contributing to a heart attack and the signs of a heart attack.

Of all the major cardiovascular diseases, **coronary heart disease (CHD)** is the greatest killer, accounting for about 1 in 7 deaths in the United States (over 360,000 people). Over 700,000 new and recurrent heart attacks occur in the United States each year.[29]

A **myocardial infarction (MI)**, or **heart attack**, is a medical emergency where an area of the heart suffers permanent damage because its normal blood supply becomes blocked, leading to lack of oxygen and cell death. This condition is often brought on by **coronary thrombosis**, the formation of a clot that blocks blood flow, or from an atherosclerotic narrowing that blocks a coronary artery (an artery supplying the heart muscle with blood). When a clot, or **thrombus**, becomes dislodged and moves through the circulatory system, it is called an **embolus**. Whenever blood does not flow readily, there is a corresponding decrease in oxygen flow to tissue below the blockage.

If the blockage is extremely minor, an otherwise healthy heart will adapt over time, enlarging existing blood vessels and growing new ones to reroute needed blood through other areas. This system, called **collateral circulation**, is a form of self-preservation that allows an affected heart muscle to cope with damage.

When a heart blockage is more severe, however, the body is unable to adapt on its own, and outside life-saving support is critical. The hour Immediately after a heart attack is the most crucial period.

It is important to know and recognize the symptoms of a heart attack so that help can be obtained immediately (Table 11.2). Ignoring symptoms or delays in seeking treatment can have fatal consequences. Become familiar with heart attack symptoms, and know how to summon emergency help at home, work, and school.

Skills for Behavior Change

What to Do When a Heart Attack Hits

People often miss the signs of a heart attack, or they wait too long to seek help, which can have deadly consequences. Knowing what to do in an emergency could save your life or somebody else's.

- **Keep a list of emergency rescue service numbers next to your telephone and in your pocket, wallet, or purse. Be aware of whether your local area has a 9-1-1 emergency service.**
- **Expect the person to deny the possibility of anything as serious as a heart attack, particularly if that person is young and appears to be in good health. If you're with someone who appears to be having a heart attack, don't take no for an answer; insist on taking prompt action.**
- **If you are with someone who suddenly collapses, perform cardiopulmonary resuscitation (CPR). See www.heart.org for information on new AHA chest-compression-only recommendations. If you're trained and willing, use conventional CPR methods.**

Source: Adapted from American Heart Association, "Warning Signs of Heart Attack, Stroke, and Cardiac Arrest," 2016, www.heart.org/HEARTORG/Conditions/911-Warnings-Signs-of-a-Heart-Attack_UCM_305346_SubHomePage.jsp

Check Yourself

- **What is a heart attack, and what are its causes?**
- **What should you do if someone shows signs of a heart attack?**

TABLE 11.2 Common Heart Attack Symptoms and Signs

Sign or Symptom	Gender Who Most Commonly Experiences It
Crushing or squeezing chest pain	More common in men
Pain radiating down arm, neck, or jaw	More common in men
Chest discomfort or pressure with shortness of breath, nausea/vomiting, or lightheadedness	Women more likely to feel pressure than pain. Shortness of breath, nausea, and lightheadedness common in both women and men
Shortness of breath without chest pain, discomfort in back, neck, or jaw or in one or both arms	More common in women
Unusual weakness	More common in women
Unusual fatigue	More common in women
Sleep disturbances	More common in women
Indigestion, flulike symptoms	More common in women

Source: American Heart Association, "Symptoms of Heart Attack in Women," 2012, www.heart.org.

Cardiovascular Disease, Cancer, and Diabetes

11.5

11.6 List the major factors contributing to stroke and the signs of a stroke.

The brain relies on a continuous supply of oxygen delivered via blood in order to survive. A **stroke** (or *cerebrovascular accident*) occurs when blood supply to the brain is interrupted, killing brain cells as a result of oxygen deprivation. Brain cells have little capacity to heal or regenerate, so while some recovery after certain types of strokes is possible, rehabilitation may be lengthy, difficult, and limited. Depression is also an issue for many survivors.

Strokes may be *ischemic* (caused by plaque or a clot that reduces blood flow) or *hemorrhagic* (caused by bulging or rupture of a weakened blood vessel). **Figure 11.4** illustrates blood vessel disorders that can lead to a stroke. An **aneurysm** is the most life-threatening hemorrhagic stroke.

Mild strokes cause temporary dizziness, weakness, or numbness. More serious interruptions in blood flow may impair speech, memory, or motor control, often affecting one side of the body. Other strokes affect heart and lung function regulation, killing within minutes.

Many major strokes are preceded days, weeks, or months earlier by **transient ischemic attacks (TIAs)**, brief interruptions of the brain's blood supply that cause temporary impairment.[30] Symptoms of TIAs include dizziness (particularly on rising), falls, blackouts, weakness, temporary paralysis or numbness, temporary memory loss, blurred vision, nausea, headache, and difficulty speaking. Some people have no obvious symptoms.

The earlier a stroke is recognized and treatment started, the more effective the treatment will be. One of the great medical successes in recent years is the decline in the death rate from strokes, which in the United States has dropped by one-third since the 1980s.[31] Greater awareness of stroke symptoms, improvements in emergency medicine protocols and medicines, and a greater emphasis on fast rehabilitation and therapy help many people survive strokes.

In addition to treatment regimens having a major impact on improved outcomes with stroke, lifestyle changes in recent decades have clearly improved the stroke profiles of Americans. Major declines in smoking, decreases in high fat diets, increased use of drugs such as statins, which reduce cholesterol, and improvements in diagnosis and emergency medicine have played a role in improving stroke risks and survival. Despite overall decreases, stroke still affects nearly 7.0 million Americans and kills 133,000 people annually, making it the fifth leading cause of death in the United States.[32] Ten percent of all strokes occur in people age 18 to 50 and are on the increase among young adults, meaning significant increases in costs associated with long treatment courses and medication.[33]

Skills for **Behavior Change**

A Simple Test for Stroke

People often ignore, minimize, or misunderstand stroke symptoms. Starting treatment within just a few hours is crucial for the best recovery outcomes. So if you suspect that someone is having a stroke, use the tool many emergency teams do to assess what is happening: Think FAST.

1. **Facial Droop.** Ask the person to smile. It is normal for both sides of the face to move equally, and it is abnormal if one side moves less easily.
2. **Arm Weakness.** Ask the person to raise both arms. It is normal if both arms move equally (or not at all). It is abnormal if one arm drifts or cannot be raised as high as the other.
3. **Speech Difficulty.** Have the patient restate a sentence such as "You can't teach an old dog new tricks." It is normal if they can say the sentence correctly, and it is abnormal if they use inappropriate words, slur, or cannot speak.
4. **Time to Act and call 9-1-1.** Don't delay if you note F, A, and S above. Time is of the essence.

Source: Centers for Disease Control, "Stroke Signs and Symptoms," April 2015, www.cdc.gov/stroke/signs_symptoms.htm.

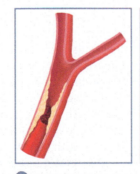
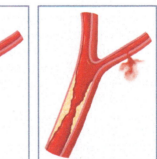
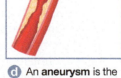

a A **thrombus** is a blood clot that forms inside a blood vessel and blocks the flow of blood at its origin.

b An **embolus** is a blood clot that breaks off from its point of formation and travels in the bloodstream until it lodges in a narrowed vessel and blocks blood flow.

c A **hemorrhage** occurs when a blood vessel bursts allowing blood to flow into the surrounding tissue or between tissues.

d An **aneurysm** is the bulging of a weakened blood vessel wall.

Figure 11.4 **Blood Vessel Disorders That Can Lead to Stroke**

Check Yourself

- What is stroke, and what are its causes?
- What should you do if someone shows signs of a stroke?

11.7 Know the signs and symptoms of angina pectoris, arrhythmias, congestive heart failure, and childhood cardiovascular defects.

Other cardiovascular diseases of concern include angina pectoris, arrhythmias, congestive heart failure, and childhood cardiovascular defects.

Angina Pectoris

Angina pectoris is a term that means "strangling of the chest." It occurs when inadequate oxygen supply to heart muscle results in chest pain or pressure. Although angina pectoris is not a heart attack, it does indicate underlying heart disease. About 10 million people in the United States suffer from mild to severe symptoms of angina—from indigestion or heartburn-like sensations to crushing chest pain.[34] Generally, the more serious the oxygen deprivation, the more severe the pain.

Mild angina cases are treated with rest. Treatments for more severe cases involve drugs that affect either the supply of blood to the heart muscle or the heart's demand for oxygen. Pain and discomfort are often relieved with *nitroglycerin*, a drug that relaxes (dilates) the veins, improving blood flow to the heart. Patients with angina caused by spasms of the coronary arteries are often given *calcium channel blockers*, which prevent calcium atoms from passing through the arteries and causing the contractions. *Beta-blockers* control potential overactivity of the heart muscle.

Arrhythmias

Over the course of a lifetime, most people experience some type of **arrhythmia**, an irregularity in heart rhythm that occurs when the electrical impulses that coordinate the heartbeat don't work properly. A person with a racing heart in the absence of exercise or anxiety may be experiencing *tachycardia*, the medical term for an abnormally fast heartbeat. On the other end of the continuum is *bradycardia*, an abnormally slow heartbeat. When a heart goes into **fibrillation**, it beats in a sporadic pattern that causes extreme inefficiency in moving blood through the cardiovascular system. If untreated, fibrillation can be fatal. The most common type of arrhythmias, preventricular contractions (PVCs)—premature heart beats in the ventricles—are on the rise among all age groups. Teens, young adults, and athletes seem particularly susceptible to PVCs.[35]

Not all arrhythmias are life-threatening. In many instances, excessive caffeine or nicotine consumption can trigger an arrhythmia episode. However, severe cases may require drug therapy or external electrical stimulus to prevent serious complications. When in doubt, it is always best to check with your health care provider.

Congestive Heart Failure

When the heart muscle is damaged and can't pump enough blood to supply body tissues, fluids may begin to accumulate in various parts of the body, most notably the lungs, feet, ankles, and legs. Acute shortness of breath and fatigue are often key symptoms of heart failure (HF) or congestive heart failure (CHF). Nearly 5.1 million adults in the United States have HF, and cases are estimated to rise to nearly 10 million by 2030.[36] Underlying causes of HF may include an injury that results in damage to heart muscle (**cardiomyopathy**), affects heart valves, or causes problems with heart rhythms. Infectious diseases, such as rheumatic fever, can damage heart valves. Bacteria and viruses can inflame blood vessels, increasing atherosclerotic plaque formation. Uncontrolled high blood pressure, coronary artery disease, diabetes, and other chronic conditions can all lead to heart failure. Certain drugs such as nonsteroidal anti-inflammatory drugs (NSAIDs) and diabetes medications also increase risks, as do chronic drug and alcohol abuse. In some cases, damage is due to cancer radiation or chemotherapy treatments.

Untreated, HF can be fatal. However, most cases respond well to treatment, which includes *diuretics* (drugs that increase urination) to relieve fluid accumulation; drugs such as *digitalis* that increase the heart's pumping action; and *vasodilators*, drugs that expand blood vessels and decrease resistance, making the heart's work easier.

Congenital and Rheumatic Heart Disease

Approximately 40,000 children are born in the United States each year with some form of **congenital cardiovascular defect** (*congenital* means that the problem is present at birth).[37] These defects may be relatively minor, such as slight *murmurs* (low-pitched sounds caused by turbulent blood flow through the heart) caused by valve irregularities, which many children outgrow. About 25 percent of those born with congenital heart defects must undergo invasive procedures to correct problems within the first year of life.[38] Underlying causes are unknown but may be related to hereditary factors; maternal diseases, such as rubella, that occurred during fetal development; or pregnant women's chemical intake (particularly binge drinking, with increased risks for mothers who binge drink and smoke and those who use methamphetamine) during pregnancy. A greater risk of having a child with a congenital cardiovascular defect is also seen among women who are diabetic, those with a high body mass index (BMI), and those with folate deficiency. With advances in pediatric cardiology, the prognosis for children with congenital heart defects is better than ever before.

Rheumatic heart disease is attributed to rheumatic fever, an inflammatory disease caused by an unresolved *streptococcal infection* of the throat (strep throat). Over time, the strep infection can affect connective tissues of the heart, joints, brain, or skin. In some cases, the infection can lead to an immune response in which antibodies attack the heart as well as the bacteria. Many operations on heart valves are related to rheumatic heart disease.

- What are the common symptoms for angina pectoris, arrhythmias, congestive heart failure, and congenital and rheumatic heart disease? What are risk factors for each?

11.8 List the cluster of factors composing metabolic syndrome.

A large cluster of factors are related to increased risk for CVD. The U.S. Burden of Disease Collaborators determined that the greatest contributor to overall CVD burden was suboptimal diet, followed by tobacco smoking, high BMI, high blood pressure, high fasting plasma glucose, and physical inactivity.[39] A growing body of research has implicated selected CVD risks and conditions such as obesity and hypertension with an increased risk for impaired cognitive function and an increased risk for Alzheimer's disease.[40] **Cardiometabolic risks** are the combined risks, which indicate physical and biochemical changes that can lead to diseases. Some risks result from choices and behaviors and are modifiable; others are inherited or are intrinsic (such as age and gender) and cannot be changed.

Over the past decade, health professionals have attempted to establish diagnostic cutoff points for a cluster of combined cardiometabolic risks, variably labeled *syndrome X*, *insulin resistance syndrome*, and, most recently, **metabolic syndrome (MetS)**. Historically, MetS is believed to increase risk for atherosclerotic heart disease by as much as three times normal rates. Women are more likely than men to have metabolic syndrome overall.[41] The highest prevalence occurs among Hispanics, followed by non-Hispanic whites and blacks.[42] As age increases, so does MetS, affecting over 18 percent of 20- to 39-year-olds to nearly 47 percent of people age 60.[43] Although different professional organizations have slightly different criteria for MetS, that of the National Cholesterol Education Program's Adult Treatment Panel (NCEP/ATPIII) is most commonly used. According to these criteria, for a diagnosis of metabolic syndrome a person would have three or more of the following risks (**Figure 11.5**):

- Abdominal obesity (waist measurement of more than 40 inches in men or 35 inches in women)
- Elevated blood fat (triglycerides greater than 150 mg/dL)
- Low levels of high-density lipoprotein ("good" cholesterol) (less than 40 mg/dL in men and less than 50 mg/dL in women)
- Blood pressure greater than 130/85 mmHg
- Fasting glucose greater than 100 mg/dL (a sign of insulin resistance or glucose intolerance)

The use of the MetS classification and other, similar terms has been important in highlighting the relationship between the number of risks a person has and that person's likelihood of developing CVD and diabetes. Groups such as the American Heart Association are giving increased attention to multiple risks and emphasizing cardiovascular health in lifestyle interventions.

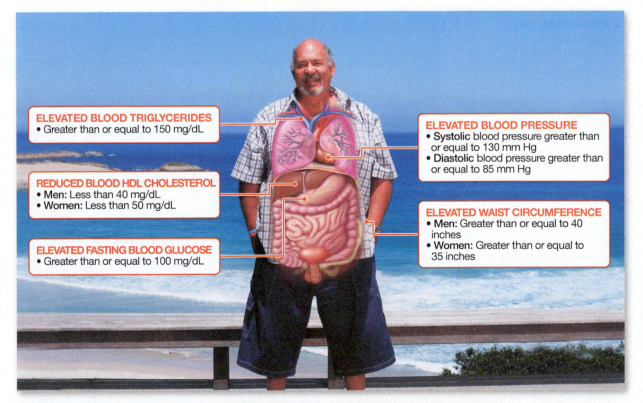

ELEVATED BLOOD TRIGLYCERIDES
- Greater than or equal to 150 mg/dL

REDUCED BLOOD HDL CHOLESTEROL
- **Men:** Less than 40 mg/dL
- **Women:** Less than 50 mg/dL

ELEVATED FASTING BLOOD GLUCOSE
- Greater than or equal to 100 mg/dL

ELEVATED BLOOD PRESSURE
- **Systolic** blood pressure greater than or equal to 130 mm Hg
- **Diastolic** blood pressure greater than or equal to 85 mm Hg

ELEVATED WAIST CIRCUMFERENCE
- **Men:** Greater than or equal to 40 inches
- **Women:** Greater than or equal to 35 inches

Figure 11.5 Risk Factors Associated with Metabolic Syndrome

- How does metabolic syndrome contribute to the risk of heart disease?

Cardiovascular Disease, Cancer, and Diabetes

11.8

CVD Risk: Modifiable Factors

11.9 Describe modifiable factors affecting CVD risk.

From the first moments of your life, you begin to accumulate risks for CVD. Your past and current lifestyle choices may haunt you as you enter your middle and later years. Behaviors you choose today and over the coming decades can actively reduce or increase your risk for CVD.

Avoid Tobacco Smoke

Cigarette smoking is the leading cause of preventable death in the United States, causing more deaths each year than HIV, alcohol abuse, motor vehicle crashes, and firearm-related deaths combined. Smokers are also 2 to 4 times more likely to develop coronary heart disease and stroke.[44] Smoking causes 90 percent of all lung cancers , 80 percent of all COPD, and a variety of other health issues.[45] Social smoking (not daily but in regular social settings) has been found to result in a major increase in CVD risk.[46] Non-smokers who are regularly exposed to secondhand smoke have a 25 to 30 percent increased risk of heart disease, with over 35,000 deaths per year.[47]

The good news is that if you stop smoking, your heart and lungs can begin to mend themselves. After 1 to 2 years, the former smoker's risk of heart disease drops significantly, respiratory symptoms such as coughing and shortness of breath begin to improve, risks of lung and other cancers drop, and among women who smoke, risks of infertility and low birth weight babies decrease significantly.[48] In short, you'll feel better, function better, and smell better! (See Chapter 7 for more information).

See It! Videos

What habits can you change now to improve your heart health? Watch **Importance of Heart Health** in the Study Area of Mastering Health.

Cut Back on Saturated Fat

Diets that are high in saturated fat and *trans* fats are widely believed to raise cholesterol levels and make the blood more viscous, which increases risk of heart attack, stroke, and atherosclerosis. Cutting back on saturated fat remains a recommended way to decrease the risk of CVD.

However, recommendations about consumption of *cholesterol*, a fat-like substance found in the bloodstream and cells, have shifted in recent years. Your body produces about 75 percent of the cholesterol found in it; the rest comes from foods in your diet. Cholesterol plays a role in the production of cell membranes and hormones and helps to process vitamin D. For decades, high levels of cholesterol have been thought to increase CVD risk. People were told to avoid foods with high cholesterol levels. However, in early 2016, surprising reversals in the "cholesterol is bad" mantra emerged with the new *Dietary Guidelines for Americans*.[49] As a result of years of study, experts eased up on recommendations focused on cutting cholesterol. Eggs and other cholesterol-rich foods are now on the "eat in moderation" list as experts put the emphasis on reducing saturated fat from high-fat meats and dairy to 10 percent of the daily diet.

Historically, clinicians have looked at total cholesterol, triglycerides, and high- and low-density lipoproteins as being key to determining CVD risks. There are two components to cholesterol: **Low-density lipoprotein (LDL)**, or "bad cholesterol," is believed to build up on artery walls. **High-density lipoprotein (HDL)**, or "good cholesterol," appears to remove such buildup. In theory, if LDL levels get too high or HDL levels get too low, cholesterol will accumulate inside arteries and lead to cardiovascular problems. However, new research indicates that raising HDL levels to prevent negative CVD outcomes may not be as beneficial as was once thought.[50]

Other blood lipid factors may increase CVD risk. *Lipoprotein-associated phospholipase A2 (Lp-PLA2)* is an enzyme that circulates in the blood and attaches to LDL; it plays an important role in plaque accumulation and increased risk for stroke and coronary events, particularly in men.[51] *Apolipoprotein B (apo B)* is a primary component of LDL essential for cholesterol delivery to cells. Some researchers believe that apo B levels may be more important to heart disease risk than total cholesterol or LDL levels.[52]

When you consume calories, the body converts any extra to **triglycerides**, which are stored in fat cells to provide energy. High

TABLE 11.3 Recommended Cholesterol Levels for Lower/Moderate-Risk Adults

Total Cholesterol Level (lower numbers are better)	
<200 mg/dL	Desirable
200–239 mg/dL	Borderline high
≥240 mg/dL	High
HDL Cholesterol Level (higher numbers are better)	
Less than <40 mg/dL (for men)	Low
≥60 mg/dL	Desirable
LDL Cholesterol Level (lower numbers are better)	
<100 mg/dL	Optimal
100–129 mg/dL	Near or above optimal
130–159 mg/dL	Borderline high
160–189 mg/dL	High
≥190 mg/dL	Very high
Triglyceride Level (lower numbers are better)	
<150 mg/dL	Normal
150–199 mg/dL	Borderline high
200–499 mg/dL	High
≥500 mg/dL	Very high

Source: Adapted from ATP III Guidelines At-a-Glance Quick Desk Reference, National Heart, Lung, and Blood Institute, National Institutes of Health. Update on Cholesterol Guidelines, 2004.

counts of blood triglycerides are often found in people who are obese or overweight or who have high cholesterol levels, heart problems, or diabetes. A baseline cholesterol test (lipid panel or lipid profile) measures triglyceride, HDL, LDL, and total cholesterol. You should have one done at age 20, with follow-ups every 5 years, then annually for men over 35 and women over 45. (See Table 11.3 for recommended levels of cholesterol and triglycerides.)

In spite of all of the education on the dangers of high cholesterol, Americans continue to have higher than recommended levels, and millions are taking cholesterol-lowering drugs. Nearly 40 percent of adults age 20 and over have cholesterol levels at or above 200 mg/dL, and nearly 14 percent have levels in excess of 240 mg/dL.[53]

Modify Other Dietary Habits

Research continues into dietary modifications that may affect heart health. The National Heart, Lung, and Blood Institute's DASH eating plan has strong evidence to back up its claims of reducing CVD risk. Eating recommendations include the following:

- Eat lots of fiber—5 to 10 milligrams per day of soluble fiber, from sources such as oat bran, fruits, vegetables, legumes, and psyllium seeds.
- Consume about 2 grams per day of **plant sterols**, which are present in many fruits, vegetables, nuts, seeds, cereals, legumes, vegetable oils, and other plant sources.
- Cut down on dietary sodium. Table salt is typically about 40 percent sodium. Excess sodium has been linked to high blood pressure, which can affect CVD risk. Sodium is hidden in many popular foods; amounts of sodium in breads, pasta sauces, pizza, pastry, processed meats such as hotdogs, and some ethnic foods are extremely high.

Several foods, including fish that is high in omega-3 fatty acids, olive oil, whole grains, nuts, green tea, and dark chocolate, have been shown to reduce the chances that cholesterol will be absorbed in the cells, reduce levels of LDL cholesterol, or enhance the protective effects of HDL cholesterol.[54]

Maintain a Healthy Weight

Overweight people are more likely to develop heart disease and stroke even if they have no other risk factors. If you're heavy, losing even 5 percent of your body weight can make a significant difference in reducing your risk for CVD and diabetes.[55] This is especially true if you're an "apple" (thicker around the upper body and waist) rather than a "pear" (thicker around the hips and thighs), are prediabetic, and/or have metabolic syndrome.

Exercise Regularly

Inactivity is a definite risk factor for CVD. Even light activity—walking, gardening, housework, dancing—is beneficial if done regularly and over the long term. Exercise can increase HDL levels, lower triglycerides levels, and reduce coronary risks in several ways.

Control Diabetes and Blood Pressure

Heart disease death rates among adults with diabetes are 2 to 4 times higher than the rates for adults without diabetes. At least

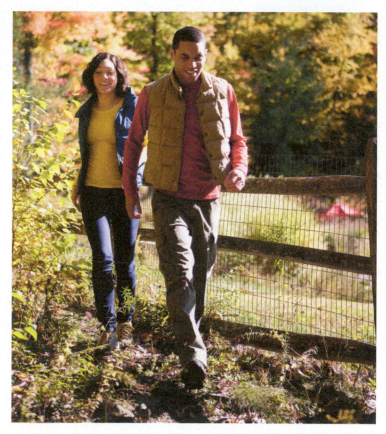

Even low-intensity activity can reduce your risk of CVD. Exercise can increase HDL levels, lower triglyceride levels, and reduce coronary risks in several ways.

65 percent of people with diabetes die of heart disease or stroke.[56]

Although blood pressure typically creeps up with age, lifestyle changes can dramatically lower CVD risk. Among the most beneficial are losing extra pounds, cutting back on sodium, exercising more, reducing alcohol and caffeine intake, and quitting smoking.

See It! Videos

Can a way of eating reduce your risk of heart disease? Watch **Mediterranean Diet Could Help Reduce Heart Disease** in the Study Area of Mastering Health.

Manage Stress and Get More Sleep

Research indicates that everyday, chronic stressors can lead to increased risk of hypertension, coronary events, strokes, and sudden cardiac death.[57] Sleep deprivation may also increase risks for these conditions.[58]

Check Yourself

- **Of the risk factors described, which are of the most concern to you? What kind of changes could you make to improve in these areas?**

CVD Risk: Nonmodifiable Factors

11.10 Identify nonmodifiable factors affecting CVD risk.

Some risk factors for CVD cannot be prevented or controlled. Among these factors are the following:

- **Race and Ethnicity.** African Americans tend to have the highest overall rates of CVD—among the highest average blood pressure rates in the world. Mexican Americans have the highest percentage of adults with cholesterol levels exceeding 200 mg/dL and the highest rates of obesity and overweight.[59] **Figure 11.6** summarizes deaths from heart disease and stroke by ethnicity.

- **Heredity.** Family history of heart disease appears to increase CVD risk significantly. Amount of cholesterol produced, tendencies to form plaque, and a host of other factors seem to have genetic links. Newer research has focused on studying the interactions between nutrition and genes (*nutrigenetics*) and the role that diet may play in increasing or decreasing risks among certain genetic profiles.[60]

- **Age.** Although CVD can affect people of all ages, the vast majority of heart attacks occur in those over age 65. Increasing age ups the risk for CVD for all.

- **Gender.** Men are at greater risk for CVD until about age 60, when women catch up and then surpass them. Women under 35 have a fairly low risk, although oral contraceptives and smoking increase risk. Hormonal factors appear to reduce risk for women, though after menopause, women's LDL levels tend to rise. Women who have heart attacks also have poorer health outcomes and higher death rates than men who have heart attacks.[61]

Inflammation and C-Reactive Protein

Inflammation—which occurs when tissues are injured, for example by bacteria, trauma, toxins, or heat—may play a major role in development of atherosclerosis because injured vessel walls are more prone to plaque formation. Cigarette smoke, high blood pressure, high LDL levels, diabetes mellitus, certain forms of arthritis, and exposure to toxins have been linked to increased risk of inflammation. However, the greatest risk appears to be from infectious disease pathogens, most notably *Chlamydia pneumoniae* (a common cause of respiratory infections), *Helicobacter pylori* (a bacterium that causes stomach ulcers), herpes simplex virus, and *cytomegalovirus* (a herpes virus that infects most Americans before age 40). For many years, *homocysteine* was believed to play a role in inflammation and CVD. Although there is still some evidence that it may play a role, the jury is out on homocysteine's role and whether there is anything that can be done to reduce risk.

During an inflammatory reaction, **C-reactive proteins (CRPs)** tend to be present in blood at high levels. A recent meta-analysis shows a strong association between C-reactive proteins in the blood and increased risks for atherosclerosis and CVD.[62] Doctors can test patients using an assay called hs-CRP; if levels are high, action could be taken to prevent progression to reduce inflammation.

A recent meta-analysis of over 38 studies with nearly 170,000 subjects has shown a strong association between C-reactive proteins in the blood and increased risks for atherosclerosis and CVD.[63] Blood tests can test these proteins using a highly sensitive assay called *hs-CRP* (high-sensitivity C-reactive protein); if levels are high, action could be taken to reduce inflammation.

The FDA recently approved a new, nonfasting blood test that predicts heart attack in people with no history of heart disease. Known as *PLAC*, the test measures activity of inflammatory enzymes in the blood, which cause plaque to form. More inflammatory enzymes mean more plaque in vessels and greater risk. The PLAC test could increase our ability to spot and treat potential heart attacks early in the process.[64]

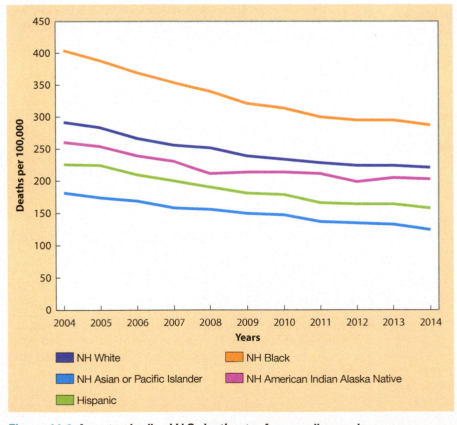

Figure 11.6 Age-standardized U.S. death rates from cardiovascular disease by race/ethnicity, 2004-2014

Source: Data are from Centers for Disease Control and Prevention, National Vital Statistics System.

Legend:
- NH White
- NH Asian or Pacific Islander
- Hispanic
- NH Black
- NH American Indian Alaska Native

- **Of the risk factors described, which is of the most concern to you and why?**

11.11 Describe techniques for diagnosing and treating CVD.

There are many options for diagnosing and treating CVD. Medications can strengthen heartbeat, control arrhythmias, remove fluids, reduce blood pressure, and improve heart function.

CVD Diagnostic Techniques

Patients may undergo a *stress test*—exercise on a stationary bike or treadmill with an **electrocardiogram (ECG)**, a record of the heart's electrical activity—or a *nuclear stress test*, which involves injecting a radioactive dye and taking images of the heart to reveal blood flow problems. In **angiography** (*cardiac catheterization*), a thin tube called a *catheter* is threaded through heart arteries, a dye is injected, and an X-ray is taken to identify blocked areas. A **positron emission tomography (PET) scan** produces three-dimensional images of the heart as blood flows through it. In **magnetic resonance imaging (MRI)**, magnetic fields are used to image the body to help identify damage, congenital defects, and disease. *Ultrafast computed tomography (CT)*, a form of sophisticated X-ray, is used to evaluate bypass grafts, diagnose ventricular function, and identify irregularities. *Coronary calcium score* is derived from another type of ultrafast CT used to diagnose calcium levels in heart vessels that may increase risk for heart attack. There is a risk from the high levels of radiation used in CT scans. Check with your health care provider about risks and benefits of any proposed diagnostic test or treatment.

Surgical Options

Coronary bypass surgery has helped many patients survive coronary blockages or heart attacks. In a coronary artery bypass graft (CABG, referred to as a "cabbage"), a blood vessel from another site in the patient's body is removed and implanted in the heart to "bypass" blocked coronary arteries so that blood supply is retained for the heart tissue.

In an **angioplasty**, a catheter is threaded through blocked heart arteries. The catheter has a balloon at the tip, which is inflated to flatten fatty deposits against arterial walls, allowing blood to flow more freely. Other surgical options include laser angioplasty and *atherectomy*, a procedure that removes plaque. Many people who undergo angioplasty receive a **stent**, a steel mesh tube inserted to keep the artery open. Although stents are highly effective, inflammation and tissue growth in the area may increase after the procedure, and in about 30 percent of patients, the treated arteries become clogged again within 6 months.[65] Newer stents are usually medicated to reduce this risk.

Drug Therapies

Because the pain reliever aspirin also has blood-thinning qualities, physicians sometimes recommended a low dose of aspirin to help prevent heart attacks, or improve outcome when a heart attack

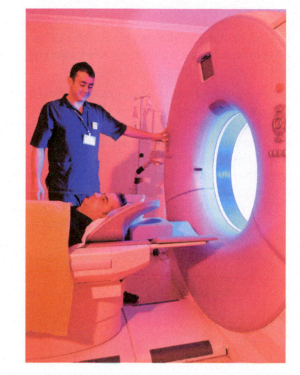

Magnetic resonance imaging is one of several methods used to detect damage, abnormalities, or defects in the heart.

occurs. However, the benefits of an aspirin regimen for otherwise healthy adults remains questionable. New research indicates an increased risk of gastrointestinal bleeding and stroke in people who take aspirin daily.[66] Research also shows that once a patient has taken aspirin regularly, stopping this regimen may increase his or her risk for a heart attack.[67]

Clot-busting therapy with **thrombolysis** can be performed within the first 1 to 3 hours after a heart attack or stroke. Thrombolysis involves injecting an agent such as *tissue plasminogen activator (tPA)* to dissolve the clot and restore some blood flow, thereby reducing the amount of tissue that dies from ischemia.

Cardiac Rehabilitation and Recovery

Every year, more than 1 million Americans survive heart attacks. Millions more have a number of medical interventions to help them survive and thrive. Rehabilitation may include exercise training and classes on nutrition and CVD risk management. Not all patients choose to participate. They may lack insurance, fear an exercise-induced attack, or have other concerns. However, the benefits far outweigh the risks.

Check Yourself

- **How is CVD commonly diagnosed and treated?**

Learning Outcome

11.12 Define the term *cancer,* know the difference between benign and malignant tumors, and understand what metastasis is.

Cancer is the name given to a large group of diseases characterized by the uncontrolled growth and spread of abnormal cells. When something interrupts normal cell programming, uncontrolled growth and abnormal cellular development result in a **neoplasm**, a new growth of tissue serving no physiological function. This neoplasmic mass often forms a clump of cells known as a **tumor**.

Not all tumors are **malignant** (cancerous); in fact, most are **benign** (noncancerous). Benign tumors are generally harmless unless they grow to obstruct or crowd out normal tissues. A benign tumor of the brain, for instance, may become life-threatening if it grows enough to restrict blood flow and cause a stroke. The only

way to determine whether a tumor is malignant is through **biopsy**, or microscopic examination of cell development.

Benign tumors generally consist of ordinary-looking cells enclosed in a fibrous shell or capsule that prevents their spreading to other body areas. In contrast, malignant tumors are usually not enclosed in a protective capsule and can therefore spread to other organs (**Figure 11.7**). This process, known as **metastasis**, makes some forms of cancer particularly aggressive in their ability to overwhelm bodily defenses. Malignant tumors frequently metastasize throughout the body, making treatment extremely difficult. Unlike benign tumors, which merely expand to take over a given space, malignant cells invade surrounding tissue, emitting clawlike protrusions that disturb the RNA and DNA within normal cells. Disrupting these substances, which control cellular metabolism and reproduction, produces **mutant cells** that differ in form, quality, and function from normal cells.

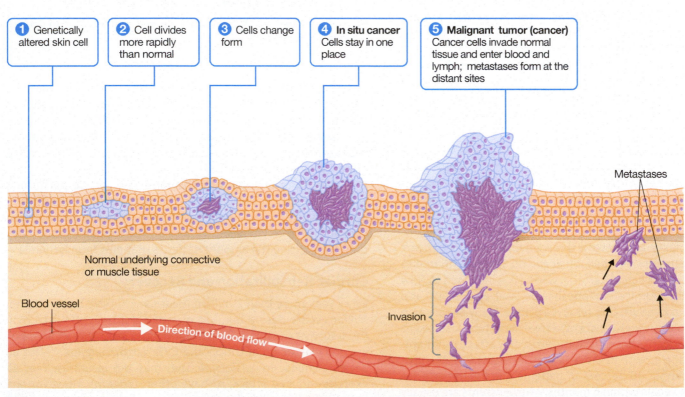

1 **Genetically altered skin cell**

2 **Cell divides more rapidly than normal**

3 **Cells change form**

4 **In situ cancer** Cells stay in one place

5 **Malignant tumor (cancer)** Cancer cells invade normal tissue and enter blood and lymph; metastases form at the distant sites

Metastases

Normal underlying connective or muscle tissue

Blood vessel

Direction of blood flow

Invasion

Figure 11.7 Metastasis

A mutation to the genetic material of a skin cell triggers abnormal cell division and changes cell formation, resulting in a cancerous tumor. If the tumor remains localized, it is considered in situ cancer. If the tumor spreads, it is considered a malignant cancer.

Mastering Health & Nutrition

Metastasis

Check Yourself

- **What is cancer?**
- **What is the difference between benign tumors and malignant tumors?**

11.13 Types and Sites of Cancer

11.13 List the major types and most common sites of cancer.

The word *cancer* refers not to a single disease, but to hundreds of different diseases. They are grouped into four broad categories based on the type of tissue from which the cancer arises:

- **Carcinomas.** Epithelial tissues (tissues covering body surfaces and lining most body cavities) are the most common sites for cancers; cancers occurring in epithelial tissue are called *carcinomas*. These cancers affect the outer layer of the skin and mouth as well as the mucous membranes. They metastasize initially through the circulatory or lymphatic system and form solid tumors.
- **Sarcomas.** Sarcomas occur in the mesodermal, or middle, layers of tissue—for example, in bones, muscles, and general connective tissue. In the early stages of disease, they metastasize primarily via the blood. These cancers are less common but generally more virulent than carcinomas. They also form solid tumors.
- **Lymphomas.** Lymphomas develop in the lymphatic system—the infection-fighting regions of the body—and metastasize through the lymphatic system. Hodgkin's disease is an example. Lymphomas also form solid tumors.
- **Leukemias.** Cancer of the blood-forming parts of the body, particularly the bone marrow and spleen, is called leukemia. A nonsolid tumor, leukemia is characterized by an abnormal increase in the number of white blood cells that the body produces.

Figure 11.8 shows the most common sites of cancer and the estimated number of new cases and deaths from each type in 2017.

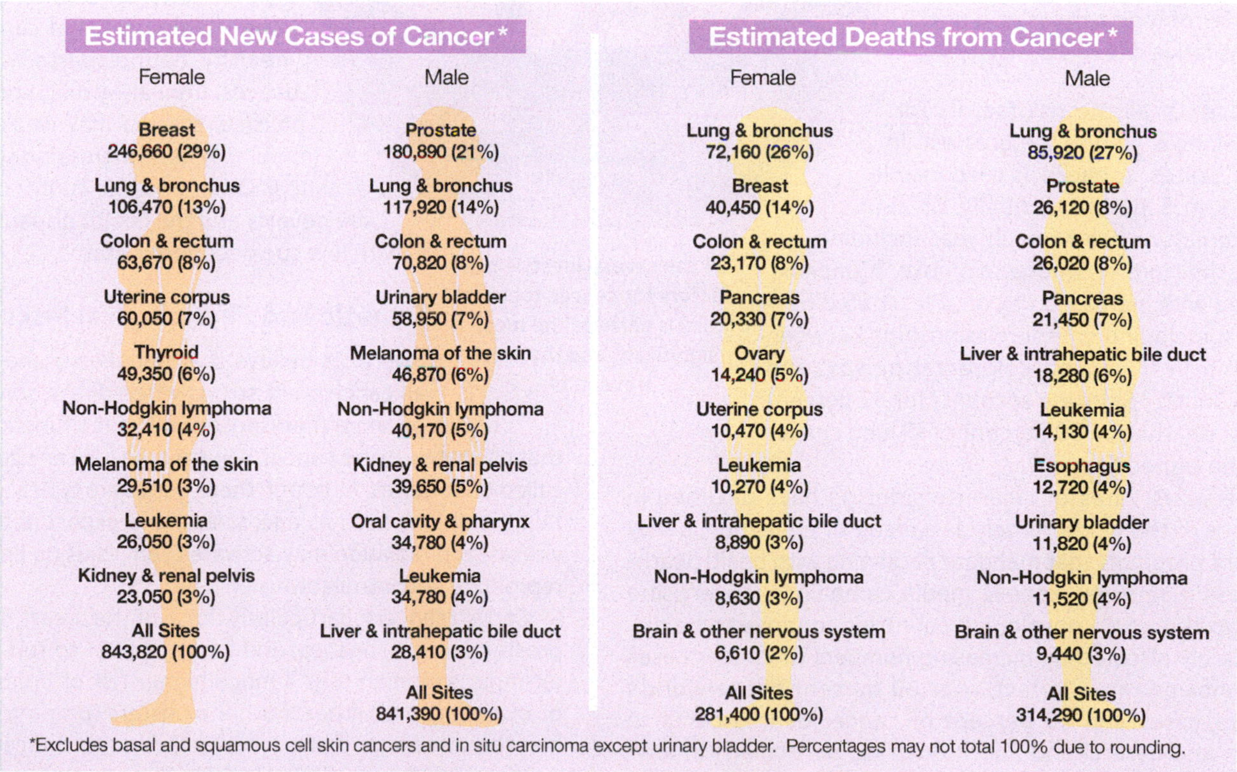

Estimated New Cases of Cancer*		Estimated Deaths from Cancer*	
Female	Male	Female	Male
Breast 246,660 (29%)	Prostate 180,890 (21%)	Lung & bronchus 72,160 (26%)	Lung & bronchus 85,920 (27%)
Lung & bronchus 106,470 (13%)	Lung & bronchus 117,920 (14%)	Breast 40,450 (14%)	Prostate 26,120 (8%)
Colon & rectum 63,670 (8%)	Colon & rectum 70,820 (8%)	Colon & rectum 23,170 (8%)	Colon & rectum 26,020 (8%)
Uterine corpus 60,050 (7%)	Urinary bladder 58,950 (7%)	Pancreas 20,330 (7%)	Pancreas 21,450 (7%)
Thyroid 49,350 (6%)	Melanoma of the skin 46,870 (6%)	Ovary 14,240 (5%)	Liver & intrahepatic bile duct 18,280 (6%)
Non-Hodgkin lymphoma 32,410 (4%)	Non-Hodgkin lymphoma 40,170 (5%)	Uterine corpus 10,470 (4%)	Leukemia 14,130 (4%)
Melanoma of the skin 29,510 (3%)	Kidney & renal pelvis 39,650 (5%)	Leukemia 10,270 (4%)	Esophagus 12,720 (4%)
Leukemia 26,050 (3%)	Oral cavity & pharynx 34,780 (4%)	Liver & intrahepatic bile duct 8,890 (3%)	Urinary bladder 11,820 (4%)
Kidney & renal pelvis 23,050 (3%)	Leukemia 34,780 (4%)	Non-Hodgkin lymphoma 8,630 (3%)	Non-Hodgkin lymphoma 11,520 (4%)
All Sites 843,820 (100%)	Liver & intrahepatic bile duct 28,410 (3%)	Brain & other nervous system 6,610 (2%)	Brain & other nervous system 9,440 (3%)
	All Sites 841,390 (100%)	All Sites 281,400 (100%)	All Sites 314,290 (100%)

*Excludes basal and squamous cell skin cancers and in situ carcinoma except urinary bladder. Percentages may not total 100% due to rounding.

Figure 11.8 Leading Sites of New Cancer Cases and Deaths, 2017 Estimates

Source: Data from American Cancer Society, *Cancer Facts and Figures* (Atlanta, GA: American Cancer Society; 2017). Note that percentages do not add up to 100, owing to omissions of certain rare cancers as well as rounding of statistics.

- What are the major types of cancer?
- What sites are the most common sites of cancer?

Risk Factors for Cancer

11.14 List lifestyle, genetic, environmental, and medical risk factors for cancer.

Specific risk factors for cancer fall into two major classes: hereditary risk and acquired (environmental) risk. Hereditary factors cannot be changed, whereas environmental factors are potentially modifiable.

Lifestyle Risks for Cancer

Anyone can develop cancer at any age or time. However, nearly 78 percent of cancers are diagnosed at age 55 and above.[68] *Lifetime risk* refers to the probability that an individual, over the course of a lifetime, will develop cancer or die from it. In the United States, men have a lifetime risk of about 42 percent, while women have a 33 percent risk.[69]

Relative risk is a measure of the strength of the relationship between risk factors and a particular cancer. Basically, it compares your risk of cancer if you engage in certain known risk behaviors with that of someone who does not. For example, men and women who smoke have 25 times the risk of lung cancer of a nonsmoker—a relative risk of 25.[70]

Tobacco Use Of all the risk factors for cancer, smoking is among the greatest. In the United States, tobacco is responsible for nearly 1 in 5 deaths annually, or about 480,000 premature deaths each year, including 42,000 deaths from secondhand smoke.[71] Smoking is associated with increased risk of at least 15 different cancers, including causal relationships between smoking and liver cancer, colorectal polyps, and colorectal cancer.[72] Smoking accounts for 32 percent of all cancer deaths and 80 percent of all lung cancer deaths in the United States.[73]

Over the years, rates of cigarette smoking have declined in many regions of the world, largely as a result of education, policy development programs that mandate packaging with health warnings and less glamorous appeal, media campaigns, advertising bans, and taxation. Still, developing countries continue to be disproportionately affected by increasing numbers of cancer cases and high smoking rates. In fact, over 60 percent of the world's total cancer cases and 70 percent of cancer deaths occur in Africa, Asia, and Central and South America, particularly in low- and middle-income countries.[74] Lung cancer continues to be the leading cause of cancer deaths globally.[75]

Alcohol Countless studies have implicated alcohol as a risk factor for cancer, particularly for oral cavity and pharynx, esophagus, colorectal, liver, larynx, and female breast cancer. There is

Of the several lifestyle risk factors for cancer, tobacco use is perhaps the most significant and the most preventable.

increasing evidence that moderate to high levels of drinking are associated with some other cancers such as pancreas and prostate cancer and melanoma.[76] Both men and women who binge-drink (more than 8 drinks per week for women and 15 drinks per week for men) significantly increase their risks of cancer.[77]

Poor Nutrition, Physical Inactivity, and Obesity Obesity may be a key contributor in 1 of 5 cancer deaths.[78] Dietary choices and physical activity are some of the most important modifiable determinants of cancer risk. Several studies indicate a relationship between a high BMI and death rates from cancers of the esophagus, colon, rectum, liver, stomach, kidney, pancreas, and others, as well as a high risk of endometrial cancer among younger women age 18 to 25 with higher BMIs and rapid weight gain.[79] Numerous other studies support the link between various forms of cancer and obesity.[80] The higher the BMI, the greater the cancer risk.[81]

Stress and Psychosocial Risks While a recent large meta-analytic study found no relationship between job strain and risk for colorectal, lung, breast, or prostate cancer, people who are under chronic, severe stress or who suffer from depression or other persistent emotional problems do show higher rates of cancer than their healthy counterparts.[82] Sleep disturbances, unhealthy diet, and emotional or physical trauma may weaken the body's immune system, increasing susceptibility to cancer. Other possible contributors to cancer are poverty and the health disparities associated with low socioeconomic status.

Genetic and Physiological Risks

Scientists believe that between 5 and 10 percent of all cancers are strongly hereditary; some people may be more predisposed to the malfunctioning of genes that ultimately cause cancer.[83] Suspected cancer-causing genes are called **oncogenes**. Although these genes are typically dormant, certain conditions such as age, stress, and exposure to carcinogens, viruses, and radiation may activate them, causing cells to grow and reproduce uncontrollably.

Certain cancers, particularly those of the breast, stomach, colon, prostate, uterus, ovaries, and lungs, appear to run in families. For example, a woman runs a much higher risk of breast cancer and/or ovarian cancer if her mother or sisters (primary relatives) have had the disease or if she inherits the breast cancer susceptibility genes (*BRCA1* or *BRCA2*). Hodgkin disease and certain leukemias show similar familial patterns. The complex interaction of hereditary predisposition, lifestyle, and environment on the development of cancer makes it a challenge to determine a single cause. Even among people who are predisposed to genetic mutations, avoiding risks may decrease the chances of developing cancer.

Reproductive and Hormonal Factors Having a higher than average number of fertile or menstrual cycle years (early menarche, late menopause), not having children or having them later in life, recent use of birth control pills or hormone replacement therapy, and opting not to breast-feed all appear to increase risks of breast cancer.[84] While the above factors appear to play a significant role in increased risk for non-Hispanic white women, they do not appear to have as strong an influence on Hispanic women, who may have more protective reproductive patterns (an overall lower age at first birth and a greater number of births). Hispanic women also use less hormone replacement therapy and have a lower utilization rate for mammograms, making comparisons difficult.[85]

Inflammation Risks

Inflammatory processes in the body are thought to play a significant role in the development of cancer—from initiation and promoting cancer cells to paving the way for these cells to invade, spread, and weaken the immune response. According to some researchers, 90 percent of cancers are caused by cellular mutations and environmental factors that occur as a result of inflammation, including chronic infections (up to 20 percent); tobacco smoking and particulates such as asbestos (30 percent);[86] and dietary factors and obesity (35 percent).[87] Inflammation appears to be a key factor in colorectal cancer, with gastrointestinal tract inflammatory problems having a higher risk of cancer development.[88]

Occupational and Environmental Risks

Several substances are known to cause cancer when exposure levels are high or prolonged. Asbestos, nickel, chromate, benzene, arsenic, and vinyl chloride are **carcinogens** (cancer-causing agents), as are certain dyes and radioactive substances, coal tars, inhalants, and possibly some herbicides and pesticides.

Radiation Ionizing radiation—radiation from X-rays, radon, cosmic rays, and ultraviolet radiation (primarily UVB radiation)—is has been proven to cause human cancer. Virtually any part of the body can be affected by ionizing radiation, but bone marrow and the thyroid are particularly susceptible. Radon exposure in homes can increase the risk for lung cancer, especially in cigarette smokers. To reduce the risk of harmful effects, diagnostic medical and dental X-rays are set at the lowest dose levels possible.

Nonionizing radiation produced by radio waves, cell phones, microwaves, computer screens, televisions, electric blankets, and other products has been an issue of great concern in recent years, though research to date has not proven excess risk.

Some forms of cancer have strong genetic bases. Daughters of women with breast cancer have an increased risk of developing the disease.

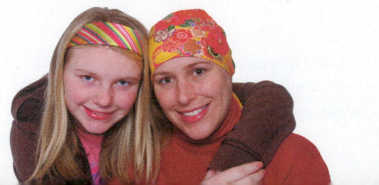

Chemicals in Foods Much of the concern about chemicals in food centers on possible harm from pesticide and herbicide residue. Continued research is essential, and scientists and consumer groups stress the importance of a balance between chemical use and the production of high-quality food products.

Infectious Disease Risks

Over 10 percent of all cancers in the United States and 15 to 20 percent worldwide are caused by infectious agents such as viruses, bacteria, or parasites.[89, 90] Infections are thought to influence cancer development in several ways, most commonly through chronic inflammation, suppression of the immune system, or chronic stimulation.

Hepatitis B, Hepatitis C, and Liver Cancer Viruses such as the ones that cause chronic forms of hepatitis B and C chronically inflame liver tissue, which may make it more hospitable for cancer development. Global increases in both hepatitis B and C rates and liver cancer indicate an association.

Human Papillomavirus and Cervical Cancer Every year in the United States, nearly 28,500 men and women get cancer linked to *human papillomavirus (HPV)* infection, which causes most cervical, vulvar, vaginal, anal, and oropharyngeal cancers in females and most oropharyngeal, anal, and penile cancers in males. HPV vaccinations can prevent infection as well as linked cancers.[91]

***Helicobacter pylori* and Stomach Cancer** *Helicobacter pylori* is a bacterium found in the stomach lining of approximately 30 percent of Americans.[92] It causes irritation, scarring, and ulcers, damaging the lining of the stomach and leading to cellular changes that may lead to cancer. More than half of all cases of stomach cancer may be linked to *H. pylori* infection. Treatment with antibiotics has been effective in treating and reducing risk of new stomach cancers.[93]

Medical Factors

Some medical treatments can increase a person's risk for cancer. Several studies have indicated that Hormone Replacement Therapy (HRT) used for relieving women's menopausal symptoms increases risk of breast and ovarian cancer; hence, the use of estrogen therapy has declined dramatically. However, recent research indicates that while women may have a slightly increased risk of these cancers, women on HRT therapy for many years have no greater risk of dying than those not on HRT. If you are concerned, talk with your doctor.[94] (Some chemotherapy drugs have been shown to increase risks for other cancers; weighing the benefits against the harms of these treatments is always necessary.

Check Yourself

- **What are some major lifestyle, genetic, environmental, and medical risk factors for cancer?**

- **What are your risks for cancer? What lifestyle changes can you make to mitigate these risks?**

11.15 Identify the major factors contributing to lung cancer.

While breast cancer is the most commonly diagnosed cancer in women, lung cancer is actually the number one cause of cancer death; in fact, lung cancer has killed more women than breast cancer for decades and is the leading cause of cancer deaths for both men and women in the United States. It killed an estimated 155,870 Americans in 2017, accounting for about 1 of 4 all cancer deaths.[95] About 2 of 3 people diagnosed with **lung cancer** are 65 of age or older, while fewer than 2 percent are younger than 45 years old. Risks begin to rise around age 40 and continue to climb thereafter.[96]

Detection, Symptoms, and Treatment

Symptoms of lung cancer include a persistent cough, blood-streaked sputum, voice change, chest or back pain, and recurrent attacks of pneumonia or bronchitis. CT scans, molecular markers in saliva, and newer biopsy techniques have improved the screening accuracy for lung cancer.

Treatment of lung cancer depends on the type and stage of cancer. Surgery, radiation therapy, chemotherapy, and targeted biological therapies are all options. If the cancer is localized, surgery is usually the treatment of choice. If it has spread, surgery is combined with radiation, chemotherapy, and other targeted drug treatments.

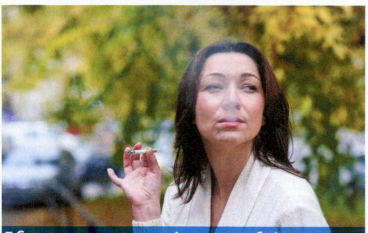

If my mom quits smoking now, will it reduce her risk of cancer, or is it too late?

It's never too late to quit. Stopping smoking at any time will reduce your risk of lung cancer, in addition to the numerous other health benefits that are gained. Studies of women have shown that within 5 years of quitting, their risk of death from lung cancer had decreased by 21 percent when compared with people who had continued smoking.

20–40% is the percentage of cancers that could be prevented if people quit smoking, avoided heavy drinking, kept a healthy weight, and got just half an hour per day of moderate exercise.

Unfortunately, fewer than 15 percent of lung cancer cases are diagnosed at the early, localized stages, since symptoms don't present until the cancer is well advanced. This is one reason that lung cancer is particularly deadly: While nearly half of people diagnosed with the earliest stage lung cancers survive for at least 5 years, those diagnosed in later stages have 5-year survival rates ranging between 1 and 14 percent.[97]

Risk Factors and Prevention

Tobacco use is the number one factor that leads to lung cancer; over 80 percent of cases occur among smokers.[98] On a positive note, as rates of tobacco use have declined in many countries, so have the rates of lung cancer. However, smoking continues to be a habit more common among people with less education and lower incomes, meaning that the most disadvantaged people in society tend also to have a high risk for this disease. Risks for cancer increase dramatically on the basis of the quantity of cigarettes smoked and the number of years smoked, often referred to as *pack-years*. The higher the number of pack-years, the greater the risk of developing cancer. Quitting smoking reduces the risk of developing lung cancer.[99] Exposure to industrial substances or radiation also highly increases the risk for lung cancer.

Between 15 and 20 percent of all lung cancers occur among *never smokers*—people who have avoided using tobacco. Never smokers' lung cancer is believed to be related to exposure to radon gas, secondhand smoke, asbestos, indoor wood-burning stoves, and aerosolized oils caused by cooking with oil and deep fat frying.[100] Unfortunately, because health care providers often don't think of lung cancer when a never smoker presents with a cough, patients are often put on antibiotics or cough suppressants as therapy. By the time they recognize that it's really lung cancer, their cancer is likely to be more advanced and treatment more challenging.

- What is lung cancer, and what are its causes?
- How can you protect yourself against lung cancer?
- What are the symptoms and treatment of lung cancer?

11.16 Identify the major factors contributing to colorectal cancer.

Colorectal cancers (cancers of the colon and rectum) are the thirdmost commonly diagnosed cancer in both men and women, as well as the second leading cause of cancer deaths in men and the third leading cause of death in women. [101] In 2017, an estimated 95,520 cases of colon cancer and 39,910 cases of rectal cancer were diagnosed in the United States, and 50,260 deaths were attributed to colon or rectal cancer.[102]

While rates of colon cancer appear to be declining in people over age 50, they are increasing among those under age 50, largely driven by increased rates of rectal cancer.[103] Younger men and women have approximately a 1 in 300 risk of developing colon and rectal cancer from birth to age 49, and the risk increases to about 1 in 21 to 22 later in life.[104]

Detection, Symptoms, and Treatment

Because colorectal cancer tends to spread slowly, the 5-year survival rate for cases that are diagnosed in the early, localized stages is over 90 percent, compared to 14 percent if it has spread to other areas of the body.[105] However, because early stages are often asymptomatic, many cases are diagnosed at later stages when the cancer is more difficult to treat. As the disease progresses, bleeding from the rectum, blood in the stool, and changes in bowel habits are the major warning signals.

An excellent way to catch colorectal cancers early is through screening tests. Most people should begin having colonoscopies at age 50. Virtual colonoscopies and fecal DNA testing are newer, less invasive diagnostic techniques that have shown promise. The most basic screening test—the at-home *fecal occult blood test*—simply detects blood in stool, which is a warning sign that cancer may be present.

However, although several early detection options are available (see Module 11.22), and rates of screening have increased, 35 percent of whites, 38 percent of blacks, 46 percent of Hispanics, and 51 percent of Asians over the age of 50 have not been screened. Screening rates were lowest among the uninsured (25 percent) and immigrants who had resided in the United States fewer than 10 years (34 percent).[106]

Treatment for colorectal cancer typically consists of radiation or surgery. Chemotherapy, although not used extensively in the past, is today a possibility.

Risk Factors and Prevention

Anyone can get colorectal cancer, but people who are older than age 50, who are obese, who have a family history of colon and rectal cancer, who have a personal or family history of polyps (benign growths) in the colon or rectum, or who have inflammatory bowel

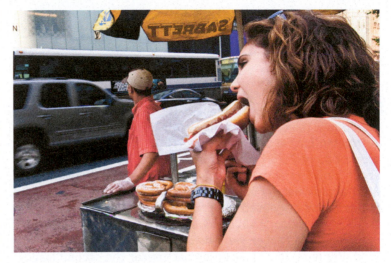

The consumption of red meat and processed meats is a risk factor for colorectal cancer, as is obesity. Food additives, particularly sodium nitrate, are used to preserve and give color to red meat and to protect against pathogens, particularly *Clostridium botulinum*, the bacterium that causes botulism. Concern about the carcinogenic properties of nitrates, which are often used in hot dogs, hams, and luncheon meats, has led to the introduction of meats that are nitrate-free or contain reduced levels of the substance.

problems such as colitis are at increased risk. A history of diabetes also seems to increase risk.

Other possible risk factors include diets that are high in fat or low in fiber, high consumption of red and processed meats, smoking, a sedentary lifestyle, a high level of alcohol consumption, and low intake of fruits and vegetables. New research shows an alarming increase in colorectal cancer among young adults age 20 to 49.[107]

Regular exercise, a diet with lots of fruits and other plant foods, a healthy weight, and moderation in alcohol consumption appear to be among the most promising prevention strategies.

Some studies indicate that taking NSAIDs and consumption of certain vitamins and minerals, including calcium, folic acid, selenium, and vitamin E, may also help. However, studies on these diet- and drug-related factors are conflicting, so further research must be done.[108]

- What is colorectal cancer, and what are its causes?

- What can you do to protect against colorectal cancer?

11.17 Breast Cancer

Learning Outcome

11.17 Identify the major factors contributing to breast cancer.

Breast cancer is a group of diseases that cause uncontrolled cell growth in breast tissue, particularly in the glands that produce milk and the ducts that connect those glands to the nipple. Cancers can also form in the connective and lymphatic tissues of the breast.

Women have a 1 in 8 lifetime risk of being diagnosed with breast cancer.[109] For women from birth to age 49, the chance is about 1 in 53; rates are significantly higher after menopause.[110] In 2017, approximately 252,710 women and 2,500 men in the United States will be diagnosed with invasive breast cancer for the first time.[111] In addition, 63,500 new cases of *in situ* breast cancer, a more localized cancer, were diagnosed.[112] Over 40,600 women (and 450 men) died, making breast cancer the second leading cause of cancer death for women.[113]

Detection

The earliest signs of breast cancer are usually observable on mammograms, often before lumps can be felt. However, mammograms are not foolproof, and there is debate about the age at which women should start having them done regularly. Hence, regular breast self-examination (BSE) can also be useful (see below for information on BSE). A newer form of MRI, though not recommended as a screening tool per se, appears to be even more accurate than mammograms, particularly in women with genetic risks for tumors or those who have suspicious areas of the breast or surrounding tissue that warrant a clearer image. If you are referred for a breast MRI, be sure to go to a facility where a breast biopsy can be performed if there are any areas that need further investigation.[114]

Symptoms

If a breast cancer grows large enough, it can produce the following symptoms: a lump in the breast or surrounding lymph nodes, thickening, dimpling, skin irritation, distortion, retraction or scaliness of the nipple, nipple discharge, or tenderness.

Breast Awareness and Self-Examination

For decades, the BSE was endorsed by many health organizations as an important cancer detection method. However, in more recent years, studies have shown that BSEs did not lead to earlier detection of cancer and sometimes increased worry and resulted in further invasive or unnecessary testing. Therefore, the

U.S. Preventive Services Task Force no longer strongly promotes doing the BSE on a monthly basis. However, it still recommends that women "learn how to do them, and if you desire, do them to know your body and be able to recognize changes."[115] Figure 11.9 depicts how to do a BSE.

To do a BSE, begin by standing in front of a mirror to inspect your breasts, looking for their usual symmetry. Some breasts are not symmetrical, and if this is not a change for yours, it is okay. Raise and lower both arms while checking that the breasts move evenly and freely. Next, inspect the skin, looking for areas of redness, thickening, or dimpling, which might have the appearance of an orange peel. Look for any scaling on the nipple.

To feel for lumps, raise one arm above your head while either standing or lying. This will flatten out the breast, making it easier to feel the tissue. Using the index, middle, and fourth fingers of your opposite hand, gently push down on the breast tissue and move the fingers in small circular motions, varying pressure from light to more firm. Start at one edge of the breast and move upward and then downward, working your way across the breast until all of the breast tissue has been covered. Often, breast tissue will feel dense and irregular, and this is usually normal. It helps to do regular BSEs to become familiar with what your breast tissue feels like; then, if there is a change, you will notice. Cancers usually feel like a dense or firm little rock and are very different from normal breast tissue.

Next, lower the arm, reach into the top of the underarm, and pull downward with gentle pressure, feeling for any enlarged lymph nodes. To complete the exam, squeeze the tissue around the nipple. If you notice discharge from the nipple and you have not recently been breastfeeding, consult your health care provider. Likewise, if you notice any asymmetry, skin changes, scaling on the nipple, or new lumps in the breast, you should see your health care provider for evaluation.

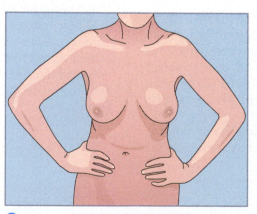

❶ Face a mirror and check for changes in symmetry.

❷ Either standing or lying down, use the pads of the three middle fingers to check for lumps. Follow an up and down pattern on the breast to ensure all tissue gets inspected.

Figure 11.9 Breast Self-Examination

Treatment

Treatments for breast cancer range from a lumpectomy to radical mastectomy to various combinations of radiation or chemotherapy. Among nonsurgical options, promising results have been noted in women using *selective estrogen-receptor modulators (SERMs)* such as tamoxifen and raloxifene, particularly women whose cancers appear to grow in response to estrogen. These drugs, as well as new *aromatase inhibitors*, work by blocking estrogen. The 5-year survival rate for people with localized breast cancer has risen from 80 percent in the 1950s to over 90 percent today.[116] However, these statistics vary dramatically according to the stage of the cancer when it is first detected and whether it has spread. The survival rate for black women is 11 percent lower overall than that for white women, largely because of the stage of the cancer at diagnosis.[117]

Risk Factors and Prevention

The incidence of breast cancer increases with age. Although there are many possible risk factors, the ones that are well supported by research are family history of breast cancer, menstrual periods that started early and ended late in life, weight gain after the age of 18, obesity after menopause, recent use of oral contraceptives or postmenopausal hormone replacement therapy, never bearing children or bearing a first child after age 30, consuming two or more drinks of alcohol per day, and physical inactivity. Other factors that increase risk include smoking, having dense breasts, type 2 diabetes, high bone mineral density, shift work and sleep deprivation, dietary risks, and exposure to high-dose radiation.[118] Although the *BRCA1* and *BRCA2* gene mutations are rare and occur in less than 1 percent of the population, they account for approximately 5 to 10 percent of all cases of breast cancer.[119] (For more

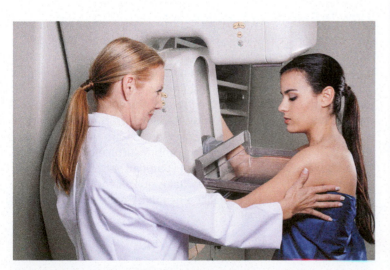

Early detection through mammography and other techniques greatly increases a woman's chance of surviving breast cancer.

What are some of the challenges facing cancer survivors?

The journey through cancer survivorship is not always smooth. Even after the 5-year benchmark has been reached, living a full, positive life in cancer's wake can be a major challenge. There may be physical, emotional, and financial issues to cope with for years after diagnosis and treatment. Survivors may find themselves struggling with access to health insurance and life insurance, financial strains, difficulties with employment, and the toll on personal relationships. Survivors also have to live with the possibility of a recurrence. However, cancer survivors can and do live active, productive lives despite these challenges.

information on who is at risk for inherited breast cancer, see http://ww5.komen.org/BreastCancer/InheritedGeneticMutations.html.)

International differences in breast cancer incidence correlate with variations in diet, especially fat intake, although a causal role for these dietary factors has not been firmly established. Sudden weight gain has also been implicated. Research also shows that regular exercise, particularly at higher than recommended rates, can reduce risk of breast cancer, colon cancer, diabetes, and CVD.[120]

Check Yourself

- What is breast cancer, and what are its causes?
- What can you do to protect against breast cancer?

11.18 Identify the major factors contributing to prostate and testicular cancer.

Prostate Cancer

After skin cancer, prostate cancer is the most frequently diagnosed cancer in American males with approximately 151,360 new cases in 2017.[121] It is the third leading cause of cancer deaths in men, killing an estimated 26,730 men in 2017.[122] However, with improved screening and early diagnosis, 5-year survival rates are nearly 100 percent for all but the most advanced cases, which have a much more bleak outcome, with only 29 percent surviving.[123]

Detection, Symptoms, and Treatment The prostate is a muscular, walnut-sized gland that surrounds part of a man's urethra, the tube that transports urine and sperm out of the body. The prostate is a part of the reproductive system, its primary function being to produce seminal fluid. Symptoms of prostate cancer may include weak or interrupted urine flow; difficulty starting or stopping urination; feeling the urge to urinate frequently; pain on urination; blood in the urine; or pain in the low back, pelvis, or thighs. Many men have no symptoms in the early stages.

Men over age 40 should have an annual digital rectal prostate examination. Another screening method for prostate cancer is the **prostate-specific antigen (PSA)** test, a blood test that screens for an indicator of prostate cancer. However, the U.S. Preventive Services Task Force recommends that otherwise asymptomatic men no longer receive the routine PSA test because, overall, it does not save lives and may lead to unnecessary treatments. If you have a family history or other symptoms, consult your health care provider.

Risk Factors and Prevention Increasing age is one of the biggest risks for prostate cancer, as are African ancestry and a family history of prostate cancer. Over 97 percent of cases occur in men over the age of 50.[124] Genetics may account for between 5 and 10 percent of prostate cancers overall. Black men in the United States and Caribbean men of African descent have the highest documented prostate cancer incidence rates in the world. They are also more likely to be diagnosed at more advanced stages than other racial groups.[125] Having a father or brother with prostate cancer more than doubles a man's risk of getting prostate cancer. Men who have had several relatives with prostate cancer, especially those with relatives who developed prostate cancer at younger ages, are also at higher risk.[126]

Eating more fruits and vegetables, particularly those containing lycopene, a pigment found in tomatoes and other red fruits, may lower the risk of prostate cancer death.[127] Diets that are high in processed meats or dairy and obesity appear to increase risks.[128] The best advice is to follow recommendations for a balanced diet and to maintain a healthy weight.

Testicular Cancer

Testicular cancer is one of the most common types of solid tumors found in young adult men, affecting nearly 8,720 young men in 2017.[129] Over one-half of all cases occur between the ages of 20 and 34, with steady increases in this group in the last few years.[130]

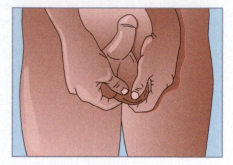

Figure 11.10 Testicular Self-Examination

However, with a 95 percent 5-year survival rate, it is one of the most curable forms of cancer, particularly if caught in localized stages. Men with undescended testicles appear to be at greater risk, and some studies indicate a genetic influence. Risk is also higher if you are white, if you have HIV or AIDS, or if a primary relative (father or brother, in particular) has had testicular cancer.[131]

Testicular Self-Examination

Testicular tumors first appear as an enlargement of the testis or thickening in testicular tissue. Some men report a heavy feeling, a dull ache, or pain that extends to the lower abdomen or groin area. Testicular self-examinations have long been recommended for teen boys and young men to perform monthly as a means of detecting testicular cancer (see **Figure 11.10**). However, recent studies discovered that findings from monthly self-exams result in testing for noncancerous conditions and thus are not cost-effective. For this reason, the U.S. Preventive Services Task Force has dropped its recommendation for monthly testicular self-exams. Regardless, most cases of testicular cancer are discovered through self-exam, and there is currently no other screening test for the disease.

How To Examine Your Testicles

The testicular self-exam is best done after a hot shower, which will relax the scrotum and make the exam easier. Standing in front of a mirror, hold the testicle with one hand while gently rolling its surface between the thumb and fingers of your other hand. Feel underneath the scrotum for the tubes of the epididymis and blood vessels that sit close to the body. Repeat with the other testicle. Be attentive for any lump, thickening, or pea-like nodules and any areas that may be painful over the entire surface of the scrotum. When done, wash your hands with soap and water. Doing regular self-exams will help you to know what is normal for you and to note any deviation from that. Consult a health care provider if you note anything that is unusual.

- **What are prostate and testicular cancer, and what are their causes?**

11.18 Cardiovascular Disease, Cancer, and Diabetes

11.19 Skin Cancer

Learning Outcome

11.19 Identify the major factors contributing to skin cancer.

Skin cancer is the most common form of cancer in the United States today, with millions of cases occurring each year. The exact number of cases remains in question, since skin cancer incidence isn't reported to cancer registries as other types of cancer are. The good news is that most cases are either **basal cell carcinoma** or **squamous cell carcinoma**, which are highly treatable and not life-threatening. Most skin cancer deaths—nearly 10,000 in 2017—are caused by a much more serious form of skin cancer known as **malignant melanoma**, which affects over 87,000 people in the United States each year.[132] The majority of these deaths are in white men over the age of 50, with only rare cases among African Americans.

Detection, Symptoms, and Treatment

Basal and squamous cell carcinomas typically develop on the face, ears, neck, arms, hands, and legs as warty bumps, colored spots, or scaly patches. Bleeding, itchiness, pain, and oozing may occur. Although surgery may be necessary to remove these carcinomas, they seldom spread and are typically not life threatening.

In striking contrast is melanoma, an invasive killer that may appear as a skin lesion. Typically, the lesion's size, shape, or color changes, and it spreads to regional organs and throughout the body. If melanoma has not yet penetrated the underlying layers of skin, chances of survival are over 98 percent. However, if it is diagnosed after deeper layers of skin have been penetrated and it has spread to other organs, the survival rate falls to 17 percent.[133] **Figure 11.11** shows melanoma compared to basal cell and squamous cell carcinomas. The *ABCDE rule* can help you remember the warning signs of melanoma:

- **Asymmetry.** One half does not match the other half.
- **Border irregularity.** Edges are uneven, notched, or scalloped.
- **Color.** Pigmentation is not uniform. Melanomas may vary in color from tan to deeper brown, reddish black, black, or deep bluish black.

- **Diameter.** Diameter is greater than 6 millimeters (about the size of a pea).
- **Evolving.** Size, symmetry, shape, color, border, or other characteristics change over time.

Depending on the type, stage, and location of the cancer, treatment options include surgery, laser treatments, topical chemical agents, *electrodessication* (tissue destruction by heat), and *cryosurgery* (tissue destruction by freezing). For melanoma, treatment may involve surgical removal of the regional lymph nodes, radiation, or chemotherapy.

Risk Factors and Prevention

Anyone who overexposes himself or herself to ultraviolet (UV) radiation without adequate protection is at risk for skin cancer. This usually comes from sun exposure, but people who use tanning booths or beds are also at risk. The risk is greatest for people who:

- Have fair skin and light eyes;
- Always burn before tanning or burn easily and peel readily;
- Don't tan easily but spend lots of time outdoors;
- Use no or low-SPF (sun protection factor) or expired sunscreens;
- Have had skin cancer or have a family history of skin cancer;
- Experienced severe sunburns during childhood.

Preventing skin cancer is a matter of limiting exposure to harmful UV rays. The skin responds to exposure to these rays by increasing its thickness and the number of pigment cells (melanocytes), which produce darker, tanned skin. Ultraviolet light damages the skin's immune cells, lowering the normal immune protection of skin and priming it for cancer. Photodamage also causes wrinkling by impairing collagens that keep skin soft and pliable.

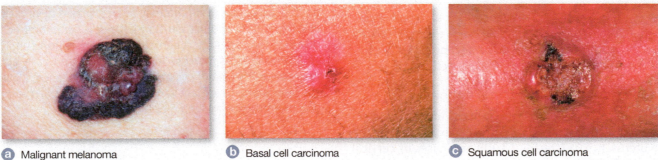

(a) Malignant melanoma   (b) Basal cell carcinoma   (c) Squamous cell carcinoma

Figure 11.11 Types of Skin Cancers
Preventing skin cancer includes keeping a careful watch for any new, pigmented growths and for changes to any moles. The ABCD warning signs of melanoma (a) include *asymmetrical* shapes, irregular *borders*, *color* variation, and an increase in *diameter*. Basal cell carcinoma (b) and squamous cell carcinoma (c) should be brought to your health care provider's attention but are not as deadly as melanoma.

Check Yourself

- **What is skin cancer, and what are its causes?**
- **What can you do to protect against skin cancer?**

11.20 Know the signs and symptoms of ovarian and uterine cancers, leukemia, and lymphoma.

Ovarian Cancer

Ovarian cancer is the fifth leading cause of cancer deaths for women, with nearly 23,000 diagnoses in 2017 and just over 14,000 deaths.[134] Ovarian cancer causes more deaths than any other cancer of the reproductive system because women tend not to discover it until the cancer is at an advanced stage, when the 5-year survival rate is only 29 percent.[135] Women under the age of 45 are much more likely to survive 5 years than are women age 65 or older. The average 5 year survival rate when all stages are combined is only 46 percent.[136]

A woman with ovarian cancer may complain of feeling bloated, having pain in the pelvic area, feeling full quickly, or feeling the need to urinate more frequently. Some may experience persistent digestive disturbances; other symptoms include fatigue, pain during intercourse, unexplained weight loss, unexplained changes in bowel or bladder habits, and incontinence. If these vague symptoms persist for more than a week or two, prompt medical evaluation is a must.

Early-stage treatment for ovarian cancer typically includes surgery, chemotherapy, and occasionally radiation. Depending on the patient's age and desire to bear children, one or both ovaries, fallopian tubes, and the uterus may be removed.

Primary relatives (mother, daughter, sister) of a woman who has had ovarian cancer are at increased risk. A family or personal history of breast or colon cancer is also associated with increased risk. Women who have never been pregnant are more likely to develop ovarian cancer than are those who have given birth to a child. The more children a woman has had, the less risk she faces. The use of postmenopausal estrogen replacement therapy may increase a woman's risk. Use of talcum powder, smoking, and obesity are other risk factors.[137] Using birth control pills, adhering to a low-fat diet, having multiple children, and breastfeeding appear to reduce the risk of ovarian cancer.[138]

To protect yourself from ovarian cancer, get a complete pelvic examination. Women over 40 should have a cancer-related checkup every year. Uterine ultrasound or a blood test is recommended for those with risk factors or unexplained symptoms.

Cervical and Endometrial (Uterine) Cancer

Most uterine cancers develop in the body of the uterus, usually in the endometrium. The rest develop in the cervix, located at the base of the uterus. In 2017, nearly 13,000 new cases of cervical cancer and over 60,000 cases of endometrial cancer were diagnosed in the United States, with nearly 15,000 combined deaths.[139] As more women have regular **Pap test** screenings—a procedure in which cells taken from the cervical region are examined for abnormal activity—rates of these cancers should decline even further. Pap tests are very effective for detecting early-stage cervical cancer, though less effective for detecting cancers of the uterine

lining. Women have a lifetime risk of 1 in 161 for being diagnosed with cervical cancer and a 1 in 36 risk of being diagnosed with uterine corpus cancer.[140] Early warning signs of uterine cancer include bleeding outside the normal menstrual period or after menopause or persistent unusual vaginal discharge.

Risk factors for cervical cancer include early age at first intercourse, multiple sex partners, cigarette smoking, and certain sexually transmitted infections, including HPV (the cause of genital warts) and herpes. For endometrial cancer, age, estrogen, and obesity are strong risk factors. Risks are increased by treatment with tamoxifen for breast cancer, metabolic syndrome, late menopause, never bearing children, history of polyps in the uterus or ovaries, history of other cancers, and race, white women being at higher risk.[141]

Leukemia and Lymphoma

Leukemia is a cancer of the blood-forming tissues that leads to proliferation of millions of immature white blood cells. These abnormal cells crowd out normal white blood cells (which fight infection), platelets (which control hemorrhaging), and red blood cells (which carry oxygen to body cells). This results in symptoms such as fatigue, paleness, weight loss, easy bruising, repeated infections, nosebleeds, and other forms of hemorrhaging.

Leukemia can be acute or chronic and can strike both sexes and all age groups. An estimated 62,130 new cases were diagnosed in the United States in 2017.[142] Chronic leukemia can develop over several months or years and have few symptoms in the early stages. It is usually treated with radiation and chemotherapy. Other methods of treatment include bone marrow and stem cell transplants.

Lymphomas, a group of cancers of the lymphatic system that include Hodgkin's disease and non-Hodgkin lymphoma, are among the fastest growing cancers, with an estimated 80,500 new cases in 2017.[143] Much of this increase has occurred in women. The cause is unknown; however, a weakened immune system is suspected, particularly one that has been exposed to viruses such as HIV, hepatitis C, and Epstein-Barr virus or is compromised through diseases like lupus, or rheumatoid arthritis. Interestingly, Hodgkin's disease rates increase in adolescence and early adulthood, decrease in the middle years, and like many cancers, increase in the later years. Treatment varies by type and stage; chemotherapy and radiotherapy are commonly used.

- What are the signs and symptoms of ovarian and uterine cancers, leukemia, and lymphoma?

11.20

Cardiovascular Disease, Cancer, and Diabetes

11.21 Mindfulness-Based Interventions for Cancer Patients

11.21 Describe some mindfulness-based interventions that have proven effective in helping people deal with cancer diagnosis, treatment, and long-term survival.

Imagine that you have just noticed a lump somewhere on your body. After probing, scans, and a biopsy, your worst fear becomes reality: You have cancer. You are scared and feel alone. Facing such a diagnosis, many people go through similar stages of emotional turmoil: They feel pain and anxiety during treatment, and even if they're cleared of cancer, fear remains. Is the cancer really gone, or is it still lurking?

Coping with Cancer Takes More Than Just Medicine

Increasingly, cancer experts realize that people need help battling that alien entity in their bodies—the one that is beating them up physically and emotionally, sapping their strength when they need it most. Some efforts have focused on *mindfulness-based* *interventions (MBIs)* for cancer survivor care.[144] MBIs have consistently proven effective in helping people deal with diagnosis, treatment, and life as survivors. They help individuals cope with loss of control, uncertainty about the future, and fear of recurrence. In addition, these interventions can help with psychological and physiological realities of treatment, including pain, anxiety, anger, sleeplessness, fatigue, and depression.

MBI participants learn skills to help them refocus on the things that are important to them in the present moment. Through meditation, *mindfulness-based stress reduction (MBSR)*, yoga, and other spirituality-based techniques, survivors can move through the stages of grieving for themselves and focus outward again.

MBSR programs are typically 8 weeks long with sessions that last for 2 to 3 hours each week, usually in small groups. *Mindfulness-based cancer recovery (MBCR)* programs that focus specifically on the unique challenges of coping with cancer survivorship are also available and results are promising. Most cancer treatment programs include MBSR, relaxation, and meditation programs for survivors and family members.

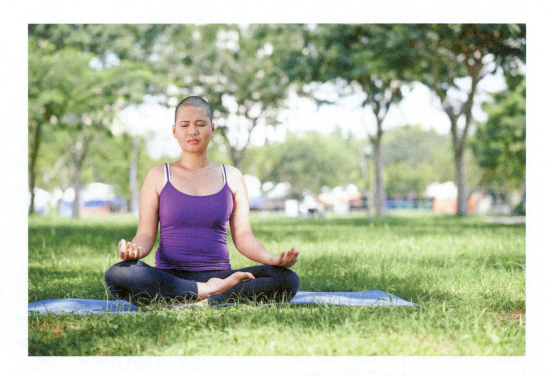

Check Yourself

- Name some of the mental health issues that arise during cancer treatment, and describe some mindfulness based interventions that can help patients cope with these challenges.

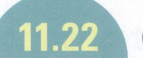
for Cancer Patients

11.22 **Describe several common cancer detection and treatment options.**

Detecting Cancer

Magnetic resonance imaging (MRI) uses a powerful electromagnet to detect tumors by mapping the vibrations of atoms in the body on a computer screen. The **computerized axial tomography (CAT) scan** uses X-rays to examine parts of the body. *Prostatic ultrasound* (a rectal probe that uses ultrasonic waves to produce an image of the prostate) is being investigated as a means to increase early detection of prostate cancer, combined with the PSA blood test. Mammography is a specialized X-ray technique that can detect abnormalities in the breast. New 3D mammogram machines offer significant improvements in imaging and breast cancer detection, but with the tradeoff that they deliver nearly double the radiation risk of conventional mammogram equipment. Finally, if scans detect possible cancer, very often a biopsy (removal of suspected abnormal tissue) is done so that the sample can be analyzed for cell type by a laboratory. Table 11.4 shows screening recommendations for selected cancers.

Cancer Treatments

Surgery to remove the tumor and surrounding tissue may be performed alone or with other treatments. The surgeon may operate using traditional surgical instruments or a laser, laparoscope, or other tools.

Stereotactic radiosurgery, also known as **gamma knife surgery**, uses a targeted dose of gamma radiation to zap tumors without any blood loss. **Radiotherapy** (use of radiation) and **chemotherapy** (use of drugs) are also used to kill cancerous cells. Radiation is most effective in treating localized cancer because it can be targeted to a particular area. Side effects of radiotherapy include fatigue, changes to skin in the affected area, and slightly greater chances of developing another type of cancer.

Chemotherapy may be used to shrink a tumor before or after surgery or radiation therapy or on its own. Powerful drugs are administered, usually in cycles so that the body can recover from their effects. Side effects, which may include nausea, hair loss, fatigue, and increased chance of bleeding, bruising, infection, and anemia, fade after treatment. Other effects, such as loss of fertility, may be permanent. Long-term damage to the cardiovascular and other body systems from radiotherapy and chemotherapy can be significant.

Participation in clinical trials (people-based studies of new drugs or procedures) has provided hope for many. Deciding whether to participate in a clinical trial can be difficult. Despite the risks, which should be carefully considered, thousands of clinical trial participants have benefited from treatments that would otherwise have been unavailable to them.

77% of cancers are diagnosed in adults age 55 or older.

Before beginning any form of cancer therapy, be a vigilant and vocal consumer. Read and seek information from cancer support groups. Check the skills of your surgeon, radiation therapist, and doctor in terms of clinical experience and interpersonal interactions. Look at Oncovin and other websites supported by the National Cancer Institute and the American Cancer Society to check out clinical trials, reports on treatment effectiveness, experimental therapies, and so forth. And although you might like and trust your family health care provider, it is always a good idea to seek consultation or advice from larger cancer facilities.

Newer Treatments

Surgery, chemotherapy, and radiation therapy remain the most common cancer treatments. However, newer techniques may be more effective for certain cancers or certain patients, and exciting new advances offer promising options for individuals. See https://

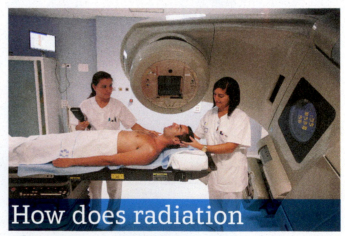

How does radiation therapy work?

Radiation therapy is often used to target and destroy cancerous tumors. The machine in this photograph emits gamma rays, which are typically used to treat localized secondary cancers, and also provide pain relief for otherwise untreatable cancers. Gamma rays are less powerful than the X-rays emitted from linear accelerators, another machine frequently used in radiation therapy.

11.4 Screening Guidelines for Early Cancer Detection in Average Risk and Asymptomatic People

Cancer Site	Screening Procedure	Age and Frequency of Test
Breast	Mammogram	The National Cancer Institute recommends that women in their forties and older have mammograms every 1 to 2 years. Women who are at higher-than-average risk of breast cancer should talk with their health care provider about whether to have mammograms before age 40 and how often to have them.
Cervix	Pap test (Pap smear)	Women should begin having Pap tests 3 years after they begin having sexual intercourse or when they reach age 21 (whichever comes first). Most women should have a Pap test at least once every 3 years.
Colon and rectum	*Fecal occult blood test:* Sometimes cancer or polyps bleed. This test can detect tiny amounts of blood in the stool. *Sigmoidoscopy:* Checks the rectum and lower part of the colon for polyps. *Colonoscopy:* Checks the rectum and entire colon for polyps and cancer.	People age 50 and older should be screened. People who have a higher-than-average risk of cancer of the colon or rectum should talk with their health care provider about whether to have screening tests before age 50 and how often to have them.
Prostate	Prostate-specific antigen (PSA) test	Some groups encourage yearly screening for men over age 50, and some advise men who are at a higher risk for prostate cancer to begin screening at age 40 or 45. Others caution against routine screening. Currently, Medicare provides coverage for an annual PSA test for all men age 50 and older.

Source: National Cancer Institute, National Institutes of Health, "What You Need to Know about Cancer Screening," www.cancer.gov; National Cancer Institute, "Fact Sheet, Prostate-Specific Antigen (PSA) Test," www.cancer.gov.

www.cancer.gov/research/areas/treatment/immunotherapy-using-immune-system for more information on the various types of immunotherapy and other treatments.

- **Immunotherapy.** Immunotherapy is designed to enhance the body's disease-fighting systems and use the immune system to actually fight cancer. Essentially, immunotherapy increases the strength of immune response against tumors or counteract cancer cell signals that suppress immune response.
- **Biological therapies.** *Cancer-fighting vaccines* alert the body's immune defenses to cells gone bad. Rather than preventing disease as other vaccines do, they help people who are already ill.
- **Gene therapies.** Viruses may carry genetic information that makes the cells they infect (such as cancer cells) susceptible to an antiviral drug. Scientists are also looking at ways to transfer genes that increase immune response to the cancerous tumor or that confer drug resistance to bone marrow so higher doses of chemotherapeutic drugs can be given.
- **Angiogenesis inhibitors.** Some compounds may stop tumors from forming new blood vessels, a process called *angiogenesis.* Without adequate blood supply, tumors either die or grow very slowly.
- **Disruption of cancer pathways.** Steps in the *cancer pathway* include oncogene actions, hormone receptors, growth factors, metastasis, and angiogenesis. Preliminary studies are underway to design compounds that inhibit actions at each of these steps.

- **Smart drugs.** *Targeted smart-drug therapies* attack only the cancer cells, not the entire body.
- **Enzyme inhibitors.** An enzyme inhibitor, *TIMP2*, shows promise for slowing metastasis of tumor cells. A metastasis suppressor gene, *NM23*, has also been identified.
- **Neoadjuvant chemotherapy.** This method uses chemotherapy to shrink the tumor before surgically removing it.
- **Stem cell transplants.** Transplants of healthy stem cells from donor bone marrow are used to treat cancers of the blood when a patient's bone marrow has been destroyed by disease, chemotherapy, or radiation.

Check Yourself

- What are the screening recommendations for several common cancers?
- Have you been screened for any cancers for which you might be at risk? Why or why not?
- What are some traditional and new treatments for cancer?

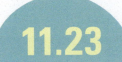

What Is Diabetes?

11.23 Explain the development of diabetes, distinguish between type 1 and type 2 diabetes, and describe the overall world trend in diabetes incidence.

Diabetes mellitus is actually a group of diseases, each with its own mechanism but all characterized by a persistently high level of glucose (sugar) in the blood. High blood glucose levels (known as **hyperglycemia**) can lead to widespread damage in the body. Serious health conditions related to diabetes include heart disease, stroke, failure of wounds on extremities to heal (leading to infection and amputations), nerve damage, kidney failure, liver damage, and blindness. (See Module 11.24 for more on complications.)

In 2015, diabetes was the primary cause of death for over 79,000 Americans.[145] An estimated 1.6 million deaths were directly caused by diabetes worldwide that same year.[146]

In a healthy person, carbohydrates from foods are broken down into a monosaccharide called *glucose*, which is the preferred fuel most body cells use to conduct many other necessary metabolic functions. Whenever a surge of glucose enters the bloodstream from the digestive system, the **pancreas**, an organ just beneath the stomach, secretes a hormone called **insulin**. This stimulates cells to take up glucose from the bloodstream.

Insulin also assists in the conversion of any excess glucose into the molecule glycogen, which is then stored in the liver and muscles. The average adult has 5 to 6 grams of glucose in the blood at any given time, which is enough to provide energy for about 15 minutes of activity. If blood glucose becomes depleted, the body draws on its glycogen reserves.

Type 1 Diabetes

Type 1 diabetes (insulin-dependent diabetes) is an autoimmune disease in which the immune system attacks and destroys insulin-making cells in the pancreas. By reducing or stopping insulin production, cells cannot take up glucose, and blood glucose levels become permanently elevated.

Type 1 diabetes used to be called *juvenile diabetes* because it most often appears during childhood or adolescence. Only about 5 percent of diabetic cases are type 1. European ancestry, a genetic predisposition, and certain viral infections all increase the risk. People with type 1 diabetes require daily insulin injections (or regular infusions from an insulin pump) and must carefully monitor their diet and exercise levels.

See It! Videos

Could fewer, larger meals be better for people with diabetes? Watch **Two Meals a Day Could Help Diabetics Control Blood Sugar** in the Study Area of Mastering Health.

54% increase in type 1 and 2 diabetes between 2015 and 2030?

Type 2 Diabetes

Type 2 diabetes (non-insulin-dependent diabetes) accounts for 90 to 95 percent of all cases. In type 2, either the pancreas does not make enough insulin or the body cells become resistant to

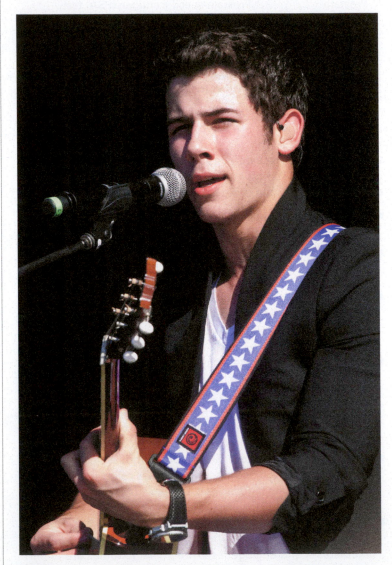

Singer and pop star Nick Jonas is one of the 5 to 10 percent of diabetics diagnosed with type 1 diabetes.

39.9% or

84.1 million people in the United States aged 18 and over are prediabetic

its effects and don't efficiently use available insulin (**Figure 11.12**), a condition referred to as **insulin resistance**.

Unlike type 1 diabetes, which can appear suddenly, type 2 diabetes usually develops slowly. In the early stages, cells begin to resist the effects of insulin. One contributor to insulin resistance is an overabundance of free fatty acids in fat cells (common in obese individuals). These free fatty acids inhibit cells' glucose uptake and diminish the liver's ability to self-regulate conversion of glucose into glycogen.

As blood levels of glucose gradually rise, the pancreas attempts to compensate by producing more insulin. Over time, more and more pancreatic insulin-producing cells sustain damage and become nonfunctional. As insulin output declines, blood glucose levels rise enough to warrant diagnosis of type 2 diabetes.

Diabetes Trends in the United States and the World

According to the WHO, the number of people with diabetes rose from 108 million in 1980 to 422 million in 2014.[147] About half of those with the disease are found in just five countries: China, India, the United States, Brazil, and Indonesia. Over 30 million Americans have the disease.[148] In contrast, the lowest diabetes rates are in Switzerland, the Netherlands, Denmark, Austria, and Belgium.[149]

Rates of diabetes have risen the fastest in low- and middle-income nations, where access to prevention and treatment may be lacking. In general, your chance of developing the disease starts out relatively low when you are young and steadily increases with both your age and weight.

The WHO projects that by 2030, diabetes will become the seventh leading cause of death worldwide. In the United States, some researchers believe that as many as 1 in 3 adults with be diabetic by the year 2050.[150] In addition to the physical and emotional toll the disease takes, the combined economic burden from diabetes was estimated at over $245 billion in 2012.[151]

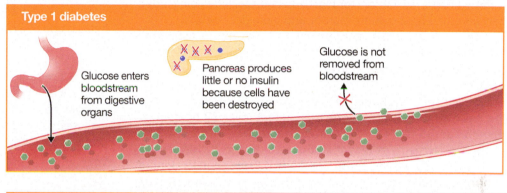

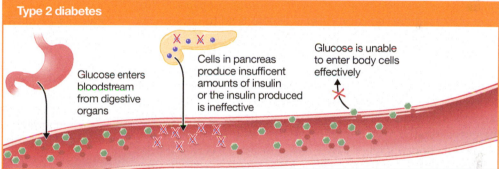

Figure 11.12 Diabetes: What It Is and How It Develops
In a healthy person, a sufficient amount of insulin is produced and released by the pancreas and used efficiently by the cells. In type 1 diabetes, the pancreas makes little or no insulin. In type 2 diabetes, either the pancreas does not make sufficient insulin or cells are resistant to insulin and thus are not able to use it efficiently.

Mastering Health & Nutrition

How Diabetes Develops

Check Yourself

- What is the role of glucose and insulin in diabetes?

- What is the difference between type 1 and type 2 diabetes?

- Why do you think diabetes rates have increased so dramatically in the United States?

Diabetes: Risk Factors, Symptoms, and Complications

Risk Factors

Nonmodifiable risk factors for type 2 diabetes include being older, certain ethnicities, genetic factors, and biological factors.

The Centers for Disease Control and Prevention estimates that almost 10 percent of the U.S. population have diabetes and that 25 percent of them don't know it. Another 86 million have **prediabetes**, *with elevated blood glucose levels that are rising, but are not yet high enough to be classified as diabetic.*[152] Increasing age and weight are risk factors; in fact, over 22 percent of people age 65 to 74 in the United States have prediabetes.[153] According to the most recent study, rates of type 2 diabetes are up significantly among youth age 10 to 19, particularly among minorities. Rates among Hispanics, Native Americans, Asian/ Pacific Islanders, non-Hispanic blacks, and non-Hispanic whites have increased dramatically.[154] Females also tend to have higher rates than males.

Having a close relative with type 2 diabetes is another significant risk factor. Most experts support the theory that type 2 diabetes is caused by the complex interaction between environmental factors, lifestyle, and genetic susceptibility. Although numerous potential genes have been identified as likely culprits in increased risk, the mechanisms by which inherited diabetes develops remain poorly understood.

Body weight, dietary choices, level of physical activity, sleep patterns, and stress level are all modifiable risk factors. In adults, a BMI of 25 or greater increases risks, with significantly higher risks for each 5 kg/m^2 increase.[155] Excess weight around the waistline— a condition called *central adiposity*—is a significant risk factor for older women and younger adults.[156] People with type 2 diabetes who lose weight and increase their physical activity can significantly improve their blood glucose levels.

Inadequate sleep may contribute to the development of both obesity and type 2 diabetes, possibly because sleep-deprived people tend to engage in less physical activity.[157] People who are routinely sleep-deprived are also at higher risk for *metabolic syndrome*, a cluster of risk factors that include poor glucose metabolism.[158] A recent review of the accumulated research indicates that the risk for type 2 diabetes increases among people who are experiencing trauma or stressful working conditions; those with chronically high inflammation levels; those with a history of depression; and those with confrontational personalities.[159] In addition, diabetes is more common among people with low socioeconomic status (SES) and in racial and ethnic minorities, independent of current SES.[160]

Prediabetes

An estimated 86 million Americans age 20 or older—37 percent of the adult population—have a set of symptoms known as **prediabetes**, a condition in which blood glucose levels are higher than normal but not high enough to be classified as diabetes.[161] If this condition is not addressed, diabetes will eventually strike. Prediabetes is one of a cluster of six conditions linked to overweight and obesity that together constitute a dangerous health risk known as metabolic syndrome (MetS) (see Module 11.8). A person with MetS is five times more likely to develop type 2 diabetes than is a person without the syndrome.[162]

If you have already been diagnosed with prediabetes or type 2 diabetes, you can follow the tips in the Skills for Behavior Change box to halt or slow the progression of your condition. Even if you have never had your blood glucose tested, these steps could reduce your risk.

Gestational Diabetes

A third type of diabetes, **gestational diabetes**, is a state of high blood glucose during pregnancy, thought to be associated with metabolic stresses that occur in response to changing hormonal levels. As many as 18 percent of pregnancies are affected by gestational diabetes, posing added risks for the mother and developing fetus.[163] Between 40 and 50 percent of women with gestational diabetes may progress to type 2 diabetes if they fail to make significant lifestyle changes.[164]

Symptoms of Diabetes

Common symptoms of diabetes are similar for type 1 and type 2:

- **Thirst and excessive urination.** Kidneys filter excessive glucose by diluting it with water. This can pull too much water from the body and result in dehydration and increased need to urinate.
- **Weight loss.** Because so many calories are lost in the glucose that passes into urine, a person with diabetes often feels hungry. Despite eating more, he or she typically loses weight.
- **Fatigue.** When glucose cannot enter cells, fatigue and weakness become inevitable.
- **Nerve damage.** High glucose levels damage the smallest blood vessels of the body, leading to numbness and tingling.
- **Blurred vision.** High blood glucose levels can dry out the cornea or damage microvessels in the eye.
- **Poor wound healing and increased infections.** High levels of glucose can affect ability to ward off infection and overall immune function.

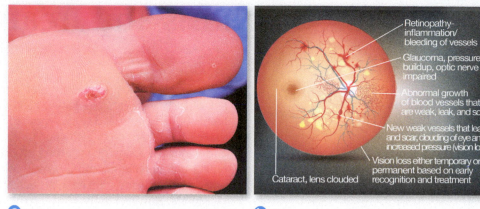

a Diabetics are prone to wounds that don't heal on the feet as nerves may be damaged, healing impaired, and sensation diminished. Blisters, infections, and other irritants can easily progress to more serious problems.

b Uncontrolled diabetes can damage the eye, causing swelling and rupture of blood vessels.

Figure 11.13 Complications of Uncontrolled Diabetes: Amputation and Eye Disease

Diabetes Complications

Poorly controlled diabetes can lead to a variety of complications that are described in **Figure 11.13**:

- **Diabetic coma.** In the absence of glucose, body cells break down stored fat for energy. This produces acidic molecules called *ketones*, excessive amounts of which dangerously elevate blood acid. The diabetic slips into a coma and, without prompt medical intervention, can die.
- **Cardiovascular disease.** Because many diabetics are also overweight or obese, hypertension is often present. Blood vessels become damaged and essential nutrients and other substances are not transported as effectively.
- **Kidney disease.** Kidneys become scarred by their extraordinary workload and by high blood pressure in their blood vessels. More than 247,000 Americans are currently living with kidney failure due to diabetes.[165]
- **Amputations.** More than 60 percent of non-trauma-related amputations of legs, feet, and toes are due to diabetes. Each year, nearly 73,000 non-trauma-related lower-limb amputations are performed on people with diabetes.[166]
- **Eye disease and blindness.** Nearly 7.7 million people over the age of 40 have *early-stage retinopathy*, which could lead to blindness without treatment.[167]
- **Infectious diseases.** People with diabetes have increased risk of poor wound healing and greater susceptibility to infectious diseases, particularly influenza and pneumonia.
- **Other complications.** People with diabetes may have gum and tooth disease, foot neuropathy, and chronic pain that makes walking, driving, and simple tasks more difficult. In addition, people with diabetes are more likely to suffer from depression, making intervention and treatment more difficult.

Skills for **Behavior Change**

Key Steps to Begin Reducing Your Risk for Diabetes

- Eat smaller portions, and choose foods with less fat, salt, and added sugars. Keep calories equal to energy expended. Eat more fruits, vegetables, and complex carbohydrates, and make sure you consume lean protein.
- Get your body moving. Aim for at least 30 minutes of moderate activity 5 days a week.
- Quit smoking; in addition to cancer and heart disease, smoking increases blood glucose levels.
- Reduce or eliminate alcohol consumption. Alcohol is high in calories and can interfere with blood glucose regulation.
- Get enough sleep.
- Inoculate yourself against stress. Learn to take yourself less seriously; find time for fun; develop a strong support network; and use relaxation skills, yoga, meditation, and other mindfulness strategies.
- If you have a family history of diabetes or several risk factors, get regular checkups.

Source: Centers for Disease Control and Prevention, "National Diabetes Prevention Program," 2016, https://www.cdc.gov/diabetes/prevention/lifestyle-program/experience/index.html.

Check Yourself

- Name three possible complications of poorly controlled diabetes.
- What factors put someone at greatest risk for type 2 diabetes?
- What are common symptoms of type 1 and type 2 diabetes?

11.25 Diabetes: Diagnosis and Treatment

Learning Outcome

11.25 Explain how diabetes is diagnosed and treated.

Diagnosing and Monitoring Diabetes

Generally, a physician orders one of the following blood tests to diagnose prediabetes or diabetes:

- The *fasting plasma glucose (FPG) test* requires the patient to fast overnight; a small sample of blood is then tested for glucose concentration. An FPG level greater than or equal to 100 mg/dL indicates prediabetes, and a level greater than or equal to 126 mg/dL indicates diabetes (**Figure 11.14**).
- The *oral glucose tolerance test (OGTT)* requires the patient to drink a fluid containing concentrated glucose. Blood is drawn for testing 2 hours later. A reading greater than or equal to 140 mg/dL indicates prediabetes, and a reading greater than or equal to 200 mg/dL indicates diabetes.
- The *A1C* or *glycosylated hemoglobin test (HbA1C)* gives the average value of a patient's blood glucose over the past 2 to 3 months instead of at one moment in time. In general, an A1C of 5.7 to 6.4 means that the patient is at high risk for diabetes or is prediabetic. If the A1C is 6.5 or higher, diabetes may be diagnosed.[168] *Estimated average glucose (eAG)* shows how AIC numbers correspond to the blood glucose numbers people are used to seeing. For example, someone with an A1C value of 6.1 would be able to look at a chart and see that his or her average blood glucose was around 128—a high level that should encourage healthy lifestyle modifications.

People with diabetes need to check their blood glucose level several times throughout each day to make sure they stay within their target range. To check blood glucose, the person must prick a fingertip to obtain a drop of blood. A handheld glucose meter is then used to evaluate the blood sample.

Treating Diabetes

Lifestyle changes can prevent or delay the development of type 2 diabetes by up to 58 percent.[169] For people with type 2 diabetes, such lifestyle changes can prevent or delay need for medication or insulin injections.

Weight loss significantly lowers risk of progressing from prediabetes to diabetes. A loss of as little as 5 to 7 percent of current body weight and regular physical activity significantly lower the risk of progressing to diabetes.[170]

A low-fat, reduced-calorie diet aids weight loss. Researchers have studied a variety of foods for their effect on blood glucose levels. A diet high in whole grains reduces risk of type 2 diabetes.[171] Eating high-fiber foods—berries, vegetables, beans, nuts, and seeds—may reduce diabetes risk.[172] Eating low-carbohydrate diets also appears to reduce overall CVD risks and may have a significant effect on preventing and controlling type 2 diabetes. In addition, consumption of fish that is high in omega-3 fatty acids is linked with decreased progression of insulin resistance. However, newer research has called this connection between high fish intake and risk reduction into question.[173] More research is necessary.

It is important for people with diabetes to prevent surges in blood sugar after they eat. The **glycemic index (GI)** compares foods with the same amount of carbohydrates and determines how quickly and how much each raises blood glucose levels. Foods that are low on the GI have far less effect on blood glucose than those that are high on the GI. A food's **glycemic load (GL)** is defined as its GI (potential to raise blood glucose) multiplied by the grams of carbohydrates it provides, divided by 100. By learning to combine high- and low-GI foods to avoid surges in blood glucose, diabetics can help control their average blood glucose levels throughout the day. Eating smaller amounts, several times a day, from low GI sources is an important part of glucose control.

In late 2016, the American Diabetes Association changed their exercise recommendations for diabetes prevention, calling for based on information found in source light activity every 30 minutes during long sitting stretches. Rather than prescribing 90

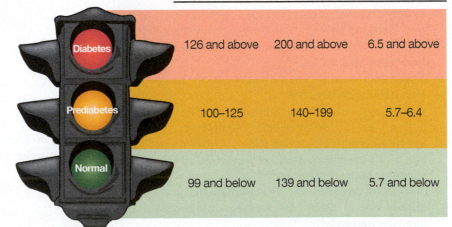

	FPG Levels	OGTT Levels	A1C Levels
Diabetes	126 and above	200 and above	6.5 and above
Prediabetes	100–125	140–199	5.7–6.4
Normal	99 and below	139 and below	5.7 and below

Figure 11.14 Blood Glucose Levels in Prediabetes and Untreated Diabetes
The fasting plasma glucose (FPG) test measures levels of blood glucose after a person fasts overnight. The oral glucose tolerance test (OGTT) measures levels of blood glucose after a person consumes a concentrated amount of glucose. The A1C or glycosylated hemoglobin test (HbA1C) gives the average value of a patient's blood glucose over the past 2 to 3 months.
Source: American Diabetes Association, "Diagnosing and Learning about Prediabetes," June 9, 2015, www.diabetes.org/diabetes-basics/diagnosis.

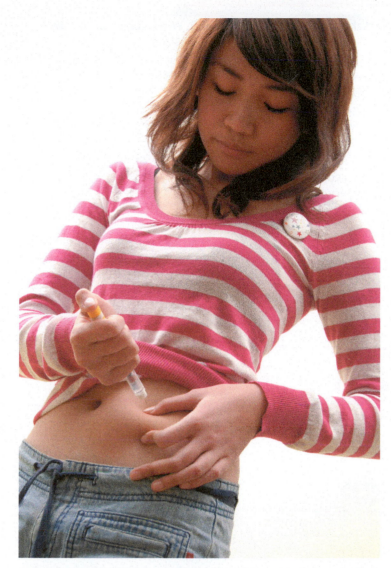

Some type 2 diabetics can control their condition with changes in diet and lifestyle habits or with oral medications. However, some type 2 diabetics and all type 1 diabetics require insulin injections or infusions.

Losing

5–7%

of body weight can cause significant reductions in blood glucose levels and help prevent diabetes.

Currently, there is much discussion about whether people with prediabetes should use the drug metformin, along with lifestyle intervention and counseling, as an early intervention. Although sources indicate potential benefits, metformin is not without risks, particularly for individuals with a history of gastrointestinal, cardiovascular, or kidney problems.[175]

People who undergo gastric or bariatric surgery have shown remarkable reductions in blood glucose and diabetes symptoms more than 2 years after surgery.[176] Those who combined gastric bypass or sleeve gastrectomy with intensive medical therapy had similar outcomes.[177] In many cases, former diabetics can stop taking some medications, and their diabetes symptoms stop altogether. Consensus is growing about potential short- and long-term benefits of these more drastic methods.[178] However, gastric bypass surgeries are not without risks, which can include death and serious complications.

With type 1 diabetes, the pancreas cannot produce adequate insulin, making added insulin essential. People with type 2 diabetes whose blood glucose cannot be controlled with other treatments also require insulin. Insulin cannot be taken in pill form because it is a protein and therefore would be digested in the gastrointestinal tract. It must therefore be inserted into the fat layer under the skin, from which it is absorbed into the bloodstream.

Today, many diabetics use an *insulin infusion pump* rather than injections. The pump, which is small and easily hidden by clothes, delivers insulin in minute amounts throughout the day through a catheter inserted under the skin.

minutes of exercise over several days, getting people up and moving at more regular intervals is key to glucose control.[174] Exercise increases sensitivity to insulin. The more muscle mass you have and the more you use your muscles throughout the day, the more efficiently cells use glucose, meaning less glucose circulating in the bloodstream.

When lifestyle changes fail to control type 2 diabetes, one of several oral medications may be prescribed, each of which influences blood glucose in a different way: reducing the liver's glucose production, slowing absorption of carbohydrates from the small intestine, increasing pancreatic insulin production, or increasing cells' insulin sensitivity.

Drugs known as SGLT2 inhibitors cause the kidneys to actually excrete more glucose, which lowers the levels of glucose circulating in the body.

All diabetes drugs have side effects and contraindications; however, each person must balance risks of medications with risks of elevated blood glucose.

Check Yourself

- **What tests are commonly used to diagnose diabetes?**

- **What are some of the treatments for diabetes?**

- **How do people with diabetes monitor their blood glucose level?**

Summary

LO 11.1 The cardiovascular system consists of the heart and circulatory system, a network of vessels that supplies the body with nutrients and oxygen.

LO 11.2–11.7 Cardiovascular diseases include atherosclerosis, coronary artery disease, peripheral artery disease, coronary heart disease, stroke, hypertension, angina pectoris, arrhythmias, congestive heart failure, and congenital and rheumatic heart disease.

LO 11.8–11.10 Many risk factors for cardiovascular disease can be modified, such as cigarette smoking, high blood cholesterol and triglyceride levels, hypertension, lack of exercise, a diet high in saturated fat, obesity, diabetes, and emotional stress. Some risk factors, such as age, gender, and heredity, cannot be modified.

LO 11.11 Coronary bypass surgery is an established treatment for heart blockage; however, increasing numbers of angioplasty procedures and stents are being used with great success. Drug therapies can be used to prevent and treat CVD.

LO 11.12 Cancer is a group of diseases characterized by uncontrolled growth and spread of abnormal cells. These cells may create tumors.

LO 11.13–11.14 Cancers are grouped into four categories: carcinomas, sarcomas, lymphomas, and leukemias. Lifestyle factors that increase risks for cancer include smoking, obesity, poor diet, lack of exercise, and stress. Biological risk factors include inherited genes, age, and gender. Infectious agents that may cause cancer are chronic hepatitis B and C, human papillomavirus, and genital herpes.

LO 11.15–11.20 Common cancers include those of the lung, breast, colon and rectum, skin, prostate, testis, ovary, and uterus; leukemia; and lymphomas.

LO 11.21 Early diagnosis of cancer improves survival rate. Surgery or biopsies may aid in diagnosis. Treatment options include chemotherapy, radiation, and immunotherapies.

LO 11.22 Mindfulness-based interventions such as meditation and yoga can help people with cancer cope with loss of control, uncertainty about the future, pain, fatigue, and depression.

LO 11.23 Diabetes mellitus is characterized by a persistently high level of glucose in the blood. In type 1 diabetes, the immune system attacks insulin-making cells in the pancreas, leading to dangerously elevated glucose levels. In type 2 diabetes, the pancreas doesn't make sufficient insulin, or the cells don't use it efficiently.

LO 11.24 Factors that increase risk for type 2 diabetes include increasing age, higher weight, certain ethnicities (notably African American and Hispanic groups), genetics, and lifestyle. Prediabetes may eventually lead to diabetes if health risks are not addressed.

LO 11.25 Treatments for diabetes include improving lifestyle factors, taking medications, undergoing weight-loss surgery, and receiving insulin.

Pop Quiz

Visit Mastering Health to personalize your study plan with Chapter Review Quizzes and Dynamic Study Modules.

LO 11.6 1. A stroke results
a. when the heart stops beating.
b. when cardiopulmonary resuscitation has failed to revive a stopped heart.
c. when blood flow in the brain has been compromised by either blockage or hemorrhage.
d. when blood pressure rises above 120/80 mmHg.

LO 11.8 2. Which of the following is *correct* about metabolic syndrome?
a. It is decreasing among the general population both in the United States and globally.
b. It lowers your risk of cardiovascular disease.
c. It includes high fasting blood glucose, obesity, high triglyceride levels, hypertension, and other risks.
d. It is a nonmodifiable risk factor for CVD.

LO 11.9 3. The "bad" type of cholesterol found in the bloodstream is known as
a. high-density lipoprotein (HDL).
b. low-density lipoprotein (LDL).
c. total cholesterol.
d. triglycerides.

LO 11.9 4. What does a person's cholesterol level indicate?
a. The formation of fatty substances, called *plaque*, which can clog the arteries
b. The level of triglycerides in the blood, which can increase the risk of coronary disease
c. Hypertension, which leads to thickening and hardening of the arteries
d. The level of C-reactive proteins in the blood, indicating inflammation

LO 11.12 5. When cancer cells have metastasized,
a. they have grown into a malignant tumor.
b. they have spread to other parts of the body.
c. the cancer is retreating, and cancer cells are dying off.
d. the tumor is localized and considered *in situ.*

LO 11.12 6. A cancerous neoplasm is a
a. type of biopsy.
b. form of benign tumor.
c. type of treatment for a tumor.
d. malignant group of cells or tumor.

LO 11.14 7. "If you are male and smoke, your chances of getting lung cancer are 25 times greater than those of a nonsmoker." This statement refers to a type of risk assessed statistically, known as
a. relative risk.
b. comparable risk.
c. cancer risk.
d. genetic predisposition.

LO 11.19 8. The most serious and life-threatening type of skin cancer is
a. basal cell carcinoma.
b. squamous cell carcinoma.
c. melanoma.
d. lymphoma.

LO 11.22 9. Which of the following is true of type 2 diabetes?
a. It is an autoimmune disorder.
b. It is correlated with obesity and a sedentary lifestyle.
c. It usually appears suddenly.
d. It is also referred to as insulin-dependent diabetes.

LO 11.22 10. By 2050, experts predict more than _____ Americans will have diabetes.
a. 1 in 3
b. 1 in 10
c. 1 in 100
d. 1 in 200

Answers to these questions can be found on page A-1. If you answered a question incorrectly, review the module identified by the Learning Outcome. For even more study tools, visit Mastering Health.

Think About It

LO 1 1. List the different types of CVD. Compare and contrast their symptoms and prevalence. Why do some populations have higher rates than others? What are your risk factors, if any?

Infectious Conditions

12

ASSESS YOURSELF: STIs: Do You Really Know What You Think You Know? Find out in the Study Area at Mastering Health.

Disease-causing agents, or **pathogens**, are found throughout our world. New varieties arise constantly; others have existed for as long as there has been life on this planet. Infectious diseases such as the common cold are **endemic**, meaning that they are present at expected prevalence rates in virtually all populations on Earth. When the number of cases of a disease suddenly increases with higher than projected endemic numbers, it becomes an **epidemic**; such as bubonic plague, for example, which killed up to one-third of the population of Europe in the 1300s. A **pandemic**, or global epidemic, of influenza killed more than 20 million people in many countries of the world in 1918. Today, new, resistant forms of older organisms—such as H1N1 flu and *methicillin-resistant*

Staphylococcus aureus, or MRSA, a staph infection—defy current pharmacological weapons and show pandemic trends.

Despite constant bombardment by pathogens, however, our immune systems are remarkably adept at protecting us. Exposure to invading microorganisms actually helps build resistance to pathogens. Millions of *endogenous microorganisms* live in and on our bodies, usually in peaceful coexistence. *Exogenous microorganisms*, in contrast, are those that don't normally inhabit the body. When they do, they are apt to produce infection or illness. The more easily these pathogens can gain a foothold and sustain themselves, the more **virulent**, or aggressive, they may be in causing disease.

12.1 Infection, Risk Factors, and the Role of Mindfulness

12.1 Explain the process of infection and defenses against pathogens, and list common risk factors for infection.

Most diseases are **multifactorial**, caused by the interaction of several factors inside and outside a person. For a disease to occur, the person, or *host*, must be *susceptible*, which means that the immune system must be in a weakened condition (**immunocompromised**); an *agent* capable of *transmitting* a disease must be present; and the *environment* must be *hospitable* to the pathogen. Although all pathogens pose a threat if they gain entry and begin to grow in the body, the chances that they will do so are actually quite small.

Your body constantly protects against and defends you from pathogens that could make you ill. To gain entry into your body, pathogens must overcome the body's elaborate defenses , mechanisms that keep organisms from entering, weaken organisms that breach these barriers, and control or destroy organisms that pose threats. **Figure 12.1** summarizes some of the body's defenses against invasion.

Cropped at Bottom

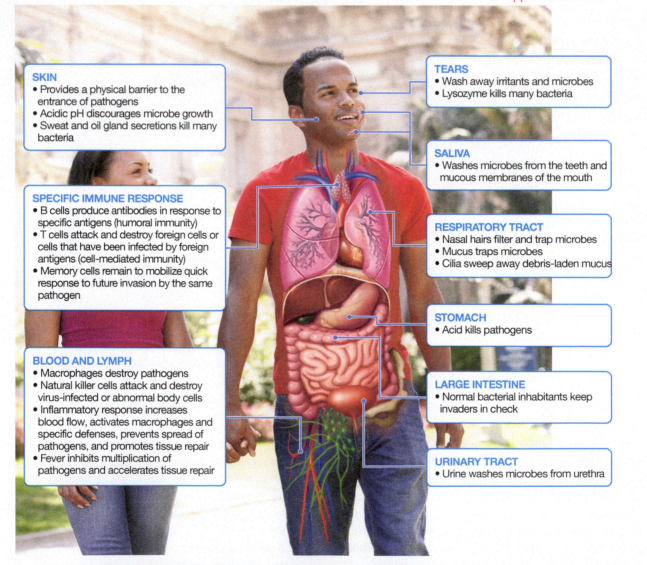

SKIN
- Provides a physical barrier to the entrance of pathogens
- Acidic pH discourages microbe growth
- Sweat and oil gland secretions kill many bacteria

SPECIFIC IMMUNE RESPONSE
- B cells produce antibodies in response to specific antigens (humoral immunity)
- T cells attack and destroy foreign cells or cells that have been infected by foreign antigens (cell-mediated immunity)
- Memory cells remain to mobilize quick response to future invasion by the same pathogen

BLOOD AND LYMPH
- Macrophages destroy pathogens
- Natural killer cells attack and destroy virus-infected or abnormal body cells
- Inflammatory response increases blood flow, activates macrophages and specific defenses, prevents spread of pathogens, and promotes tissue repair
- Fever inhibits multiplication of pathogens and accelerates tissue repair

TEARS
- Wash away irritants and microbes
- Lysozyme kills many bacteria

SALIVA
- Washes microbes from the teeth and mucous membranes of the mouth

RESPIRATORY TRACT
- Nasal hairs filter and trap microbes
- Mucus traps microbes
- Cilia sweep away debris-laden mucus

STOMACH
- Acid kills pathogens

LARGE INTESTINE
- Normal bacterial inhabitants keep invaders in check

URINARY TRACT
- Urine washes microbes from urethra

Figure 12.1 The Body's Defenses against Disease-Causing Pathogens
In addition to the defenses listed, many of the body's defensive secretions and fluids, such as earwax, tears, mucus, and blood, contain enzymes and other proteins that can kill some invading pathogens or prevent or slow their reproduction.

Mastering Health & Nutrition Chain of Infection

Preventing Pathogens from Entering the Body

Pathogens can enter the body via several routes of transmission. They may be transmitted by *direct contact* between infected persons, such as during sexual relations, kissing, or touching, or by *indirect contact*, such as by touching an object that an infected person has touched. You may also **autoinoculate** yourself, or transmit a pathogen from one part of your body to another. For example, you may touch a herpes sore on your lip, then transmit the virus to your eye by touch.

Dogs, cats, livestock, and wild animals can spread **zoonotic diseases** through bites or feces or by carrying infected insects into living areas. Although *interspecies transmission* of diseases (diseases passed from humans to animals and vice versa) is fairly rare, it is increasing in frequency with some pathogens.

Risk Factors You Can Control

With all these pathogens floating around, how can you avoid getting sick? Fortunately, there are ways to take care of yourself. Too much stress, inadequate nutrition, a low fitness level, lack of sleep, misuse or abuse of legal and illegal drugs, poor personal hygiene, and high-risk behavior significantly increase the risk for many diseases. College students often are at higher risk because of many of the above factors, in addition to the fact that alcohol and other drugs, increasing numbers of sexual experiences, and close living conditions all create higher risk for exposure to pathogens. You can make changes in your community to clean up toxins, set policies on contaminant levels, and reduce the likelihood of exposure to pathogens or toxins. The chain of infection between pathogen, environment, and host presents multiple opportunities for individuals and communities to intercede and break the chain, preventing and controlling disease transmission.

Risk Factors You Typically Cannot Control

Unfortunately, some factors that make you susceptible to a certain disease are either hard to control or completely beyond your control:

- **Heredity.** One of the key factors influencing disease risk is genetics. It is often unclear whether hereditary diseases are due to inherited genetic traits or to inherited insufficiencies in the immune system. It is possible that we inherit the quality of our immune system, which would make some people naturally more resistant to disease and infection.
- **Aging.** People under age 5 and over age 65 are often more vulnerable to infectious diseases because body defenses that we take for granted are either not fully developed or not as effective as they once were. Thinning of the skin, reduced sweating, and other physical changes can make older adults more vulnerable to disease. In addition, as people age, certain **comorbidities** (diseases that occur at the same time) overwhelm the body's ability to ward off enemies and increase the risk of infection. In these situations, **opportunistic infections** can cause illness.
- **Environmental conditions.** A growing body of research points to climate change as a major contributor to infectious diseases.

As temperatures rise, insect populations may increase, potentially increasing cases of mosquito-borne diseases such as *West Nile virus, malaria, dengue fever,* and *chikungunya virus.* Dwindling water supplies where there is little water turnover or flow contribute to pathogen growth. When animals move to new environments in search of water and congregate near water sources, they are exposed to new species of animals with a new set of pathogens. In these environments, disease spreads quickly. Scientists argue that changing environmental conditions, such as drought, flooding, fires, and other natural and human-caused events, may increase disease spread and hasten the chances of interspecies transmission in humans.[1] Chronic exposure to toxic chemicals in pesticides, herbicides, mercury, and lead and other threats such as radiation exposure can damage the immune system and increase disease susceptibility.

- **Organism virulence and resistance.** Even tiny amounts of a particularly virulent organism may make the hardiest of us ill. Other organisms have mutated and become resistant to the body's defenses and to medical treatments. **Drug resistance** occurs when pathogens grow and proliferate in the presence of chemicals that would normally slow growth or kill them.

Mindfulness: A New Ally in Bolstering Defenses

Although several lifestyle variables and their potential positive effects on immune system functioning are discussed throughout this book—including factors such as a healthy diet, exercise, stress reduction, and sleep—an emerging body of research indicates that mindfulness strategies may provide another weapon in your arsenal against infectious diseases. A recent systematic review of the accumulated research indicates that mindfulness may in fact, have a positive effect on immune functioning. Although promising, more research is necessary to determine the exact mechanisms that play a role in bolstering body defenses.[2] Another recent study indicates that adversity early in life is associated with higher risks of diseases overall in adulthood. Long-term adversity may result in cumulative pathologies, including inflammation, autoimmune diseases, allergies, and asthma, as well as alterations in immune function related to higher stress and sleep disturbances.[3] If adversity leads to impaired immune functioning, perhaps mindfulness strategies that help reduce negative consequences of adversity could also reduce risk. Another new study analyzes the accumulated research showing the link between emotions and the immune system, indicating that infectious diseases can affect emotions and that emotions can alter immune function. Mindfulness and other anxiety- and stress-relieving strategies appear to have great potential for reducing the risks of disease initiation and progress.[4]

Check Yourself

- **What are three common routes of infection?**
- **What are some ways in which your body fights off infection?**
- **List three risk factors for infection that are typically beyond your control.**

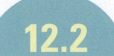 **Your Immune System**

Learning Outcome

12.2 **Explain how the immune system defends against invasion by pathogens.**

The immune system is able to quickly recognize and destroy **antigens**—outside or foreign substances capable of causing disease. An antigen can be a virus, a bacterium, a fungus, a parasite, a toxin, or a tissue or cell from another organism. *Immunity* is a condition of being able to resist a particular disease by counteracting the substance that produces the disease.

How the Immune System Works

As soon as an antigen breaches the body's initial defenses, the body responds by forming substances called **antibodies** that are matched to that specific antigen, much as a key is matched to a lock. The body analyzes the antigen, considers its size and shape, verifies that the antigen is not part of the body itself, and then produces a specific antibody to destroy or weaken it. This process is part of a complex system called *humoral immune responses*. **Humoral immunity** is the body's major defense against many bacteria and the poisonous substances, called **toxins**, that they produce.

In **cell-mediated immunity**, specialized white blood cells called **lymphocytes** attack and destroy the foreign invader. Lymphocytes constitute the body's main defense against viruses, fungi, parasites, and some bacteria, and they are found in the blood, lymph nodes, bone marrow, and certain glands. Other key players in this immune response are **macrophages** (a type of phagocytic, or cell-eating, white blood cell).

Two forms of lymphocytes in particular, the *B lymphocytes* (B cells) and *T lymphocytes* (T cells), are involved in the immune response. *Helper T cells* are essential for activating B cells to produce antibodies. They also activate other T cells and macrophages. Another form of T cell, known as the *killer T cell*, directly attacks infected or malignant cells. *Suppressor T cells* turn off or suppress the activity of B cells, killer T cells, and macrophages. After a successful attack on a pathogen, some of the attacker T and B cells are preserved as *memory T and B cells*, enabling the body to recognize and respond quickly to subsequent attacks by the same kind of organism.

Once people have survived certain infectious diseases, they become immune to those diseases, meaning that in all probability, they will not develop them again. Upon subsequent attack by the same disease-causing microorganisms, their memory T and B cells are quickly activated to come to their defense. **Figure 12.2** provides a summary of the cell-mediated immune response.

When the Immune System Misfires: Autoimmune Diseases

Although the immune response generally works in our favor, the body sometimes makes a mistake and targets its own tissue as the enemy, builds up antibodies against that tissue, and attempts to destroy it. This is known as **autoimmune disease** (*auto* means

"self"). The National Institutes of Health estimates that over 32 million Americans have *autoantibodies*—proteins made by the immune system that target the body's tissues—that can indicate autoimmunity well before the symptoms of autoimmune diseases actually appear.[5] Researchers estimate that there are over 80 different types of autoimmune diseases, many of which are chronic, debilitating, and life threatening. They can affect virtually any part of the body, and some of them may cause disability and death. Among the most common autoimmune diseases are type 1 diabetes, rheumatoid arthritis, multiple sclerosis, celiac disease, and irritable bowel syndrome.

Inflammatory Response, Pain, and Fever If an infection is localized, pus formation, redness, swelling, and irritation often occur. These symptoms are components of the body's inflammatory response, and they indicate that the invading organisms are being fought systemically. The four cardinal signs of inflammation are *redness, swelling, pain,* and *heat.*

Pain is often one of the earliest signs that an injury or infection has occurred. Pathogens can kill or injure tissue at the site of infection, leading to swelling that puts pressure on nerve endings in the area, causing pain. Although pain does not feel good, it plays a valuable role in the body's response to injury or invasion. For example, pain can cause a person to avoid activity that may aggravate the injury or site of infection, thereby protecting against further damage.

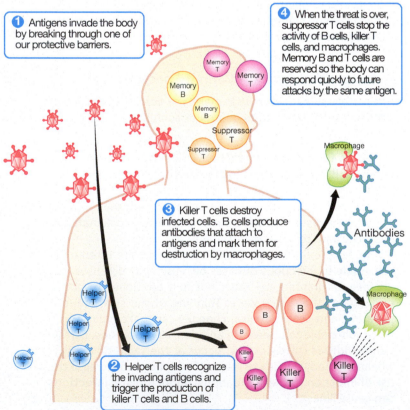

Figure 12.2 The Cell-Mediated Immune Response

1. Antigens invade the body by breaking through one of our protective barriers.

2. Helper T cells recognize the invading antigens and trigger the production of killer T cells and B cells.

3. Killer T cells destroy infected cells. B cells produce antibodies that attach to antigens and mark them for destruction by macrophages.

4. When the threat is over, suppressor T cells stop the activity of B cells, killer T cells, and macrophages. Memory B and T cells are reserved so the body can respond quickly to future attacks by the same antigen.

Another frequent indicator of infection is *fever*, or a body temperature above the average norm of 98.6°F. Fever is frequently caused by toxins secreted by pathogens that interfere with the control of body temperature. Although extremely elevated temperatures are harmful to the body, a mild fever is protective: Raising body temperature by one or two degrees destroys some disease-causing organisms. A fever also stimulates the body to produce more white blood cells, which destroy more invaders. Of course, with fevers beyond 101°F or 102°F, risks to the patient outweigh any benefits. In such cases, obtain medical treatment.

Vaccines: Bolstering Your Immunity

Once a person has been exposed to a specific pathogen, subsequent attacks activate the memory T and B cells, thus giving the person immunity. This is the principle on which **vaccination** is based.

A *vaccine* consists of killed or weakened versions of a disease-causing microorganism or an antigen similar to but less dangerous than the disease antigen. It is administered to stimulate the immune system to produce antibodies against future attacks without actually causing the disease (or by causing a very minor case of it). Vaccines typically are given orally or by injection; this form of immunity is termed *artificially acquired active immunity*, in contrast to *naturally acquired active immunity* (which is obtained by exposure to antigens in the normal course of daily life) or *naturally acquired passive immunity* (as occurs when a mother passes immunity to her fetus via their shared blood supply or to an infant via breast milk). Because of their close living quarters and frequent interactions with other people, college students face a higher than average risk of infection from diseases that are largely preventable. Vaccines that should be a priority among students include those in Table 12.1. People with certain health, job, or lifestyle risks are recommended to receive hepatitis A.[6]

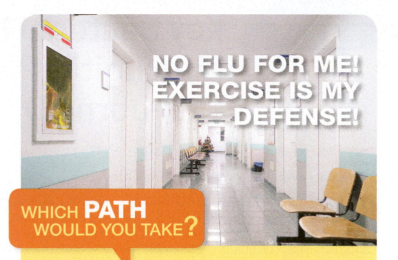

NO FLU FOR ME! EXERCISE IS MY DEFENSE!

WHICH PATH WOULD YOU TAKE?

Go to Mastering Health to play "Protecting Against Infectious Diseases" and see how your actions today affect your future health.

TABLE	
12.1	**Recommended Vaccinations for Teens and College Students***

- Tetanus, diphtheria, pertussis vaccine (Td/Tdap)
- Meningococcal vaccine (booster at age 16)
- HPV vaccine series
- Hepatitis B vaccine series
- Polio vaccine series
- Measles-mumps-rubella (MMR) vaccine series
- Varicella (chickenpox) vaccine series
- Influenza vaccine
- Pneumococcal polysaccharide (PPV) vaccine
- Hepatitis A vaccine series

*Note: These are the vaccinations that students will typically see required or recommended. Students should contact their student health center for specific recommendations.

Source: Centers for Disease Control and Prevention, "Preteen and Teen Vaccines," updated April 2016, www.cdc.gov/vaccines/who/teens/vaccines/index.html, accessed October 2017; Centers for Disease Control and Prevention, "Vaccine Information for Adults," updated January 2017, www.cdc.gov/vaccines/adults/rec-vac/index.html, accessed October 2017.

While some people are concerned about vaccinations, avoiding a potentially deadly or disabling disease outweighs any risks. If you develop minor rashes or other symptoms after being immunized, let your doctor know.

Skills for **Behavior Change**

Reduce Your Risk of Infectious Disease

- **Limit your exposure to pathogens.** Stay home if you are not feeling well, and encourage others to do the same. Don't share utensils or drinking glasses, keep your toothbrush away from those of other people. Keep hands away from your mouth, nose, eyes, and other body orifices. Keep purses and backpacks off of kitchen counters and restroom floors.
- **Exercise regularly.** Regular exercise raises the core body temperature, strengthens the immune system, and kills pathogens.
- **Get enough sleep.** Sleep allows the body time to refresh itself, produce necessary cells, and reduce inflammation. Even a single night without sleep can increase inflammatory processes and delay wound healing.
- **Optimize eating.** Enjoy a balanced, healthy diet. and eat mindfully.

Check Yourself

- How do vaccines help your body resist viruses?
- What are four steps you can take to reduce your overall chances of infection?

We can categorize pathogens into six major types: bacteria, viruses, fungi, protozoans, parasitic worms, and prions (see **Figure 12.3**). Each has a particular route of transmission and characteristic elements that make it unique. In the following pages, we discuss each of these categories and the diseases that they cause.

Bacteria (singular: *bacterium*) are simple, single-celled microscopic organisms. Although there are several thousand known species of bacteria (and many thousands more that are unknown), just over 100 of them lead to disease in humans. In many cases, it is not the bacteria themselves that cause disease, but rather the toxins that they produce. Diseases caused by bacteria can be treated with **antibiotics**. However, today's arsenal of antibiotics is becoming less effective as strains of bacteria with **antibiotic resistance** become more common. Such "superbugs" can result when successive generations of bacteria mutate to develop an ability to withstand the effects of specific drugs.

Staphylococcal Infections

Staphylococci are normally present on the skin or in the nostrils of most people at any given time and usually present no problems. However, with a cut or break in the *epidermis*, or outer layer of skin, staphylococci may enter the system and cause an **infection**. If you have suffered from acne, boils, styes (infections of the eyelids), or infected wounds, you've probably had a "staph" infection.

Although most of these infections are readily defeated by the immune system, resistant forms of staph are on the rise. One, **methicillin-resistant *Staphylococcus aureus* (MRSA)**, has come under intense scrutiny. Symptoms of MRSA infection often start with a rash or pimple-like skin irritation. Within hours, symptoms may progress to redness, inflammation, pain, and deeper wounds. If untreated, MRSA may invade blood, bones, joints, surgical wounds, heart valves, and lungs. It can be fatal.

Health care–associated or *health care–acquired MRSA (HA-MRSA)* cases arise in settings, such as hospitals or nursing homes, where invasive treatments, infectious pathogens, and weakened immune systems converge. Five to 10 percent of hospitalized patients—over 1.7 million people yearly—develop serious infections, usually from HA-MRSA, and over 99,000 die.[7] Infection with *community-acquired MRSA (CA-MRSA)* occurs during normal daily activities.

One of the most common and difficult to treat health-care associated bacterial infections in the United States is *Clostridium difficile*, or *C. diff*. Symptoms include inflammation of the colon, diarrhea, fever, pain, bloating, and nausea. Ironically, long-term use of antibiotics to treat bacterial infection is the major cause of *C. diff*, because the antibiotics also kill the good bacteria that help keep the gastrointestinal system running smoothly.[8]

Streptococcal Infections

At least five types of the **Streptococcus** microorganism are known to cause bacterial infections (see **Figure 12.3a**). Group A streptococci cause the most common diseases, such as streptococcal pharyngitis ("strep throat") and scarlet fever. One particularly virulent group of group A streptococci can lead to rare but serious diseases such as *toxic shock syndrome* or *necrotizing fasciitis* (often referred to as "flesh-eating strep"). Group B streptococci can cause illness in newborns, pregnant women, older adults,

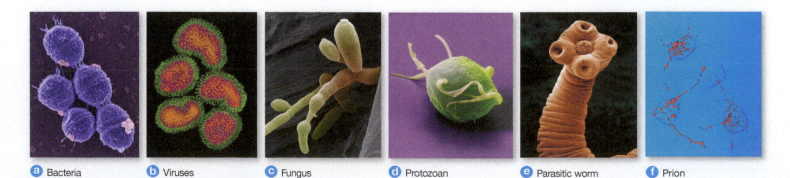

ⓐ Bacteria **ⓑ** Viruses **ⓒ** Fungus **ⓓ** Protozoan **ⓔ** Parasitic worm **ⓕ** Prion

Figure 12.3 Examples of Five Major Types of Pathogens
(a) Color-enhanced scanning electron micrograph (SEM) of *Streptococcus* bacteria, magnified 40,000×. (b) Colored transmission electron micrograph (TEM) of influenza (flu) viruses, magnified 32,000×. (c) Color SEM of *Candida albicans*, a yeast fungus, magnified 50,000×. (d) Color TEM of *Trichomonas vaginalis*, a protozoan, magnified 9,000×. (e) Color-enhanced SEM of a tapeworm, magnified 50×. (f) Prion.

and adults with illnesses such as diabetes or liver disease. Since about 1 in 4 pregnant women have *group B strep* in their rectum or vagina, the Centers for Disease Control and Prevention (CDC) recommends testing for the microorganism in the last weeks of pregnancy.[9] A form of resistant *Streptococcus pneumoniae* is a leading cause of bacterial pneumonia, ear infections, sinus infections, and bloodstream infections, or *sepsis*.

Meningitis

Meningitis is an infection and inflammation of the *meninges*, the protective membranes that surround the brain and spinal cord. Some forms of bacterial meningitis are contagious and can be spread through contact; *pneumococcal meningitis* is the most common and the most dangerous. *Meningococcal meningitis*, a virulent form of meningitis, remains prevalent on college campuses. Globally, between 5 and 10 percent of meningococcal cases are fatal, and up to 20 percent of people who are infected are left with neurological problems.[10] There were nearly 500 cases of meningococcal disease in the United States last year.[11] Children, adolescents, and young adults between 16 and 23 years of age are among the most likely to be infected.[12] The signs of meningitis are sudden fever, severe headache, and a stiff neck, particularly causing difficulty touching chin to chest. People who are suspected of having meningitis should receive immediate, aggressive medical treatment. Vaccines are available for some types of meningitis.

Pneumonia

Pneumonia is a general term for a range of conditions that result in inflammation of the lungs and difficulty breathing. It is characterized by chronic cough, chest pain, chills, high fever, fluid accumulation, and eventual respiratory failure.

Bacterial pneumonia responds readily to antibiotic treatment in the early stages but can be deadly in more advanced stages. Pneumonias caused by viruses, fungi, chemicals, or other substances in the lungs are more difficult to treat. Vulnerable populations include children; the poor; people displaced by war, famine, and natural disasters; older adults; people who are occupationally exposed to chemicals and particulates that damage the lungs; and those suffering from other illnesses.

Tuberculosis (TB)

Only HIV/AIDS is a greater infectious killer than **tuberculosis (TB)** in the global population.[13] With over 10.4 million new cases of TB and 1.8 million deaths from the disease in 2015, an astounding one-third of the world's population is infected with TB.[14] Although infection rates have decreased dramatically in the United States since the 1950s, there were still nearly 9,300 new cases of TB in 2016.[15] During the past 20 years, overcrowding and poor sanitation in some developing nations kept the disease alive. Failure to isolate active cases of TB and fully treat them, an increase in TB infections in the United States resulting from immigration and international travel, and a weakened public health infrastructure that funded less screening kept the disease from disappearing in North America.

Symptoms of TB include persistent coughing, weight loss, fever, and spitting up blood. People who are at highest risk include the poor, especially children, and the chronically ill; people in crowded prisons and homeless shelters who continuously inhale infected air.

The current recommended treatment for TB involves taking four drugs for 6 to 9 months; however, a 12-dose regimen is available for high-risk populations.[17] The lengthy, difficult treatment, along with barriers to obtaining drugs and care in many developing areas, leads to missed doses and treatments that end before the cure and thus breed drug-resistant bacteria.

Multidrug-resistant TB (MDR-TB) is a form of TB that is resistant to at least two of the best anti-TB drugs. An even more dangerous form, **extensively drug-resistant TB (XDR-TB)**, is extremely difficult to treat. These newer strains of tuberculosis are reaching epidemic proportions in over 58 countries.[18]

Tick-borne Bacterial Diseases

Certain tick-borne diseases have become major health threats in the United States. The most noteworthy include two bacterially-caused diseases. **Lyme disease** is a major threat to pets and humans in many regions of the U.S. Symptoms range from none; to a rash or bull's eye lesion and flulike symptoms; to chronic arthritis, blindness, and long-term disability. **Ehrlichiosis** has flulike symptoms that may progress quickly to respiratory difficulties and even death. Fortunately, antibiotics given early in the disease course are effective in preventing any serious threats.

Rickettsia are bacteria that multiply within small blood vessels, causing vascular blockage and tissue death. Rickettsia require an insect vector (carrier) for transmission to humans. Two common forms of human rickettsial disease are *Rocky Mountain spotted fever (RMSF)*, carried by a tick, and *typhus*, carried by a louse, flea, or tick. These produce similar symptoms, including high fever, weakness, rash, and coma; both can be life threatening.

Ticks can also transmit viruses and other pathogens, such as the **Powassan virus**. Related to *West Nile virus*, powassan attacks the brain of those who have been bitten by ticks carrying the virus, causing encephalitis and life-threatening symptoms. **Babesiosis**, a tick-borne disease caused by a protozoan, causes flulike symptoms including aches, headache, fatigue, nausea, and anemia. Older adults and people with weakened immune systems are at greatest risk of complications.

For all insect-borne diseases, the best protection is to stay indoors at dusk and early morning to avoid high levels of insect activity. If you must go out, wear protective clothing or use insecticides containing natural oils, pyrethrins, or DEET (diethyl toluamide). If you are traveling where insect-borne diseases are prevalent, use bed nets and other protective measures.

Ticks are a vector for several devastating bacterial diseases.

Check Yourself

- List three illnesses or conditions that can result from bacterial infection.

- What can you do to reduce your risk of bacterial infections?

Viral Infections: Mono, Hepatitis, Herpes, Mumps, Measles, and Rubella

12.4 Identify the causes and symptoms of common viral infections.

Viruses are the smallest known pathogens, approximately 1/500th the size of bacteria. Essentially, a virus consists of a protein structure that contains either *ribonucleic acid (RNA)* or *deoxyribonucleic acid (DNA)*. Viruses are incapable of carrying out any life processes on their own. To reproduce, viruses must invade a host cell, inject their own DNA and RNA into it, take it over, and force the cell to make copies of itself containing the virus. The new viruses then erupt out of the host cell and seek other cells to invade. Hundreds of viruses are known to cause diseases in humans.

Viral diseases can be difficult to treat because many viruses can withstand heat, formaldehyde, and large doses of radiation. Some viruses have **incubation periods** (the length of time required to develop fully and cause symptoms in their hosts) that last for years, which delays diagnosis. Drug treatment for viral infections is also limited. Drugs that are powerful enough to kill viruses generally kill the host cells too, although some medications block stages in viral reproduction without damaging the host cells.

Infectious Mononucleosis

Caused primarily by the Epstein-Barr virus, **mononucleosis** is most widespread among people between the ages of 15 and 24; college students and people living in close quarters are among those at highest risk. By adulthood, most people have been infected, many without ever showing symptoms.[19] Because saliva seems to be a key route of transmission, "mono" has often been referred to as "the kissing disease." However, sharing eating utensils, drinking vessels, towels, or cosmetics, or even coughing can spread the virus. Body fluids, including blood, genital secretions, and mucus, can also spread the disease. Common symptoms include intense fatigue, headache, fever, aches and pains, sore throat, rashes, and swollen lymph nodes. Anything that weakens the immune system, such as high stress, lack of sleep, poor diet, or too much alcohol or drug use, can increase risk. A simple blood test can determine whether you have mono. Rest, balanced nutrition, stress management, and healthy lifestyle are the best treatments.

Hepatitis

Hepatitis is a virally caused inflammation of the liver. Symptoms include fever, headache, nausea, loss of appetite, skin rashes, pain in the upper right abdomen, dark yellow-brown urine, and jaundice. There are several known forms of hepatitis (A, B, C, D, and E); hepatitis A, B, and C have the highest rates of incidence.

Hepatitis A (HAV) is contracted by eating food or drinking water contaminated with human feces. Since vaccinations became available, U.S. HAV rates declined until 2013, when they again began to increase. In 2015, there were nearly 2,800 reported new cases of HAV.[20] Handlers of infected food, children at day care centers, people who have sexual contact with HAV-positive individuals, or those traveling to regions where HAV is endemic are at higher risk, as are people who ingest seafood from contaminated water or use contaminated needles. Fortunately, individuals infected with hepatitis A don't become chronic carriers, and vaccines for the disease are available.

Hepatitis B (HBV) is spread through unprotected sex; sharing needles or accidental needlesticks; or, for newborns, an infected mother. HBV can lead to chronic liver disease or liver cancer. Numbers of HBV cases have declined rapidly since vaccines became available, and needle exchange programs are believed to be an important part of risk reduction for HBV and HCV infection, as well as HIV infection, in the past decade.[21] Rates are also on the decline in the United States; however, an estimated 20,000 cases are reported each year, and nearly 1.4 million people are chronic carriers.[22] Globally, HBV is the 15th leading cause of death, with 240 million chronically infected.[23]

Hepatitis C (HCV) infections are becoming epidemic as resistant forms of the virus emerge. Some cases can be traced to blood transfusions or organ transplants. An estimated 33,900 new cases of HCV occurred in 2015, and the estimated number of chronic cases of HCV may be as high as 3.5 million.[24] Of those infected, 75 to 85 percent will develop chronic hepatitis C, and 60 to 70 percent will develop chronic liver disease.[25] Between 5 and 20 percent of those who develop chronic liver disease will develop cirrhosis of the liver.[26] One in five of those with chronic HCV will die from cirrhosis or liver cancer.[27] For a complete listing of current treatment guidelines and promising new treatments, see http://www.hcvguidelines.org.[28]

To prevent spread of HBV and HCV, use latex condoms every time you have sex; don't share personal care items that might have blood on them, such as razors or toothbrushes; get a blood test for HBV; never share needles; and if you are having body art done, go only to reputable artists or piercers who follow established sterilization and infection control protocols.

Herpes Viruses

Herpes viruses are among the more common viruses infecting humans; painful, blistering rashes or weeping sores are hallmarks of these infections. These diseases are easily transmitted via physical contact and can become chronic problems.

Caused by the *herpes varicella zoster virus (HVZV)*, **chickenpox** produces symptoms of fever and fatigue 13 to 17 days after exposure, followed by skin eruptions that itch, blister, and produce a clear fluid. The virus is present in these blisters for approximately 1 week. Although a vaccine is available, many parents incorrectly assume that the vaccine is not necessary and that contracting the disease will ensure lifelong immunity.

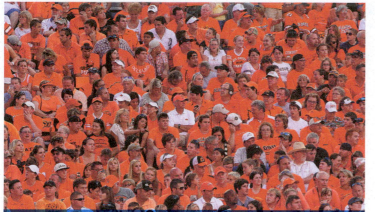

Why does it matter if people opt out of recommended vaccines?

Vaccinations are key in protecting us from infectious diseases, yet many people opt out for religious or philosophical reasons. College students and those who live or routinely hang out in crowded areas, ride on public transportation, travel internationally, attend major sporting events or concerts, or spend time in hospitals or other places where sick people congregate are more likely to come in contact with those who are sick. Keeping up-to-date on your vaccines is a big part of being responsible and protecting yourself and others.

One in three people in the United States will develop **shingles**, a painful, blistering rash that causes extreme pain when the chickenpox virus reactivates later in life. Usually, shingles occurs when the immune system is taxed as a result of stress, disease, or injury. Shingles affects over 1 million people in the United States, most of whom are over the age of 60.[29] The best way to prevent shingles is to get a shingles vaccine, particularly if your immune system is compromised or you are over 60.

Herpes gladiatorum is caused by the herpes simplex type 1 virus. It shows itself as a blistered rash on the face, neck, or torso. Herpes gladiatorum is also referred to as "mat pox" or "wrestler's herpes" because it is highly contagious and easily spread via mats used in a yoga studio or gym or through body-to-body contact.

Herpes infections that are sexually transmitted are discussed later in this chapter.

Mumps

Since the introduction of a vaccine, reported cases of **mumps** have declined, but in the last decade, several outbreaks have occurred in the United States and globally, largely because parents' unsubstantiated fears of vaccine complications have kept many school-aged children from being vaccinated.

Approximately half of all mumps infections produce only minor symptoms, and about one-third of infected people never show any. The most common symptom is the swelling of the parotid (salivary) glands. One of the greatest dangers associated with mumps is the potential for sterility in men who contract the disease in young adulthood. Some victims also suffer hearing loss.

Measles and Rubella

Measles is a highly contagious viral disorder that often affects young children, but it is increasing among young people today, particularly on college campuses. Young adults might not have been fully vaccinated in childhood, as their parents may have thought measles was no longer a problem in the United States. People who refuse vaccination put the immunocompromised and others at risk, as babies are typically not vaccinated until after 1 year of age. Increased incidences of these and other vaccine-preventable diseases seen between 2015 and 2016 are reason for significant concern in many regions of the country.

Symptoms of measles include an itchy rash and a high fever. Measles can be life threatening, causing high fever, pneumonia, encephalitis, and other complications. Symptoms tend to be worse for individuals under 5 years of age and those age 20 and over.

Rubella (German measles) is a milder viral infection that causes rashes, usually on upper extremities, and is believed to be spread by inhalation. Rubella is a threat to the very young and the unborn, as it is known to cause blindness, deafness, heart defects, and cognitive impairments in fetuses and newborns. Infections in children who have not been immunized against measles can lead to fever-induced problems such as rheumatic heart disease, kidney damage, and neurological disorders.

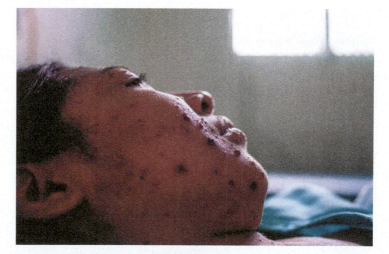

Measles can strike at any age, including the college years, especially if people have not been vaccinated.

12.4 Infectious Conditions

Check Yourself

- List three illnesses or conditions that can result from viral infection.

- What can you do to reduce your risk of viral infections?

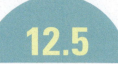
Viral Infections: The Cold and Flu

Learning Outcome

12.5 Identify the causes and symptoms of the common cold and influenza.

The Common Cold

Colds are the main reason for missed work and missed school in the United States, with millions of cases each year.[30] Colds can be caused by over 200 viruses, although most are caused by the rhinovirus or the coronavirus.[31] Colds are endemic (always present to some degree). Otherwise healthy people carry cold viruses in their noses and throats most of the time; these are held in check until the host's resistance is lowered. It is possible to "catch" a cold from airborne droplets of a sneeze or from skin-to-skin or mucous membrane contact, though the hands are the greatest avenue for virus transmission. Covering your nose and mouth with a tissue or handkerchief or your arm when sneezing is better than using your bare hand and then touching other objects.

To avoid a cold, bolster your immune system with a healthy diet, exercise, stress reduction, sleep, and other health-promoting behaviors. Wash your hands with soap and water and keep your hands away from your eyes, nose, and mouth. If you have a cold, stay away from others; if others have a cold, avoid close contact with them and wash your hands often. Throw used tissues in the trash, and disinfect TV remotes and other objects that you have been touching. Opt for disposable tissues rather than re-usable handkerchiefs. Wash your hands immediately after flossing to avoid spreading virus to other household surfaces. Contrary to popular belief, you cannot catch a cold from getting a chill, but a prolonged chill may lower your immune system's resistance to a pathogenic virus if one is present.

Influenza

In otherwise healthy people, **influenza**, or flu, is usually not life threatening (see **Figure 12.3b** and **Figure 12.4** for differences between cold and flu). However, for individuals over age 65, under age 5, or with respiratory problems or heart disease, flu can be very serious. Estimates of death rates from flu range from 3,000 to 49,000 per year.[32] Treatment is *palliative*—focused on symptom relief rather than cure. Signs of flu include body aches, fatigue, and fever.

Flu Vaccine The best way to avoid the flu is to get an annual vaccination. Because there are numerous and constantly mutating flu strains, vaccines are formulated every year for the few strains that are most likely to be prevalent in an upcoming season. If researchers predict strains correctly, vaccines are thought to be 70 to 90 percent effective in healthy adults for about a year.[33] Flu shots take 2 to 3 weeks to become effective, so people at risk should get these shots in the fall before the flu season begins. Some options for low- or no-cost vaccines are campus health centers, public health departments, pharmacies and big box stores, and community centers.

If you have had a severe reaction to past flu shots, have a severe allergy to chicken eggs, are running a fever, or have other health problems, consult with your doctor before having a shot. Other options include a high-dose shot if you are over age 65 or at risk or the Flublok shot if you are allergic to the eggs used to produce vaccines. Another popular option, the nasal spray FluMist, is under investigation to make sure it is effective.[34]

If you think that you have been exposed to the flu or have early symptoms, ask your doctor about antiviral sprays, capsules, or powders to reduce symptoms and prevent complications.

SYMPTOMS	COLD	FLU
Fever	Rare	Usual; high (100–102°F, occasionally higher, especially in children); lasts 3–4 days
Headache	Rare	Common
General aches and pains	Slight	Usual; often severe
Fatigue, weakness	Sometimes	Usual; can last up to 2–3 weeks
Extreme exhaustion	Never	Usual; at the beginning of the illness
Stuffy nose	Common	Sometimes
Sneezing	Usual	Sometimes
Sore throat	Common	Sometimes
Chest discomfort, cough	Common; mild to moderate, hacking cough	Common; can become severe
TREATMENT	Antihistamines, decongestants, nonsteroidal anti-inflammatory medicines	Antiviral medicines—see your doctor
PREVENTION	Wash your hands often with soap and water; avoid close contact with anyone with a cold	Annual vaccination; antiviral medicines—see your doctor
COMPLICATIONS	Sinus congestion, middle ear infection, asthma	Bronchitis, pneumonia; can worsen chronic conditions; can be life threatening

Figure 12.4 Is It a Cold or the Flu?

Source: Adapted from National Institutes of Health, National Institute of Allergy and Infectious Diseases. "Is it a Cold or the Flu?" August 2014. http://www .jointcommission.org/assets/1/6/Cold_or_flu.pdf. Accessed August 2017.

Check Yourself

- **What are the causes, symptoms, and treatment for the common cold and influenza?**

12.6 Other Pathogens

12.6 Describe how fungi, protozoans, parasitic worms, and prions cause infection.

Bacteria and viruses account for many, but not all, common diseases. Other organisms can also infect a host. Among these are fungi, protozoans, parasitic worms, and prions.

Fungi

Our environment is inhabited by hundreds of species of **fungi**, which are multicellular or unicellular organisms that obtain food by infiltrating the bodies of other organisms, both living and dead (see **Figure 12.3c**). Many fungi, such as edible mushrooms, penicillin, and the yeast used to make bread, are useful to humans, but some species can produce infections. Candidiasis (vaginal yeast infection), ringworm, jock itch, and toenail fungus are common fungal diseases.

With most fungal diseases, keeping the affected area clean and dry and treating it promptly with appropriate medications (often available over the counter) will generally bring relief. Fungal diseases are typically transmitted via physical contact, so avoid going barefoot in public showers, hotel rooms, and other areas where fungus may be present.

Coccidioidomycosis, also known as *valley fever*, is an infection that occurs when humans or pets inhale soil-dwelling fungal spores. In the last decade, rates have soared in desert regions of Mexico, Central and South America, and the southwestern United States. New cases are now being seen as far away as the Pacific Northwest, Minnesota and Wisconsin, and New Hampshire.[35] Because early symptoms of headache, aches, and fever are common to many ordinary diseases, cases often go unreported and can quickly progress to pneumonia, meningitis, or other life-threatening complications. As many as 40 percent of cases require hospitalization and have symptoms lasting weeks or months.[36] The best means of prevention is to avoid actions that stir the soil and cause spores to be aerosolized. Staying indoors during dust storms may also help to reduce risks.

Protozoans

Protozoans are single-celled organisms that cause diseases such as African sleeping sickness and malaria (see **Figure 12.3d**). Although prevalent in nonindustrialized countries, they are largely controlled in the United States. The most common protozoan disease in the United States is *trichomoniasis*, discussed later in the chapter. A common waterborne protozoan disease, *giardiasis*, can cause intestinal pain and discomfort weeks after infection. Protection of water supplies is the key to prevention.

Parasitic Worms

Parasitic worms are the largest of the pathogens. Ranging in size from small pinworms to large tapeworms (see **Figure 12.3e**), most are more a nuisance than a threat. Of special note are worm infestations associated with eating raw fish such as sushi. Eating raw fish can lead to infection with herring worms, round worms, and other parasites. Symptoms ranging from nausea and vomiting to severe pain and cramping may occur as worms invade the intestines and the immune system fights back. Medicines can be prescribed to kill worms. In severe cases, surgery may be required to remove them. You can prevent worm infestations by cooking fish and other foods to temperatures sufficient to kill the worms and their eggs. Worms can also be contracted through close contact with pets at home and poor pet and human hygiene. Preventive measures include getting your pets checked and wearing shoes in parks or public places where animal feces are present.

Prions

A **prion** is a self-replicating, protein-based agent that can infect humans and animals (see **Figure 12.3f**). One such prion is believed to be the underlying cause of spongiform diseases such as *bovine spongiform encephalopathy (BSE)* or "mad cow disease" found in beef cattle in various regions of the world. If humans eat contaminated meat from cattle with BSE, they may develop a mad cow–like disease known as *variant Creutzfeldt-Jakob disease (vCJD)*. Symptoms of vCJD include loss of memory, tremors, and muscle spasms, also known as tics. Within a fairly short time, depression, difficulty walking, seizures, and severe dementia can lead to death in both cows and humans.[37] An increasing number of infected cattle have been found in the United States and globally. To date, there have been four cases of vCJD in the United States.[38] Improved surveillance and reporting are necessary to determine whether more cases have occurred. In the meantime, because infected brain tissue and spinal tissue of cattle have been implicated in global infections, these animal parts from high-risk older cattle are restricted from the human food chain.[39]

- What are three illnesses or conditions that can result from fungi, protozoans, parasitic worms, or prions?

- What can you do to reduce your risk of these illnesses or conditions?

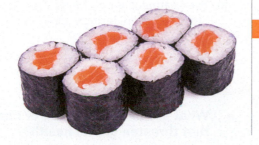

Eating raw fish, such as sushi, can increase your risk of infection from parasitic worms.

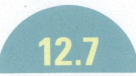

12.7 Emerging Diseases

Learning Outcome

12.7 Explain the problem of emerging and resurgent diseases.

Although our immune systems are adept at responding to challenges, microbes and other pathogens appear to be gaining ground. Rates of many infectious diseases have rapidly increased over the past decade, owing to a combination of human overpopulation, inadequate health care, increasing poverty, environmental degradation, and drug resistance.

West Nile Virus

In 2016, there were 2,038 cases of West Nile virus in the United States. Over 56 percent of infected individuals have the *neuroinvasive* type, which has more serious symptoms of meningitis or encephalitis that can lead to disability and death, and 44 percent have the non-neuroinvasive type, with headache and other flulike symptoms that are less severe.[40] Today, only Alaska and Hawaii remain free of the disease in the United States.

West Nile virus is spread by infected mosquitoes, so the best way to avoid infection is through mosquito eradication programs, wearing mosquito repellent, and avoiding mosquito-infested areas altogether, especially at peak mosquito feeding times. There is no vaccine or specific treatment.

Avian (Bird) Flu

Avian influenza is an infectious disease of birds, with strains that are capable of crossing the species barrier to cause severe illness in humans who come into contact with bird droppings or fluids. Bird flu appears to have originated in Asia and spread via migrating bird populations.[41] Although the virus has yet to mutate into a form highly infectious to humans, outbreaks in which people contract the disease from birds in rural areas of the world (where people often live in close proximity to poultry and other animals) have occurred. By the end of 2016, the World Health Organization had recorded 859 cumulative cases of bird flu in humans with 453 deaths, an indication of the severity of this disease.[42]

Escherichia coli O157:H7

Escherichia coli O157:H7 is one of over 170 types of *E. coli* bacteria that can infect humans. Most *E. coli* organisms are harmless and live in the intestines of healthy animals and humans.

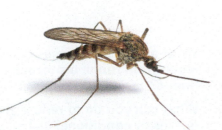

Mosquitoes spread many diseases, including West Nile virus and malaria.

E. coli O157:H7, however, produces a lethal toxin and can cause severe illness or death. It can live in the intestines of healthy cattle and then can contaminate food products at slaughterhouses. Eating ground beef that is rare or undercooked, drinking unpasteurized milk or juice, or swimming in sewage-contaminated water or public pools can also cause infection.

A symptom of *E. coli* O157:H7 infection is nonbloody diarrhea, usually 2 to 8 days after exposure; however, asymptomatic cases have been noted. Children, older adults, and people with weakened immune systems are particularly vulnerable to serious side effects such as kidney failure, intestinal damage, or death.

Ebola Virus Disease

Ebola virus disease (EVD) is a rare, often fatal disease that is ravaging parts of Central and West Africa, with over 8,000 cases reported in September 2014 and death rates of 50 to 90 percent. Fruit bats, chimpanzees, and other animals are natural hosts and spread the disease to humans, who spread it to others via contact with infected body fluids or surfaces such as sheets and clothing. Once a person has been infected, blood clotting ability diminishes, leading to internal and external bleeding. Without rehydration, organ failure and death can occur. Body rash, vomiting, diarrhea, fever, pain, and headache are early symptoms. No vaccines for Ebola are currently available, although two are being tested.

Malaria

Today, approximately 50 percent of the world's population, mostly those living in the poorest countries, are at risk for malaria. The disease is transmitted by mosquitoes carrying a parasite. There were 212 million cases of malaria and an estimated 235,000 to 639,000 deaths in 2015, even though mortality rates have dropped significantly in the last decade.[43] Most deaths occur among poor and vulnerable children and pregnant women in the African region (92%), followed by the Southeast Asian region (6%) and the Eastern Mediterranean region (2%).[44]

Travelers from malaria-free regions entering areas where there is malaria transmission are highly vulnerable, as they have little or no immunity and often receive a delayed or wrong malaria diagnosis when they return home.[45] Mosquito nets and use of insect repellents are particularly important to prevention, as is removal of standing water in outdoor areas. Natural disasters that leave standing water in which mosquitoes can flourish pose increased risks. Resistance to chloroquine, once a widely used and highly effective treatment, is now found in most regions of the world, and other treatments are losing their effectiveness at alarming rates.

Check Yourself

- **What are three emerging or resurgent diseases that threaten global health?**

12.8 Antibiotic Resistance

Learning Outcome

12.8 Explain the phenomenon of antibiotic resistance.

Antibiotics are supposed to wipe out bacteria that are susceptible to them. However, many common antibiotics are becoming ineffective against resistant strains of bacteria. Here's how this happens: Bacteria and other microorganisms that cause infections and diseases can evolve rapidly, developing ways to survive drugs that had once been able to kill or weaken them. Through this process, some of the bacteria and microorganisms are becoming "superbugs" that cannot be stopped with existing medications.

Antibiotic Resistance on the Rise

Antibiotic resistance is a problem today for several reasons:[46]

- **Overuse of antibiotics in food production.** About 70 percent of antibiotics produced today are ingested by animals or fish living in crowded feedlots or fish farms to encourage their growth and fight off disease. Water runoff and sewage from feedlots can contaminate the water in rivers and streams with antibiotics. Antibiotic-resistant bacteria may also spread beyond farms via dried particles of animal manure that disperse in the wind.
- **Improper use of antibiotics by humans and unnecessary prescriptions.** Humans also contaminate waterways and soil through dumping their unused prescription drugs down the toilet or tossing them into the garbage. Furthermore, the CDC estimates that one-third to one-half of the 150 million antibiotic prescriptions written each year are unnecessary, resulting in bacterial strains that are tougher than the drugs used to fight them. Growing awareness of the problem has led patients and doctors to be more careful in their requests for and dispersal of antibiotics.
- **Misuse and overuse of antibacterial soaps and other cleaning products.** Preying on the public's fear of germs and disease, the cleaning products industry adds antibacterial ingredients to many soaps and household cleaners. Just how much these products contribute to overall resistance is difficult to assess; as with antibiotics, the germs these products do not kill may become stronger than before.

What Can You Do?

You can take the following steps to prevent antibiotic resistance[47]:

- **Be responsible with medications.** Use antibiotics only when they are prescribed for you, and take them only for the disease for which they are intended. Ask your doctor whether there is an older-generation antibiotic that still works to treat

the illness, and save the newer drugs for the most difficult problems.
- **Finish the entire course of a drug as prescribed.** Antibiotic regimens are designed to kill entire colonies of bacteria if taken exactly as prescribed. If you stop early, the hardiest bacteria may survive, leading to increased chances of drug-resistant pathogens.
- **Use regular soap when washing your hands.** Research suggests that antibacterial agents contained in soaps may actually kill normal bacteria found on the skin that does not cause disease, thus creating an environment for resistant, mutated bacteria that are impervious to antibacterial cleaners and antibiotics to colonize the skin.
- **Avoid food that has been treated with antibiotics.** Buy organic meat and poultry, particularly products with labels that say that they have not been fed antibiotics or hormones. If you buy farmed fish, choose fish grown in U.S. coastal waters, where there is less likelihood of questionable fish-feeding practices and less chance of contaminated water and antibiotics or growth hormones.

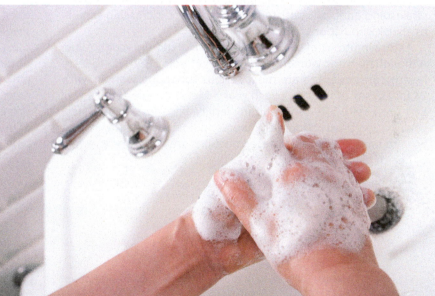

To prevent the spread of infectious disease, wash your hands! But use regular soap, not antibacterial products. Antibacterial soaps may actually encourage the development of antibiotic resistance.

Check Yourself

- How do bacteria become resistant to antibiotics?
- What can you do to prevent antibiotic resistance?

12.9 Sexually Transmitted Infections

12.9 Explain risk factors for sexually transmitted infections and identify actions that can prevent their spread.

There are more than 20 known types of **sexually transmitted infections (STIs)**, sometimes called sexually transmitted diseases (STDs). The term STI describes a condition that has visible symptoms or that alters key functions of the body. Some STIs, especially *chlamydia*, *gonorrhea*, and *syphilis*, are increasing at alarming rates, particularly among young adults with the highest overall numbers of reported cases ever reported in the United States occurring in 2016.[48]

Huge disparities in rates exist by age, race, income, and gender.[49] Sexually transmitted infections affect people of all backgrounds and socioeconomic levels, but they disproportionately affect women, minorities, and infants.[50] Young people age 15 to 24 acquire half of all new STIs, making this age group the most at risk group for STIs overall and putting campuses where the majority of students are in this demographic, at risk.[51] More virulent strains and antibiotic-resistant forms indicate increasing threats to at-risk populations.

Early symptoms of an STI are often mild and unrecognizable. Although men and women both feel the effects of STIs, long-term health consequences are most serious for young women, with 24,000 cases of infertility each year.[52] Men can face sterility too. Left untreated, STIs can result in sterility, blindness, central nervous system destruction, disfigurement, and even death. Infants born to mothers carrying these infections are at risk for a variety of health problems.

What's Your Risk?

Several reasons have been proposed to explain the present high rates of STIs. The first relates to the moral and social stigmas associated with these infections. Shame and embarrassment often keep infected people from seeking treatment. Unfortunately, the infected usually continue to be sexually active, thereby infecting unsuspecting partners. People who are uncomfortable discussing sexual issues may also be less likely to use, and ask their partners to use, condoms to protect against STIs and pregnancy or to take other precautions that could reduce their risks. Detailed fact sheets about many of the major STIs are provided at this CDC website: https://www.cdc.gov/std/healthcomm/fact_sheets.htm

Another reason proposed for the STI epidemic is our casual attitude about sex. Bombarded by media that glamorizes sex, many people take sex partners without considering the consequences. Others are pressured into sexual relationships they don't really want or aren't ready for. Generally, the more sex partners a person has, the greater the risk for contracting an STI.

Ignorance—about the infections, their symptoms, and the fact that someone can be asymptomatic but still infected—is also a factor. A person who is infected but asymptomatic can unknowingly spread an STI to others who also ignore or misinterpret symptoms. By the time either partner seeks medical help, one or both of them may have infected several others. In addition, many people mistakenly believe that certain sexual practices—oral sex, for example—carry no risk for STIs. In fact, oral sex practices among young adults may be responsible for increases in herpes and other STIs. **Figure 12.5** shows the continuum of risk for various sexual behaviors. The **Skills for Behavior Change** offers tips for ways to practice safer sex.

High-risk behaviors	Moderate-risk behaviors	Low-risk behaviors	No-risk behaviors
Unprotected vaginal, anal, and oral sex—any activity that involves direct contact with bodily fluids, such as ejaculate, vaginal secretions, or blood—are high-risk behaviors.	Vaginal, anal, or oral sex with a latex or polyurethane condom and a water-based lubricant used properly and consistently can greatly reduce the risk of STI transmission. Dental dams used during oral sex can also greatly reduce the risk of STI transmission.	Mutual masturbation, if there are no cuts on the hand, penis, or vagina, is very low risk. Rubbing, kissing, and massaging carry low risk, but herpes can be spread by skin-to-skin contact from an infected partner.	Abstinence, phone sex, talking, and fantasy are all no-risk behaviors.

Figure 12.5 Continuum of Risk for Various Sexual Behaviors
Different behaviors have different levels of risk for various sexually transmitted infections; however, no matter what, any sexual activity involving direct contact with blood, semen, or vaginal secretions is high risk.

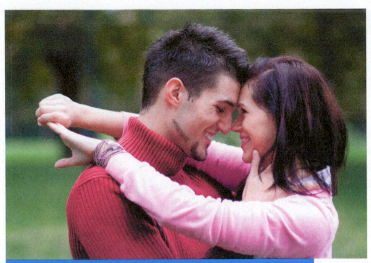

How can I tell if someone I'm dating has an STI?

You can't tell whether people have an STI just by looking at them. It isn't something broadcast on a person's face, and many people with STIs are themselves unaware of the infection because it could be asymptomatic. The only way to know for sure is to go to a clinic and get tested. In addition, partners need to be open and honest with each other about their sexual histories, and practice safer sex.

Routes of Transmission

STIs are generally spread through some form of intimate sexual contact. Vaginal intercourse, oral–genital contact, hand–genital contact, and anal intercourse are the most common modes of transmission. Less likely but still possible modes of transmission include mouth-to-mouth contact and contact with fluids from body sores that may be spread by the hands. Although each STI is a different infection caused by a different pathogen, all STI pathogens prefer dark, warm, moist places, especially the mucous membranes lining the reproductive organs. Most of these pathogens are susceptible to light and excess heat, cold, and dryness, and many die quickly on exposure to air. Like other communicable infections, STIs have both pathogen-specific *incubation periods* and periods of time during which transmission is most likely, called *periods of communicability*.

Where to Go for Help

If you are concerned about your own risk or that of a friend, arrange a confidential meeting with a health professional at your college health service or community STI clinic. He or she will provide you with the information that you need to decide whether you should be tested for an STI. If the student health service is not an option for you, seek assistance through your local public health department or community STI clinic.

Skills for Behavior Change

Safe Is Sexy

The following behaviors will help you reduce your risk of contracting a sexually transmitted infection (STI) when considering a sexual encounter:

- Avoid multiple sexual partners.
- Remember that oral sex is *not* safe sex. While the risks of contracting an STI are lower with oral sex than with vaginal or anal intercourse, the risk is still not zero. It is entirely possible to contract HIV from oral sex, as well as herpes, gonorrhea, syphilis, genital warts, and other diseases.
- Just say NO to casual sex. Know what you will say ahead of time. An example might be, "No. Sorry. I'm attracted to you (or I "like you") but I don't have sex with anyone I don't know well."
- Insist on using a latex condom or a dental dam.
- Get tested. If no partner tests, NO SEX!
- Avoid injury to body tissue, including abrasions and microscopic tears during sexual activity. Don't be afraid to say, "That hurts. Stop."
- Make handwashing a habit, insisting that both you and your partner wash hands before sex, petting, or masturbation and afterward. As a rule, use a full stream of water and soap and count to 20 while washing hands before and after sexual encounters. Urinate after sexual relations and, if possible, wash your genitals.
- Abstinence is the only way to be 100 percent sure you don't transmit or contract an STI.
- Get vaccinated for HPV, hepatitis B, and hepatitis C.
- If you contract an STI, ask your health care provider for advice on notifying past or potential partners.

Sources: American College of Obstetricians and Gynecologists, *How to Prevent Sexually Transmitted Infections*, Frequently Asked Questions, https://www.acog.org/Patients/FAQs/How-to-Prevent-Sexually-Transmitted-Infections-STIs; American Sexual Health Association, "Reduce Your Risk," 2017 http://www.ashasexualhealth.org/stdsstis/reduce-your-risk.

Check Yourself

- How are STIs transmitted?
- What can you do to protect yourself against STIs?

12.10 Define HIV/AIDS and explain its transmittal and treatment.

Acquired immunodeficiency syndrome (AIDS) is a significant global health threat. Approximately 78 million people worldwide have become infected with **human immunodeficiency virus (HIV)**, the virus that causes AIDS, and 35 million have died from diseases associated with the syndrome.[53] Today, between 30-43 million people worldwide are living with HIV, with as many as 2.1 million new infections and 1.1 million deaths in 2016.[54]

Initially, people were diagnosed as having AIDS only when they developed blood infections, the cancer known as Kaposi's sarcoma, or other indicator diseases common in male AIDS patients. The CDC has expanded the indicator list to include pulmonary tuberculosis, recurrent pneumonia, and invasive cervical cancer. Perhaps the most significant indicator today is a drop in the level of the body's master immune cells, the CD4 cells (also called helper T cells), to one-fifth the level in a healthy person.

How HIV Is Transmitted

HIV typically enters one person's body via another person's infected body fluids (e.g., semen, vaginal secretions, blood), often through a break in the mucous membranes of the genital organs or the anus. After initial infection, HIV multiplies rapidly, progressively destroying helper T cells (which call the rest of the immune response to action), weakening the body's resistance to disease. HIV cannot be transmitted through casual contact, such as sharing food utensils, musical instruments, or toilet seats. Research also provides overwhelming evidence that insect bites do not transmit HIV.

High-Risk Behaviors AIDS is not a disease of gay people or minority groups; rather, it is related to high-risk behaviors such as having unprotected sexual intercourse and sharing needles. **Figure 12.6** shows the breakdown of new HIV diagnoses for the most-affected populations.

The majority of HIV infections arise from the following high-risk behaviors:

- **Exchange of body fluids.** The greatest risk factor is the exchange of HIV-infected body fluids, including blood, semen, and vaginal secretions, during vaginal or anal intercourse.
- **Injecting drugs.** A significant percentage of AIDS cases in the United States results from sharing or using HIV-contaminated needles and syringes. Although users of illegal drugs are commonly considered the only members of this category, others may also share needles—for example, people with diabetes who inject insulin or athletes who inject steroids.

Mother-to-Child (Perinatal) Transmission Transmission from mother to child can occur during pregnancy, during labor and delivery, or through breastfeeding. Without antiretroviral treatment, approximately 15 to 45 percent of HIV-positive pregnant women will transmit the virus to their infant.[55] With appropriate interventions during pregnancy, labor, birth, and breastfeeding, transmission rates can be lowered to 5 percent.[56]

Body Piercing and Tattooing Body piercing and tattooing can be done safely, but dangerous pathogens can be transmitted with any puncture of the skin. Unsterile needles can transmit HIV, as well as other diseases. If you opt for tattooing or body piercing, take the following safety precautions:[57]

- Look for clean, well-lighted work areas and inquire about sterilization procedures.
- Packaged, sterilized needles should be used once, then discarded. A piercing gun cannot be sterilized properly. Watch that the artist uses new needles and tubes from a sterile package.
- Immediately before piercing or tattooing, the body area should be carefully sterilized. The artist should wash his or her hands and put on new latex gloves for each procedure.
- Leftover tattoo ink should be discarded after each procedure. Do not allow the artist to reuse ink that has been used for other customers. Used needles should be disposed of in a "sharps" container.

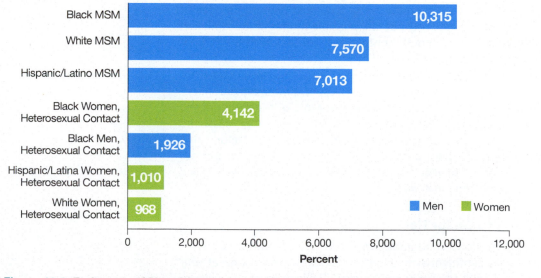

Figure 12.6 Estimates of New HIV Diagnoses in the United States for Most Affected Subpopulations, 2015

MSM: men who have sexual contact with men.

Source: CDC, "HIV Diagnoses in the United States: At a Glance," June 9, 2017, https://www.cdc.gov/hiv/statistics/overview/ataglance.html

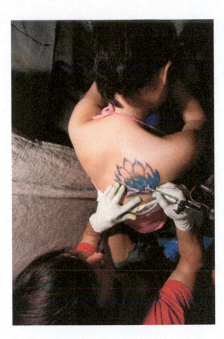

Like any activity that involves bodily fluids, tattooing carries some risk of disease transmission.

Symptoms of HIV/AIDS

A person may go for months or years after infection with HIV before any significant symptoms appear, and incubation time varies greatly from person to person. Without treatment, it typically takes an average of 8 to 10 years for the virus to cause the slow, degenerative changes in the immune system that are characteristic of AIDS. During this time, the person may experience *opportunistic infections* (infections that gain a foothold when the immune system is not functioning effectively). Colds, sore throats, fever, tiredness, nausea, night sweats, and other generally non–life-threatening pre-AIDS symptoms may occur. As HIV progresses, wasting syndrome, swollen lymph nodes, and neurological problems may occur. A diagnosis of AIDS, the final stage of HIV infection, is made when the infected person has either a dangerously low CD4 (helper T cell) count (below 200 cells per cubic milliliter of blood) or has contracted one or more opportunistic infections characteristic of the disease, such as Kaposi's sarcoma, tuberculosis, recurrent pneumonia, or invasive cervical cancer.

Testing for HIV

Today, we know that nearly a third of the new cases of HIV are transmitted by people who have undiagnosed HIV. Because of this and the multiple ways in which HIV is transmitted, the CDC recommends that everyone between the ages of 13 and 64 get tested for HIV at least once as part of their routine health care and more often if there are risk factors. The sooner you start antiretroviral therapy after diagnosis, the smaller the chance of spreading the disease and the better the chance of a better treatment result.[58]

There are three major types of HIV tests: *Antibody tests, Antigen/Antibody Tests* and *Nucleic Acid Tests (NATs)*.

Antibody Tests detect antibodies, proteins that your immune system makes in response to HIV. Rapid tests and home tests are typically antibody tests and they can tell you if you have been infected; however you need to understand how they work. For example if the *window period* – the amount of time needed for

sufficient antibodies to be detectable is 14-84 days after infection and you get a test on day 34 or even on day 65, you may test negative, even though a test on day 84 shows you are positive! Newer rapid antibody tests provides results from blood in 30 minutes, and an oral quick test kit can provide results within 20 minutes. The Home Access HIV Testing Kit requires a finger prick of blood to be sent to a lab. Results are generally available anonymously after 24 hours. Be sure to check the reported accuracy rates of any test you choose.

Antigen/Antibody tests detect both HIV antibodies and *antigens*- those foreign substances that trigger an immune response. Infection with HIV triggers the production of p24, an HIV antigen which is detectable earlier. That antigen then triggers an *antibody* response which is detectable through testing a bit later in the infection cycle. There are also rapid antigen/antibody tests available; however they are considerably more expensive than regular antibody tests.

Nucleic Acid Tests (NATs) and HIV p24 Antigen Test These newer, quicker, more costly tests look for the actual HIV virus (NATs) and antigens for the virus (HIV p24) .

If you are wondering about the tests and whether they are right for you, check out this website: https://www.cdc.gov/hiv/basics/testing.html

Treatments and Prevention

New drugs have slowed the progression from HIV to AIDS and have prolonged life expectancies. Since the 1990s, the U.S. death rate from AIDS has dropped nearly 83 percent.[59] However, the average cost for the medicines ranges from $4,000 to $48,000 per year. These costs do not include regular testing and doctor's visits.[60]

Current treatments combine selected drugs, especially protease inhibitors and reverse transcriptase inhibitors. *Protease inhibitors* (e.g., amprenavir, ritonavir, and saquinavir) act to prevent the production of the virus in chronically infected cells and seem to work best in combination with other therapies. Other drugs, such as AZT, ddI, ddC, d4T, and 3TC, inhibit the HIV enzyme *reverse transcriptase* before the virus has invaded the cell, thereby preventing the virus from infecting new cells. Drug options change frequently, and no combination has proven effective for all people.[61]

There is currently no vaccine to prevent HIV, and there is no cure. People at high risk who aren't HIV positive can reduce their risk of infection by taking Truvada, a daily combination pill. However, Truvada is not 100 percent effective. The key to its effectiveness is taking it consistently, using condoms and other prevention strategies, and getting regular medical checkups.[62]

Of course, the simplest answer is abstinence. If you don't exchange body fluids, you won't get the disease. If you do decide to be intimate, the next best option is to use a condom.

Check Yourself

- What are three common routes of transmission for HIV?

- What can you do to prevent the spread of HIV and to protect yourself against it?

12.11 Sexually Transmitted Infections: Chlamydia and Gonorrhea

Learning Outcome

12.11 List the symptoms and treatment of chlamydia and gonorrhea.

Two of the most common sexually transmitted infections are chlamydia and gonorrhea.

Chlamydia

Chlamydia, an infection caused by the bacterium *Chlamydia trachomatis* that often presents no symptoms, is the most commonly reported STI in the United States. In 2016, nearly 1.6 million chlamydia infections were reported; the vast majority (over 2/3 of all cases) in young adults aged 15-24. Experts believe that the actual number may be closer to 3 million cases annually.[63] Significant numbers of state and local health departments have lost funding in recent years, with shortages in staff, available hours, and affordable diagnosis and treatment. This, at a time when numbers of STIs are rising at unprecedented rates. Although often without obvious symptoms in early stages, untreated chlamydia can take a toll on men, women, and children of all ages, with pain, potential reproductive complications and other problems.

Signs and Symptoms In men, early symptoms may include painful and difficult urination; frequent urination; and a watery, pus-like discharge from the penis. Symptoms in women may include a yellowish discharge, spotting between periods, and occasional spotting after intercourse. However, many people with chlamydia display no symptoms and therefore do not seek help until the disease has done secondary damage. Women are especially likely to be asymptomatic; many do not realize they have the disease.

Complications Men can suffer injury to the prostate gland, seminal vesicles, and bulbourethral glands, and they can suffer from arthritis-like symptoms and inflammatory damage to the blood vessels and heart. Men can also experience *epididymitis*, inflammation of the area near the testicles.

In women, chlamydia-related inflammation can injure the cervix or fallopian tubes, causing sterility, and it can damage the inner pelvic structure, leading to **pelvic inflammatory disease (PID)**. If an infected woman becomes pregnant, she has a high risk for miscarriage and stillbirth. Chlamydia may also be responsible for one type of *conjunctivitis*, an eye infection that affects not only adults but also infants, who can contract the disease from an infected mother during delivery (**Figure 12.7**). Untreated conjunctivitis can cause blindness.

Women with chlamydia are also at greater risk for **urinary tract infections (UTIs)**. A woman's urethra is much shorter than a man's, making it easier for bacteria to enter the bladder. In addition, a woman's urethra is closer to the anus than is a man's, allowing bacteria to spread into her urethra and cause an infection. Symptoms of a UTI in women include a burning sensation during urination and lower abdominal pain. A UTI can be diagnosed through a urine test and treated by antibiotics.

Men can also get UTIs, although they are rarer. One form most commonly caused by *Chlamydia trachomatis* is *nongonococcal urethritis*. Infections should be taken seriously. If you have a milky penile discharge and/or burning during urination, contact your health care provider.

How Is it Transmitted? When someone has chlamydia they can transmit it to others through sexual contact with the mouth, penis, vagina, or anus, regardless of whether ejaculation has occurred. It can also be spread from the mother to her baby during childbirth, putting the newborn at risk for a variety of health problems. Once you are treated, you can get it again; in fact it is easily transmittable and if one partner has it and is treated, and they have had sex with a partner, they can pass it back and forth in a ping-pong type effect between successful treatments.

Diagnosis and Treatment A sample of urine or fluid from the vagina or penis is collected to identify the presence of the bacteria. Unfortunately, chlamydia tests are not a routine part of many health clinics' testing procedures. If detected early, chlamydia is easily treatable with antibiotics.

Gonorrhea

Gonorrhea is also on the rise in the United States, with an estimated 820,000 new infections each year; only half of which are reported.[64]. Over two-thirds of reported cases occur in 15- to 24-year-olds.[65]

Caused by the bacterial pathogen *Neisseria gonorrhoeae*, gonorrhea primarily infects the linings of the urethra, genital tract, pharynx, and rectum. It may spread to the eyes or other body regions by the hands or through body fluids, typically during vaginal, oral, or anal sex.

Signs and Symptoms In men, a typical symptom is a white, milky discharge from the penis accompanied by painful, burning urination 2 to 9 days after contact (**Figure 12.8**). Epididymitis, swelling (inflammation) of the epididymis, can also occur as a symptom of infection. However, some men with gonorrhea are asymptomatic.

In women, the situation is just the opposite: Most women do not experience any symptoms, but if a woman does experience symptoms, they can include vaginal discharge or a burning sensation on urinating.[66] The organism can remain in the woman's vagina, cervix, uterus, or fallopian tubes for long periods with no apparent symptoms other than an occasional slight fever. Thus a

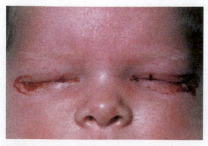

Figure 12.7 Conjunctivitis in a Newborn's Eyes
Untreated chlamydia and gonorrhea in a pregnant woman can be passed to her child during delivery, causing the eye infection conjunctivitis.

woman can be unaware that she has been infected and that she is infecting her sex partners.

Complications In a man, untreated gonorrhea may spread to the prostate, testicles, urinary tract, kidney, and bladder. Blockage of the vasa deferentia due to scar tissue may cause sterility. In some cases, the penis develops a painful curvature during erection. If gonorrhea goes undetected in a woman, it can spread to the fallopian tubes and ovaries, causing sterility or, at the very least, severe inflammation and PID. The bacteria can also spread through the blood, leading to arthritis and problems with bones and joints, as well as cardiovascular and brain issues—problems.[67] If an infected woman becomes pregnant, the infection can be transmitted to her baby during delivery, potentially causing blindness, joint infection, or a life-threatening blood infection.

Diagnosis and Treatment Diagnosis of gonorrhea is similar to that of chlamydia, requiring a sample of either urine or fluid from the vagina or penis to detect the presence of the bacteria. Chlamydia and gonorrhea often occur at the same time, but different antibiotics are needed to treat each infection separately. If detected early, gonorrhea, like chlamydia, is treatable with antibiotics, but antimicrobial resistance is posing an even greater threat.

Complications of STIs: PID in Women, Epididymitis in Men

If left untreated, many STIs can lead to serious complications for both men and women. Pelvic inflammatory disease (PID) can be caused by *Neisseria gonorrhoeae* or *Chlamydia trachomatis*. Pelvic inflammatory disease is a catchall term for a number of infections of the uterus, fallopian tubes, and ovaries and difficulties becoming pregnant are complications resulting from an untreated STI. Symptoms of PID vary but generally include lower abdominal pain, fever, unusual vaginal discharge, painful intercourse, painful urination, and irregular menstrual bleeding. The vague symptoms associated with chlamydial and gonococcal PID can cause a delay seeking medical care, thereby increasing the risk of permanent damage and scarring that can lead to infertility and other complications. In the United States, approximately 1 million women develop PID every year. It is estimated that 1 in 8 sexually active adolescent girls will develop PID before the age of 20.[68]

Epididymitis is most common among young men ages 19 to 35.[69] Epididymitis is most commonly caused by the spread of

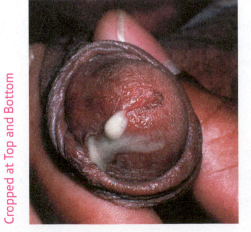

Figure 12.8 Gonorrhea One common symptom of gonorrhea in men is a milky discharge from the penis, accompanied by burning sensations during urination. These symptoms will cause most men to seek diagnosis and treatment. By contrast, women with gonorrhea are often asymptomatic, so they may not be aware that they are infected.

Neisseria gonorrhoeae or *Chlamydia trachomatis* from the urethra or the bladder. Symptoms can include blood in the semen, swollen groin area, discharge from the urethra, discomfort in the lower abdomen or pelvis, and pain during ejaculation or during urination. A physical examination along with other medical tests, including a testicular scan and tests for chlamydia and gonorrhea, can diagnose epididymitis. Treatment usually involves pain medications and anti-inflammatory medications.

Skills for **Behavior Change**

Communicating About Safer Sex

At no time in your life is it more important to communicate openly than when you are starting an intimate relationship. The following will help you communicate with your partner about potential sexual risks:

- Plan to talk before you find yourself in an awkward situation.
- Select the right moment and place for both of you to discuss safer sex; choose a relaxing environment in a neutral location, free of distractions.
- Remember that you have a responsibility to your partner to disclose your own health status. You also have a responsibility to yourself to stay healthy and celibate if you find out that you have any form of sexually transmitted diseases.
- Be direct, honest, and determined in talking about sex before you become involved. Don't let the conversation drift off or lose focus.
- Discuss the issues without sounding defensive or accusatory. Reassure your partner that your reasons for desiring abstinence or safer sex arise from respect and caring and not distrust.
- Analyze your own beliefs and values ahead of time. Know where you will draw the line on certain actions, and be very clear with your partner about what you expect.
- Decide what you will do if your partner does not agree with you. Anticipate potential objections or excuses, and prepare your responses accordingly.

Consider asking the following questions: Have you been tested for STIs? How long ago? Results? Have you had sex with someone since that last test? With how many people? Do you know whether that person or those individuals was positive for any STIs? Would you be willing to get a test before we consider having sex? Do you have any symptoms right now that make you wonder if you might have an STI?

Source Adapted from Queensland Health, "Talking to Your Partner about Sex," 2010, www.health.qld.gov.au and American Sexual Health Association. "Talking about Sex." 2017. http://www.ashasexualhealth.org/sexual-health/talking-about-sex/

Check Yourself

- What are the primary signs of chlamydia? Of gonorrhea?
- How does PID affect women? How does epididymitis affect men?

12.12 Sexually Transmitted Infections: Syphilis

Learning Outcome

12.12 **List the symptoms and treatment of syphilis in men and women.**

Syphilis is caused by a bacterium, the spirochete *Treponema pallidum*. Although nearly wiped out a decade ago, syphilis has been on an epidemic rise in the U.S. in recent years. The incidence of syphilis is highest in adults age 20 to 39 and is particularly high among women, African Americans, and men who have sex with men. There were nearly 88,000 reported new cases of syphilis in 2016, up significantly from the 17,375 cases in 2013.[70] Because it is extremely delicate and dies readily on exposure to air, dryness, or cold, *T. pallidum* is generally transferred only through direct sexual contact or from mother to fetus. The incidence of syphilis in newborns has continued to increase in the United States.[71]

Signs and Symptoms

Syphilis is known as the "great imitator" because its symptoms resemble those of several other infections. However, some people experience no symptoms at all. Syphilis can occur in four distinct stages:[72]

- **Primary syphilis.** The first stage of syphilis, particularly for men, is often characterized by the development of a **chancre** (pronounced "shank-er"), a sore located most frequently at the site of initial infection that usually appears 3 to 4 weeks after initial infection (see **Figure 12.9**). In men, the site of the chancre tends to be the penis or scrotum; in women, the site of infection is often internal: on the vaginal wall or high on the cervix, where the chancre is not readily apparent and the likelihood of detection is not great. Whether or not it is detected, the chancre is oozing with bacteria, ready to infect an unsuspecting partner. In both men and women, the chancre will disappear in 3 to 6 weeks.
- **Secondary syphilis.** If the infection is left untreated, secondary symptoms may appear a month to a year after the chancre disappears. These symptoms include a rash or white patches on the skin or on the mucous membranes of the mouth, throat, or genitals. Hair loss may occur, lymph nodes may enlarge, and the victim may develop a slight fever or headache. In rare cases, sores develop around the mouth or genitals. As during the active chancre phase, these sores contain infectious bacteria, and contact with them can spread the infection.
- **Latent syphilis.** After the secondary stage, if the infection is left untreated, the syphilis spirochetes begin to invade body organs, causing lesions called *gummas*. The infection now is rarely transmitted to others, except during pregnancy, when it can be passed to the fetus.

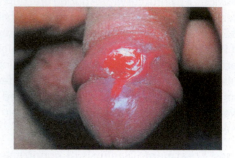

Figure 12.9 Syphilis
A chancre on the site of the initial infection can be a symptom of primary syphilis. However, a chancre does not always appear, and if it does, it might not look this obvious.

- **Tertiary/late syphilis.** Years after syphilis has entered the body, its effects become all too evident if it is still untreated. Late-stage syphilis indications include heart and central nervous system damage, blindness, deafness, paralysis, premature senility, and, ultimately, dementia.

Complications

Pregnant women with syphilis can experience complications such as premature births, miscarriages, and stillbirths. An infected pregnant woman may transmit the syphilis to her unborn child. The infant will then be born with *congenital syphilis*, which can cause death; severe birth defects such as blindness, deafness, or disfigurement; developmental delays; seizures; and other health problems. Because in most cases the fetus does not become infected until after the first trimester, treatment of the mother during this time will usually prevent infection of the fetus.

Diagnosis and Treatment

Syphilis can be diagnosed with a blood test or by collecting a sample from the chancre. Syphilis can easily be treated with antibiotics, usually penicillin, for all stages except the late stage.

Check Yourself

- **What are the four stages of untreated syphilis?**
- **How is syphilis diagnosed and treated?**

12.12

Infectious Conditions

12.13 List the symptoms and treatment of both types of herpes simplex virus.

Herpes is a general term for a family of infections characterized by sores or eruptions on the skin that are caused by the herpes simplex virus. The herpes family of diseases is not transmitted exclusively by sexual contact; kissing or sharing eating utensils can also transmit the infection.

There are two types of herpes simplex virus: HSV-1 and HSV-2. About 50 to 60 percent of American adults have HSV-1, which usually appears as cold sores on their mouths (see **Figure 12.10**) and sometimes causes genital herpes infections.[73] Only about 1 in 6 Americans are believed to have HSV-2; however, exact numbers are difficult to assess.[74] Both types can infect any area of the body.[75] Herpes simplex virus remains in nerve cells for life and can flare up when the body's ability to maintain itself is weakened.

Herpes infections range from mildly uncomfortable to extremely serious. **Genital herpes** affects approximately 16 percent of the population age 14 to 49 in the United States, with over 776,000 new cases overall each year in the United States.[76] People may get genital herpes by having sexual contact with others who don't know they are infected or who are having outbreaks of herpes without any sores. A person with genital herpes can also infect a sex partner during oral sex. The virus is spread rarely, if at all, by touching objects such as a toilet seat.

Signs and Symptoms

The precursor phase of a herpes infection is characterized by a burning sensation and redness at the site of infection. This phase is quickly followed by the second phase, in which a blister filled with a clear fluid containing the virus forms. A person with herpes who picks at this blister or otherwise spreads this fluid with fingers, lipstick, or some other object can autoinoculate other body parts. Particularly dangerous is the possibility of spreading the infection to the eyes, which can cause blindness.

Over a period of days, the blister will crust over, dry up, and disappear, and the virus will travel to the base of an affected nerve supplying the area and become dormant. Only when the person becomes overly stressed, when diet and sleep are inadequate, when the immune system is overworked, or when excessive exposure to sunlight or other stressors occur will the virus become reactivated (at the same site) and begin the blistering cycle again. Each time a sore develops, it casts off (sheds) viruses that can be highly infectious. However, a herpes site also can shed the virus when no overt sore is present, particularly during the interval between the earliest symptoms and blistering.

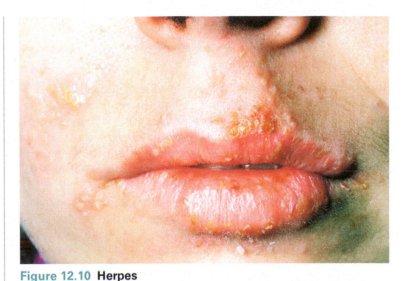

Figure 12.10 Herpes
Both genital and oral herpes can be caused by either herpes simplex virus type 1 or type 2.

Complications

Genital herpes is especially serious in pregnant women because the baby can be infected while passing through the vagina during birth. Many physicians recommend cesarean deliveries for women infected with genital herpes. Additionally, women with a history of genital herpes appear to have a greater risk of developing cervical cancer and may have regular flare-ups during the menstrual cycle or in times of high stress.

Diagnosis and Treatment

Diagnosis of herpes can be determined by collecting a sample from the suspected sore or by performing a blood test. Although there is no cure for herpes at present, antiviral medications can prevent or shorten outbreaks. Certain prescription drugs such as *acyclovir*, and over-the-counter medications such as Abreva can be used to treat symptoms. The effectiveness of other treatments, such as L-lysine, is largely unsubstantiated. Other drugs, such as *famciclovir* (FAMVIR), may reduce viral shedding between outbreaks, potentially reducing risks to the infected person's sex partners. One that has been particularly promising in two species of animals is in final trials. Stay tuned!. Although vaccines are being tested, there is currently no commercially available vaccine that is protective against genital herpes.[77]

- **What are the primary signs of and treatments for herpes?**

Sexually Transmitted Infections: Human Papillomavirus and Genital Warts

Learning Outcome

12.14 **List the various problems caused by human papillomavirus.**

Human papillomavirus (HPV) is one of a group of over 150 related viruses—each given a number indicating its type. HPV is the type that causes **genital warts** (also known as *venereal warts* or *condylomas*). HPV infections are so common that most sexually active men and women will have at least one form of HPV during their lives.[78] More than 40 types can infect the genital or anal areas of humans via skin-to-skin contact, making vaginal, anal, and oral sex all risky behaviors.[79] While genital warts are the most common result of the infection, HPV can also lead to cervical cancer and to cancer of the vulva, penis, anus, vagina, back of the throat, and tongue. Because HPV is often asymptomatic in the early stages, the risk of infection is great, particularly among people who are immunocompromised, such as those with HIV or AIDS.

See It! Videos

Learn more about the surprising prevalence of oral HPV. Watch **Oral HPV** in the Study Area of Mastering Health.

Signs and Symptoms The typical incubation period of HPV is 6 to 8 weeks after contact. People infected with low-risk types of HPV may develop genital warts, a series of bumps or growths on the genitals, ranging in size from small pinheads to large cauliflower-like growths (see **Figure 12.11**). Warts on the penis may be flat and difficult to see. Cancer may develop years after sexual contact and be symptomless for years.

Complications Cervical cancers often result from HPV infection, particularly infection with HPV-16 and HPV-18.[80] Cervical cancer may be detected at its earliest stages through a Pap test. HPV tests can also identify women at risk for rare cervical cancers (adenocarcinomas) that Pap tests might miss.[81] Ask your doctor whether your Pap test includes an HPV test and, if not, discuss whether one might be right for you.

In addition, HPV may also pose a threat to a fetus that is exposed to the virus during birth. Cesarean deliveries may be considered in serious cases. Human papillomavirus can cause cancers—called *oropharyngeal cancers*—around the tonsils or the base of the tongue, with oral sex as the suspected culprit. Over 9000 people are diagnosed with oropharyngeal cancer each year, men being about four times more likely to develop it than women.[82]

Diagnosis and Treatment Diagnosis of genital warts from low-risk types of HPV is determined through a visual examination. High-risk types can be diagnosed in women through microscopic analysis of cells from a Pap smear or by collecting a sample from the cervix to test for HPV DNA. There is currently no HPV DNA test for men.

Treatment is available only for the low-risk forms of HPV that cause genital warts. Most warts can be treated with topical medications or can be frozen with liquid nitrogen and then removed, but large warts may require surgical removal.

HPV Vaccines

There are two vaccines—Cervarix and Gardasil—that can help to prevent HPV infection.[83] Both Cervarix and Gardasil are very effective against high-risk HPV types 16 and 18, which cause 70 percent of cervical cancer cases. However, only Gardasil protects against low-risk HPV types 6 and 11. These HPV types cause 90 percent of cases of genital warts in females and males, so Gardasil is approved for use with males as well as females.[84]

HPV vaccines are recommended for 11- and 12-year-old girls but can be given to girls as young as 9 years old. Vaccination is also recommended for girls and women age 13 to 26 who have not yet been vaccinated.[85] Gardasil is also licensed, safe, and effective for males age 9 to 26. The CDC recommends Gardasil for all boys 11 or 12 years of age and for males age 13 to 21 who did not get any or all of the three recommended doses when they were younger.[86]

Note that neither Cervarix nor Gardasil protects against all types of HPV, so about 30 percent of cervical cancers will not be prevented. It will be important for women to continue getting screened for cervical cancer through regular Pap tests. Also, the vaccines do not prevent other STIs.[87]

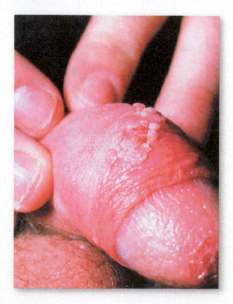

Figure 12.11 Genital Warts
Genital warts are caused by certain types of the human papillomavirus.

Check Yourself

- **How can women guard themselves against HPV-linked cervical cancer?**

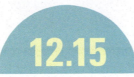

12.15 Other Sexually Transmitted Infections

12.15 List the symptoms and treatment of other common STIs.

Several other sexually transmitted infections have less serious effects than infections such as HIV and syphilis but nevertheless should be avoided.

Candidiasis (Moniliasis)

Most STIs are caused by pathogens that come from outside the body; however, the yeast-like fungus *Candida albicans* is a normal inhabitant of the vaginal tract in most women. (See Figure 12.3c for a micrograph of this fungus.) Only when the normal chemical balance of the vagina is disturbed will these organisms multiply and cause the fungal disease **candidiasis**, also sometimes called *moniliasis* or a *yeast infection*.

Signs and Symptoms   Symptoms of candidiasis include severe itching and burning of the vagina and vulva and a white, cheeselike vaginal discharge. When this microbe infects the mouth, whitish patches form, and the condition is referred to as *thrush*. Thrush infection can also occur in men and is easily transmitted between sex partners. Symptoms of candidiasis can be aggravated by contact with soaps, douches, perfumed toilet paper, chlorinated water, and spermicides.

Diagnosis and Treatment   Diagnosis of candidiasis is usually made by collecting a vaginal sample and analyzing it to identify the pathogen. Antifungal drugs applied on the surface or by suppository usually cure candidiasis in just a few days.

Trichomoniasis

Unlike many STIs, **trichomoniasis** is caused by a protozoan, *Trichomonas vaginalis*. (See Figure 12.3d for a micrograph of this organism.) An estimated 3.7 million new cases occur in the United States each year, although only about one-third of people who contract trichomoniasis experience symptoms. The good news is that it is one of the most curable STIs if diagnosed and treated.[88] The "trich" organism can be spread by sexual contact and by contact with items that have discharged fluids on them.

Signs and Symptoms Symptoms of trichomoniasis among women include a foamy, yellowish, unpleasant-smelling discharge accompanied by a burning sensation, itching, and painful urination. Most men with trichomoniasis do not have any symptoms, though some men experience irritation inside the penis, mild discharge, and a slight burning after urinating.[89]

Diagnosis and Treatment Diagnosis of trichomoniasis is determined by collecting fluid samples from the penis or vagina to test for the presence of the protozoan. Treatment includes oral

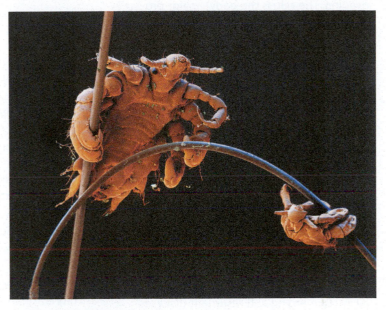

Figure 12.12 Pubic Lice
Pubic lice, also known as "crabs," are small, parasitic insects that attach themselves to pubic hair.

metronidazole, usually given to both sex partners to avoid the possible "ping-pong" effect of repeated cross-infection typical of STIs.

Pubic Lice

Pubic lice, often called "crabs," are small parasitic insects that are usually transmitted during sexual contact (see **Figure 12.12**). More annoying than dangerous, they move easily from partner to partner during sex. They have an affinity for pubic hair and attach themselves to the base of these hairs, where they deposit their eggs (nits). Within 2 weeks, the nits develop into adults that lay eggs and migrate to other body parts.

Signs and Symptoms Symptoms of pubic lice infestation include itchiness in the area covered by pubic hair, bluish-gray skin color in the pubic region, and sores in the genital area.

Diagnosis and Treatment Diagnosis of pubic lice involves an examination by a health care provider to identify the eggs in the genital area. Treatment includes washing clothing, furniture, and linens that may harbor the eggs. It usually takes 2 to 3 weeks to kill all larval forms.

- Describe symptoms and treatment of candidiasis and trichomoniasis.

- How are pubic lice transmitted and treated?

Summary

LO 12.1–12.2 Your body has several defense systems to keep pathogens from invading. The skin is the body's major protection. The immune system creates antibodies to destroy antigens. Fever and pain play a role in defending the body. Vaccines bolster the body's immune system against specific diseases, and mindfulness may bolster overall immune function.

LO 12.3–12.6 The major classes of pathogens are bacteria, viruses, fungi, protozoans, parasitic worms, and prions. Bacterial infections include staphylococcal infections, streptococcal infections, meningitis, pneumonia, tuberculosis, and tick-borne diseases. Major viral infections include the common cold; influenza; hepatitis; the herpes viruses, including chickenpox, shingles, and herpes gladiatorum; mumps; measles; and rubella.

LO 12.7 Emerging and resurgent diseases such as avian flu, West Nile virus, and malaria pose significant threats for future generations. Many factors contribute to these risks. Possible solutions focus on a public health approach to prevention.

LO 12.8 Many bacteria are evolving to become "superbugs" that are resistant to antibiotics. Being responsible with medications and using regular (not antibacterial) soap can prevent antibiotic resistance.

LO 12.9 Sexually transmitted infections (STIs) are spread through sexual intercourse, oral–genital contact, anal sex, hand–genital contact, and sometimes mouth-to-mouth contact.

LO 12.10 Acquired immunodeficiency syndrome (AIDS) is caused by the human immunodeficiency virus (HIV). Globally, HIV/AIDS has become a major threat to the world's population. Anyone can get HIV by engaging in high-risk sexual activities that include exchange of body fluids, by having received a blood transfusion before 1985, and by injecting drugs (or having sex with someone who does). You can reduce your risk for contracting HIV significantly by not engaging in risky sexual activities or IV drug use.

LO 12.11–12.15 STIs include chlamydia, gonorrhea, syphilis, herpes, human papillomavirus (HPV) and genital warts, candidiasis, trichomoniasis, and pubic lice.

306

Sexual transmission may also be involved in some urinary tract infections (UTIs).

Pop Quiz

Visit Mastering Health to personalize your study plan with Chapter Review Quizzes and Dynamic Study Modules.

LO 12.1 1. Jennifer touched her viral herpes sore on her lip and then touched her eye. She ended up with the herpes virus in her eye as well. This is an example of
a. acquired immunity.
b. passive spread.
c. autoinoculation.
d. self-vaccination.

LO 12.2 2. Which of the following do *not* assist the body in fighting disease?
a. Antigens   c. Lymphocytes
b. Antibodies   d. Macrophages

LO 12.2 3. An example of passive immunity is
a. inoculation with a vaccine containing weakened antigens.
b. when the body makes its own antibodies to a pathogen.
c. the antibody-containing part of the vaccine that came from someone else.
d. when lymphocytes attack and destroy a foreign invader.

LO 12.4 4. Which of the following is a *viral* disease?
a. Hepatitis
b. Tuberculosis
c. Malaria
d. Streptococcal infection

LO 12.5 5. Because colds are always present to some degree throughout the world, they are said to be
a. globally acquired.
b. vector-borne.
c. endemic.
d. resistant to antibiotics.

LO 12.6 6. Which of the following diseases is caused by a prion?
a. Shingles
b. Listeria
c. Mad cow disease
d. Trichomoniasis

LO 12.10 7. Which of the following is a true statement about HIV?
a. Drugs can prolong life expectancies for individuals with HIV.
b. An infected mother cannot pass the virus to her baby.

c. You can get HIV from a public restroom toilet seat.
d. HIV symptoms usually appear immediately after initial infection.

LO 12.11 8. Pelvic inflammatory disease (PID) is a(n)
a. sexually transmitted infection.
b. type of urinary tract infection.
c. infection of a woman's fallopian tubes or uterus.
d. disease that both men and women can get.

LO 12.11 9. The most widespread sexually transmitted bacterium is
a. gonorrhea.   c. syphilis.
b. chlamydia.   d. chancroid.

LO 12.12 10. Which of the following STIs cannot be treated with antibiotics?
a. Chlamydia   c. Syphilis
b. Gonorrhea   d. Herpes

Answers to these questions can be found on page A-1. If you answered a question incorrectly, review the module identified by the Learning Outcome. For even more study tools, visit Mastering Health.

Think About It!

LO 12.1–12.8 1. What are three lifestyle changes you could make right now that would reduce your risk of developing an infectious disease? How can you help to reduce antibiotic resistance in the world?

LO 12.1–12.2 2. What are pathogens, antigens, and antibodies? Discuss noncontrollable and controllable risk factors that can make you more or less susceptible to infectious pathogens in your immediate surroundings.

LO 12.3–12.5 3. What are some differences between bacteria and viruses?

LO 12.9 4. What are the key risk factors for STI infections? What kind of behaviors should you avoid to lower your risk of contracting a sexually transmitted infection?

LO 12.10–12.15 5. Identify five STIs and their symptoms. How are the STIs transmitted? What are their potential long-term effects?

LO 12.10 6. Why are women more susceptible to HIV infection than men? What implication does this have for prevention, treatment, and research?

Violence and Unintentional Injuries

The World Health Organization defines **violence** as "the intentional use of physical force or power, threatened or actual, against oneself, another person, or against a group or community, that either results in or has a high likelihood of resulting in injury, death, psychological harm, maldevelopment or deprivation."[1] The U.S. Public Health Service categorizes violence resulting in injuries into either intentional injuries or unintentional injuries. **Intentional injuries**—those committed with general intent to harm—typically include assaults, homicides, and self-directed injuries and suicides. **Unintentional injuries** are those committed without intent to harm and usually occur as a result of incidents such as vehicle accidents or fires.

Unfortunately, violent and abusive interactions are especially common problems for younger (and often otherwise healthy) adults. Among 15- to 34 year olds:[2]

- Unintentional injuries, particularly from motor vehicle crashes, are the number one cause of death.
- Suicide and homicide are the second and third leading causes of death.

This chapter discusses common instances of both violence and unintentional injuries, identifying steps you can take to reduce your risk as well as strategies for managing a violent or injurious situation should one occur.

Crime Rates and Causes of Violence

13.1   Describe the basic crime trend in the United States for the past few decades, and list individual and social factors contributing to violence.

How crime affects you personally has a great deal to do with your gender, ethnicity, socioeconomic status, and location. For instance, male homicide victims are more likely to be killed by strangers, while female homicide victims are more likely to be killed by someone they know. Women also make up the majority of victims of sexual assault crimes. Understanding the broad crime trends can help us understand contributors and provide a rationale for interventions. Unemployment, discrimination and hate, gun legislation, political agendas, drug and alcohol abuse, mental illness, cuts to social service programs and health insurance, and a host of other factors contribute to increased tensions, hopelessness, disenfranchisement and anger—all catalysts for violence.

The Federal Bureau of Investigation (FBI) found that overall crime, particularly certain types of violence, steadily increased from the 1970s through the early 2000s. After that, the crime rate declined, falling more than 10 percent between 2012 and 2014.[3] However, in 2015, violent crime rose 1.7% overall, and it increased by 5.3% in the first half of 2016, according to the FBI (**Figure 13.1**).[4] During this recent period, the Bureau of Justice Statistics (BJS) reported little change in violent crime.[5] However, because the BJS

56% of crime against college students occurred on campus, with an additional 28% in residence halls.

statistics don't include homicides and crimes against businesses— which FBI statistics do include—the numbers are bound to be different. Even with the recent uptick in certain crimes, overall rates today are still significantly lower than they were in the 1990s.

It also bears noting that crime statistics only capture *reported* instances of violence and injuries. It is estimated that over half of all violent victimizations are not reported to the police. Even though over 23 percent of college women will be raped or sexually assaulted before they graduate, 95 percent of them never report these crimes.[6] Typical reasons for not reporting crime include concerns over privacy, fear of retaliation, embarrassment or shame, lack of support, perception that the crime was too minor or that they were somehow at fault, or uncertainty that it was a crime.

Violence at Schools

In the past decade, gun violence in schools and universities has accelerated. Often, these tragedies involve a lone shooter with automatic or semiautomatic weapons. Sandy Hook Elementary School captured national attention in 2012 when the unthinkable occurred: 26 children and adults were murdered. In 2018, 17 people were gunned down at Marjory Stoneman Douglas High School in Florida. Gun control is a hot-button issue in the United States. Some believe that more controls won't stop violent individuals from committing crimes. Others believe that by expanding controls on weapon sales, restricting sale of guns to the mentally ill and people with a history of criminal violence, and regulation of certain automatic weapons and ammunition, public safety would improve. Meanwhile, school authorities at all levels—in public and private schools, colleges and universities—have been forced to reevaluate campus safety, changing their protocols and safety plans to account for these types of violent incidents.

More recently, violence related to political demonstrations and counterprotests has erupted on college campuses and in surrounding communities. From the violence that erupted in August 2017 between white nationalists and left-leaning groups in Charlottesville, Virginia, near the University of Virginia to the mask-wearing "antifa" (anti-fascist)

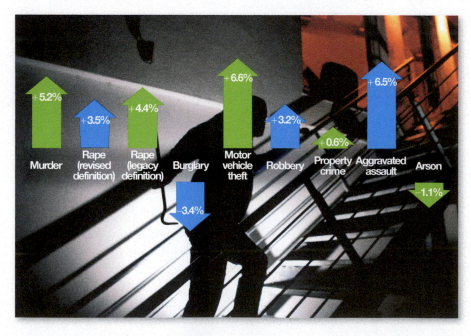

Figure 13.1 Changing Crime Rates
FBI statistics show reported violent crimes increased by 6.2% in 2015 and 5.3% in 2016. Rates of crimes vary by type of crime, location, sex, and other variables. The most violent crimes are on the increase overall.

Source: Federal Bureau of Investigation, "Crime in the United States, 2016: Preliminary Semiannual Uniform Crime Report, January–June 2016," accessed March 2017, www.fbi.gov.

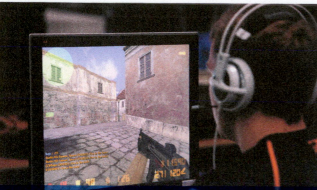

Does violence in the media cause violence in real life?

Arguably, Americans today—especially children—are exposed to more depictions of violence than ever before, but research has not shown a clear link between a person's exposure to violent media and his or her propensity to engage in violent acts.

protestors who several times battled with right-wing activists on the University of California Berkeley campus and nearby locations, tensions are clearly on the rise. Issues surrounding freedom of speech, peaceful versus violent protesting, outsider interference, and police responses have been raised in each of these incidents, with very different opinions about each. Each side blamed the other, and both sides blamed the police. Differences in race, religion, sexual orientation, ideology, values, and a host of beliefs and biases have sparked significant injury and death in recent years, leading to the potential for major emotional and psychological distress on campus and in surrounding communities.

While tensions flare around students and the media provides a steady dose of "downer news," rates of interpersonal violence on campus continue to rise along with increases in mental health problems. Relationship violence is one of the most prevalent, yet hidden problems on college campuses. In the most recent American College Health Association survey, 10.9 percent of women and 6.4 percent of men reported having been emotionally abused in the past 12 months in an intimate relationship.[7] Over 6.6 percent of women and 2.4 percent of men reported having been stalked, and 2.0 percent of women and 1.8 percent of men reported having been involved in a physically abusive relationship.[8] Nearly 1 percent of men and 2.7 percent of women reported having been in a sexually abusive relationship.[9]

Factors Contributing to Violence

Aggressive behavior and anger are often key aspects of violent interactions. **Primary aggression** is goal-directed, hostile self-assertion that is destructive in nature. **Reactive aggression** is more often part of an emotional reaction brought about by frustration. Several factors increase the likelihood of violent acts:[10]

- **Community contexts.** Persistent poverty, particularly environments where unsafe housing, neighborhoods, schools, and workplaces predominate, increase risks of exposure to drugs, guns, and gangs. Inadequately staffed police and social services add to the risks.[11]
- **Societal factors.** Policies and programs that seek to remove inequality and disparity and to discourage discrimination decrease risks. Social and cultural norms that support male dominance over women and violence as a means of settling problems increase risks.[12]
- **Religious beliefs and differences.** Extreme religious beliefs can lead people to think that violence against others is justified.
- **Political differences.** Civil unrest and differences in political party affiliations and beliefs have historically been triggers for violent acts.
- **Breakdowns in the criminal justice system.** Overcrowded prisons and inadequate availability of mental health services can encourage repeat offenses and future violence.
- **Stress, depression, or other mental health issues.** People who are in crisis, are depressed, feel threatened, or are under stress are more apt to be highly reactive, striking out at others, displaying anger, or acting irrationally.

How Much Impact Do the Media Have?

Although the media are blamed for playing a role in the escalation of violence, this association has been challenged. While early studies seemed to support a link between excessive exposure to violent media and subsequent violent behavior, much of this research has been criticized for methodological problems such as poor or inconsistent measures of violence, biased subject selection, and sample size issues.[13]

A new meta-analysis by the American Psychological Association indicates that violent media may increase risks of aggression and desensitize people when violence occurs. However, there is less evidence that violent videos increase risks for violent criminal activity. Other researchers continue to point out that exposure to violent videos has neither long- nor short-term effects on either positive or negative behaviors.[14]

13.1

Violence and Unintentional Injuries

Check Yourself

- Have crime rates trended up or down in the United States since the 1990s? What types of violence are typically encountered on campus these days?

- What are three factors that might make a person prone to violence?

13.2 Identify and define the various types of interpersonal violence.

Intentional injuries have three basic categorizations: *interpersonal*, *collective*, and *self-directed*.[15] **Interpersonal violence** includes acts inflicted against one individual by another or a small group of others; homicide, hate crimes, domestic violence, child abuse, elder abuse, and sexual victimization all fit into this category.

Homicide

Homicide, defined as murder or non-negligent manslaughter, is the thirteenth leading cause of death in the United States but the second leading cause of death for people age 15 to 24. Overall, it is among the top five leading causes of death for people age 1 to 44.[16] Nearly half of all homicides occur among people who know one another.[17] In two-thirds of these cases, the perpetrator and the victim are friends or acquaintances; in one-third, they are family members.[18] Homicide rates reveal clear disparities across race, gender, and age. Homicides are the fifth leading cause of death for African American males, the sixth leading cause of death for Native Americans, and the ninth leading cause of death in Latino populations.[19]

The rates of homicide in the United States are higher than those in many other developed nations (Table 13.1). As Figure 13.2 shows, handguns are consistently responsible for more murders than any other single type of weapon. Thirty percent of the world's mass shootings, the most in the world, occur in the United States, which has a mere 5 percent of the world's population.[20] Today, 35 percent of American homes have a gun on the premises higher rates than any other country in the world. Nearly 300 million privately owned guns have been registered—and millions more are unregistered and/or illegal. Some sources have reported that the ready availability of guns in the home or surroundings increases the risk of suicide, in particular, and also of homicide.[21] However, gun rights advocates argue that people in high-risk areas are more likely to have guns for protection and although the numbers of homicides are higher in those homes, the number might have been even higher without the guns. They also say that the problem lies not with guns, but with the people who own them; they point to countries such as Canada, with similar numbers of guns as in the United States, but with much lower gun-related crime rates. Mental health issues and alcohol are also huge factors in homicide deaths. People who seek more gun control typically contend that those with a history of mental illness and/or alcohol and other drug abuse should not have guns.

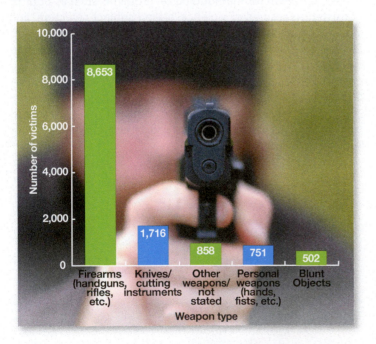

Figure 13.2 Homicide in the United States by Weapon Type, 2014.
The vast majority of murders in the United States are committed by using firearms, far outweighing all other weapons combined.
Source: Data from Federal Bureau of Investigation, "Crime in the United States, 2015, Expanded Homicide Data Table 8—Murder Victims by Weapon—2011–2015," 2015, https://ucr.fbi.gov/crime-in-the-u.s/2015/crime-in-the-u.s.-2015/tables/expanded_homicide_data_table_8_murder_victims_by_weapon_2011-2015.xls.

Hate and Bias-Motivated Crimes

A **hate crime** is a violent, intimidating, or destructive act committed against people or property. Hate crimes are motivated by the offender's bias against the race, ethnicity, religion, disability, sexual orientation, and/or gender (or gender identity) of the target victim or victims. Hate crimes may include vandalism, slurs, verbal threats, intimidation, or physical violence. *Bias-related crime*, sometimes referred to as **ethnoviolence,** describes violence based on prejudice and discrimination among ethnic groups in the larger society.

1 in 370 is the lifetime odds of dying in an assault by a firearm. For comparison, the odds of dying as a passenger in a motor vehicle crash are 1 in 647.

Prejudice is an irrational attitude of hostility directed against an individual; a group; a race; or the supposed characteristics of an individual, group, or race. **Discrimination** constitutes actions that deny equal treatment or opportunities to a group of people, often based on prejudice. Often prejudice and discrimination stem from a fear of change and a desire to blame other people when forces such as the economy and crime seem to be out of control. In 2017, vandalism of Jewish cemeteries and attacks against Muslims made headline news. In August 2017, a white supremacist drove his vehicle into a crowd of antiracist protestors in Charlottesville, Virginia, killing one person and injuring 19 others.

The BJS conducts an anonymous crime victimization survey each year; data from these surveys show that U.S. residents were subjected to about 250,000 hate crime events each year in the period between 2004 and 2015.[22]

Numerous studies over the years show that at least half of hate crimes go unreported to authorities. This is likely why the official FBI statistics on hate crimes, which count only crimes reported to authorities, were mostly flat throughout much of this period while the BJS reports showed increases. Fear of retaliation keeps many hate crimes hidden. Figure 13.3 illustrates the annual rate of bias-motivated crimes.

Common reasons given to explain bias-related and hate crimes include (1) *thrill seeking* by multiple offenders through a group attack, (2) fear or *feeling threatened* that others will take their jobs or property or best them in some way, (3) *retaliating* for some real or perceived insult or slight, and (4) lack of understanding and *fearing the unknown or differences*. For other people, hate crimes are a part of their mission in life, because of either religious zeal or distorted moral beliefs.

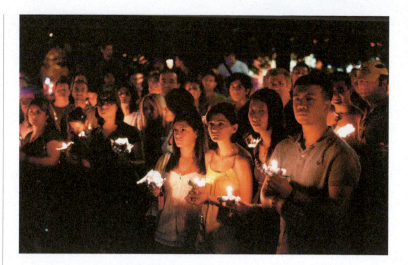

TABLE 13.1	Intentional Homicide Counts and Rates per 100,000 Population: Selected Countries	
Rate per 100,000	**Country**	**Number of Homicides**
1.5	Saudi Arabia	472
1.58	France	1017
1.68	Canada	604
4.88	United States	15,690
11.31	Russian Federation	16,232
16.35	Mexico	20,762
26.74	Brazil	55,574
34.27	South Africa	18,673
43.21	Jamaica	1207
108.64	El Salvador	6,656

Source: Data from United Nations Office on Drugs and Crime, "UNODC Homicide Rates and Counts, 2000–2015," August 2017, https://data.unodc.org/#state:0.

Campuses have responded to reports of hate crimes by offering courses that emphasize diversity, zero tolerance for violations, training faculty appropriately, and developing policies that enforce punishment for hate crimes.

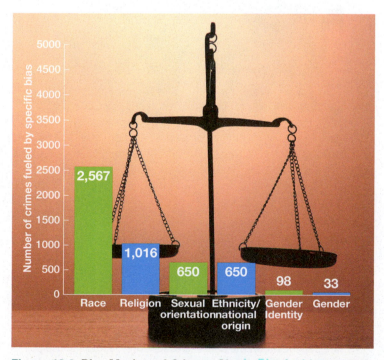

Figure 13.3 Bias-Motivated Crimes, Single-Bias Incidence, 2015
Source: Data from Federal Bureau of Investigation, "Hate Crime Statistics, 2015," Table 1, www.fbi.gov, November 2016.

Check Yourself

- What factors are correlated with increased homicide rates in the United States?

- Why do you think hate crimes and racial unrest appear to be growing issues in the United States today?

13.3 Explain how personal and social factors can lead to domestic violence and child or elder abuse.

Sadly, victims of violence and abuse may find that the perpetrators of these crimes are their own spouse, partner, parent, or child. Why do people commit acts of violence against their own loved ones?

Domestic Violence

Domestic violence refers to the use of force to control and maintain power over another person in the home environment. It can occur between parent and child, between spouses or intimate partners, or between siblings or other family members. The violence may involve emotional abuse; verbal abuse; threats of physical harm; and physical violence ranging from slapping and shoving to beatings, rape, and homicide.

Intimate partner violence (IPV) describes physical, sexual, or psychological harm done by a current or former partner or spouse; it can occur among heterosexual or same-sex couples and does not require sexual intimacy. Over the course of a year, millions of women and men are victims of rape, physical and psychological abuse, stalking, and other offenses by an intimate partner. Homicide committed by a current or former intimate partner is the leading cause of death of pregnant women in the United States.[23] Nearly 75 percent of all murder-suicides were perpetrated by an intimate partner, and 96 percent of the dead were women.[24]

Nearly half of all women and men in the United States have experienced psychological aggression by an intimate partner in their lifetime. Psychological abusers seek to intimidate and debase their partners, thereby gaining control over the partner and the relationship. People who have experienced this violence are more likely to have depression, difficulty in intimate relationships, frequent headaches, chronic pain, difficulty with sleeping, activity limitations, poor physical health, irritable bowel syndrome, and other health problems.[25]

A wide range of individual, relational, community, policy, and legal and societal factors contribute to the risk of becoming an IPV victim or perpetrator.[26] Why do people stay in abusive relationships? Women, particularly those with small children and those who are financially dependent on their partners, often have few options. Others fear retaliation against themselves or their children. Some hope that the situation will change with time, and others stay because cultural or religious beliefs forbid divorce. Finally, some women still love the abusive partner and are concerned about what will happen to him if they leave.

In the 1970s, psychologist Lenore Walker developed a theory called the *cycle of violence* that explained predictable, repetitive patterns of psychological and/or physical abuse in abusive relationships.[27] Over the years, Walker's initial work has been criticized for its lack of scientific rigor, anecdotal approach, and seeming overstatement of selected patterns as universal truths. In her most recent book, *The Battered Woman Syndrome*, Walker responds to many of her early critics with improved quantitative analysis, reviews of recent research, and an extensive list of experts in the field of violence.[28]

The cycle of violence continues to be important to understanding why people stay in otherwise unhealthy relationships. The cycle consists of three major phases:

1. **Tension building.** This phase typically occurs before the overtly abusive act and includes breakdowns in communication, anger, psychological aggression and violent language, growing tension, and fear.
2. **Incident of acute battering.** At this stage, the batterer usually is trying to "teach her a lesson"; when he feels that he has inflicted enough pain, he stops. When the acute attack is over, he may respond with shock and denial about his own behavior or blame the woman for "making" him do it.

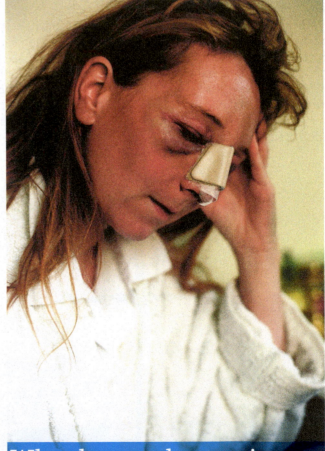

Why do people stay in abusive relationships?

People who stay with their abusers may do so because they are dependent on the abuser, because they fear the abuser, or even because they love the abuser. In some cultures, women may not be free to leave an abusive relationship because of restrictive laws, religious beliefs, or social mores.

3. Remorse/reconciliation. During this "honeymoon" period, the batterer may be kind, loving, and apologetic, swearing that he will never act violently again and will work to change his behavior. However, when things that triggered past abuse resurface, the cycle starts over.

For a woman caught in this cycle, it is often very hard to summon the resolution to extricate herself. Most need effective outside intervention. No single reason explains why people tend to be abusive in relationships. Alcohol abuse is often associated with such violence; marital dissatisfaction is also a predictor. Numerous studies also point to differences in communication patterns between abusive and nonabusive relationships. Stress, mental health issues, economic uncertainty/frustration, jealousy, issues of power/control and gender roles, and issues with self-esteem are among common rationale given for IPV.[29]

Child Abuse and Neglect

Children living in families in which domestic violence or sexual abuse occurs are at great risk for damage to personal health and well-being. **Child maltreatment** is defined as any act or series of acts of commission or omission by a parent or caregiver that results in harm, potential for harm, or threat of harm to a child.[30] **Child abuse** refers to **acts of commission**, which are deliberate or intentional words or actions that cause harm, potential harm, or threat of harm to a child. The abuse may be sexual, psychological, physical, or any combination of these. **Neglect** is an *act of omission*, meaning a failure to provide for a child's basic needs for food, shelter, clothing, medical care, education, or proper supervision. **Figure 13.4** shows the rates of abuse and neglect among children of different ages.

Sexual abuse of children by adults or older children includes sexually suggestive conversations; inappropriate kissing, touching, or petting; oral, anal, or vaginal intercourse; and other kinds of sexual interaction. As with other crimes that carry social stigma, reliable statistics on child abuse can be difficult to find. Recent studies indicate that the rates of sexual abuse in children are on the increase. Girls are at greater risk than young boys, though young boys are abused in significant numbers.[31]

There were nearly 685,000 reported cases of child abuse and neglect in 2015. Seventy-five percent of these cases were for neglect, 17% were for physical abuse, and 8.4 percent were for sexual abuse. Many more cases are unsuspected and go unreported.[32] The shroud of secrecy surrounding this problem makes it likely the number of actual cases is grossly underestimated. Ninety percent of child sexual abuse victims know their perpetrator; nearly 70 percent of children are abused by family members, usually an adult male.[33]

Victims of child abuse have a higher risk of depression, unintended pregnancy, sexually transmitted diseases, suicide, drug and alcohol abuse, and an overall lowered life expectancy, particularly among those who are repeatedly victimized.[34]

There is no single profile of a child abuser. Frequently, the perpetrator is a young adult in his or her mid-twenties without a high school diploma, living at or below the poverty level, depressed, socially isolated, with a poor self-image, and having difficulty

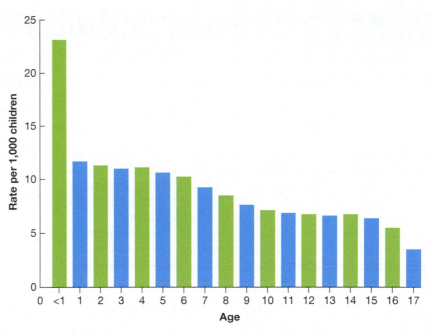

Figure 13.4 Child Abuse and Neglect Victims by Age, 2015
Source: U.S. Department of Health and Human Services, Administration on Children, Youth and Families, "Child Maltreatment, Exhibit 3-F, Victims by Age," 2015.

coping with stressful situations. In many instances, the perpetrator has experienced violence and is frustrated by life.

Not all violence against children is physical. Health can be severely affected by psychological violence—assaults on personality, character, competence, independence, or general dignity as a human being. Negative consequences of this kind of victimization can include depression, low self-esteem, and a pervasive fear of offending the abuser.

See It! Videos
Should strangers step in to prevent partner abuse? Watch **Will Anyone Confront Abusive Boyfriend?** in the Study Area of Mastering Health.

Elder Abuse

By 2030, the number of people in the United States over the age of 65 will exceed 71 million—nearly double their number in 2000. Each year, hundreds of thousands of adults over the age of 60 are abused, neglected, or financially exploited as they enter the later years of life, and these statistics are likely an underestimate.[35] Many victims fail to report abuse because they are embarrassed or because they don't want the abuser to get in trouble or retaliate by putting them in a nursing home or escalating the abuse. A variety of social services focus on protecting our seniors, just as we endeavor to protect other vulnerable populations.

Check Yourself

- How does the cycle of violence explain why people stay in dangerous or unhealthy relationships?

- What steps can be taken to reduce child abuse and elder abuse?

13.4 Sexual Victimization

13.4 Identify the types and prevalence of rape and sexual assault.

The term *sexual victimization* refers to any situation in which an individual is coerced or forced to comply with or endure another's sexual acts or overtures. It can run the gamut from harassment to stalking to assault and rape. As with all forms of violence, both men and women are susceptible to sexual victimization.

Sexual victimization and sexual violence can have devastating and far-reaching effects on people of any age. Fear, sexual avoidance, sleeplessness, anxiety, and depression are just a few of the long-term consequences for victims.[36]

Sexual Assault and Rape

Sexual assault is any act in which one person is sexually intimate with another person without that person's consent. This may range from touching to forceful penetration and may include, for example, ignoring indications that intimacy is not wanted, threatening force or other negative consequences, and actually using force.

Considered the most extreme form of sexual assault, **rape** is usually defined as "penetration without the victim's consent." However, a new, clarified definition of rape endorsed by the FBI specifies the following: "Penetration, no matter how slight, of the vagina or anus with any body part or object, or oral penetration by a sex organ of another person, without the consent of the

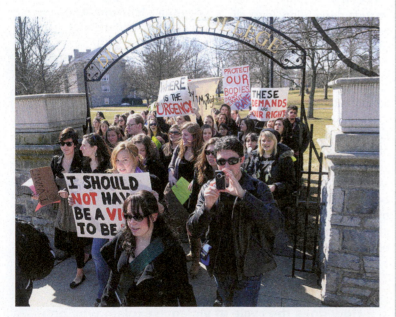

The reluctance to report sexual assault on campus and the difficulty of pursuing criminal proceedings in the campus environment can create turmoil in victims' lives while too rarely leading to punishment of offenders.

Over

23% of undergraduate women have been sexually assaulted one or more times during their undergraduate years.

victim. This includes the offenses of rape, sodomy, and sexual assault with an object." Incidents of rape generally fall into one of two types. An **aggravated rape** is any rape involving one or multiple attackers, strangers, weapons, or physical beatings. A **simple rape** is a rape perpetrated by one person whom the victim knows and does not involve a physical beating or use of a weapon. Most rapes are classified as simple rape, but that terminology should not be taken to mean that a simple rape is any less violent or criminal.

Nearly 1 in 5 women and 1 in 59 men in the United States have been raped at some time in their lives, and nearly 80 percent of female rape victims experience their first rape before the age of 25.[37] By most indicators, reported cases of rape appear to have declined in the United States since the early 1990s, even as reports of other forms of sexual assault have increased. This decline is thought to be due to shifts in public awareness and attitudes about rape, combined with tougher crime policies, major educational campaigns, and media attention. These changes enforce the idea that rape is a violent crime and should be treated as such. However, numerous sources indicate that rape is among the most underreported crimes, particularly on college campuses.[38]

The terms *date rape* and *acquaintance rape* have been used interchangeably in the past. However, most experts now believe that the term *date rape* is inappropriate because it implies a consensual interaction in an arranged setting and may minimize the crime of rape when it occurs. **Acquaintance rape** refers to any rape in which the rapist is known to the victim. Acquaintance rape is more common when drugs or alcohol have been consumed by the offender and/or victim, making the campus party environment a high-risk venue. Alcohol is frequently involved in rape, as are a growing number of rape-facilitating drugs such as Rohypnol and gamma-hydroxybutyrate (GHB).

Rape on U.S. Campuses Over 23 percent of college students are sexually assaulted as undergraduates.[39] In 1992, Congress passed the Campus Sexual Assault Victim's Bill of Rights, known as the Ramstad Act, which gave victims the right to call in off-campus authorities to investigate campus crimes and required universities to develop educational programs. The 2014 Campus Sexual Violence Elimination Act requires colleges and universities to report cases of stalking, intimate partner violence, dating violence, and sexual assault on annual campus crime reports. Notification

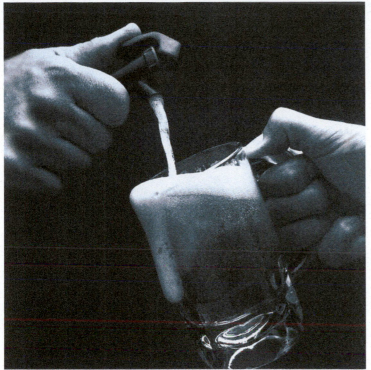

A lot of campus rapes start here.

Whenever there's drinking or drugs, things can get out of hand. So it's no surprise that many campus rapes involve alcohol.

But you should know that under any circumstances, sex without the other person's consent is considered rape. A felony, punishable by prison. And drinking is no excuse.

That's why, when you party, it's good to know what your limits are. You see, a little sobering thought now can save you from a big problem later.

What does *acquaintance rape* mean?

The term *date rape* was formerly applied to a sexual assault occurring in the context of a dating relationship. The term has fallen out of favor because the word *date* implies something reciprocal or arranged, thus minimizing the crime. The term *acquaintance rape* is now more commonly used, referring to any rape in which the rapist is known to the victim, even if only minimally. Acquaintance rape is particularly common on college campuses, where alcohol and drug use can impair young people's judgment and self-control.

▶ **Mastering Health & Nutrition** Acquaintance Rape on Campus

procedures, options for victims and accused perpetrators, and consequences—including loss of federal support if schools don't conduct campus climate surveys and assess their prevention activities—are all included in the new act's provisions.[40] Despite these changes, in 2014, many colleges and universities that were not receiving federal funds did not report campus violence. In fact,

as many as 500 of them reported no rapes or sexual assaults at all, prompting considerable national concern in the media.[41]

In 2014, California became the first state in the nation to implement a "yes means yes" law, changing the definition of sexual consent to require "an affirmative, conscious, and voluntary agreement to engage in sexual activity."[42] If one party is unable to give consent because of intoxication or other factors, the perpetrator could be prosecuted for sexual assault. Beyond changing definitions, the law requires schools who receive funding from the state to develop policies around numerous situations related to sexual assault.[43]

Marital Rape Although its legal definition varies within the United States, **marital rape** can be any unwanted intercourse or penetration (vaginal, anal, or oral) obtained by force or threat of force or when the spouse is unable to consent. This problem has undoubtedly existed since the origin of marriage as a social institution, though it is noteworthy that marital rape did not become a crime in all 50 states until 1993. Even more noteworthy is the fact that 30 states still allow exemptions from marital rape prosecution, meaning that the judicial system may treat it as a lesser crime.[44]

Social Contributors to Sexual Violence

Certain societal assumptions and traditions can promote sexual violence, including the following:

- **Trivialization.** Many people think that rape committed by a husband or intimate partner doesn't count as rape.
- **Blaming the victim.** In spite of efforts to combat this type of thinking, there is still the belief that a scantily clad woman "asks" for sexual advances.
- **Pressure to be macho.** Males are taught from a young age that showing emotions is a sign of weakness. This portrayal often depicts men as aggressive and predatory and females as passive targets.
- **Male socialization.** Many people still believe that "boys will be boys" and being sexually predatory is natural for men.
- **Male misperceptions.** Some men mistakenly believe that when a woman says "no," she does not necessarily mean it, or is even signaling that she wants to be seduced.
- **Situational factors.** Dates in which the one person makes all the decisions, pays for everything, and generally controls the entire situation are more likely to end in an aggressive sexual scenario. Alcohol and other drugs increase the risk and severity of assaults.

Check Yourself

- What are three types of rape and sexual abuse?
- What are two social contributors to sexual violence?

13.5 Explain the definitions of, and ways to address, sexual harassment and stalking.

Sexual harassment and stalking are two common forms of sexual violence, even when they do not involve physical harm.

Sexual Harassment

Sexual harassment is defined as unwelcome sexual conduct that is related to any condition of employment or evaluation of student performance. Unwelcome sexual advances, requests for sexual favors, and other verbal or physical conduct of a sexual nature constitute sexual harassment when any of the following occurs:[45]

- Submission to such conduct is made either explicitly or implicitly a term or condition of an individual's employment or education.
- Submission to or rejection of such conduct by an individual is used as the basis for employment or education-related decisions affecting that individual.
- Such conduct is sufficiently severe or pervasive that it has the effect, intended or unintended, of unreasonably interfering with an individual's work or academic performance because it has created an intimidating, hostile, or offensive environment and would have such an effect on a reasonable person of that individual's status.

Commonly, people think of harassment as involving only faculty members or people in power who use sex to exhibit control of a situation. However, peers can harass one another, too. Sexual harassment may include unwanted touching; unwarranted

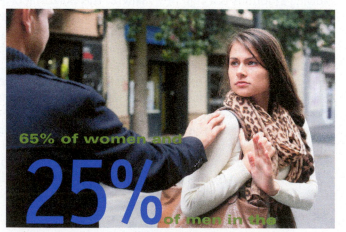

65% of women and 25% of men in the United States have experienced street harassment, including whistling, leering, vulgar gestures, and sexually explicit comments.

Source: Stop Street Harassment, "Unsafe and Harassed in Public, A National Street Harassment Survey," Spring 2014, http://www.stop-streetharassment.org/wp-content/uploads/2012/08/National-Street-Harassment-Report-November-29-20151.pdf.

sex-related comments or subtle pressure for sexual favors; deliberate or repeated humiliation or intimidation based on sex; and gratuitous comments, jokes, questions, or remarks about clothing or bodies, sexuality, or past sexual relationships.

Most schools and companies have sexual harassment policies in place, as well as procedures for dealing with harassment problems. If you feel you are being harassed, take the following steps:

- **Tell the harasser to stop.** Be clear and direct. Tell the person that if it continues, you will report it. If the harassing is via phone or Internet, block the person.
- **Document the harassment.** Make a record of each incident. If the harassment becomes intolerable, a record of exactly what occurred (and when and where) will help you make your case. Save copies of all communication from the harasser.
- **Try to make sure you are never alone with the harasser.** Witnesses to harassment can ensure appropriate validation of the event.
- **Complain to a higher authority.** Talk to legal authorities or your instructor, adviser, or counseling center psychologist about what happened.
- **Remember that you have not done anything wrong.** You will likely feel awful after being harassed (especially if you have to complain to superiors). However, feel proud that you are not keeping silent.

Stalking

Stalking can be defined as conduct directed at a person that would cause a reasonable person to feel fear. This may include repeated visual or physical proximity, nonconsensual written or verbal communication, and implied or explicit threats. The most common stalking behaviors included unwanted phone calls and messages, spreading rumors, spying on the victim, and showing up at the same places as the victim without having a reason to be there.[46] Technology such as security cameras, tracking and GPS devices that can provide location, spyware, and inexpensive devices can instill fear and cause people to modify normal behavior.[47] College students are 200% more likely to be stalked than the general public, and 18- to 24-year-olds are the most likely to be stalked overall.[48]

Like sexual harassment, stalking is an underreported crime. Often, students do not think a stalking incident is serious enough to report, or they worry that the police will not take it seriously.

See It! Videos

What are the repercussions of sexual assault? Watch **Sexual Assaults on College Campuses: 95 Colleges Under Federal Investigation** in the Study Area of Mastering Health.

Check Yourself

- How can sexual harassment be prevented and controlled?

Learning Outcome

13.6 List the factors associated with terrorism and gang violence.

Collective violence is violence perpetrated by groups against other groups; it includes violent acts related to political, governmental, religious, cultural, or social clashes. Gang violence and terrorism are two forms of collective violence that have become major threats in recent years.

Gang Violence

Gang violence is increasing in many regions of the world; U.S. communities face escalating threats from gang networks engaged in drug trafficking, sex trafficking, shootings, beatings, thefts, carjackings, and the killing of innocent victims caught in the crossfire. There are over 33,000 gangs in the United States, with membership in excess of 1.4 million.[49] Gangs are believed to be responsible for 48 percent of violent crime overall in the United States and as much as 90 percent in some locations.[50]

Why do young people join gangs? Often, gangs give members a sense of self-worth, companionship, security, and excitement. In other cases, gangs provide economic security through drug sales, prostitution, and other types of criminal activity. Friendships with delinquent peers, lack of parental monitoring, negative life events, and alcohol and drug use appear to increase risks for gang affiliation. Other risk factors include low self-esteem, academic problems, low socioeconomic status, alienation from family and society, a history of family violence, and living in gang-controlled neighborhoods.[51] Since it becomes difficult to leave gangs once a youth becomes involved, prevention strategies appear to offer the most promise.

Terrorism

Numerous terrorist attacks around the world have revealed the vulnerability of all nations to domestic and international threats. In the United States, this was particularly apparent on September 11, 2001, when terrorist attacks on the World Trade Center and the Pentagon revealed the vulnerability of our nation to domestic and international threats. More than 16 years later, threats against our airlines, mass transportation systems, cities, national monuments, and population fuel fears of looming terrorist attacks. Effects on our economy, travel restrictions, additional security measures, and military buildups are but a few of the examples of how terrorist threats have affected our lives. As defined in the U.S. Code of Federal Regulations, **terrorism** is the "unlawful use of force or violence against persons or property to intimidate or coerce a government, the civilian population, or any segment thereof in furtherance of political or social objectives."[52]

In 2002, the Centers for Disease Control and Prevention (CDC) established the Office of Public Health Preparedness and Response. This group monitors potential public health problems such as bioterrorism, chemical emergencies, radiation emergencies, mass casualties, national disaster, and severe weather; develops plans for mobilizing communities in the case of emergency; and provides information about terrorist threats.[53] In addition, the Department of Homeland Security works to prevent future attacks, and the FBI and other government agencies have prepared a set of procedures and guidelines to ensure citizens' health and safety.

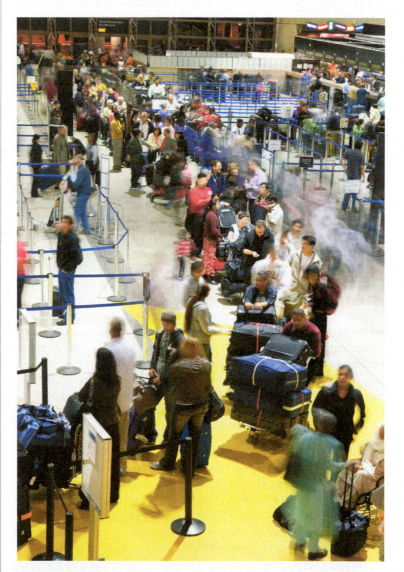

The threat of terrorism has affected many aspects of our daily lives. From increased security at airports to restrictions on public transit, steps taken to protect against terrorism have changed how we conduct our day-to-day activities.

Check Yourself

- What is collective violence?
- What factors contribute to collective violence?

13.7 How to Avoid Becoming a Victim of Violence

13.7 List strategies to prevent violence against yourself and others.

After a violent act has been committed against someone we know, we may acknowledge the horror of the event, express sympathy, and go on with our lives, but it may take the brutalized person months or years to recover both physically and emotionally. For this reason, preventing a violent act is far better than recovering from it. Both individuals and communities can play important roles in the prevention of violence and intentional injuries. Assaults and threats can arise from in-person encounters, or they may develop from online encounters.

Social Networking Safety

Posting personal information online, such as your phone number, class schedule, and e-mail address, poses a threat to personal safety and puts you at greater risk for identify theft or even stalking. Additionally, posting negative messages about employers or colleagues can have damaging consequences; hiring and firing decisions have been influenced by information that employees and job applicants made publicly available on Facebook and Twitter. Using social media sites for dating or hookups poses addition risks; in addition to the vulnerabilities involved in exchanging personal information with strangers, underage users may pose as adults, leading to claims of inappropriate sexual contact with minors and other criminal offenses on the part of people interacting with them online.

To safely enjoy the benefits and avoid the risks of social networking sites, you'll need to practice a little caution and use some common sense. The following tips will help you to remain safe, protect your identity, and feel free to express yourself without fear of repercussions:

- Don't post anything on the Web that you wouldn't want someone to access on the Web or elsewhere and read. Your address, phone numbers, banking information, calendar, family secrets, and other information should be kept off the sites.
- Don't post compromising pictures, videos, or other things that you wouldn't want your mother, coworkers, or boss to see.
- If you plan to meet a stranger in person whom you've met only online, always bring a trusted friend along or, at the very least, notify a close friend of where you will be and when you will return. Arrange a ride home with a friend in advance, and choose a well-established, public place to meet during daylight hours. Don't give your address or traceable phone numbers to the person you are meeting.
- When you get rid of phones or other devices, make sure you wipe them of your data and close all accounts in your name.

- Avoid banking or accessing sensitive personal financial documents when using public WiFi servers. Change passwords often and pay particular attention to the URL you are accessing while banking or in other accounts. The first URL posted for logging in, may not be the real website. Make sure your cell phone is not posting your location publically.
- Change your passwords and security questions often, and don't write them all down where someone can find them.

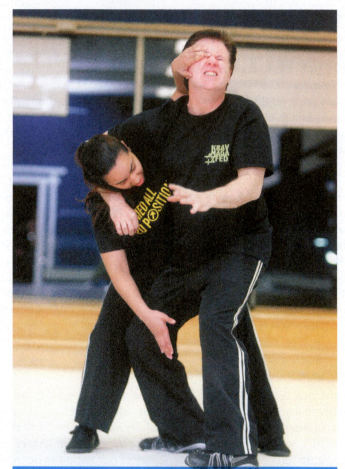

How can I protect myself from becoming a victim of violence?

One of the best ways to protect yourself from violence is to avoid situations or circumstances that could lead to it. Another way to protect yourself is to learn self-defense techniques. College campuses often offer safety workshops and self-defense classes to arm students with the physical and mental skills that may help them to repel or deter an assailant.

Self-Defense against Rape and Personal Assault

Assault can occur no matter what preventive actions you take, but commonsense self-defense tactics can lower the risk. Self-defense is a process that includes increasing your awareness, developing self-protective skills, taking reasonable precautions, and having the good judgment necessary to respond quickly to changing situations. Because rape on campus often occurs in social or dating settings, it is important to know ways to avoid and extract yourself from potentially dangerous situations. The **Skills for Behavior Change** box identifies practical tips for preventing dating violence.

Most attacks by unknown assailants are planned in advance. Many rapists use certain ploys to initiate their attacks. Examples include asking for help; offering help; staging a deliberate "accident," such as bumping into you; or posing as a police officer or other authority figure. Sexual assault frequently begins with a casual, friendly conversation.

Listen to your feelings, and trust your intuition. Be assertive and direct to someone who is starting to get out of line or becoming threatening. Stifle your tendency to be nice, and don't fear making a scene. Use the following tips to let a potential assailant know that you mean what you say and are prepared to defend yourself:

- **Speak in a strong voice.** State, "Leave me alone!" rather than questions such as "Will you please leave me alone?" Avoid apologies and excuses. Sound like you mean it.
- **Maintain eye contact with a would-be attacker.** Eye contact keeps you aware of the person's movements and conveys an aura of strength and confidence.
- **Stand up straight, act confident, and remain alert.** Walk as if you own the sidewalk.

If you are attacked, act immediately. Draw attention to yourself and your assailant. Scream, "Fire!" Research has shown that passersby are much more likely to help if they hear the word *fire* rather than just a scream.

What to Do If a Rape Occurs

If you are a rape victim, report the attack. This gives you a sense of control. Follow these steps:

- Call 9-1-1.
- Do not bathe, shower, douche, clean up, or touch anything that the attacker may have touched.
- Save the clothes you were wearing, and do not launder them. They will be needed as evidence. Bring a clean change of clothes to the clinic or hospital.
- Contact the rape assistance hotline in your area, and ask for advice on therapists or counseling if you need additional help or advice.

If a friend is raped, here's how you can help:

- Believe the rape victim. Don't ask questions that might appear to imply that she or he is at a fault in any way for the assault.
- Recognize that rape is a violent act and that the victim was not looking for this to happen.

- Encourage your friend to see a doctor immediately because she or he may have medical needs but feel too embarrassed to seek help. Offer to go with your friend.
- Encourage your friend to report the crime.
- Be understanding, and let your friend know that you will be there for her or him.
- Recognize that this is an emotional recovery, and it may take months or years for your friend to bounce back.
- Encourage your friend to seek counseling.

One of the most important things you can do is to be supportive. Don't put your friend on the defensive with questions such as "Why didn't you leave?" or "What were you thinking by taking that drink?" Better options for questions might be "What happened? What do you feel that you want to do now? Is there anyone in particular you want to call or talk to? Is there anything I can do for you?"

Skills for **Behavior Change**

Reducing Your Risk of Dating Violence

- **Before your date, think about your values; set personal boundaries before you walk out the door.**
- **If a situation feels as though it is getting out of control, stop and talk, speak directly, and don't worry about hurting feelings. Be firm.**
- **Watch your alcohol consumption. Drinking might get you into situations you would otherwise avoid.**
- **Do not accept beverages or open-container drinks from anyone you do not know well and trust. At a bar or a club, accept drinks only from the bartender or wait staff.**
- **Never leave a drink or food unattended. If you get up to dance, have someone you trust watch your drink, or take it with you.**
- **Go out with several couples or in groups when dating someone new.**
- **Stick with your friends. Agree to keep an eye out for one another at parties, and have a plan for leaving together and checking in with one another. Never leave a bar or party alone with a stranger.**
- **Pay attention to your date's actions. If there is too much teasing and all the decisions are made for you, it could mean trouble. Trust your intuition.**
- **Practice what you will say to your date if things go in an uncomfortable direction. You have the right to express your feelings, and it is OK to be assertive. Do not be swayed by arguments such as "What about my feelings?," "You were leading me on," and "If you really cared about me, you would."**

Check Yourself

- **What are three things you can do to reduce your risk of personal assault?**

- **How can you support a friend who has been raped or assaulted?**

13.8 Describe how college campuses are responding to the threat of violence.

Prevention and Early Response Efforts

Campuses are reviewing the effectiveness of emergency messaging systems, including mobile phone alert systems. The REVERSE 9-1-1 system uses database and geographic information system (GIS) mapping technologies to notify campus police and community members in the event of problems, and other systems allow administrators to send out alerts in text, voice, e-mail, or instant message format. Some schools program the phone numbers, photographs, and basic student information for all incoming first-year students into a university security system so that in the event of a threat, students need only hit a button on their phones, whereupon campus police will be notified, and tracking devices will pinpoint their location.

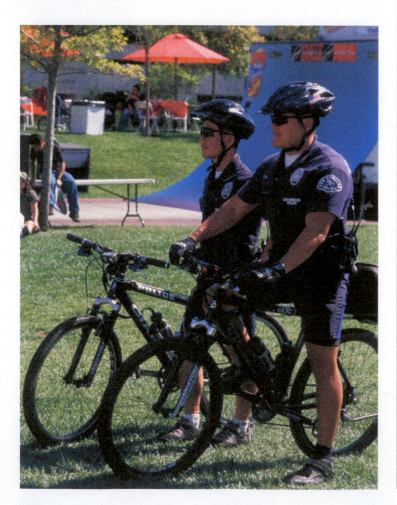

Changes in the Campus Environment

Administrators are asking key questions about the safety of the campus environment. Campus lighting, parking lot security, call boxes for emergencies, removal of overgrown shrubbery along bike paths and walking trails, and stepped-up security are increasingly on the radar of campus safety personnel. Buildings themselves are designed with better lighting and more security provisions, and in some cases security cameras have been installed in hallways, classrooms, and public places throughout campus. Safe rides are provided for students who have consumed too much alcohol; campus leaders have become more involved in campus safety issues; and health promotion programs have stepped up their violence prevention efforts through seminars on acquaintance rape, sexual assault, harassment, and other topics.

Hazing, which can be defined as "any activity expected of someone joining or participating in a group that humiliates, degrades, abuses, or endangers them regardless of a person's willingness to participate," can contribute to an atmosphere of violence and intimidation on campus. The issue of hazing has become headline news, with several deaths reported over the last few years. Currently, hazing is considered a crime in 39 states.

Most colleges and universities have policies against hazing, but few students ever report it. Typically, hazing involves forcing students to consume excessive alcohol; dress in humiliating garb; undergo forced sleep deprivation; endure verbal abuse from group members; or be subjected to physical abuse in the form of beatings, heat or cold exposure, or forced sexual acts. According to a national study, 55 percent of college students involved in clubs, teams, and organizations experience hazing, and 9 out of 10 students who experience hazing in college do not realize that they've been hazed.[54]

In 95 percent of cases in which students identified their experience as hazing, they did not report the events to campus officials.[55] One reason for this seems to be that more students perceive positive rather than negative outcomes of hazing, for example, feeling a sense of accomplishment or belonging. Students also report that school administrators do little to prevent hazing beyond maintaining a "hazing is not tolerated" stance. If schools are to have an impact on the prevalence of hazing on their campuses, they need to implement broader prevention and intervention efforts and work to educate their campus community on the physical and legal perils of hazing.

Campus Law Enforcement

Campus law enforcement has changed over the years by increasing both numbers of its members and its authority to prosecute student offenders. Campus police are responsible for emergency responses to situations that threaten safety, human resources, the general campus environment, traffic and bicycle riders, and other dangers. They have the power to enforce laws with students in the same way those laws are handled in the general community. In fact, many campuses now hire state troopers or local law enforcement officers to deal with campus issues rather than maintain a separate police staff.

Coping in the Event of Campus Violence

Although schools have worked tirelessly to prevent violence, it can and does still occur. There is no fix for traumatic events, but several strategies can be helpful. In the event of a campus-wide tragedy, members of the campus community should be allowed to mourn. Memorial services and acknowledgment of grief, fear, anger, and other emotions are critical to healing. Students, faculty, and staff should also be involved in planning to prevent future problems—it can help to impart a feeling of control. To cope with emotional trauma, students should seek out resources in their community, such as support groups, therapists, and trusted family members or friends. Journaling or writing about feelings can also help.

Community Strategies for Preventing Violence

You can take a number of steps to ensure your personal safety (see **Skills for Behavior Change**). However, it is also necessary to address issues of violence and safety at a community level. The CDC's Injury Response initiatives include community interventions designed to prevent violence before it begins:

- Inoculate children against violence in the home. Teaching young people the principles of respect and responsibility is fundamental to the health and well-being of future generations.
- Develop policies and laws that prevent violence. Enforce laws so that offenders know you mean business in your settings.
- Develop skills-based educational programs that teach the basics of interpersonal communication, elements of healthy relationships, anger management, conflict resolution, appropriate assertiveness, stress management, and other health-based behaviors.
- Involve families, schools, community programs, athletics, music, faith-based organizations, and other community groups in providing experiences that help young people to develop self-esteem and self-efficacy.
- Promote tolerance and acceptance, and establish and enforce policies that forbid discrimination. Offer diversity training and mandate involvement.
- Improve community services focused on family planning, mental health services, day care and respite care, and alcohol and substance abuse prevention.
- Make sure walking trails, parking lots, and other public areas are well lit, unobstructed, and patrolled regularly to reduce threats.
- Improve community-based support and treatment for victims, and ensure that individuals have choices available when trying to stop violence in their lives.

Skills for **Behavior Change**

Stay Safe On All Fronts

You can take a number of steps to protect yourself from assault. Follow these tips to increase your awareness and reduce your risk of a violent attack.

OUTSIDE ALONE

- Carry a cell phone, and keep it turned on, but stay off it. Be aware of what is happening around you. Don't walk to your car in a dark parking lot while chatting or texting with others. Stay alert.
- If you are being followed, don't go home. Head for a location where there are other people. If you decide to run, run fast and scream loudly to attract attention.
- Vary your routes, Walk or jog with others.
- Park near lights. Avoid dark areas where someone could hide.
- Carry pepper spray or other deterrents. Consider using your campus escort service.
- Tell others where you are going and when you expect to be back.

IN YOUR CAR

- Lock your doors. Do not open your doors or windows to strangers.
- If someone hits your car while you are driving, drive to the nearest gas station or other public place. Call the police or road service for help, and stay in your car until help arrives.
- If a car appears to be following you, do not drive home. Drive to the nearest police station.

IN YOUR HOME

- Install deadbolts on all doors and locks on all windows. Don't leave a spare key outside. Consider installing a home alarm system.
- Lock doors when at home, even during the day. Close blinds and drapes whenever you are away and in the evening when you are home.
- Rent apartments that require a security code or clearance to gain entry. Avoid easily accessible apartments such as first-floor units. When you move into a new residence, pay a locksmith to change the keys and locks.
- Don't let repair people in without asking for identification; have someone with you when repairs are made.
- If you return to find that your residence has been broken into, don't enter. Call the police. If you encounter an intruder, it is better to give up your money than to fight back.

IN PUBLIC PLACES-ACTIVE SHOOTER

- Stay alert. Pay attention to unusual actions or suspicious behaviors. If there is an active shooter, follow the new "Run, Hide, Fight" guidelines. See the FBI video "How to Survive an Active Shooter: Run, Hide, Fight" at https://www.youtube.com/watch?v=mnTXQbmXFw8.

Check Yourself

- What is being done on your campus to reduce the risk of violence from sexual assaults, potential shooters, and/or terrorist threats? What is being done about other forms of violence?

Reducing Your Risk on the Road

13.9 List the major causes of motor vehicle accidents, and explain how to stay safe on the road.

In 2016, over 40,200 Americans died of injuries sustained in motor vehicle crashes (MVCs), a 6 percent increase over the previous report's time period.[56]

Factors Contributing to Motor Vehicle Crashes

Factors that are within your control—distracted driving, impaired driving, speeding, and vehicle safety issues such as failure to wear your seat belt—contribute to the great majority of vehicle crashes.

Distracted Driving Four types of activities constitute distracted driving: looking at something other than the road, hearing something not related to driving, manipulating something other than the steering wheel, and thinking about something other than driving. Examples typically include using a cell phone, eating and drinking, talking with passengers, adjusting your music or navigation system, reading, personal grooming, playing with a pet, tending to a child, changing clothes, picking up something you dropped, and daydreaming. Distracted driving kills at least over 3.000 people per year and injures over 420,000 more.[57]

Distracted driving was a factor in 76 percent of rear-end crashes and 89 percent of road-departure crashes, the majority of which involved cell phone usage.[58] At any given time during daylight hours, nearly 550,000 passenger vehicles are driven by someone using a handheld cell phone and many of them are texting.[59] Despite clear statistics to the contrary, a recent study indicated that 20 percent of drivers age 18 to 20 and nearly 30 percent of drivers age 21 to 34 said that texting does not affect their driving. Highway safety experts estimate that when traveling at 55 mph, the average text takes the driver's eyes off the road long enough to cross a football field.[60] Currently, 46 states ban texting while driving, and 14 states ban all handheld cell phone use of any kind while driving.[61]

Texting and other distractions triple your risk of getting into a crash. The next time you're tempted to text, make a call, or even swat an insect while driving, pull over. Handle the distraction. Then rejoin traffic when you have finished.

Impaired Driving In 2015, there were 10,265 people killed in alcohol impaired crashes. These alcohol impaired crashes made up nearly nearly one-third of all motor vehicle fatalities in the United States.[62] Of alcohol-impaired drivers involved in fatalities, 7 percent had a previous conviction for driving while impaired (DWI), and another 24 percent had a history of license suspension or revocation.[63] People age 21 to 24 have the highest percentage of alcohol-impaired drivers involved in fatal crashes.[64]

After alcohol, marijuana is the drug most often linked to impaired driving.[65] Marijuana use reduces attention, increases weaving in and out of traffic, and slows reaction time.[66] A recent study of fatal crashes in Colorado shows increases in the number of fatal crashes since the legalization of marijuana.[67] Prescription drugs, mainly opioids and sedatives, are also common factors in MVC fatalities.[68]

Public health and law enforcement agencies are cooperating on measures to keep impaired drivers off the road:

- Designated driver programs, including public funding of "safe rides"
- Strict enforcement of laws defining impaired driving and the legal drinking age
- Measures to prevent repeat offenses, including mandatory alcohol or drug abuse treatment, ignition interlock systems that prevent vehicle operation by anyone with a blood alcohol concentration above a specified level, stricter testing for and punishment of drivers who abuse prescription medicines and/or drive when sleep impaired, and license revocation

Vehicle Safety Issues Always wear a seat belt in a car. Forty-nine percent of all people killed in MVCs in 2014 were not wearing seat belts at the time.[69] If you're transporting an infant or child, follow state laws governing the use and location of age-appropriate safety seats.

When buying, look for vehicles with the highest crash safety ratings, side and knee airbags, antilock brakes, traction and stability controls, impact-absorbing crumple zones, strong compartment and roof supports, automatic braking for impending frontal crashes, and blind spot assistance. Unfortunately, people who don't have the financial resources to drive vehicles with all of these safety features—and that group often includes college students—are at increased risk during MVCs.

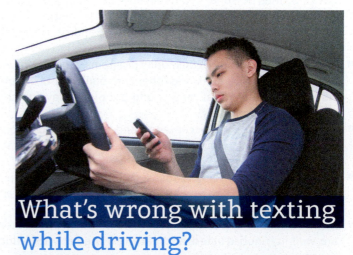

What's wrong with texting while driving?

Texting or talking on a cell phone while driving puts you at a greater risk of being in a motor vehicle accident. It also increases the risk of injury and death to other drivers, passengers, and pedestrians and is illegal in many states.

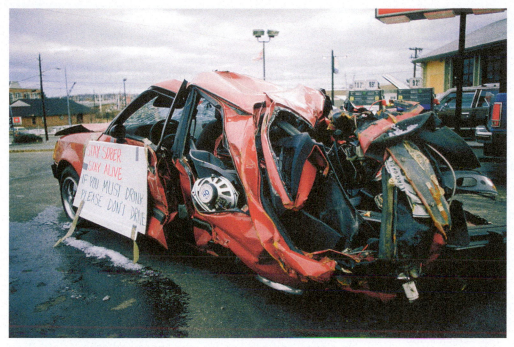

Driving under the influence of alcohol greatly increases the risk of being involved in a motor vehicle crash. Of all drivers between the ages of 21 and 24 involved in fatal crashes, nearly 1 out of 3 were legally drunk.

Many college students drive small cars because they are more affordable and use less gas, but the laws of physics make small cars more dangerous. All cars sold in the United States must meet U.S. Department of Transportation standards for crash worthiness. However, in 2012, there were nearly four times as many deaths per vehicle among minicars as compared to very large cars, and 23 of the top 26 cars with the lowest rates of driver deaths were midsize or larger.[70]

What about motorcycles? Per vehicle mile traveled, motorcyclists are about 27 times more likely than passenger car occupants to die in an MVC and 5 times more likely to be injured. [71]

Many motorcyclists who have been involved in accidents have avoided severe injuries because they were wearing a helmet. Although the benefits of helmets and protective clothing are well established, only 19 states have full helmet requirements for anyone riding a motorcycle.[72] To find out your state requirements, go to www.iihs.org.

Risk-Management Driving Techniques

Although you can't control what other drivers are doing, you can reduce your risk of injury:

- Don't manipulate electronic devices or talk on a cell phone while driving, even if the phone is hands-free.
- Don't drink and drive. Take a taxi or Uber, or arrange for someone to be the designated driver.
- Don't drive when tired or in a highly emotional or stressed state.
- Never tailgate. The rear bumper of the car ahead of you should be at least 3 seconds worth of distance away, making stopping safely possible. Increase the distance when visibility is reduced, speed is increased, or roads are slick.

- Scan the road ahead of you and to both sides. Stay alert.
- Drive with your low-beam headlights on, *day and night*, to make your car more visible to other drivers.
- Anticipate the actions of others as much as you can; be on the alert for unsignaled lane changes, sudden braking, or other unexpected maneuvers.
- Obey all traffic laws.
- Whether you're the driver or a passenger, always wear a seat belt.

Road Rage

The National Highway Traffic Safety Administration (NHTSA) defines aggressive driving as "the operation of a motor vehicle in a manner that endangers or is likely to endanger persons or property."[73] An extreme version of such behavior is *road rage*, which is believed to be a leading cause of highway deaths. Although you cannot control or predict the behavior of other people, there are steps you can take to avoid becoming a victim of road rage:

- **Avoid eye contact and engagement with other drivers.** If you're driving or in public and someone tries to get a reaction from you, avoid confrontation and remove yourself from the situation.

See It! Videos

Are you at risk of falling asleep at the wheel? Watch **Dozing and Driving: 1 in 24 Asleep at Wheel** in the Study Area of Mastering Health.

- **Don't antagonize other drivers.** Slowing down in traffic to bug someone who is obviously in a hurry, honking your horn, flashing your high beams, or other passive-aggressive gestures can upset even the most mild-mannered people.
- **If someone follows you after a nasty interaction, either in a car or on foot, do not immediately go home or to your workplace.** Head for the nearest police station or busy area. Never isolate yourself.
- **Take names.** If you don't know the person, try to memorize a mental description or get a license plate number. Report offenders even if you're afraid of getting involved.
- **Stay calm.** Think before opening your mouth, and practice stress-management techniques whenever possible.

Check Yourself

- **What are three factors linked to increased risk of motor vehicle accidents?**

- **What can you do to stay safe on the road?**

13.10 Safe Recreation

Learning Outcome

13.10 Explain how to stay safe while biking, skateboarding, skiing, snowboarding, swimming, and boating.

Recreational activities among young people that commonly involve injury include biking, skateboarding, snow sports, and swimming and boating. By following some basic guidelines while enjoying these activities, you can have fun and be safe.

Bike Safety

The NHTSA reports that 818 bicyclists died in traffic collisions in 2015, and 45,000 were injured.[74] Most fatal collisions occur at nonintersections (60 percent) between 4:00 p.m. and midnight. Alcohol plays a significant role in bicycle deaths and injuries; in about one-third of all fatal crashes between motor vehicles and bicycles, either the driver or the cyclist was drunk.[75]

Wearing a properly fitted bicycle helmet has been estimated to reduce the risk of head injury by half (**Figure 13.5**).[76] In addition, consider the following suggestions:

- Wear a helmet approved by the American National Standards Institute (ANSI) or the Snell Memorial Foundation.
- Watch the road, and listen for traffic sounds. Never listen to an MP3 player or talk on a cell phone, even hands free, while cycling.
- Don't drink and ride.
- Follow all traffic laws, signs, and signals.
- Ride with the flow of traffic.
- Wear light or brightly colored, reflective clothing that is easily seen at dawn, dusk, and during full daylight.

- Avoid riding after dark. If you must ride at night, use a front light and a red reflector or flashing rear light, as well as reflective tape or other markings on your bike and clothing.
- Know and use proper hand signals.
- Keep your bicycle in good condition.
- Use bike paths whenever possible.
- Stop at stop signs and traffic lights.

Safe Skateboarding

According to the U.S. Consumer Product Safety Commission (CPSC), skateboard-related injuries are commonly due to riding in traffic, trick riding, excessive speed, and consumption of alcohol. Lack of protective equipment, poor board maintenance, riding on irregular road surfaces, inexperience, and overconfidence also play a role. Following are skateboard safety tips from the CPSC:

- Wear an approved helmet, padded clothes, special skateboarding gloves, and padding for your knees and other joints. Padding should be snug but loose enough to allow movement.
- Between uses, check your board for loose, broken, sharp, or cracked parts, and have it repaired if necessary.
- Examine the surface where you'll be riding for holes, bumps, and debris.
- Never skateboard in the street.
- Never hitch a ride from a car, bicycle, or other vehicle while on a skateboard.
- Practice complicated stunts in specially designed areas, wearing protective padding.
- Don't speed.
- Don't ride alone.
- Don't drink and ride.

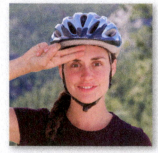 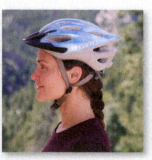 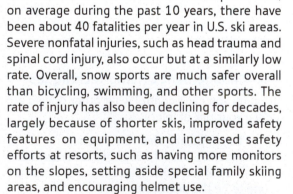

❶ The helmet should sit level on your head and low on your forehead—one or two finger-widths above your eyebrows.

❷ The sliders on the side straps should be adjusted to form a "V" shape under, and slightly in front of, your ears. Lock the sliders if possible.

❸ The chin strap buckle should be centered under your chin. Tighten the strap until it is snug, so that no more than two fingers fit under the strap.

Figure 13.5 Fitting a Bicycle Helmet
When your helmet fits correctly, opening your mouth wide in a yawn should cause the helmet to pull down on your head. Also, you should not be able to rock the helmet back more than the width of two fingers above the eyebrows or forward into your eyes.

▶ **Mastering Health & Nutrition** Biking Safety

Safety in the Snow

The National Ski Areas Association reports that, on average during the past 10 years, there have been about 40 fatalities per year in U.S. ski areas. Severe nonfatal injuries, such as head trauma and spinal cord injury, also occur but at a similarly low rate. Overall, snow sports are much safer overall than bicycling, swimming, and other sports. The rate of injury has also been declining for decades, largely because of shorter skis, improved safety features on equipment, and increased safety efforts at resorts, such as having more monitors on the slopes, setting aside special family skiing areas, and encouraging helmet use.

As with bicycles, wearing a helmet and protective goggles and carrying a GPS locator In areas where avalanches are common are good practices. It's also important to keep skis and snowboards in good condition and to choose trails according to your ability. Pay attention to the locations of others; if you stop, move to the side of the trail. Observe all posted signs and warnings.

Water Safety

According to the latest statistics, 3,406 Americans die each year by drowning, making it the fifth leading cause of unintentional injury death among Americans of all ages.[77] Children age 1 to 4 have the highest rate of drowning, but young Americans aged 15 to 24 experience the most drownings.[78] People who survive near-drownings may experience severe brain damage.[79]

Swimming The vast majority of adults who drown are not wearing life jackets (88 percent) and are under the influence of alcohol (70 percent).[80] Most drownings occur during water recreation—swimming, diving, or just simply having fun—in unorganized or unsupervised areas, such as ponds or pools without lifeguards present. Many drowning victims were strong swimmers.

All swimmers should take the following precautions:

- Don't drink alcohol before or while swimming.
- Don't swim alone, even if you are a skilled swimmer. You never know what might happen.
- Never leave a child unattended, even in extremely shallow water.
- Before entering water, check the depth. Most neck and back injuries result from diving into water that is too shallow.
- Never swim in a river with currents too swift for easy, relaxed swimming or in muddy or dirty water that obstructs your view of the bottom. Water that is discolored and choppy or foamy may indicate a rip current.
- If you're caught in a rip current, swim parallel to the shore. Once you are free of the current, swim toward the shore.
- Learn cardiopulmonary resuscitation (CPR).

Boating In 2013, the U.S. Coast Guard received reports of 2,620 injured boaters and 560 deaths.[81] About 77 percent of these boating fatalities were drownings, and among those who drowned, 84 percent were not wearing a **personal flotation device**—that is, a lifejacket.[82]

About one-third of all boating fatalities involve alcohol.[83] When boat operators are drinking, both collisions with other boats and falls overboard are much more likely. If someone who has been drinking falls overboard, he or she is more likely to drown or to die of hypothermia. Unfortunately, the "designated driver" concept does not apply to boating—intoxicated passengers often cause or contribute to boating accidents. The U.S. Coast Guard and every state have "Boating under the Influence" (BUI) laws that carry stringent penalties, including fines, license revocation, and even jail time.[84]

Consider the following safety tips from the American Boating Association[85]:

- Before leaving home, let other people know where you are going, who will be with you, and when you expect to return.
- Check the weather. Listen to small craft warnings and advisories regarding high winds, storms, and other environmental factors.

Do I really have to wear a helmet while I'm skateboarding?

The majority of skateboarding injuries occur among people who have been practicing the sport for more than a year, often when they attempt a stunt beyond their level of skill. Wearing a helmet, no matter how experienced a skateboarder you are, will help protect you in case of a fall.

- Even for short trips, make sure the vessel doesn't leak, has enough fuel (if powered), and has proper safety equipment.
- Make sure you have enough life jackets for all on board that they are easily accessible. Encourage everyone on board to wear one at all times. When a boat sinks or capsizes, there is typically not enough time to grab and don a life jacket. When someone falls overboard, it may take time for the boat to return to the spot, and the person in the water might be unconscious or unable to stay afloat without a life jacket.
- Carry an emergency radio and cell phone.
- Don't drink alcohol before you leave, and don't bring any aboard.

The U.S. Coast Guard recommends that before setting out, you put on your life jacket. Most modern life jackets are thin and flexible and can be worn comfortably all day. Children must wear a life jacket once the vessel is under way, unless they are below deck. Wear a life jacket not only when sailing or motor boating, but also when canoeing, kayaking, and rafting.

Check Yourself

- **What are three strategies that can help keep you safe when biking or skateboarding? In the snow? On the water?**

13.11 Avoiding Injury from Excessive Noise

Learning Outcome

13.11 List factors contributing to noise-induced hearing loss and explain how to protect your hearing.

Our modern society is too often filled with excessive noise. Take a look at **Figure 13.6**, which shows the decibel (dB) levels of common sounds. In general, noise levels above 85 dB (about as loud as a diesel truck) increase risks for hearing loss. An estimated 48 million U.S. teens and adults have some degree of hearing loss.[86] This represents about 20 percent of the adult population. Moreover, hearing loss becomes more common with each decade we age, and some populations are at greater risk than others.

Noise-induced hearing loss results when exposure to high-decibel (high-dB) noise, usually over time, damages sensory receptors in the cochlea, or inner ear. Loud music in a short period such as a concert, high levels of noise exposure for prolonged periods in occupational settings and sudden bursts of noise from a single event, such as a large caliber gunshot in close proximity, can result in either temporary or permanent hearing loss.

One of the highest rates of sudden noise-induced hearing loss is among teens and young adults; nearly 10 percent of these groups show signs of hearing loss. Loud music played through headsets, mobile devices, and multiple car speakers is directly related to auditory loss. Students in professional music programs in college appear to have an increased risk.[87] The precise decibel level, frequency, and duration of exposure that might correlate with hearing loss are under investigation.[88]

Another source of hearing impairment is frequent concert attendance. Most rock musicians use earplugs when performing or rehearsing, and their audiences would be wise to do the same. Hearing loss may result from one evening in front of huge speakers at a rock concert. Sporting events, such as stock car races and football games, can also be very loud. If you can't hear the person standing next to you at a concert or sporting event, then you should put in earplugs or look for a quieter spot. In addition, you should rest your ears between nights out partying or attending loud events.

What can you do to avoid hearing loss while still enjoying your music? Keep the volume below 80 dB—a level at which you can carry on a conversation—and you won't need to limit time spent listening to music. If you're listening through ear buds or headphones and a friend nearby can hear your music, it's definitely too loud. And though debate continues over the relative safety of over-the-ear headphones versus ear buds, headphones seem to be safer.[89]

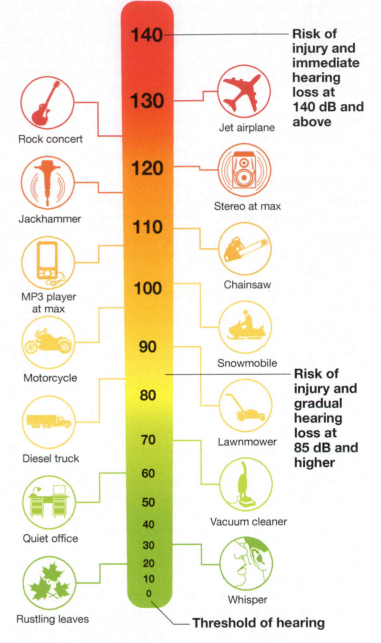

Figure 13.6 Noise Levels of Various Sounds (dB)
Decibels increase logarithmically, so each increase of 10 dB represents a tenfold increase in loudness.

Source: Adapted from National Institute on Deafness and Other Communication Disorders, "How Loud Is Too Loud?" Updated July 2011, www.nidcd.nih.gov.

Check Yourself

- **What are three things you can do to avoid hearing loss?**

13.12 Safety at Home

13.12 List steps to take to prevent and address common household safety hazards.

Poisoning

A **poison** is any substance that is harmful when ingested, inhaled, injected, or absorbed through the skin. In 2015, 55 poison control centers in the United States logged more than 2.1 million calls for poisonings of humans, 50,000 for poisonings of dogs, and 5,000 for poisonings of cats.[90] Following are some things you can do to prevent poisoning:[91]

- Read and follow all usage and warning labels before taking medications or working with chemicals, including household products.
- Never share or sell prescription drugs and don't take anyone else's prescription drugs!
- Never take more than one medication at the same time without the approval of your health care provider. Mixing medications can result in poisoning.
- When working with chemicals, wear a protective mask, and make sure the area in which you work is well ventilated. Wear gloves and other protective clothing, and wear eyeglasses or an eye guard if splashing could occur.
- Keep medications, dietary supplements, and alcohol out of sight of children, preferably in a locked cabinet.
- Program the 24-hour national poison control number into your phone: 1-800-222-1222.

If you suspect that you have ingested or inhaled a poison or you are with someone who has collapsed, call 9-1-1. If the victim is not breathing and you are trained in CPR, provide CPR until paramedics arrive. If the victim is awake and alert, dial the poison control hotline (1-800-222-1222). Follow the instructions given. If you go to a hospital emergency room, bring the suspected poison if possible.

Falls

Falls are the third most common cause of death from unintentional injury in the United States, causing 31,959 deaths in 2014.[92] About 20 percent of people who fall suffer serious injury, such as a hip fracture or a head injury. Following are some things you can do to reduce your risk of falls:

- Use slip proof mats on all small rugs.
- Train pets to stay away from your feet.
- Install slip-proof mats, treads, or decals in showers and tubs.
- Wear supportive shoes. Flip-flops and loose shoes can trip you.

Fire

In 2014, nearly 3500 Americans died in fires.[94] Although fire-related deaths are not common on college campuses in the United States, 85 fatal campus fires occurred between 2000 and 2015, claiming 118 lives.[95] Smoke alarms were missing or disconnected

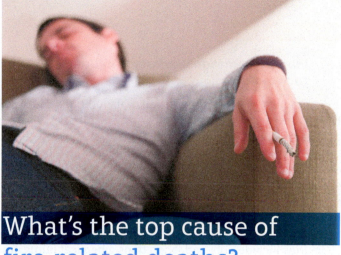

What's the top cause of fire-related deaths?

If you fall asleep with a lit cigarette, bedding and clothing can quickly ignite. If you can't quit, take it outside.

in 58 percent of these fatal fires, and alcohol was also a major factor; at least one of the students involved was legally drunk at the time.[96] Following are some things you can do to prevent fires:

- Extinguish cigarettes in ashtrays. Never smoke in bed.
- Place lamps away from drapes, linens, and paper.
- Keep kitchen cloths and sleeves away from stove burners.
- Keep candles away from combustibles. Never leave candles unattended.
- Avoid overloading electrical circuits with appliances and cords.
- Have the proper fire extinguishers and make sure they are easily accessible.
- Replace batteries in smoke alarms and test the alarms periodically.

If a fire breaks out, your priority is to get out *as soon as possible*. First, feel the door handle. If it's hot, don't open the door. Go to a window, open it wide, and call for help. Hang a sheet from the window to alert rescuers. Call 9-1-1. If smoke is entering your room, seal cracks under and around the door with blankets or towels. Stay low—there's less smoke close to the floor.

If the door handle is not hot, open the door cautiously. If the hallway is clear, get out, yelling, "Fire!" and knocking on doors as you leave. If you encounter smoke, stay low. Crawl if necessary. If you pass a fire alarm, pull it. Always use stairs, never an elevator. Once you're outside, call 9-1-1.

- What are two things each that you can do to prevent household poisoning, falls, and fire?

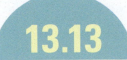

13.13 Avoiding Workplace Injury

Learning Outcome

13.13 Identify common workplace injuries and how to avoid them.

American adults spend most of their waking hours on the job. Although most job situations are pleasant and productive, others pose hazards. Transportation incidents make up the largest number of fatal work injuries (more than 25%). Workers in material moving, construction, and mining and those in the service industry are at high risk of fatal injuries. Farmers, fishery workers, and loggers are also at high risk.[97]

Although on-the-job deaths capture media attention, workers may also be seriously injured or disabled at their jobs. Common work injuries include cuts and lacerations, chemical burns, fractures, sprains, and strains (often of the back), and repetitive motion disorders. Many work injuries are due to overexertion, poor body mechanics, or repetitive motion, which means that they are largely preventable. We discuss these problems and share some prevention strategies here.

Protect Your Back

Low back pain, usually as a result of injury, is the major cause of disability for people age 20 to 45 in the United States; this age groups suffers more frequently and severely from this problem than older people do.[98] It is one of the most commonly experienced chronic ailments among college students. In a recent survey, 12.7 percent of college students reported having seen their doctor in the previous year because of back pain.[99]

Most injuries to the back are in the lumbar spine area (lower back); strengthening core muscle groups and stretching muscles to avoid cramping and spasms reduce risks. Frequently, sports injuries, stress on spinal bones and tissues, the sudden jolt of a car accident, or other obvious causes are the culprits. Other times, sitting too long in the same position or hunching over your computer while pulling an all-nighter can leave you with pain so severe that you can't stand up or walk comfortably. Carrying heavy backpacks is another frequent source of lower back pain.

Avoid typical risks by using common sense when engaging in activities that could injure your back. Get up and stretch intermittently while working in a static position. Good posture can also reduce back problems.

Other measures you can take to reduce the risk of back pain include the following:

- Invest in a high-quality, supportive mattress.
- Avoid wearing high-heeled shoes, which tilt the pelvis forward.
- Control your weight. Extra weight puts increased strain on your knees, hips, and back.
- Warm up and stretch before exercising or lifting heavy objects.
- When lifting something heavy, use proper form (**Figure 13.7**). Do not bend from the waist or take the weight load on your back.
    - Buy a desk chair with good lumbar support.
    - Move your car seat forward so that your knees are elevated.
    - Engage in regular exercise, particularly core exercises that strengthen and stretch abdominal muscles and back muscles.
    - Downsize your backpack.

Maintain Alignment While Sitting

Think back over your day. How many hours have you sat glued to a computer or book? Were you slouching, hunched over, or sitting up straight? Your answers are probably reflected in the degree of aching and stiffness you may be feeling right now. So how can you maintain healthy alignment while you work? Try these strategies:

1. Sit comfortably with your feet flat on the floor or on a footrest and your knees level with your hips. Raise or lower your chair or move to a different chair to achieve this position.

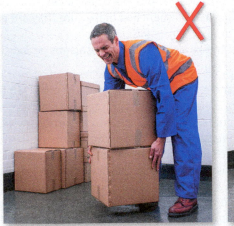

ⓐ Attempting to lift a heavy object by bending at your waist is a common cause of back injury.

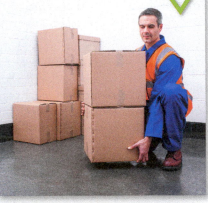

ⓑ Start as close to the object as possible, with it positioned between your knees as you squat down. Keep your feet parallel, or stagger one foot in front of the other. Keep the object close to your body as you stand, using your legs, not your back, to lift.

Figure 13.7 Lifting a Heavy Object

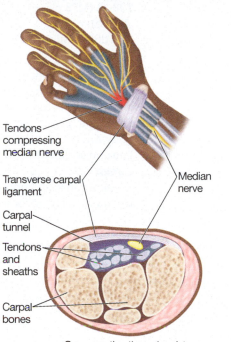

Tendons
compressing
median nerve

Transverse carpal
ligament

Median
nerve

Carpal
tunnel

Tendons
and
sheaths

Carpal
bones

Cross-section through wrist

Figure 13.8 Carpal Tunnel Syndrome
The carpal tunnel is a space beneath the transverse carpal ligament and above the carpal bones of the wrist. The median nerve and the tendons that allow you to flex your fingers run through this tunnel. Carpal tunnel syndrome occurs when repetitive use prompts inflammation of the tissues and fluids of the tunnel. This, in turn, compresses the median nerve.

2. Your middle back should be firmly against the back of the chair. The small of your back should be supported too. If you can't feel the chair back supporting your lumbar region, try placing a small cushion or rolled towel behind the curve of your lower back.

3. Keep your shoulders relaxed and straight, not rolled or hunched forward.

4. Your forearms should be at a 90 degree angle with your upper arms. Adjust your position or the position of your device to achieve this angle.

5. Ideally, you should be looking straight ahead, not peering down at the device's screen or your book.

Avoid Repetitive Motion Disorders

It's the end of the term, and you've finished the last of several papers. After hours of nonstop typing, your hands are numb, and you feel pain that makes the thought of typing one more word unbearable. You may be suffering from one of several **repetitive motion disorders (RMDs)**, sometimes called *overuse syndrome*, *cumulative trauma disorders*, or *repetitive stress injuries*. These refer to a family of soft tissue injuries that begin with inflammation and gradually become disabling.

RMDs include carpal tunnel syndrome, bursitis, tendonitis, and ganglion cysts, among others. Twisting of the arm or wrist, over-exertion, and incorrect posture or position are usually contributors. The areas that are most likely to be affected are the hands, wrists, elbows, and shoulders, but the neck, back, hips, knees, feet, ankles, and legs can be affected too. Over time, RMDs can cause permanent damage to nerves, soft tissue, and joints. Usually, RMDs are associated with repeating the same task and gradually irritating the area in question. Certain sports (tennis, golf, and others), gripping the wheel while driving, keyboarding or texting, and a number of technology-driven activities can also result in RMDs.

Because many of these injuries occur in everyday work, play, and athletics, they are often not reported to national agencies that keep track of injury statistics. Nevertheless, cases of repetitive motion problems are widespread.

One of the most common RMDs is **carpal tunnel syndrome (CTS)**, an inflammation of the soft tissues and fluids within the "tunnel" through the carpal bones of the wrist (**Figure 13.8**). This puts pressure on the median nerve, which runs down the forearm through the tunnel. Symptoms include numbness, tingling, and pain in the fingers and hands.

Carpal tunnel syndrome typically results from spending hours typing at a computer keyboard or using a mouse, flipping groceries through computerized scanners, or manipulating other objects in jobs "made simpler" by technology.

The risk for CTS can be reduced by proper design of workstations, protective wrist pads, and worker training. Physical therapy and occupational therapy are important parts of treatment and recovery.

Strategies for avoiding repetitive motion disorders include the following:[100]

- If you are doing repetitive activities such as taking notes in class by hand, reduce your force and relax your grip. There are pens available that offer oversized grips and free-flowing ink, which lessen the strain on your hand.
- Take frequent breaks to stretch your hands and wrists.
- Keep your hands and fingers warm. A cold environment can lead to stiffness and hand pain. You may need to wear fingerless gloves if you can't control your environment.

Check Yourself

- **What are two strategies to protect your back?**

- **What workplace factors contribute to repetitive motion disorders?**

- **What can you do to maintain healthy alignment in your study and work areas?**

Study Plan

Summary

LO 13.1 Overall, crime rates in the United States are down since the 1990s. Factors that contribute to violence include economic difficulties, parental influence, cultural beliefs, discrimination, political differences, substance abuse, stress, excessive fear, anger.

LO 13.2–LO 13.5 Interpersonal violence includes homicide, domestic violence, child abuse, elder abuse, and sexual victimization.

LO 13.6 Forms of collective violence, including gang violence and terrorism, result in fear, anxiety, and issues of discrimination.

LO 13.7 Recognizing how to protect yourself, knowing where to get help, and having honest, straightforward dialogue in dating situations can reduce the risk of violence.

LO 13.8 Shootings and acts of violence on campuses have resulted in a groundswell of activities designed to protect students. Preventing violence means community activism; prioritizing mental and emotional health; and skills training in anger management, coping, parenting, and other areas.

LO 13.9 Distracted or driving impaired driving and road rage are factors in many motor vehicle accidents. A well-designed and well-maintained vehicle can reduce the likelihood and severity of accidents, as can simple risk-management techniques.

LO 13.10 Basic safety practices—including wearing appropriate safety gear and staying sober—can help people stay safe during sports and recreation.

LO 13.11 High-decibel noise can lead to hearing loss. Keep earphone volume to a reasonable level and use earplugs or distance yourself from speakers to protect hearing at concerts and similar events.

LO 13.12 To stay safe at home, know how to prevent—and what to do in the event of—poisoning, fire, and injury.

LO 13.13 In the workplace, proper ergonomics can help to prevent injuries and repetitive motion disorders.

Pop Quiz

Visit Mastering Health to personalize your study plan with Chapter Review Quizzes and Dynamic Study Modules.

LO 13.2 1. An example of an intentional injury is
a. a car crash.
b. noise-induced hearing loss.
c. drowning.
d. road rage.

LO 13.4 2. In a class, students were discussing sexual assault. One student commented that some women dress too provocatively. The social assumption that this student made is
a. minimization.
b. trivialization.
c. blaming the victim.
d. "boys will be boys."

LO 13.4 3. Rape by a person the victim knows and that does not involve a physical beating or use of a weapon is called
a. simple rape.
b. sexual assault.
c. simple assault.
d. aggravated rape.

LO 13.5 4. Which of the following is an example of stalking?
a. Making intimate, sexually implied comments to another person
b. Repeated visual, physical, or virtual seeking out of another person
c. Unwelcome sexual conduct by the perpetrator
d. Sexual abuse of a child

LO 13.5 5. When Sofia began her new job with all male coworkers, her supervisor told her that he enjoyed having an attractive woman in the workplace, and he winked at her. His comment constitutes
a. acquaintance rape.
b. sexual assault.
c. sexual harassment.
d. sexual battering.

LO 13.9 6. Which of the following is *not* a good response to another driver's road rage?
a. Avoid eye contact.
b. Memorize the person's license plate number.
c. Drive home immediately.
d. Drive to the nearest police station.

LO 13.10 7. The majority of skateboarding accidents happen to riders who
a. are new to the sport.
b. have more than a year's experience.
c. are trying out new equipment.
d. are skating on public property.

LO 13.11 8. Above what decibel level do risks for hearing loss increase?
a. 70 dB (vacuum cleaner)
b. 85 dB (diesel truck engine)
c. 108 dB (MP3 player at maximum volume)
d. 130 dB (jet airplane engine)

LO 13.13 9. Which of the following is a common factor in repetitive motion disorders?
a. An incorrectly aligned computer workstation setup
b. Keeping a heavy object close to your body when lifting it off the ground
c. Looking straight ahead at a computer screen
d. Keeping hands and fingers too warm when you're typing for long periods

Answers to these questions can be found on page A-1. If you answered a question incorrectly, review the module identified by the Learning Outcome. For even more study tools, visit Mastering Health.

Think About It!

LO 13.1 1. What forms of violence do you think are most significant or prevalent in the United States today? How do you think violence affects students at your school?

LO 13.4 2. Have you known anyone personally who has been sexually assaulted on campus? What actions were taken to help the person cope with the assault? What campus services, if any, were used?

LO 13.9–13.12 3. Think about an unintentional injury that affected you. What led up to it? What could have been done to prevent it? How much control did you have over the situation and how much was it affected by other people?

Environmental Health

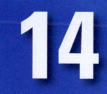

14

ASSESS YOURSELF: What Are You Doing to Preserve the Environment? **Find out in the Study Area at** Mastering **Health.**

"2014 was the planet's warmest year on record. Now, one year doesn't make a trend, but this does—14 of the 15 warmest years on record have all fallen in the first 15 years of this century."
—Barack Obama, Excerpt from January 2015 State of the Union Address

While the rising global temperature records mentioned by President Obama show a trend, it gets worse: 2015 and 2016 were the hottest years ever recorded in North America and in many regions of the world. (See https://youtube/s3RWTTtPg8E?t=49.) The global population has grown more in the past 50 years than at any other time in history. Polar ice caps are melting at rates that defy even the direst predictions, and threats of rising sea levels loom. According to one report, we have lost 58 percent of the world's mammals, fish, birds, amphibians, and reptiles in the last 40 years.[1] Clean water is becoming increasingly scarce, fossil fuels are dwindling quickly, and solid and hazardous wastes are growing in proportion to population.

Have we passed the point of being able to restore the balance between humans and nature? We must understand the factors that contribute to our global environmental crisis, and know what actions individuals, communities, and political powers need to take to bring the environmental health of planet Earth back into balance. This chapter gives an overview of these factors and actions.

14.1 List factors affecting population growth and overpopulation.

The human population has nearly tripled since 1950, from 2.5 billion people to over 7 billion. The United Nations projects that the world's population will grow to 9.8 billion by 2050, given recent jumps in **fertility rates**—the average number of births per woman in a specific country or region.[2] Add increases in overall survival, life expectancy at birth, and other variables, and the population may swell to over 12 billion by 2100.[3] Tomorrow's population will be significantly larger and more industrialized, will consume more resources, and will produce even more waste than previous generations unless population growth is controlled and major changes in environmental policy and behavior occur.[4]

Factors Affecting Population Growth

A number of factors have led to the world population's increase. Key among them are changes in fertility and mortality rates. Many countries have shown consistent declines in fertility rates in recent years, and in fact, their populations are likely to decrease. Countries whose populations are shrinking include Japan, Italy, and South Korea. However, other countries, particularly those in the most impoverished areas, continue to have high rates of fertility. Although lower fertility rates means slowing population growth, sheer population size can lead to major increases, even if fertility rates remain constant or decline (Table 14.1).[5] China, with 1.4 billion people, and India, with 1.3 billion people, are the two most populous countries, making up 37 percent of the world's

TABLE 14.1 Selected Total Fertility Rates Worldwide, 2015

Country	Number of Children Born per Woman*
Niger	7.6
Somalia	6.4 ↓
India	1.8 ↓
Mexico	2.3 ↓
United States	1.8 ↓
Australia	1.8 ↓
Canada	1.6
China	1.6 ↓
Russia	1.8
European Union	1.6 ↑

*Indicates the average number of children that would be born per woman if all women lived to the end of their childbearing years and bore children according to a given fertility rate at each age.

↓↑ Denotes change from 2015 fertility rates. If no arrow, no change.

Source: Data from Population Reference Bureau, "World Population Data Sheet," 2016, http://www.prb.org/pdf16/prb-wpds2016-web-2016.pdf.

population.[6] Of the world's ten largest nations, Nigeria is growing at the fastest rate, although India is adding more people per year than any other country.[7]

With a current population of over 326 million and a net gain of one person every 8 seconds, the United States is among the largest and fastest-growing industrialized nations.[8] It also has one of the largest **ecological footprints**—a measure of the biologically productive land and water area an individual or a population occupies and uses—exerting a greater impact on many of the planet's resources than do most other nations.[9]

Historically, in countries where women have little education and little control over reproductive choices, and where birth control is either not available or frowned upon, pregnancy rates continue to rise. As women become more educated, obtain higher socioeconomic status, work more outside of the home, and have more control over reproduction, fertility rates decline. Many countries have enacted strict population control measures or have encouraged their citizens to limit the size of their families. Proponents of *zero population growth* believe that each couple should produce only two offspring, allowing the population to stabilize.

Mortality rates from chronic and infectious diseases have declined as a result of improved public health infrastructure, increased availability of drugs and vaccines, a decline in infant mortality, better disaster preparedness, and other factors. As people live longer, they use more of the Earth's resources too.

Measuring the Impact of People

Population growth is not the only way in which humans are increasing their demands on the earth. As affluence increases in a population, so does its use of resources. People who used to walk or ride bicycles can now afford to buy a car (or two). Those same people can now move to a larger home and purchase more goods and services.

Today, experts are analyzing the **carrying capacity of the earth**—the largest population that can be supported indefinitely, given the resources available in the environment. At what point will we be unable to restore the balance between humans and nature? Since 1996, the global demand for natural resources has doubled. Currently, an estimated 1.6 planets' worth of resources are necessary to meet resource demands. By 2030 it will take the equivalent of two planets to meet the demand for resources, and by 2100, we may need more than four planets to support human needs! Simply put, we are running out of the natural resources necessary to sustain us, and the problem is growing at an unprecedented rate.[10]

Evidence of the effects of unchecked population growth is everywhere:

- **Impact on other species.** Changes in the **ecosystem** are resulting in the mass destruction of many species and their habitats.[11] Over 477 vertebrae species have gone extinct since 1900, declining over 100 times faster than normal rates of extinction. This has prompted some scientists to predict the *sixth mass extinction of living creatures*, similar to the fifth extinction, which occurred with the demise of the dinosaurs.[12] Habitat destruction and fragmentation, which occurs as humans encroach on or pollute a natural area, is a major contributor to species extinction.

  According to a recent report by the International Union for the Conservation of Nature, nearly 25 percent of Earth's 6,000 mammal species are threatened or extinct.[13] Over 20,000 African elephants, black rhinos, and walruses are slaughtered each year for their tusks and horns—far more than are born.[14] About one-third of amphibian species are threatened or extinct, and many have chemically induced ailments or genetic mutations that will hasten their demise.[15] Rapid declines in plant species and habitat are also reasons for concern.[16]

- **Impact on ecosystems.** Aquatic ecosystems are heavily contaminated by chemical and human waste. Our oceans are 30 percent more acidic than they were just 200 years ago, largely because of human-generated pollutants and an increase in carbon dioxide in the atmosphere, some of which is then absorbed into the ocean.[17] These changes in ocean conditions have led to a dramatic decline in marine populations. Coral reefs that support aquatic life have declined by over 50 percent in the last 27 years, with virtual dead zones stretching for miles.[18]

- **Impact on the food supply.** Globally, oceans are being fished 250 percent faster than they can regenerate; scientists project a global collapse of all fish species by 2050 and major food shortages.[19] Even though increasing amounts of the earth's surface are being used for agriculture, drought, erosion, and natural disasters make growing food ever more difficult, and food shortages and famine occur in many regions of the world with increasing frequency.[20]

- **Land degradation and contamination of drinking water.** The per capita availability of freshwater is declining rapidly, and contaminated water remains the greatest single environmental cause of human illness. Unsustainable land use and climate change are increasing land degradation, including erosion, toxic chemical infiltration, nutrient depletion, deforestation, and other problems. Fracking and other processes place additional pressure on increasingly scarce ground and surface water reserves.[21]

- **Energy consumption.** "Use it *and* lose it" is an apt saying for our greedy use of nonrenewable **fossil fuels** (oil, coal, natural gas). Based on total population use, the United States is the largest consumer of liquid fossil fuels and natural gas and among the top four consumers of nuclear power, coal, and hydroelectric power.[22] Although the use of alternative energy sources, such as solar and wind, are on the rise, they still only account for a small portion of energy production.

  When ranked on a per person basis, Qatar ranks first in carbon emissions at 14.58 metric tons per person, and the United States ranks twelfth with 4.9 metric tons per person.[23] In many developing regions of the world, movement toward greater industrialization and citizen affluence has also resulted in skyrocketing demand for limited fossil fuels.

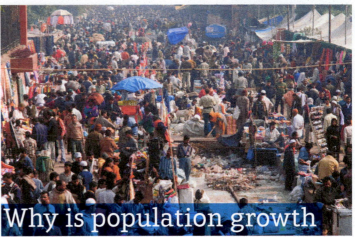

Why is population growth an environmental issue?

Every year, the global population grows by 115 million, but Earth's resources are not expanding. Population increases are believed to be responsible for most of the current environmental stress.

Strategies for Curbing Population Growth: Several strategies have been put forward to help slow population growth internationally. Examples include:

- Ensuring universal access for both men and women to contraception options.
- Educating and ensuring full and equal participation of women in the education, social economic, policy and development planning of their countries, as well as in family planning decisions.
- Educate and motivate men to accept more responsibility for unprotected sex and unplanned pregnancies. Emphasize long term consequences of unprotected sex in terms of risks to baby, economic costs, impact on society and parents, as well as environmental threats.
- Integrate lessons on population, development, and impact on the immediate and global environment in terms of available resources, human burden, and long term consequences.
- End policies that reward parents financially based on the number of children they have.
- The legal and ethical responsibilities of each parent toward the care and support of all of their children should be established. Individual decisions to have children that are not appropriately supported physically, mentally, and emotionally should not be the responsibilities of others.
- Emphasize that marriage and sexual acts should be entered into with the free and full consent of both parties.

Check Yourself

- **Consider each of the above proposals. Which do you think might have the most impact? What are the pros and cons of each?**

14.2 Air Pollution

Learning Outcome

14.2 Identify the major factors contributing to air pollution.

The term *air pollution* refers to the presence of substances (suspended particles and vapors) not found in perfectly clean air. Natural events, living creatures, and toxic by-products have always polluted the environment. What is new is the vast array of **pollutants**, their concentrations, and their potential interactive effects.

Air pollutants are either *naturally occurring* or *anthropogenic* (human caused). Naturally occurring air pollutants include particulate matter, such as ash from volcanic eruptions. Anthropogenic sources include those caused by *stationary sources* (e.g., power plants, factories, and refineries) and *mobile sources* such as vehicles. According to the Environmental Protection Agency (EPA), mobile sources are the major contributors of key air pollutants such as carbon monoxide (CO), sulfur oxide (SO_x), and nitrogen oxide (NO_x).

Today, carbon dioxide (CO_2) constitutes 82 percent of all greenhouse gases.[24] In the United States, fossil fuels used to generate electricity contribute 37 percent of greenhouse gases, followed by transportation at 31 percent and industry at 15 percent.[25]

Components of Air Pollution

Congress passed the Clean Air Act in 1970 and has amended it several times since then. The act established standards for six of the most widespread air pollutants that seriously affect health: *sulfur dioxide, particulates, carbon monoxide, nitrogen dioxide, ground-level ozone,* and *lead.*

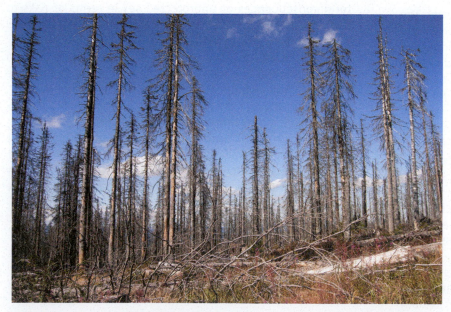

Acid deposition has many harmful effects on the environment. Because its toxins seep into groundwater and enter the food chain, it also poses health hazards to humans.

When the AQI is in this range:	... air quality conditions are	... as symbolized by this color:
0 to 50	Good	Green
51 to 100	Moderate	Yellow
101 to 150	Unhealthy for sensitive groups	Orange
151 to 200	Unhealthy	Red
201 to 300	Very unhealthy	Purple
301 to 500	Hazardous	Maroon

Figure 14.1 Air Quality Index (AQI)

The EPA provides individual AQIs for ground-level ozone, particle pollution, carbon monoxide, sulfur dioxide, and nitrogen dioxide. All AQIs are presented using the general values, categories, and colors shown in this figure.

Source: U.S. Environmental Protection Agency, "Air Quality Index: AQI Basics," August 2016, https://airnow.gov/index.cfm?action=aqibasics.aqi

Photochemical Smog

Smog is a brownish haze produced by the photochemical reaction of sunlight with hydrocarbons, nitrogen compounds, and other gases in vehicle exhaust. It is sometimes called *ozone pollution* because ozone is a main component of smog. Smog tends to form in areas that experience a **temperature inversion**, in which a cool layer of air is trapped under a layer of warmer air, preventing the air from circulating. Smog is more likely to occur in valley areas surrounded by hills or mountains, such as Los Angeles and Mexico City. The most noticeable adverse effects of smog are difficulty breathing, burning eyes, headaches, and nausea. Long-term exposure poses serious health risks, particularly for children, older adults, pregnant women, and people with chronic respiratory disorders.

Air Quality Index

The Air Quality Index (AQI) is a measure of how clean or polluted the air is on a given day and whether there are any health concerns related to air quality. The AQI focuses on health effects that can happen within a few hours or days after breathing polluted air.

The AQI scale is from 0 to 500: The higher the AQI value, the greater the level of air pollution and associated health risks. An AQI value of 100 generally corresponds to the national air quality standard for the pollutant, which is the level the EPA has set to protect public health. AQI values below 100 are generally considered satisfactory. When AQI values rise above 100, air quality is considered unhealthy at certain levels for specific groups of people and at higher levels for everyone. As shown in **Figure 14.1**, the EPA has divided

334

the AQI scale into six categories with corresponding color codes. National and local weather reports generally include information on the day's AQI.

Acid Deposition

Acid deposition (formerly called *acid rain*) refers to wet (rain, snow, sleet, fog, cloud water, and dew) and dry (acidifying particles and gases) acidic components that fall to the earth.[26] Sulfur dioxide (SO_2) and NO_x cause damage to plants, aquatic animals, forests, and humans over time. In the United States, roughly two-thirds of all sulfur dioxide and one-fourth of all nitrogen oxides come from electric power generation that relies on burning fossil fuels.[27] When coal-powered plants, oil refineries, and other facilities burn these fuels, the sulfur and nitrogen in the emissions combine with oxygen and sunlight to become SO_2 and NO_x.

Acid deposition gradually acidifies ponds, lakes, and other bodies of water. Once the acidity reaches a certain level, plant and animal life cannot survive.[28] Ironically, acidified lakes and ponds become a clear, deep blue, giving the illusion of beauty and health. Besides acidifying bodies of water, acid deposition destroys millions of trees every year. Much of the world's forestlands is now experiencing damaging levels of acid deposition.[29]

Acid deposition aggravates and may even cause bronchitis, asthma, and other respiratory problems, and people with emphysema or heart disease may suffer from exposure.[30] It may also be hazardous to fetuses. Acid deposition can cause metals such as aluminum, cadmium, lead, and mercury to **leach** out of the soil. If these metals make their way into water or food supplies, they can cause cancer in humans.

Although there have been substantial reductions in SO_2 and NO_x emissions from power plants that use the fossil fuels coal, gas, and oil in the last decade, full recovery is still years away.

Ozone Layer Depletion

The ozone layer forms a protective stratum in Earth's stratosphere—the highest level of our atmosphere, 12 to 30 miles above Earth's surface. The ozone layer protects our planet and its inhabitants from ultraviolet B (UVB) radiation, a primary cause of skin cancer. Such radiation damages DNA and weakens immune systems.

In the 1970s, instruments developed to test atmospheric contents indicated that chemicals used on Earth, especially **chlorofluorocarbons (CFCs)**, which are used in products such as refrigerants and hairsprays, were contributing to the ozone layer's rapid depletion. When released into the air through spraying or off-gassing, CFCs migrate into the ozone layer, where they

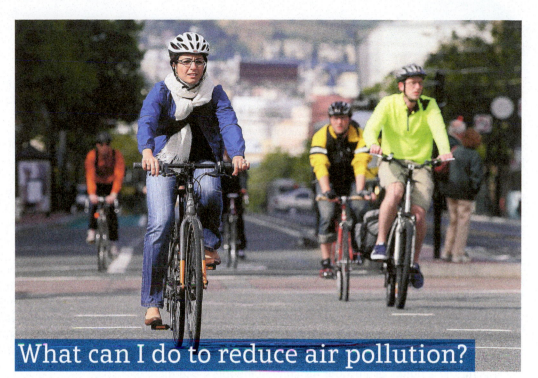

What can I do to reduce air pollution?

Much of the rise in air pollution is directly related to excess carbon dioxide (CO_2) released from burning carbon-containing fossil fuels. When you drive your car, for example, the burning of fossil fuels emits CO_2 into the atmosphere. Making small changes such as driving less, riding your bike more, taking public transportation, or carpooling can help reduce your contribution to air pollution in the environment.

decompose and release chlorine atoms. These atoms cause ozone molecules to break apart and ozone levels to be depleted.

The U.S. government banned the use of aerosol sprays containing CFCs in the 1970s. The discovery of an ozone "hole" over Antarctica led to treaties whereby the United States and other nations agreed to further reduce the use of CFCs and other ozone-depleting chemicals. Today, more than 197 United Nations countries have agreed to basic protocols designed to preserve and protect the ozone layer.[31] Although the ban on CFCs is believed to be an important step in slowing the depletion of the ozone layer, more research is needed to determine the effectiveness of CFC replacements.

See It! Videos

How far does China's extreme smog extend from its capital Beijing? Watch **China Smog Creates What Some Call a Kind of Respiratory Nuclear Winter** in the Study Area of Mastering Health.

Check Yourself

- **What are four factors contributing to air pollution?**

- **How can you as an individual reduce air pollution? What types of government policy interventions could reduce air pollution?**

14.3 Indoor Air Pollution

Learning Outcome

14.3 Identify pollutants that affect indoor air quality.

Mounting evidence indicates that air pollution levels within homes and other buildings, where we spend 90 percent of our time, may be two to five times higher than outdoor pollution levels.[32] Potentially dangerous chemical compounds can increase risks of cancer, contribute to respiratory problems, reduce the immune system's ability to fight disease, and increase problems with allergies and allergic reactions.

Age, preexisting medical conditions, and respiratory function can affect your risk of being affected by indoor air pollution. People with allergies may be particularly vulnerable, as may those living in newer airtight, energy-efficient homes. Health effects may develop over years of exposure or may occur in response to toxic levels of pollutants.

Preventing indoor air pollution involves *source control* (eliminating or reducing contaminants), *ventilation improvements* (increasing the amount of outdoor air coming indoors), and *air cleaners* (removing particulates from the air).[33]

Sources of Indoor Air Pollution

The main sources of indoor air pollution are as follows.

Environmental Tobacco Smoke Perhaps the greatest source of indoor air pollution is *environmental tobacco smoke (ETS)*, also known as secondhand smoke, which contains carbon monoxide and cancer-causing particulates. The level of carbon monoxide in cigarette smoke in enclosed spaces has been found to be 4,000 times higher than that allowed in the clean air standard established by the EPA.[34] The only effective way to eliminate ETS is to enact strict no-smoking policies. Many U.S. cities ban smoking in public places, at worksites, and in automobiles where children are present.

Home Heating If you rely on a wood-burning stove or an oil- or gas-fired furnace for home heating, make sure your heating appliance is properly installed, vented, and maintained. In wood stoves, burning properly seasoned wood reduces particulates. Thorough cleaning and maintenance can prevent carbon monoxide buildup in the home. Inexpensive home monitors are available to detect high carbon monoxide levels.

Asbestos **Asbestos** is a mineral compound used to insulate vinyl flooring, roofing materials, heating pipe coverings, and many other products in buildings constructed before 1970. When bonded to other materials, asbestos is relatively harmless, but if its tiny fibers become loosened and airborne, they can embed themselves in the lungs, leading to cancer of the lungs, stomach, and chest lining and other life-threatening lung diseases. If asbestos is detected in the home, it must be removed or sealed off by a professional.

Formaldehyde **Formaldehyde** is a colorless, strong-smelling gas released from building materials, furniture, or new carpet in a process called *off-gassing*. Off-gassing is highest in new products, but the process can continue for many years.

Exposure to formaldehyde can cause respiratory problems, dizziness, fatigue, nausea, and rashes. Long-term exposure can lead to central nervous system disorders and cancer. Ask about the formaldehyde content of products you are considering for your home, and avoid those that contain it.

Radon **Radon** is an odorless, colorless, radioactive gas found in soil. It can penetrate homes through cracks or other openings in the basement or foundation. Radon is a major nontobacco cause of lung cancer from air and drinking water exposure; it also has a synergistic effect with smoking exposure.[35]

The EPA estimates that as many as 1 in 3 U.S. homes may have elevated radon levels.[36] Homes below the third floor should be tested for radon, ideally every 2 years or on moving into a new home. Inexpensive test kits are available in hardware stores.

Lead **Lead** is a metal pollutant sometimes found in paint, batteries, soils, drinking water, pipes, dishes, and other items. Recently, toys produced in China have been recalled because of unsafe levels of lead in their paint.

Millions of homes in the United States, particularly those built before 1980, are likely to have lead in paint and pipes. Older public schools are also at risk. Cities throughout the country are struggling to ensure that water and painted surfaces in buildings do not result in increased health risks.[37]

Mold Molds are fungi that live both indoors and outdoors. They produce tiny reproductive spores that continually waft through air.

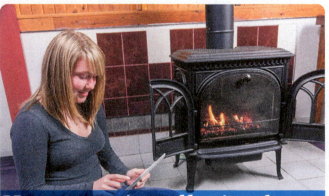

How can air pollution be a problem indoors?

The air within homes can be 2 to 5 times more hazardous than outside air. Indoor air pollution comes from wood stoves, furnaces, cigarette smoke, asbestos, formaldehyde, radon, lead, mold, and household chemicals.

These spores can irritate lungs and cause other health problems. For ways to reduce mold exposure, see Skills for Behavior Change.

Sick Building Syndrome **Sick building syndrome (SBS)** occurs when occupants of a building experience acute health effects linked to time spent in a building but no specific illness or cause can be identified.[38] Poor ventilation is a primary cause of SBS. Other causes include faulty furnaces; pet dander; mold; volatile organic compounds from products such as hairspray, cleaners, and adhesives; and heavy metals such as lead. Symptoms include eye irritation, sore throat, queasiness, and worsened asthma.

Indoor air pollution and SBS are increasing concerns in the classroom and workplace. Many U.S. schools have unsatisfactory indoor air quality, often because of poor ventilation, construction techniques that block outside air, and the use of synthetic construction materials.[39] Poor air quality can trigger allergies, asthma, and other health problems.[40]

Air Pollution and Asthma

Asthma is a long-term, chronic inflammatory disorder that causes tiny airways in the lung to spasm in response to triggers. Symptoms include wheezing, difficulty breathing, shortness of breath, and coughing. Although most asthma attacks are mild, severe attacks can trigger potentially fatal contractions of the bronchial tubes.

Asthma falls into two types: extrinsic and intrinsic. The more common form, *extrinsic* or *allergic asthma*, is associated with allergic triggers; it tends to run in families and typically develops in childhood. *Intrinsic* or *nonallergic asthma* may be triggered by anything except an allergy. Environmental factors can increase your risk of developing asthma, such as exposure to environmental tobacco smoke, mold and mildew, animal dander, dust mites, and pollen.[41]

Asthma rates have increased markedly in the last 20 years. Many blame increasing pollution rates, especially in poor and nonwhite communities, as well as triggers such as dust mites in mattresses, chemicals in carpets and furniture, and airtight modern buildings.

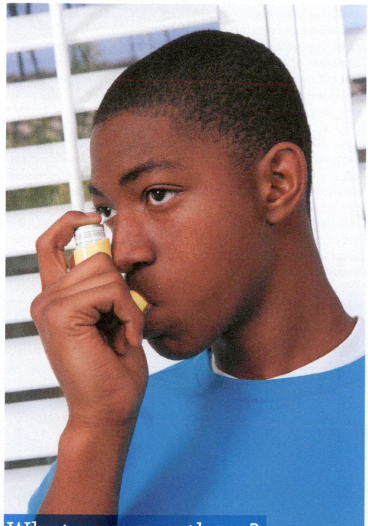

What causes asthma?

Asthma is caused by inflammation of the airways in the lungs, restricting airflow and leading to wheezing, chest tightness, shortness of breath, and coughing. In most people, asthma is brought on by contact with allergens or irritants in the air; some people also have exercise-induced asthma. People with asthma can generally control their symptoms through the use of inhaled medications, and most asthmatics keep a "rescue" inhaler of bronchodilating medication on hand to use in case of a flare-up.

Skills for **Behavior Change**

Be Mold Free

- Keep the humidity level in your home between 40 and 60 percent.
- Use a dehumidifier in damp rooms or basements.
- Be sure your home has adequate ventilation, including exhaust fans in the kitchen and bathrooms. If there are no fans, open windows.
- Buy paints with mold-resistant properties or add mold inhibitors.
- In the bathroom, wipe down shower doors, keep surfaces dry, and, if necessary, use environmentally safe mold-killing products. Do not carpet bathrooms and basements or other rooms that are routinely damp.
- Many antimold products commonly used in outdoor areas are extremely toxic; pets and wildlife may wander through these after they've been applied. Use them sparingly or not at all.
- Wash rugs used in entryways and other areas where moisture can accumulate.
- Get rid of mattresses and furniture that have been exposed to excessive moisture.
- Dry clothing thoroughly before putting it away.
- When buying a house, don't skimp on mold inspections. Check for mold growth regularly, especially in rental units where landlords might not pay attention to these risks.

Check Yourself

- What are four common indoor air pollutants and their sources? Which ones concern you the most?

14.4 Describe how greenhouse gas buildup contributes to climate change.

Climate change refers to a shift in typical weather patterns across the world. These changes can include fluctuations in seasonal temperatures, rainfall or snowfall amounts, and the occurrence of catastrophic storms. **Global warming** is a type of climate change in which average temperatures increase. Over 97 percent of scientists now agree that the planet is warming, driven largely by the burning of fossil fuels.[42] Over the last 100 years, the average temperature of the earth has increased by 1.5°F, and it is projected to rise another 2°F to 11.5°F in the next 100 years.[43]

According to the National Aeronautics and Space Administration, the National Oceanic and Atmospheric Administration, and the National Research Council, climate change poses major risks to lives, and excess **greenhouse gases** (water vapor, carbon dioxide, methane, nitrous oxide, and ozone) are key culprits.[44] Excess carbon dioxide (CO_2) accounts for 82 percent of human-caused greenhouse gases in the United States.[45,46]

The *greenhouse effect* is a natural phenomenon in which greenhouse gases form a layer in the atmosphere that acts like glass in a greenhouse, allowing solar heat to pass through, then trapping some of that heat close to the surface, where it warms the planet. The natural greenhouse effect is important for keeping the planet warm enough for life, but human activities have increased greenhouse gases in the atmosphere, resulting in the **enhanced greenhouse effect**, which is raising the planet's temperature higher than normal by trapping excess heat (**Figure 14.2**).

Scientific Evidence of Climate Change

Climate is influenced by changes in naturally occurring greenhouse gases as well as solar output and the earth's orbit. However, evidence points to unusual changes in climate in recent years that go beyond predictable natural causes:[47]

- Global sea levels rose 6.7 inches in the last 100 years, mostly in the last decade.
- 2016 was the warmest year globally since records have been kept beginning in 1880.
- 16 of the 17 warmest years on record have occurred since 2001. Since 1981, 20 of the warmest years ever have occurred.
- Greenland is losing 36 to 60 cubic miles of ice per year, and Antarctica is losing 36 cubic miles of ice per year.
- Glaciers are receding at unprecedented and rapid rates.

Multiple reconstructions of the earth's climate history show that quantities of greenhouse gases in the atmosphere went up dramatically around the time of the Industrial Revolution—when humans began burning fossil fuels on a large scale—and correlates very closely with temperature increases.[48] Studies also indicate that large changes in climate can occur within decades rather than centuries or thousands of years.[49]

Reducing the Threat of Global Warming and Moving toward Sustainable Development

Climate change problems are largely rooted in our energy, transportation, and industrial practices.[50] Rapid deforestation contributes to the rise in greenhouse gases. Trees take in carbon dioxide, transform it, store the carbon for food, and release oxygen into the air. When cut, these trees release CO_2 into the air. Some research indicates that deforestation through logging, agriculture, and other activities add more CO_2 than all cars and trucks on the world's roads. Other sources indicate that electricity generation, transportation, and industry are the major contributors to CO2 [subscript] and other greenhouse gas emissions, with land use and deforestation contributing to the problem.[51]

Most experts agree that to slow climate change, reducing consumption of fossil fuels and using mass transportation are crucial, but clean energy, green factories, hybrid and electric vehicles, improved energy efficiency, and government regulation are also key. Several global initiatives have been developed not only to reduce climate change, but also to improve lives.

In 2012, representatives of many nations gathered in Rio de Janeiro to outline a plan for **sustainable development**—development that meets present needs without compromising future generations. In 2015, these nations created a list of 17 sustainable goals to be reached by 2030 focused on ending poverty, reducing inequality, and tackling climate change.[52] However, leaders of many nations, including the United States, France, Germany, and the United Kingdom, opted not to attend. The resulting plan included a list of general goals without the "teeth" necessary to

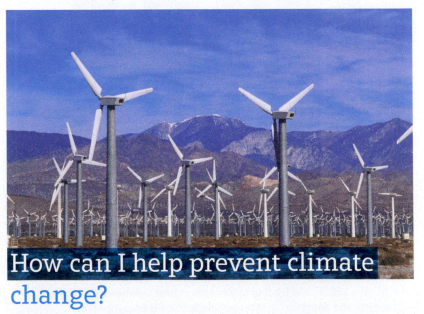

How can I help prevent climate change?

By reducing use of fossil fuels, using high-efficiency vehicles, and supporting increased use of renewable resources such as solar, wind, and water power, you can help combat climate change. For example, the National Renewable Energy Laboratory predicts that with proper development, wind power could provide 20 percent of U.S. energy needs.

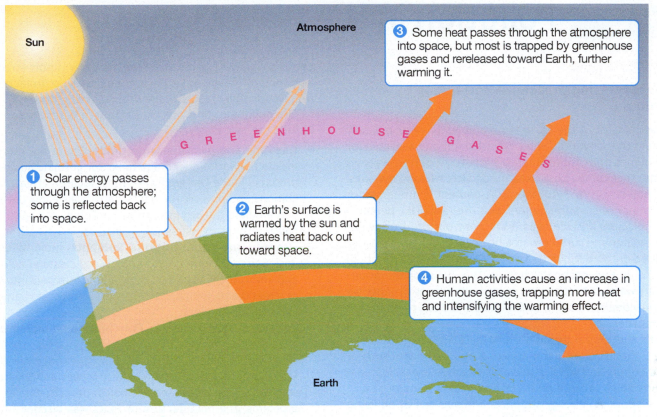

Figure 14.2 The Enhanced Greenhouse Effect
The natural greenhouse effect is responsible for making Earth habitable; it keeps the planet 33°C (60°F) warmer than it would be otherwise. An increase in greenhouse gases resulting from human activities is creating the enhanced greenhouse effect, trapping more heat and causing dangerous global climate change.
Source: ozCoasts (Geoscience Australia), "The Enhanced Greenhouse Effect (Global Warming)," 2013, www.ozcoasts.gov.au/indicators/greenhouse_effect.jsp.

▶ **Mastering Health & Nutrition** Enhanced Greenhouse Effect

motivate nations to comply with sustainable development needs.

In 2015, nearly 190 nations, accounting for over 95 percent of the world's greenhouse gas emissions, signed an agreement to work toward slowing emissions and spurring alternative energy development. The *Paris Agreement* allows countries to come up with their own **intended nationally determined contributions (INDCs)**. The U.S. goal for INDC was to reduce net greenhouse gas emissions 26 to 28 percent below 2005 levels by 2025.[53] Much of this reduction would come from obtaining compliance with existing policies, along with additional technological advances and improvements by individuals, communities, and industry.[54]

Early in 2017, President Trump said that the United States was exiting the Paris Agreement, joining just two other countries that are opposed to the agreement: Nicaragua and Syria. The pull-out by the United States has many implications for future climate change reduction policies and programs. Several states, cities, companies, and individuals, acting in defiance of the Trump administration, have stated that they intend to reduce emissions and/or provide funding for environmental initiatives.

See It! Videos

How is climate change affecting the weather during winter? Watch **Snowstorms in the Forecast** in the Study Area of Mastering Health.

Many U.S. communities have established plans to reduce their **carbon footprint**, or the amount of CO_2 emissions contributed to the atmosphere through daily life. Some already have or are considering a **carbon tax** similar to those in parts of Europe, Canada, and the United Kingdom. A carbon tax is the price a government charges for the carbon content in fuels. If you use more, you will pay more carbon tax. This provides incentives for individuals to invest in noncarbon power generation such as solar power, wind power, and hydropower—as well as to drive less and turn down the heat and air conditioning. **Cap and trade** policies set limits, or caps, on how much carbon large industrial polluters can emit. Carbon taxes and cap and trade policies are mechanisms for incentivizing green behaviors and motivating those with large carbon footprints to reduce emissions.[55] Relying more on wind, solar, and bioenergy and hybrid and electric vehicles may reduce carbon emissions. Still, major fuel-hungry industry development in poorer regions of the world may offset some of the potential decreases in future years.[56]

Check Yourself

■ **What are some possible effects of uncontained global warming?**

14.5 Identify the major factors contributing to water pollution.

Seventy-five percent of the Earth is covered with water, but only 1 to 2 percent of the world's water is freshwater and available for human consumption.[57] Approximately 1.2 percent of freshwater is surface water that comes from lakes, ground ice, swamps, marshes, rivers, and soil moisture.[58] Another 30.1 percent is groundwater from underwater wells and aquifers, and the rest (68.7 percent) is locked in glaciers and ice caps.[59] We draw our drinking water from groundwater and surface water; however, much of this water is too polluted or too difficult to reach.[60] Recent severe drought in many regions and unseasonably hot weather have forced rationing, voluntary water reduction, and community efforts to conserve water by individuals, industry, agriculture, and power generation in recent decades.

Over half the global population faces a shortage of clean water. The United Nations estimates that by 2025, two-thirds of the world's population will live in water-stressed areas, increasing competition for scarce reserves and posing a major risk to global food supplies, energy supplies, and survival of all living things.[61] See Skills for Behavior Change for tips on conserving water.

Water Contamination

Tap water in the United States is among the safest in the world. Under the Safe Drinking Water Act, the EPA sets standards for drinking water quality. However, any substance that gets into the soil can enter the water supply. Industrial pollutants and pesticides work their way into soil, then into groundwater. Underground storage tanks containing gasoline may leak.

Cities and municipalities have policies and procedures governing water treatment, filtration, and disinfection to screen out pathogens and microorganisms. However, their ability to filter out increasing amounts of chemical by-products and other substances is in question. According to a 2014 study of over 50 large wastewater sites in the United States, over half of the samples tested positive for at least 25 of the 56 prescription and over-the-counter drugs being monitored.[62] A more recent study estimates that the drinking water of over 41 million Americans in 24 major cities is contaminated with pharmaceuticals.[63] Beyond pharmaceuticals, our aging infrastructure and pipes can also lead to contamination.

Many other toxic substances also flow into our waterways. **Point source pollutants** enter a waterway at a specific location such as a ditch or pipe; the two major entry points are sewage treatment plants and industrial facilities. **Nonpoint source pollutants**—*runoff* and *sedimentation*—drain or seep into waterways from soil erosion and sedimentation, construction wastes, pesticide and fertilizer runoff, street runoff, acid mine drainage, wastes from engineering projects, leakage from septic tanks, and sewage sludge (see Figure 14.3).

The pollutants that are causing the greatest potential harm include the following[64]:

- **Gasoline and petroleum products.** There are more than 2 million underground storage tanks for gasoline and petroleum products in the United States, most located at gasoline filling stations and processing plants. Tank leaks allow petroleum to contaminate the ground and water. Fumes can spark fires and cause respiratory issues.

- **Organic solvents. Organic solvents** include chemicals designed to dissolve grease and oil; dry-cleaning fluids, paints, and antifreeze. Consumers often dump leftovers into the toilet or street drains. Industries often bury leftovers in barrels, which can corrode and leak.

- **Polychlorinated biphenyls. Polychlorinated biphenyls (PCBs)** were used for many years as insulating materials in high-voltage electrical equipment. The human body does not excrete ingested PCBs but rather stores them in fatty tissues and the liver. Exposure to PCBs is associated with birth defects, cancer, and skin problems. The manufacture of PCBs was discontinued in the United States in 1977, but some were dumped into landfills and waterways, where they continue to pose an environmental threat.

- **Dioxins. Dioxins** are found in herbicides (chemicals used to kill vegetation). They're much more toxic than PCBs; long-term effects include possible immune system damage and increased risk of infections and cancer. Short-term exposure to high concentrations of PCBs or dioxins can have severe consequences, including nausea; vomiting; diarrhea; painful rashes and sores; and chloracne, in which the skin develops painful pimples that may never go away.

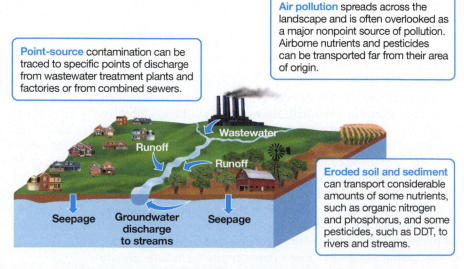

Air pollution spreads across the landscape and is often overlooked as a major nonpoint source of pollution. Airborne nutrients and pesticides can be transported far from their area of origin.

Point-source contamination can be traced to specific points of discharge from wastewater treatment plants and factories or from combined sewers.

Eroded soil and sediment can transport considerable amounts of some nutrients, such as organic nitrogen and phosphorus, and some pesticides, such as DDT, to rivers and streams.

Figure 14.3 Potential Sources of Groundwater Contamination

Source: http://www.open.edu/openlearncreate/mod/oucontent/view.php?id=80588&extra=thumbnail_idp2965248

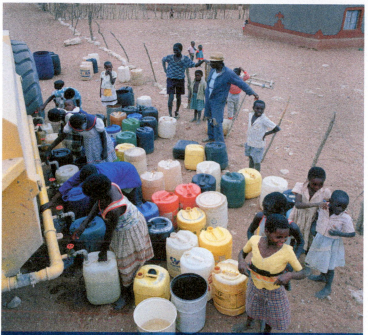

Is there really a water scarcity?

The lack of clean water and sanitation is a major global problem. *Closed basins* are regions where existing water cannot meet the agricultural, industrial, municipal, and environmental needs. The Stockholm International Water Institute estimates that 1.4 billion people live in a closed basin, and the problem is worsening.

■ **Pesticides. Pesticides** are chemicals designed to kill insects, rodents, plants, and fungi. Pesticides evaporate readily and are often dispersed by winds over a large area or carried out to sea. In tropical regions, many farmers use pesticides heavily, and the climate promotes their rapid release into the atmosphere. Pesticide residues cling to fruits and vegetables and can accumulate in the body. Potential hazards associated with exposure to pesticides include birth defects, liver and kidney damage, and nervous system disorders.

Fracking

Hydraulic fracturing of shale (*fracking*) is a method of extracting otherwise inaccessible natural gas from the ground. Most of the natural reserves of gas in North America are trapped in shale beds that have long been inaccessible to cost-effective tapping. According to some experts, these deposits could provide a significant amount of natural gas. However, the process also has many people concerned about the environmental risks to water and airborne pollutants that go with it.

In fracking, underground rock and dense soil are cracked open by pumping highly pressurized fluids into them, creating fissures that allow oil or gas to flow to the surface for extraction. Much of the fracking liquid comes up with the gas or oil and is stored in chemical pools for delivery to treatment plants. However, some

scientists and members of the public are concerned that a portion of this toxic, chemical-laden sludge can seep down and contaminate aquifers that supply drinking water to many regions of the country.

In addition to being linked to groundwater and surface water contamination, fracking is difficult to remediate. It is potentially harmful to animals, birds, and humans and leads to air quality issues and difficulties with disposal. A recent rash of earthquakes in regions of the country where shale gas is being extracted by fracking has sparked speculation that changing the internal pressures of the earth's surface via these deep wells may pose additional risks, but the potential earthquake risk remains unclear.[65] The debate continues over the use of fracking and what criteria should be used to regulate it and make it safer.

Skills for **Behavior Change**

Waste Less Water

In the Kitchen

■ **Turn off the tap while washing dishes.**
■ **Check faucets and pipes for leaks.** Leaky faucets can waste more than 3,000 gallons of water each year.
■ **Equip faucets with aerators to reduce water use by 4 percent.**
■ **Wash only full dishwasher loads;** use the energy-saving mode.

In the Laundry Room

■ **Wash only full laundry loads.**
■ **Buy or upgrade to the highest efficiency washing machine you can.**

In the Bathroom

■ **Detect and fix leaks.** A leaky toilet can waste 200 gallons of water every day.
■ **Install a high-efficiency toilet that uses 60 percent less water.**
■ **Take showers instead of baths;** save gallons of water with each shower by getting wet, shutting off water and lathering, and quickly rinsing. A long shower where you use hot water to refresh yourself wastes large amounts of water every year; water that is in short supply overall.
■ **Replace old showerheads with efficient models that use 60 percent less water.** Limit your shower time to less than five minutes. Shower in a tub with the drain closed and see how much water your showers are taking. Shorten that time.
■ **Turn off the tap while brushing your teeth** to save up to 8 gallons of water per day.

14.5

Environmental Health

Check Yourself

■ **What are three major sources of water pollution?**

■ **What are four steps that you can take to reduce water waste?**

Pollution on Land

14.6 List the major factors contributing to pollution on land.

Much of the waste that ends up polluting the water starts by polluting the land. A growing population creates more pressure on the land to accommodate increasing amounts of refuse, much of which is nonbiodegradable and some of which is directly harmful to living organisms.

Solid Waste

Each day, every person in the United States generates nearly 4.5 pounds of **municipal solid waste (MSW)**, more commonly known as *trash* or *garbage*. This totals about 258 million tons of trash each year, with organic materials making up the largest share (**Figure 14.4**).[66]

Although Americans recycle only slightly over one-third of the waste we generate, experts believe we could recycle up to 90 percent (**Figure 14.5**).[67] Currently, 34.6 percent of all MSW in the United States is recycled or composted, 12.8 percent is burned at combustion facilities, and the remaining 52.6 percent is disposed of in landfills.[68] The number of U.S. landfills has actually decreased in the past decade, but their mass has increased. As communities run out of landfill space, it is becoming common to haul garbage to other states, to dump it illegally in woods, waterways, or oceans, where it contaminates ecosystems, or to ship it to landfills in developing countries, where it becomes someone else's problem.

Communities, businesses, and individuals can adopt strategies to reduce solid waste:

- *Source reduction (waste prevention)* involves altering the design, manufacture, or use of products and materials to reduce the amount and toxicity of what gets thrown away. The most effective MSW-reducing strategy is to prevent waste from being generated in the first place.
- Several communities across the United States have placed a ban or tax on plastic bags to reduce their use in retail stores. Proponents say that plastic bags are bad for the environment because they are made from nonbiodegradable petroleum, are infrequently recycled, and are commonly discarded as litter, ending up in waterways, where they become a wildlife hazard.
- *Recycling* involves sorting, collecting, and processing materials to be reused in the manufacture of new products. This process diverts items such as paper, glass, plastics, and metals from the waste stream.
- *E-recycling* involves properly disposing of trashed computers, televisions, cell phones, and other electronic devices. The global burden of electronic waste has skyrocketed in recent years as we struggle to find sources for disposal and e-recycling.[69] Visit www.epa.gov and www.ecyclingcentral.com to find information about locations for electronic waste recycling in your state and

to learn how to reduce electronic waste in your MSW. Although there are many avenues for disposing of items such as cell phones, the best way to avoid electronic waste is not succumb to the "latest and greatest" craze in the first place—hang onto your TV, phone, or device for as long as possible.

- *Composting* involves collecting organic waste, such as food scraps and yard trimmings, and allowing it to decompose with the help of microorganisms (mainly bacteria and fungi). This process produces a nutrient-rich substance that can be used to fertilize gardens and for soil enhancement. Many communities now have yard carts that allow you to mix your food scraps in with yard trimmings.
- *Combustion with energy recovery* typically involves the use of boilers and industrial furnaces to incinerate waste and use the burning process to generate energy.

Hazardous Waste

Hazardous waste is defined as waste with properties that make it capable of harming human health or the environment. American manufacturers and individuals generate around 40 million of tons of hazardous waste each year, including commercial chemical refuse, solvents and oils, petroleum-refining by-products, and household wastes such as batteries, cleaning products, and paints.[70] Many wastes are now banned from land disposal sites or are being treated to reduce their toxicity before they become part

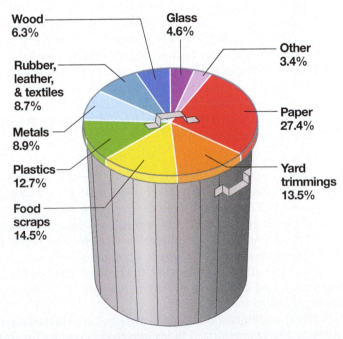

Figure 14.4 What's in Our Trash?

Source: Data from U.S. Environmental Protection Agency, "Municipal Solid Waste Generation, Recycling, and Disposal in the United States: Facts and Figures for 2012," February 2014, epa-530-F-14-001, www.epa.gov.

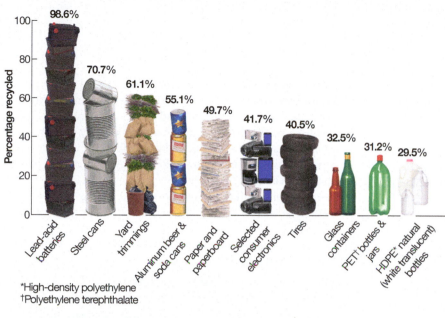

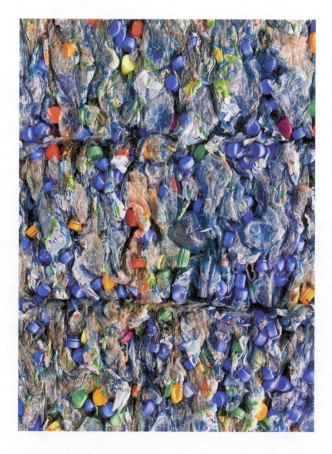

Figure 14.5 How Much Do We Recycle?

Source: EPA, "Advancing Sustainable Materials Management: 2014 Fact Sheet," June 2016, www
.epa.gov/epawaste/nonhaz/municipal/pubs/2014_advncng_smm_fs.pdf

*High-density polyethylene
†Polyethylene terephthalate

of land disposal sites. The EPA has developed protective requirements for land disposal facilities, such as double liners, detection systems for substances that may leach into groundwater, and
groundwater monitoring systems.

91%

Mass
production of plastics, which
started just 60 years ago, has
grown so rapidly that it has
created over 8 billion metric
tons of it globally—91 percent of
which is never recycled!

In 1980, the Comprehensive Environmental
Response, Compensation and Liability Act, known
as the **Superfund**, was enacted to provide funds
for cleaning up what are typically abandoned hazardous waste dump sites. Over the past three-plus
decades, the Superfund has located and assessed
tens of thousands of hazardous waste sites, worked
to protect people and the environment from contamination at the worst sites, and involved affected
communities, states, and other groups in cleanup.
More than 1700 sites have been cleared or recov-
ered and 53 proposed sites need cleanup as of July 2017.[71] To
see Superfund sites in your state, go to https://www.epa.gov/
superfund/superfund-national-priorities-list-npl.

You probably have hazardous waste sitting on a garage shelf
or under a kitchen or bathroom sink. Pesticides, paints and paint
thinners, solvents, moth killers, batteries, old gasoline cans, many
cleaning products, glues, and adhesives as well as paint and stain
removers and hot tub or pool chemicals are all examples of potential hazardous wastes.

To be a thoughtful consumer, read the labels on products
before buying them. Whenever possible, substitute less toxic,
natural products for hazardous ones. Remember to never pour old
pesticides, cleaning agents, gasoline, or solvents down the drain
or dump them on the ground.

There are many effective substitutes for harsh cleaning
products:

- To get out laundry or carpet stains, use club soda.
- To get rid of moths in your pantry or clothes, use cedar shav-
  ings or lavender.
- To clean dirty windows and surfaces, mix water with vinegar
  or ammonia.
- To clean your showers, sinks, and tubs, skip the toxic chemical
  sprays. Use a vinegar-and-water solution or baking soda. Wipe
  surfaces dry after showering to avoid buildup.

Check Yourself

- How can we reduce the amount of municipal
  solid waste generated?

- What is hazardous waste, and what are its
  dangers?

14.7 Radiation

Learning Outcome

14.7 Explain the environmental and personal risks associated with radiation.

Radiation is energy that travels in waves or particles. Many different types of radiation make up the electromagnetic spectrum. Exposure to radiation is an inescapable part of life on this planet, and only some of it poses a threat to human health.

Nonionizing Radiation

Nonionizing radiation is radiation at the lower end of the electromagnetic spectrum. This radiation moves in relatively long wavelengths and has enough energy to move atoms but not enough to remove electrons or alter molecular structure. Examples of nonionizing radiation are radio waves, TV signals, microwaves, infrared waves, and visible light.

Although many people believe that *electromagnetic fields (EMFs)* generated by electric power delivery systems increase one's risk for cancer, reproductive dysfunction, and other ailments, others point to major inconsistencies in the research and little resulting hazard to health. However, one particular form of EMF— radio frequency (RF) energy emitted by cell phones—is currently the subject of much debate and research. Cell phones emit RF energy when turned on, and in theory, all of that RF energy has the potential to penetrate the skull, neck, and upper torso. For the very young whose skulls have not yet fully hardened, the risk may be even greater.

Many countries, including the United States, use standards set by the Federal Communications Commission (FCC) for radio frequency energy based on research by several scientific groups. These groups identified a whole-body *specific absorption rate (SAR)* value for exposure to RF energy. Four watts per kilogram was identified as a level above which harmful biological effects may occur. The FCC requires wireless phones to comply with a limit of 1.6 watts per kilogram. (To find the SAR level for your phone, go to www.fcc.gov.)

After over a decade of trying to determine whether cell phone use can be linked to some type of disease, researchers have come up with very little conclusive evidence. However, much of the available research was done before cell phones were regularly used for hours each day to play games, browse the Internet, and check up on social media sites in addition to talking and texting. The U.S. Food and Drug Administration, the World Health Organization, and other major health agencies suggest a need for more research, since no long-term studies exist. A new European Cohort Study of Mobile phone use (COSMOS) will follow 250,000 people for the next 20 years to determine whether there are increased risks. This study should provide much-needed insight.[72]

In the meantime, a few small changes in behavior can greatly reduce the amount of RF energy your body absorbs:

- Limit the amount of time you spend talking on the phone. When you do make calls, use a hands-free device that keeps the phone away from your head.
- Because wireless earpieces also emit energy, use them only when you are actively engaged in a call.
- Buy a phone that emits lower RF energy than others based on its SAR level.
- Keep the phone farther away from you during the night, such as on a side table or dresser, so that it's not on your pillow.

Ionizing Radiation

Ionizing radiation is caused by the release of particles and electromagnetic rays from atomic nuclei during the normal process of disintegration. Some naturally occurring elements, such as

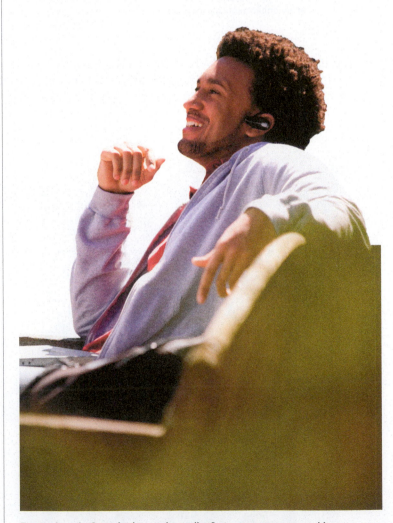

Even a hands-free device emits radio-frequency energy and its use should be limited.

uranium, emit radiation. The sun is another source of ionizing radiation, in the form of high-frequency ultraviolet rays—those against which the ozone layer protects us.

Exposure is measured in **radiation absorbed doses (rads)**, also called *roentgens*. Harm can occur with dosages as low as 100 to 200 rads, including nausea, diarrhea, fatigue, anemia, sore throat, and hair loss. At 350 to 500 rads, symptoms become more severe, and death may result because the radiation hinders bone marrow production of white blood cells that protect us from disease. Dosages above 600 to 700 rads are fatal.

Recommended maximum "permissible" dosages range from 0.5 to 5 rads per year.[73] Approximately 50 percent of the radiation to which we are exposed comes from natural and human-made sources. Natural sources include radon gas in the air and cosmic radiation. Another 45 percent comes from human-made sources such as diagnostic x-rays, nuclear medicine, and radiation therapy. The remaining 5 percent comes from nonionizing radiation.[74]

Most of us are exposed to far less radiation than the safe maximum dosage per year. The effects of long-term exposure to relatively low levels of radiation are unknown.

Nuclear Power Plants

Currently, nuclear power plants account for less than 1 percent of the total radiation to which we are exposed. However, the number of U.S. plants may increase in the next decade, so exposure levels may also increase. Proponents of nuclear energy believe that it is a safe and efficient way to generate electricity. Initial costs of building nuclear power plants are high, but actual power generation is relatively inexpensive. A 1,000-megawatt reactor produces enough energy for 650,000 homes and saves 420 million gallons of fossil fuels each year. In some areas where nuclear power plants were decommissioned, electricity bills tripled when power companies turned to hydroelectric or fossil fuel sources to generate electricity. Nuclear reactors discharge fewer carbon oxides into the air than do fossil fuel–powered generators. Advocates believe that converting to nuclear power could help slow global warming.

The advantages of nuclear energy must be weighed against the disadvantages. Disposal of nuclear waste is extremely problematic. In addition, a reactor core meltdown could pose serious threats to the immediate environment and to the world in general. A **nuclear meltdown** occurs when the temperature in the core of a nuclear reactor increases enough to melt both the nuclear fuel and its containment vessel. Most modern facilities seal the reactors and containment vessels in concrete buildings with pools of cold water on the bottom. If a meltdown occurs, the building and the pool are supposed to prevent radiation from escaping.

The International Atomic Energy Agency ranks nuclear and radiological accidents and incidents by severity on a scale of 1 to 7. To date, we have had two major nuclear disasters that resulted in a 7, the highest severity rating, meaning that there was a major release of radioactive material with widespread health and environmental consequences. The first was the 1986 reactor

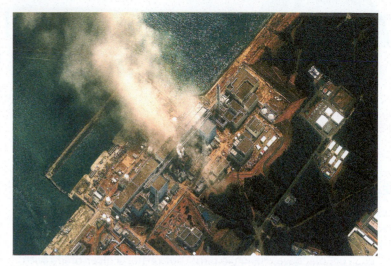

The accident at the Fukushima Daiichi plant in Japan, following an earthquake and tsunami, raised new questions about the safety of nuclear power.

core fire and explosion at the Chernobyl nuclear power plant in Ukraine, which killed thousands and left the area uninhabitable for decades.[75]

The damage to the Fukushima Daiichi Nuclear Power Station in northern Japan caused by the March 2011 earthquake and tsunami was also listed as a level 7 nuclear disaster, the worst since Chernobyl. The power station, located in the region hardest hit by the tsunami, suffered several explosions, multiple fires, radioactive gas leaks, and a partial meltdown in three of its reactors. Despite continued exposure to toxic radioactive material and risk to their lives, nuclear plant workers labored for weeks to stave off a full-scale meltdown and to minimize the destruction to the public and surrounding region by attempting to cool and repair the damaged reactors.

The Fukushima Daiichi incident reawakened worldwide fears about nuclear energy. Nonetheless, the use of nuclear power worldwide is expected to double in the next 35 years, particularly in China. Balancing the risks versus benefits of nuclear power will provide unique challenges in the future.[76]

Check Yourself

- What is the difference between ionizing radiation and nonionizing radiation?

- What are some benefits and drawbacks to the use of nuclear power?

14.8 Environmental Mindfulness and Sustainability: What You Can Do

14.8 Identify what you can do to make sustainable choices in college.

Environmental Mindfulness: It Starts With You

Today's environmental challenges are related mainly to human actions and the policies that drive international global actions. Environmental mindfulness means realizing that the earth isn't a "thing" or "place we use while here" but rather a giver of life with which we are intricately connected. Too often, we are so caught up in our own daily challenges that we don't pay attention to how our actions affect the planet. As a balm against our insecurities and self-doubts, we consume, placing value on acquisitions, obsessive shopping, beautification of our bodies and wardrobes, and having the newest and best toys and homes. Zen master Thich Nhat Hanh has described humans living in a rapidly deteriorating planet as "a group of chickens fighting desperately over a few seeds of grain, unaware that in a few hours, they will all be killed."[77] Think about how much food you waste each week as it spoils in your refrigerator. That food took precious resources to produce and we should use care in our shopping, preparation and consumption.

We all need to do more to live unselfishly and connect with what is happening around us. We need to focus less on what other people are doing and more on what *each of us* is doing as an individual, moment to moment, every day of our lives. We need to "walk the proverbial talk" about environmental concerns, to slow down, to care more by doing more to preserve and protect the planet for now and for future generations. Of course, it's not enough to just live in the moment; we need to *act* in the moment, by minimizing wasteful behaviors and doing more to tread more lightly on the earth. Do you really need the latest phone or laptop? How many pairs of unworn shoes or clothing are left sitting in your closet? Living a more minimalist lifestyle is part of living mindfully.

There are thousands of ways to do your part, reduce your footprint, and love the Earth you live with. This chapter covers dozens. Whatever ways you choose, take the time to notice what you are doing and how it might affect our scarce resources. Choose wisely and set clear goals. What steps will you take today? This week? How can you reduce, reuse, waste less, conserve more, and protect the world we all live in? It all starts with you. Pay attention, be informed, and let your actions make a difference.

Sustainability on Campus

Many campuses have established plans to reduce their carbon footprint. Creating bicycle lanes, building monitored bike garages to help prevent theft and vandalism, and holding "bike to work" days encourage students to leave cars at home. Some campuses have raised fees for parking permits to discourage cars on campus. Many colleges and universities have taken steps to "green" the campus through programs focused on recycling, moving to non-plastic cups and food containers, and reusing furniture and other items that are tossed out as students leave school in the spring, as well as buying food locally, and cutting down fossil fuels used in transportation.

As a college student, your actions and those of your friends, roommates, and school can have a lasting impact on your health and the health of the environment. Small choices you make beginning today can make a difference. Start making a positive impact by turning off lights when you leave a room or restroom and shutting off electronics when not in use. Even small charging stations add to total energy used. Find out whether your residence has a way of minimizing the amount of lights used on a floor. Sometimes lights are connected through several outlets; turning off a strand might still provide enough light but minimize the amount of energy consumed. Find out whether your administration supports the use of compact fluorescent light bulbs (CFLs), which are longer-lasting, energy-conserving bulbs that give off the same amount of light as an incandescent bulb at a fraction of the energy used. Next time you go to the store, buy a couple of CFLs for your own lighting fixtures.

Making Green Electronic Choices

When you decide to buy a new appliance, look for the Energy Star logo, indicating that the appliance meets energy-efficiency standards set by the EPA and the U.S. Department of Energy. Energy Star products can also save you money.

While you are in class, out to dinner, or in bed sound asleep, your cable box and other plugged-in-all-the-time devices are draining electricity unnecessarily, and it can add up. Also pay attention to your charging habits. Unplug your devices when they're fully charged. Turn them off (all the way, not just the screen) when not in use. Stream more, using lower-energy devices.

The global burden of e-waste (trashed computers, televisions, and other electronic devices) has skyrocketed in recent years. Although there are many avenues for disposing of electronic products, many of them end up in landfills.[78] What can you do to reduce this waste? Very simply, hang onto your devices for as long as possible. Instead of being the first with the newest technology, be proud that you are keeping your device longer and not adding to global waste. Buy less, take care of things, and waste less. When you are thinking about *e-recycling*, check out www.ecyclingcentral.com for a state-by-state listing of e-recyclers in your area.

See the Skills for Behavior Change for more ideas on sustainability.

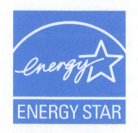

The Energy Star logo signals that an appliance meets energy conservation standards.

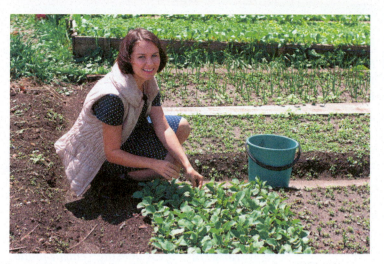
Schools can "go green" by supporting organic gardens and other sustainable activities.

Choosing a Green Location

While you can make smart consumer choices to reduce your ecological footprint, another issue to think about is the physical location of your campus and where you live. The American Lung Association periodically rates the cleanest and dirtiest U.S. cities in terms of air pollution. In the future, will students consider air pollution and other environmental factors when making their choices about schooling? Would you consider moving to or from a given city because of environmental issues?

Many "green" colleges offer sustainability programs such as organic gardens, daily meat-free meals, and bike-sharing programs. Some also have programs to protect wildlife on their property, include courses focused on sustainability in their curriculum, and take measures to divert their waste from landfills. Consider researching and getting involved with the measures toward sustainability at your school.

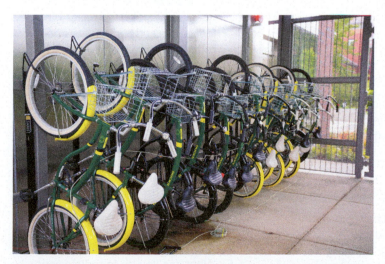
Does receiving support, such as plentiful bicycle racks, for alternative forms of transportation around campus make it more likely that you will contribute to a greener environment?

Skills for Behavior Change

Shopping To Save the Planet

Home Goods

- Look for products with less packaging or with refillable, reusable, or recyclable containers.
- Do not use caustic cleansers. Simple vinegar or a dilute mixture of water and bleach is usually just as effective and less harsh on your home and the environment.
- Buy laundry products that are free of dyes, fragrances, and sulfates. Use the smallest amount possible.
- Use soap and water to clean surfaces, not disposable cleaning cloths and spray-on shower cleaners. Avoid antibacterial soaps and cleaners because they contribute to microbial resistance.
- Buy recycled paper products when you can. Use both sides of a sheet of paper and fill it up before tossing.
- Use reusable mugs, plates, napkins, and silverware rather than disposable products. Be informed and read about the growing threat of micro-plastics in our environment.

Electronics

- Remember that your big-screen TV may be a huge energy drain, along with your old refrigerator. Replace outdated appliances when you can, and watch those energy levels.
- Buy CFLs instead of less energy-efficient incandescent bulbs. Use caution when installing and removing CFLs, and avoid breakage—CFLs contain mercury. Clear the room for at least 30 minutes after any accidental breakage.

Groceries

- Bring your own reusable, washable grocery bags to the store. (Be sure to wash bags after carrying meat in them or unpackaged produce.)
- Be a better food planner. Buy what you will use.
- Buy foods that are produced sustainably or organically or foods produced with fewer chemicals and pesticides.
- Purchase locally produced foods to reduce pollutants associated with transporting food long distances.
- Eat lower on the food chain. By eating more vegetables and nuts, legumes, and other food crops and reducing consumption of meat, dairy, and animal products, you have a smaller footprint stomping on the planet.
- Don't be picky about the looks of produce. Buy fruit and vegetables even if they don't have a perfect shape, and eat them before they rot. Consider using fruits that are slightly bruised or a little too soft for baked goods or blending them into smoothies.
- Do not buy plastic bottles of water. Purchase a hard plastic or stainless steel water bottle, and fill it from a filtered source. Wash it regularly.

Check Yourself

- What are three things you could change right now to be more environmentally responsible?
- What, if anything, prevents you from making choices that are environmentally aware?

14.8

Environmental Health

Summary

LO 14.1 Population growth is the single largest factor affecting the environment. Demand for more food, water, and energy—as well as places to dispose of waste—places great strain on Earth's resources. The United States is among the largest consumers of natural resources per person of any nation in the world. We can do more to reduce, reuse, and recycle.

LO 14.2 The primary constituents of air pollution are sulfur dioxide, particulate matter, carbon monoxide, nitrogen dioxide, ground level ozone, lead, carbon dioxide, and hydrocarbons.

LO 14.3 Indoor air pollution is caused primarily by tobacco smoke, woodstove smoke, furnace emissions, asbestos, formaldehyde, radon, lead, and mold.

LO 14.4 Pollution is depleting Earth's protective ozone layer and contributing to global warming, a type of climate change, by enhancing the greenhouse effect.

LO 14.5 Water pollution can be caused by either point sources (direct entry) or nonpoint sources (runoff or seepage). Major contributors to water pollution include petroleum products, organic solvents, polychlorinated biphenyls (PCBs), dioxins, pesticides, and lead.

LO 14.6 Solid waste pollution includes household trash, plastics, glass, metal products, and paper. Limited landfill space creates problems. Hazardous waste is toxic; improper disposal of this waste creates health hazards for people in surrounding communities.

LO 14.7 Nonionizing radiation comes from electromagnetic fields, such as those around power lines. Ionizing radiation results from the natural erosion of atomic nuclei. The disposal and storage of radioactive waste from nuclear power plants pose potential problems for public health.

LO 14.8 Living mindfully and sustainably means making smart consumer choices and reducing the amount of resources you use in daily life.

Pop Quiz

Visit Mastering Health to personalize your study plan with Chapter Review Quizzes and Dynamic Study Modules.

LO 14.1 1. The largest population that can be supported indefinitely given the resources available is known as Earth's
a. maximum fertility rate.
b. fertility capacity.
c. maximum population growth.
d. carrying capacity.

LO 14.2 2. The phenomenon that creates a barrier to protect us from the sun's harmful ultraviolet radiation rays is
a. photochemical smog.
b. the ozone layer.
c. gray air smog.
d. the greenhouse effect.

LO 14.2 3. The air pollutant that originates primarily from motor vehicle emissions is
a. particulates.
b. nitrogen dioxide.
c. sulfur dioxide.
d. carbon monoxide.

LO 14.3 4. One possible source of indoor air pollution is a gas present in some carpets and home furnishings called
a. lead.   c. radon.
b. asbestos.   d. formaldehyde.

LO 14.3 5. Which of the following substances separates into tiny fibers that can become embedded in the lungs?
a. Asbestos
b. Particulate matter
c. Radon
d. Formaldehyde

LO 14.5 6. Some herbicides contain toxic substances called
a. THMs.   c. dioxins.
b. PCPs.   d. PCBs.

LO 14.5 7. The terms *point source* and *nonpoint source* are used to describe the two general sources of
a. water pollution.
b. air pollution.
c. noise pollution.
d. ozone depletion.

LO 14.6 8. Your cereal box comes with less packaging, and your plastic water bottle now is more lightweight with less total plastic. This is an example of controlling municipal solid waste via
a. source reduction.
b. recycling.

c. composting.
d. incineration.

LO 14.7 9. Which gas is radioactive and could increase risks for cancer when it seeps into a home?
a. Carbon monoxide
b. Radon
c. Hydrogen sulfide
d. Natural gas

LO 14.7 10. What is the recommended safe level of rad exposure per year?
a. 0.5 to 5 rads   c. 100 to 200 rads
b. 5 to 100 rads   d. 200 to 350 rads

Answers to these questions can be found on page A-1. If you answered a question incorrectly, review the module identified by the Learning Outcome. For even more study tools, visit Mastering Health.

Think About It!

LO 14.1 List factors affecting population growth and overpopulation.

1. How are the rapid increases in global population and consumption of resources related? Is population control the best solution? Why or why not?

LO 14.2 Identify the major factors contributing to air pollution.

2. What are the primary sources of air pollution? What can be done to reduce air pollution?

LO 14.4 Describe how greenhouse gas buildup contributes to climate change.

3. What are the causes and consequences of global warming? What can individuals and communities do to reduce the threat of global warming?

LO 14.5 Identify the major factors contributing to water pollution.

4. What are point and nonpoint sources of water pollution? What can be done to reduce or prevent water pollution?

LO 14.6

5. How do you think communities and governments could encourage recycling efforts?

LO 14.7 Explain the environmental and personal risks associated with radiation.

6. What can you do to reduce your amount of radiation exposure? On the community level? On the national level?

Consumerism and Complementary and Integrative Health Care Choices

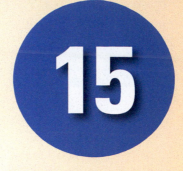

15

A variety of complementary and conventional medical therapies are available today. There are also a dwindling number of insurance options and limitations in resources. This chapter will help you understand factors you should consider in decision making; how therapies might be combined to maximize outcomes; and when they are appropriate, safe, and effective.

You have only one body. If you don't treat it with care, you will pay a major price in terms of monetary costs, pain, and other health-related limitations that may develop as you age. Throughout this book, we have emphasized the importance of healthy preventive behaviors. Learning when and how to navigate the health care system is a very important part of taking charge of your health.

15.1 Explain how to use the medical system and when to seek medical help.

As the health care industry has become more sophisticated in seeking your business, so must you become more sophisticated in purchasing its products and services. Acting responsibly in times of illness can be difficult, but the person best able to act on your behalf is you.

If you're not feeling well, the first step is deciding whether you need to seek medical advice and treatment. In some cases, self-care may be the most appropriate (and most cost-effective) option. Other times, not seeking treatment, whether because of high costs or limited insurance coverage or because you're trying to treat the illness or injury yourself, could be potentially dangerous.

Self-Care

Practicing behaviors that promote health and prevent disease can minimize your reliance on the formal medical system. Self-care consists of knowing your body, paying attention to its signals, and taking appropriate action to stop the progression of illness or injury. Common forms of self-care include the following:

- Diagnosing and treating common conditions that may not require a physician visit (such as a cold or a short bout of stomach flu)
- Proper use of over-the-counter remedies to treat minor and infrequent pain or other symptoms
- First aid for common, uncomplicated injuries
- Routine medical appointments for checking blood pressure, blood lipids, and blood glucose levels
- Assessing health care information resources and using only reputable self-help books or websites to guide your health decisions
- Eating a healthy diet, getting enough rest, and utilizing stress-reducing techniques such as meditation

In addition, a vast array of at-home diagnostic kits are now available to test for pregnancy, allergies, HIV, genetic disorders, and many other conditions. Caution is in order here. Diagnoses from these devices and kits are not guaranteed to be accurate, or you might not have the ability to understand the ramifications of what you learn without professional interpretation. Home health tests are not substitutes for regular, complete examinations by a trained practitioner.

Using self-care methods appropriately takes education and effort. Taking someone else's prescription drugs or using pills prescribed to you for an earlier illness is not safe or appropriate self-care. Neither is using unproven self-treatment methods.

When to Seek Help

Deciding which conditions warrant professional advice is not always easy. Generally, you should consult a physician if you experience *any* of the following:

- Accident or injury that includes extreme bleeding, swelling, redness, or inability to use the injured body part in a normal manner
- Sudden or severe chest pains, especially if they cause breathing difficulties
- Trauma to the head or spine accompanied by persistent headache, blurred vision, loss of consciousness, confusion, vomiting, convulsions, or paralysis
- Sudden high fever or recurring high temperature (over 102°F for children and 103°F for adults) and/or sweats
- Tingling or numbness in the face or arm accompanied by slurred speech, muscle weakness, mental confusion, severe headache, drooping face, or abrupt vision loss
- Shortness of breath, severe swelling, hives, or dizziness that develop after taking a drug, eating, or being stung or bitten by an insect
- Unexplained bleeding or loss of fluid from any body opening
- Unexplained, sudden weight loss
- Persistent or recurrent diarrhea or vomiting

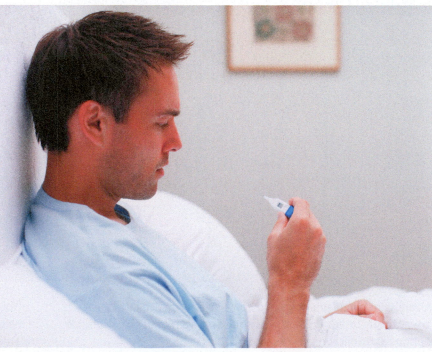

Deciding when to contact a physician can be difficult. Most people first research symptoms online and try to diagnose and treat a condition themselves.

- Blue-colored lips, eyelids, or nail beds
- Any lump, swelling, thickness, or sore that does not subside or that grows for over a month
- Any marked change or pain in bowel or bladder habits
- Yellowing of the skin or the whites of the eyes
- Any symptom that is unusual, or persists/recurs over time
- Pregnancy

The Placebo Effect

The *placebo effect* is an apparent cure or improved state of health seemingly brought about by a substance, product, or procedure that actually has no therapeutically recognized value. Patients often report improvements in a condition based on what they expect, desire, or were told would happen after receiving a treatment, even though that treatment was, for example, simple sugar pills instead of powerful drugs.

There is also a *nocebo effect*, in which a patient comes into a treatment situation with certain mental health issues and expectations that cause the patient to react negatively, or a health professional might give a patient such a bleak assessment of the problem that the patient experiences anxiety, pain, and poor outcomes. Similarly, a negative assessment of a treatment's potential efficacy may induce a failure to respond to that treatment.

Researchers are investigating how and why expectation of a treatment's effect can change a patient's experience. Evidence from pain studies suggests that use of a placebo for pain control causes the brain to release the same endogenous (natural) opioids that it releases when the study participant uses a pain medication with an active ingredient.[1] But pain is not the only factor to respond to expectation: A study of resting tremor (such as involuntary finger-tapping) in patients with Parkinson's disease found that positive or negative expectations of a treatment's effectiveness reduced or increased patient tremor when they were given the same valid medication or the same placebo.[2] Similar chemical changes on brain imaging tests were seen with placebos in studies of depression and alcohol dependency treatment.[3]

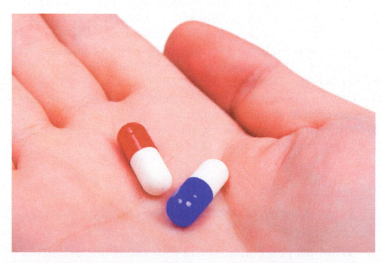

Is it a real medicine or a placebo? In some cases, it might not make a difference.

People who unknowingly use placebos when medical treatment is needed increase their risk for health problems. However, what we learn from the ways in which placebos work may someday help us harness the mind's power to treat certain diseases and conditions.

Skills for **Behavior Change**
Be Proactive in Your Health Care

Here are some tips for getting the most out of visits to your health care provider and being proactive in your health care:

- **Keep records of your own and your family's medical histories.**
- **Research your condition—causes, physiological effects, possible treatments, and prognosis. Don't rely on your health care provider for this information.**
- **Before an appointment, write down questions to ask. Bring a friend or relative along to medical visits to help you review what the health care provider says. Take notes.**
- **Ask the practitioner to explain the problem and possible treatments, tests, and drugs in a clear and understandable way. If you don't understand something, ask for clarification.**
- **Ask whether you can be prescribed generic drug equivalents that cost less rather than a brand-name medication.**
- **Ask for a written summary of any lab tests.**
- **Investigate risks and contraindications for any treatment prescribed as well as likely effectiveness. Consult only reliable sources—texts, journals, and government resources.**
- **If you have any doubt about a recommended treatment, get a second opinion from a totally different practice.**
- **If you use any complementary and integrative medicine therapy, inform your primary health care provider. It is particularly important to talk with your provider if you are thinking about replacing your prescribed treatment with one or more supplements, are currently taking a prescription drug, have a chronic medical condition, are planning to have surgery, are pregnant or nursing, or are thinking about giving supplements to children.**
- **When getting prescriptions filled, ask the pharmacist to include package inserts with details of potential drug and food interactions.**
- **Remember that *natural* and *safe* are not necessarily the same. You can become seriously ill from seemingly harmless "natural" products. Be cautious about combining herbal medications, just as you would about combining other drugs.**

Check Yourself

- **What are four instances in which you should seek medical help?**

Learning Outcome

15.2 List factors to consider in choosing a medical provider.

The most satisfied patients are those who feel that their health care provider explains diagnosis and treatment options thoroughly and demonstrates competence and caring.[4] When evaluating health care providers, consider the following questions:

- Does the provider listen and give you time to ask questions? Does the provider answer your calls?
- What professional education and training has the provider had, and from where? A *board-certified* provider has passed the national board examination for his or her specialty (e.g., pediatrics) and has been certified as competent in that specialty.
- Is the provider a specialist in family or internal medicine, or does the provider have the specialty you need?
- Is the provider affiliated with an accredited medical facility or institution? Accreditation requires that the institution verify all education, licensing, and training claims of its affiliated practitioners. Is the provider board certified?
- Is the provider open to complementary and integrative care? Is the provider willing to provide referrals?
- Does the provider explain what to expect from treatment, potential side effects of treatment, and things to watch for?
- Who will be responsible for your care when your provider is on vacation or not on call?
- Are the provider's online reviews reliable and accurate? Do they provide detailed reviews by actual patients?
- Does your insurance require that you be treated by someone in-network? You will most likely end up paying less out of pocket with an in-network provider. Also, many hospitals use *hospitalists* in their ERs who are out of network and might not be covered by your insurance. Ask whether the person you are seeing is an in-network, affiliated provider.
- Do you feel comfortable with the provider? Can you easily ask questions and express concerns?

> **See It! Videos**
>
> Knowing your medical history can keep you informed of health risks. Watch **Your Medical History** in the Study Area of Mastering Health.

Asking the right questions at the right time could save you suffering and expense. Many patients find that writing their questions down before an appointment helps.

Active participation in your treatment is the only sensible course in a health care environment that encourages **defensive medicine**, the use of medical practices designed to avert the possibility of malpractice suits. While many observers believe that defensive medicine is responsible for significant increases in health care costs, others point out that it is difficult to define what defensive medicine really is. Defensive medicine can include ordering tests or other procedures without likely benefit to avoid possible malpractice or overprescribing antibiotics or pain medications to improve patient satisfaction. However, it may also include avoidance behaviors, in which doctors limit their availability to older Medicare or Medicaid patients or patients whom they deem to be at high risk in a given procedure. In one instance, defensive medicine drives up cost; in another, patients are denied access to the best facilities or physicians, thereby reducing the likelihood of positive outcomes while keeping costs down in a practice. It can be difficult to determine whether a provider is ordering tests, procedures, and services out of concern or because he or she has economic incentives for performing more tests or procedures. Ironically, many people spend hours investigating which car or phone to purchase but take the first doctor available in a health care facility.[5] Doing your homework and checking out your options are part of individual responsibility.

Being proactive in your health care also means being means aware of the following patient rights and responsibilities:[6]

1. The right of informed consent means that before receiving any care, you should be fully informed of what is planned, the risks and potential benefits, and any possible alternative forms of treatment, including the option to refuse treatment. Your consent must be voluntary and without any form of coercion. It is critical that you read any consent forms carefully.
2. You have the right to know whether the treatment you are receiving is standard or experimental. In experimental conditions, you have the legal and ethical right to know whether any drug is being used in the research project for a purpose not approved by the Food and Drug Administration (FDA) and whether the study is one in which some people receive treatment while others receive a placebo.
3. You have the right to make decisions about the health care that is recommended by the physician.
4. You have the right to confidentiality. This means that you are not obliged to reveal the source of payment for your treatment. It also means that you have the right to make personal decisions about all reproductive matters involving your own body.
5. You have the right to receive adequate health care, to refuse treatment, and to cease treatment at any time.
6. You are entitled to have access to all of your medical records and to have those records remain confidential.
7. You have the right to continuity of health care.
8. You have the right to seek the opinions of other health care professionals about your condition.
9. You have the right to courtesy, respect, dignity, responsiveness, and timely attention to your health needs.

Check Yourself

- What should you look for when choosing a medical provider?
- What do you consider the four most important characteristics in a medical provider? Of a hospital or clinic?

15.3 Types of Allopathic Health Care Providers

15.3 Identify the main types of allopathic health care providers.

Conventional health care, also called **allopathic medicine**, is mainstream medicine, or traditional Western medical practice. Treatments are based on the premise that illness is a result of heredity (gene mutations), birth defects, functional problems or disorders, or exposure to harmful environmental agents such as infectious microorganisms, pollutants, or overabundance or underabundance of certain nutrients. In Western-style medicine, disease prevention and treatment involve vaccines, drugs, surgery, and other treatments provided by trained health care professionals.

Allopathic health care providers use **evidence-based medicine**, in which decisions about patient care are based on a combination of clinical expertise, patients' values, and current best scientific evidence.

Conventional health care is usually organized around a **primary care practitioner (PCP)**—a medical practitioner you can visit for routine ailments, preventive care, general medical advice, and referrals to specialists. The PCP for most people is a family practitioner, internist (a specialist in internal medicine), pediatrician, or obstetrician-gynecologist (OB-GYN). Some people see nurse practitioners or physician assistants who work for individual doctors or medical groups; others use nontraditional providers as their primary source of care. As a college student, you may opt to visit a PCP at your campus health center.

Doctors undergo training that includes 4 years of undergraduate work, plus another 4 years (typically) spent studying for a medical degree (MD). Some medical students then choose a specialty, such as pediatrics, cardiology, or surgery, which requires them to spend another 3 to 7 years studying that particular area of medicine.

Specialists include **osteopaths**, general practitioners who receive training similar to that of MDs but who place special emphasis on the skeletal and muscular systems. Their treatments may involve manipulation of muscles and joints. Osteopaths receive the degree of doctor of osteopathy (DO) rather than MD.

Eye care specialists can be either ophthalmologists or optometrists. An **ophthalmologist** holds a medical degree and can perform surgery and prescribe medications. An **optometrist** typically evaluates visual problems and fits glasses but is not a trained physician. If you have an eye infection, glaucoma, or other eye condition that requires diagnosis and treatment, you need to see an ophthalmologist.

Dentists are specialists who diagnose and treat diseases of the teeth, gums, and oral cavity. They attend dental school for 4 years and receive the title of doctor of dental surgery (DDS) or doctor of medical dentistry (DMD). *Orthodontists* specialize in the alignment of teeth. *Oral surgeons* perform surgical procedures to correct problems of the mouth, face, and jaw.

Nurses are highly trained and strictly regulated health professionals who provide a wide range of services, including patient education, counseling, community health and disease prevention information, and administration of medications. Registered nurses

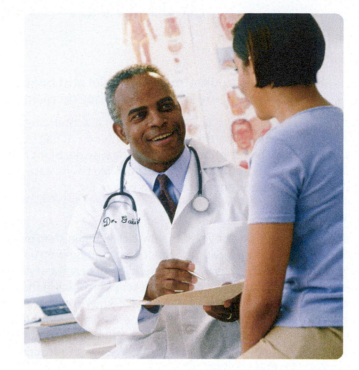

Understanding the differences among different types of health care providers is important. In some cases, you might need to see a doctor with a particular specialty; in other cases, a nurse practitioner or physician assistant may be satisfactory.

(RNs) in the United States complete either a 4-year program leading to a bachelor of science in nursing (BSN) degree or a 2-year associate degree program. Lower-level licensed practical or vocational nurses (LPNs or LVNs) complete a 1- to 2-year training program based in a community college or a hospital and then take a licensing exam.

Nurse practitioners (NPs) are nurses with advanced training obtained through either a master's degree program or a specialized nurse practitioner program. Nurse practitioners have the training and authority to conduct diagnostic tests and (in some states) to prescribe medications. They work in a variety of settings, including clinics and student health centers, and can specialize in areas such as pediatrics or acute care. Nurses and nurse practitioners may also earn the clinical doctor of nursing degree (ND), doctor of nursing science (DNS and DNSc) degrees, or a research-based PhD in nursing.

Physician assistants (PAs) examine and diagnose patients, offer treatment, and write prescriptions. Unlike a nurse practitioner, a PA must practice under a physician's supervision. Like other health care providers, PAs are licensed by state boards of medicine.

- **What is allopathic medicine?**

- **What are some of the major types of allopathic health care providers?**

Choosing Health Products: Prescription and Over-the-Counter Drugs

15.4 Explain how to determine the risks and benefits of prescription and over-the-counter medicines.

Prescription drugs can be obtained only with a written prescription from a physician, whereas over-the-counter drugs can be purchased without a prescription. Just as making wise decisions about providers is an important aspect of responsible health care, so is making wise decisions about medications.

Prescription Drugs

In about 3 out of 4 doctor visits, the physician administers or prescribes at least one medication.[7] In fact, prescription drug use has increased steadily over the past decade: over 49 percent of Americans report having used one or more prescription drugs in the previous 30 days, and more than 11 percent of Americans have used five or more.[8] Even though these drugs are administered under medical supervision, the wise consumer still takes precautions. Hazards and complications arising from the use of prescription drugs are common.

Several resources can help you determine the risks of prescription medicines and make educated decisions about whether to take a given drug. One of the best is the Center for Drug Evaluation and Research (www.fda.gov/drugs). This consumer-specific section of the FDA website provides current information on risks and benefits of prescription drugs.

Generic drugs, medications sold under their chemical name rather than a brand name, contain the same active ingredients as brand-name drugs but are less expensive. If your doctor prescribes a drug, always ask whether a generic equivalent exists and whether it would be safe and effective for you to try. There is some controversy about the effectiveness of generic drugs. Substitutions are sometimes made in minor ingredients that can affect the way the drug is absorbed, potentially causing discomfort or even allergic reactions in some patients.[9] Tell your doctor about any reactions you have to medications.

Medications Online: Buyer Beware Consumers may choose to have prescriptions filled online for convenience and to save money. Although many websites operate legally and observe the traditional safeguards for dispensing drugs, be wary of rogue websites that sell unapproved or potentially counterfeit drugs and sites that sidestep practices meant to protect consumers.

The Verified Internet Pharmacy Practice Sites (VIPPS) seal is given to online pharmacy sites that meet state licensure requirements. Follow these tips to protect yourself from fraudulent sites[10]:

- Buy only from state-licensed pharmacy sites based in the United States (preferably from VIPPS-certified sites).
- Don't buy from sites that sell prescription drugs without a prescription or that offer to prescribe a medication for the first time without a physical exam by your doctor or that require you only to answer an online questionnaire.
- Use legitimate websites that have a licensed pharmacist to answer your questions.
- Don't provide personal information, such as a Social Security number, credit card information, or medical or health history, unless you are sure the website will keep your information safe and private.

Over-the-Counter (OTC) Drugs

Over-the-counter (OTC) drugs are nonprescription substances used for self-medication. American consumers spend billions of dollars yearly on OTC preparations for relief of everything from runny noses to ingrown toenails. Despite a common belief that OTC products are safe and effective, indiscriminate use and abuse can occur with these drugs as with all others. For example, people who frequently drop medication into their eyes to "get the red out" or pop antacids every day are likely to become dependent on these remedies. Many people experience adverse side effects because they ignore the warnings on OTC drug labels or don't read them. The FDA has developed a standard label that appears on most OTC products (**Figure 15.1**).

Understanding the actions and side effects of OTC drugs is part of being a smart consumer. *Pain relievers* can be useful for counteracting localized or general pain and for reducing fever. They exist in several general formulations: *aspirin* (e.g., Bayer, Bufferin), *acetaminophen* (e.g., Tylenol), *ibuprofen* (e.g., Advil, Motrin), and *naproxen sodium* (e.g., Aleve, Naprosyn). Possible side effects include stomach problems ranging from simple upset to worsening of ulcers and liver damage with prolonged overuse. Aspirin and ibuprofen also reduce blood clotting ability (which can be a problem for people who take anticlotting medications) and, for a few users, can trigger severe allergic reactions. Finally, aspirin should not be taken by anyone under age 18 because of its association with Reye's syndrome, a rare condition that causes swelling of the brain and liver in children and teenagers who are recovering from certain infections.

Cold and allergy medicines ease symptoms in a variety of ways (but don't eliminate infection). *Antihistamines* (e.g., Claritin, Benadryl, Xyzal) dry runny noses, clear postnasal drip and sinus congestion, and reduce tears.

Be very cautious if you consider ordering medications from an online pharmacy.

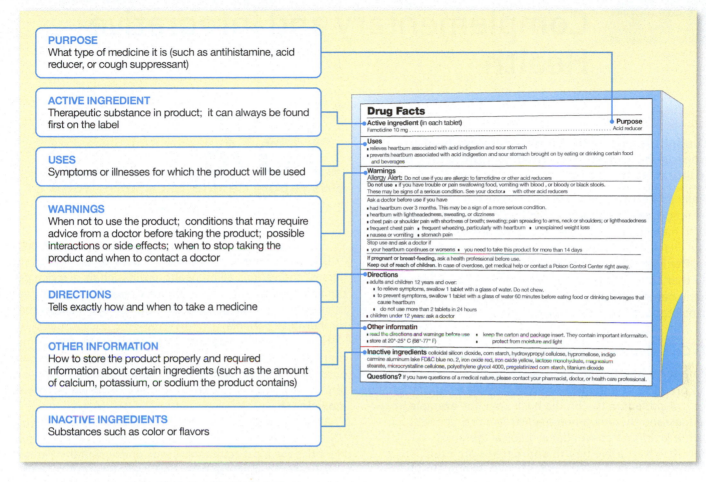

PURPOSE
What type of medicine it is (such as antihistamine, acid reducer, or cough suppressant)

ACTIVE INGREDIENT
Therapeutic substance in product; it can always be found first on the label

USES
Symptoms or illnesses for which the product will be used

WARNINGS
When not to use the product; conditions that may require advice from a doctor before taking the product; possible interactions or side effects; when to stop taking the product and when to contact a doctor

DIRECTIONS
Tells exactly how and when to take a medicine

OTHER INFORMATION
How to store the product properly and required information about certain ingredients (such as the amount of calcium, potassium, or sodium the product contains)

INACTIVE INGREDIENTS
Substances such as color or flavors

Drug Facts

Active ingredient (in each tablet) — **Purpose**
Famotidine 10 mg .... Acid reducer

Uses
▪ relieves heartburn associated with acid indigestion and sour stomach
▪ prevents heartburn associated with acid indigestion and sour stomach brought on by eating or drinking certain food and beverages

Warnings
Allergy Alert: Do not use if you are allergic to famotidine or other acid reducers
Do not use ▪ if you have trouble or pain swallowing food, vomiting with blood , or bloody or black stools. These may be signs of a serious condition. See your doctor.▪   ▪ with other acid reducers

Ask a doctor before use if you have
▪ had heartburn over 3 months. This may be a sign of a more serious condition.
▪ heartburn with lightheadedness, sweating, or dizziness
▪ chest pain or shoulder pain with shortness of breath; sweating; pain spreading to arms, neck or shoulders; or lightheadedness
▪ frequent chest pain ▪ frequent wheezing, particularly with heartburn ▪ unexplained weight loss
▪ nausea or vomiting ▪ stomach pain

Stop use and ask a doctor if
▪ your heartburn continues or worsens ▪ you need to take this product for more than 14 days

If pregnant or breast-feeding, ask a health professional before use.
Keep out of reach of children. In case of overdose, get medical help or contact a Poison Control Center right away.

Directions
▪ adults and children 12 years and over:
  ▪ to relieve symptoms, swallow 1 tablet with a glass of water. Do not chew.
  ▪ to prevent symptoms, swallow 1 tablet with a glass of water 60 minutes before eating food or drinking beverages that cause heartburn
  ▪ do not use more than 2 tablets in 24 hours
▪ children under 12 years: ask a doctor

Other informatin
▪ read the directions and warnings before use ▪ keep the carton and package insert. They contain important informaiton.
▪ store at 20°-25° C (68°-77° F) ▪ protect from moisture and light

Inactive ingredients colloidal silicon dioxide, corn starch, hydroxypropyl cellulose, hypromellose, indigo carmine aluminum lake FD&C blue no. 2, iron oxide red, iron oxide yellow, lactose monohydrate, magnesium stearate, microcrystalline cellulose, polyethylene glycol 4000, pregelatinized corn starch, titanium dioxide

Questions? If you have questions of a medical nature, please contact your pharmacist, doctor, or health care professional.

Figure 15.1 The Over-the-Counter Medicine Label
Source: Consumer Healthcare Products Association, OTC Label, www.otcsafety.org. Used with permission.

They are mild central nervous system depressants and, as such, can cause drowsiness, dizziness, and disturbed coordination in many people. *Decongestants* (e.g., Sudafed, DayQuil, Allermed) reduce nasal stuffiness due to colds. Cold medications have a wide variety of possible side effects. Some people may exhibit nervousness, restlessness, and sleep problems; others may feel drowsy or nauseated.

Antacids (e.g., Tums, Maalox) relieve "heartburn," usually by neutralizing stomach acid with a chemical base such as calcium or aluminum. Occasional use is safe, but chronic use can lead to reduced mineral absorption from food, possible concealment of an ulcer, reduced effectiveness of anticlotting medications, interference with the function of certain antibiotics (when the antacids contain aluminum), worsened high blood pressure (when the antacids contain sodium), aggravated kidney problems, and other problems.

Before you take *laxatives*, talk with your health care provider about your issues and get advice about which laxative would be best for you and would have the fewest side effects. Some are fiber-based supplements designed to relieve constipation and can be taken for longer periods of time with fewer side effects. Others are true laxatives and are not meant to be taken daily for prolonged periods. Although laxatives are safe for limited and occasional use, long-term regular use can lead to reduced absorption of minerals from food, dehydration, and even dependency.

48.5% of Americans
report taking at least one prescription drug in the past month; 21.7% report taking three or more such drugs.

Sleep aids and relaxants (e.g., Nytol, Sleep-Eze, Sominex) are designed to help relieve occasional sleeplessness. Short-term side effects include drowsiness and reduced mental alertness, dry mouth and throat, constipation, dizziness, and lack of coordination. Long-term use can lead to dependency. If you suffer from regular insomnia or other sleep problems, see your health care provider.

Check Yourself

- **What factors should you consider when ordering prescription drugs online?**

- **List the benefits and potential side effects of three OTC drugs that you use or might use in the future.**

15.5 Complementary and Integrative Health

15.5 Distinguish between complementary health approaches, alternative health approaches, and integrative medicine.

Increasingly popular for both self-care and health promotion are diverse medical systems, practices, and products that developed outside of mainstream Western, or conventional, medicine.[11] Although these complimentary, alternative, and integrative options, offer consumers a broader range of choices and research suggests that some of them may be effective, the evidence of therapeutic benefits of others is not convincing, and a few have been associated with adverse effects.

What Is Complementary and Integrative Health?

Complementary health approaches are non-mainstream practices and products commonly used together with conventional medicine.[12] A patient with chronic back pain, for example, may combine massage therapy, a non-mainstream practice, with prescription medication, a conventional medical therapy.

In contrast, **alternative health approaches** are used *in place of* conventional medicine. For example, a person might choose to follow a special diet or herbal remedy to treat cancer instead of using surgery, radiation, or other conventional treatments. The National Center for Complementary and Integrative Health (NCCIH) reports that in the United States, true alternative medicine is rare; most people who use non-mainstream approaches use them alongside conventional treatments.[13]

36% of 18- to 29-year-olds report having used some form of complementary medicine.

Doctors of medicine (MDs), doctors of osteopathy (DOs), nurses, and various allied health professionals practice conventional medicine. These practitioners may recommend massage therapy, nutrient supplements, or other complementary therapies for individual patients.

However, some practitioners incorporate complementary therapies into their conventional health care in a coordinated, purposeful way. Increasing in popularity in many health care systems today, this coordinated approach is known as **integrative medicine**.[14]

A survey conducted by the NCCIH revealed that 33 percent of U.S. adults use one or more complementary therapies.[15] Figure 15.2 identifies the most commonly used complementary therapies.

Why do so many people find complementary approaches appealing? Many people turn to these therapies to promote their general health and well-being or to relieve unrelenting symptoms associated with a chronic disease or the side effects of conventional medicine.[16] They may also be seeking a **holistic** approach, that is, care that focuses on the mind and the whole body rather than just an isolated symptom or body part. They may also desire

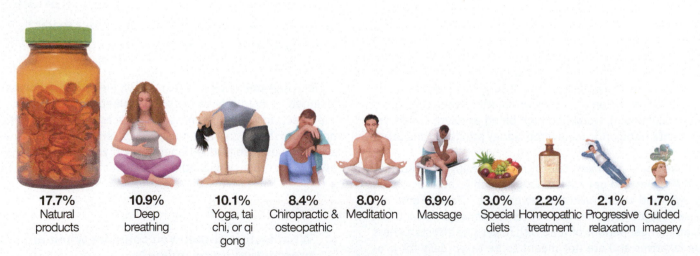

| **17.7%** Natural products | **10.9%** Deep breathing | **10.1%** Yoga, tai chi, or qi gong | **8.4%** Chiropractic & osteopathic | **8.0%** Meditation | **6.9%** Massage | **3.0%** Special diets | **2.2%** Homeopathic treatment | **2.1%** Progressive relaxation | **1.7%** Guided imagery |

Figure 15.2 **The Ten Most Common Complementary Therapies among U.S. Adults**

Source: Data from T.C. Clarke et al., "Trends in the Use of Complementary Health Approaches among Adults: United States, 2002–2012," *National Health Statistics Reports*, no. 79 (2015), February 2015, Available at www.cdc.gov/nchs/data/nhsr/nhsr079.pdf.

an approach to healing that allows them a measure of control. Mindfulness meditation, for example, has been shown to increase patients' sense of control over their symptoms and treatment and, as a result, to reduce individual health care utilization.[17]

In one study of patients who had been trained in mindfulness, annual health care utilization dropped 43 percent among patients, and the average number of annual visits to the emergency department declined from 3.6 visits to 1.7. By increasing patients' own self-care abilities, mindfulness training is thought to have the potential to substantially reduce overall health care costs.[18]

Although practitioners of most complementary health approaches spend many years in training, each approach has a different set of training standards, guidelines for practice, and licensure procedures. Moreover, there are no national standards, and states differ in their requirements.

It is important to remember that licenses or certificates do not guarantee effective or safe treatment from any provider, whether complementary or traditional. Consumers must be informed, ask questions, and make sound decisions when selecting any provider for any services.

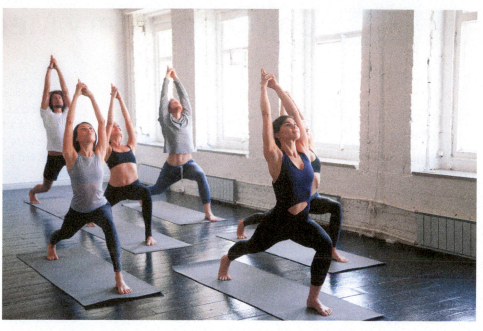

Yoga is one of the most popular complementary therapies in the United States.

When considering any complementary therapy, visit the website of the NCCIH. Its mission is to study complementary health approaches using rigorous scientific methods and to build an evidence base regarding their safety and effectiveness.

In this chapter, we group complementary health approaches into three general categories of practice: *complementary medical systems*, *mind and body practices*, and *natural products*.

Complementary medical systems include such practices as traditional Chinese medicine, Ayurveda, homeopathy, and naturopathy. These approaches to health care derived from outside of Western medicine.

Mind and body therapies include manipulative therapies such as chiropractic and massage, energy therapies such as acupuncture, acupressure, and qi gong, and meditation. In manipulative therapy, the practitioner uses massage or other techniques to align muscles and bones and to relieve pain. Energy therapies seek to balance energy in the body, promoting relaxation and pain relief.

Natural products include supplements and herbal remedies that are used for a variety of reasons.

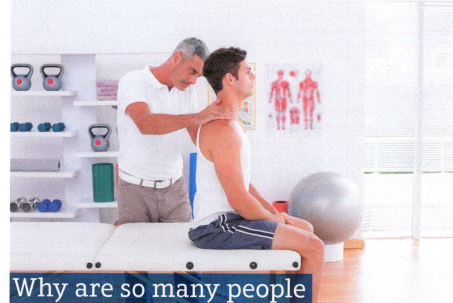

Why are so many people turning to complementary and integrative health?

People use complementary medicine for multiple reasons, and many treatments can have positive effects on a variety of physical and mental ailments. For example, chiropractic medicine has shown benefits among people with back and neck pain and headaches.

Check Yourself

- **What is the difference between complementary health approaches, alternative health approaches, and integrative medicine?**

- **What are the three categories of complementary health approaches?**

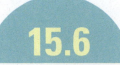

15.6 Complementary Medical Systems

Learning Outcome

15.6 Describe four complementary medical systems practiced in the United States.

Complementary medical systems reflect specific theories of physiology, health, and disease that have developed outside the influence of conventional medicine. Here, we discuss the ones that are most commonly available in the United States.

Traditional Chinese Medicine

The concept of *qi* (pronounced "chee"), or vital energy, is foundational to **traditional Chinese medicine (TCM)**. When *qi* is in balance, the person is in a state of health; an imbalance of *qi* results in disease. Diagnosis is based on personal history, observation of the body (especially the tongue), palpation, and pulse diagnosis, a detailed procedure that requires considerable skill. Techniques such as acupuncture, herbal medicine, massage, and qigong (a form of energy therapy) are among the TCM approaches to health and healing.

TCM is complex, and research into its effectiveness is limited.[19] Analyses of Chinese herbal medicines have found some of them to be contaminated by toxic heavy metals, drugs not listed on the label, and other potentially harmful ingredients. Note that herbal supplements are regulated by the FDA but not as foods or drugs. Therefore, if you are taking a dietary supplement for a specific health problem, it is always best to talk with your health care provider to determine whether these supplements are safe for your health issue.[20]

Traditional Chinese medicine practitioners within the United States must have completed a graduate program in a college or university approved by the Accreditation Commission for Acupuncture and Oriental Medicine (ACAOM). Graduate programs usually involve a 3- or 4-year clinical internship. In addition, the student must pass a national certification and licensing examination before being allowed to practice.

Ayurveda

Ayurveda (Ayurvedic medicine) is one of the world's oldest medical systems, having evolved over 3,000 years ago in India. Ayurveda seeks to integrate and balance the body, mind, and spirit to restore harmony in the individual.[21] Practitioners use various diagnostic techniques to determine which of three vital energies, or *doshas*, is dominant in the patient. Treatment plans aim to bring the doshas into balance, thereby reducing symptoms. Dietary modification and herbal remedies drawn from the botanical wealth of the Indian subcontinent are common.

Research into Ayurveda is limited, but studies have shown some of its herbal remedies to be effective for certain joint and digestive disorders.[22] However, some have been found to be tainted with lead, mercury, or arsenic.[23] Other Ayurvedic treatments are yoga, meditation, massage, steam baths, changes in sleep patterns, and controlled breathing.

Training of Ayurvedic practitioners varies. There is no national standard for certification, although professional groups are working toward creating licensing guidelines.

Homeopathy

Homeopathy (homeopathic medicine) is based on the principle that "like cures like." In other words, the same substance that in a large dose produces the symptoms of an illness—and may even be fatal—will in a small dose prompt the body's own defenses to cure the illness. Developed in the late 1700s by a German physician, homeopathy follows the "law of minimum dose," which asserts that the lower the dose of a remedy, the greater its effectiveness. Thus, homeopathic remedies, which are derived from a wide range of natural—and sometimes toxic—substances such as arsenic and belladonna, may be so diluted that no molecules of the original substance remain.[24]

The NCCIH reports that certain foundational concepts in homeopathy are at odds with foundational concepts of physics and chemistry and that little evidence supports homeopathy for treatment of any specific condition.[25]

Homeopathic training varies considerably, from diploma programs to correspondence courses. Only Arizona, Connecticut, and Nevada have homeopathic licensing boards. Requirements to practice vary from state to state.

Naturopathy

Naturopathy (naturopathic medicine) emphasizes the power of nature to restore health. Naturopathic physicians view their role as supporting the body's innate ability to maintain and restore health, typically by identifying and removing obstacles to these innate processes. They favor prevention and, when treatment is necessary, they use approaches that are holistic, natural, and minimally invasive.[26]

Specific approaches to care include diet; dietary supplements; homeopathy; spinal and soft-tissue manipulation; detoxification using fasting, juice diets, colon cleansing, or other means; and therapeutic counseling. Limited research suggests that naturopathy may be more effective than conventional medicine for certain types of chronic pain. However, the efficacy and safety of some practices may not be supported by scientific evidence.[27]

Naturopathic physicians have completed a 4-year graduate program and, in most states, have passed a licensing examination. Naturopaths who are not physicians may have received less training and typically are unlicensed.

Check Yourself

■ Describe four complementary medical systems.

Mind and Body Practices: Manipulative Therapies

Learning Outcome

15.7 Describe several mind and body practices involving manipulative therapies.

Mind and body practices are a large and diverse group of complementary health approaches that a trained practitioner or teacher often teaches or administers.[28] They include movement reeducation therapies, as well as modalities in which the practitioner directly manipulates body tissues, attempts to shift the flow of body energy, or teaches the client techniques to promote relaxation or manage stress. Several mind and body practices—including deep breathing, yoga, chiropractic, meditation, massage, progressive relaxation, and guided imagery—are among the ten most commonly used complementary therapies in the United States.

In this module, we will discuss **manipulative therapies**, which are approaches based on manipulation or movement of body tissues and structures.

Chiropractic Medicine
Chiropractic medicine has been practiced for more than 100 years and focuses on disorders of the muscular and skeletal system and the use of various modalities to reduce health effects from these disorders.[29] Many health care providers work closely with chiropractors, and many insurance companies pay for MD referrals to chiropractors.

Chiropractic medicine is based on the principle that energy flows through the nervous system. If the spine is misaligned, energy flow through the spinal cord is disrupted. Chiropractors manipulate the spine into proper alignment so that energy can flow unimpeded. Typically, chiropractors treat low back pain; neck

pain; pain in the arms, legs, and feet; and headaches. Studies suggest that chiropractic spinal manipulation is as beneficial in easing low back pain as pain relief medications and other common remedies, particularly during the first 6 weeks of transient or acute episodes. However, the evidence for other benefits is less clear, and minor adverse effects of headache, muscle stiffness, and pain may increase with manipulation.[30]

Chiropractic training typically begins with a premedical undergraduate degree followed by a 4-year chiropractic program involving intensive coursework similar to that of medical school programs, combined with hands-on clinical training. Graduates must also pass a licensing examination given by the National Board of Chiropractic Examiners. Chiropractic care is licensed and regulated in all 50 states.[31]

Massage Therapy
References to massage exist in numerous ancient texts, including those of Greece, Rome, Japan, China, Egypt, and India.[32] **Massage therapy** is soft-tissue manipulation by a trained therapist for relaxation and healing. The therapist manipulates the patient's muscles and connective tissues to loosen the fibers and break up adhesions, improve the body's circulation, and remove waste products. The NCCIH reports that research evidence supports the effectiveness of massage therapy to temporarily relieve musculoskeletal pain such as low back and neck pain, and it may help to promote relaxation and relieve depression.[33]

The course of study in massage schools varies greatly by state but typically covers sciences such as anatomy and physiology as well as massage techniques and business, ethical, and legal considerations.[34] For licensing, many states require a minimum of 500 hours of training and a passing grade on a national certification exam. Massage therapists work in private studios and health spas and in medical and chiropractic offices, nursing homes, hotels, and fitness centers with a job outlook that is very strong.[35]

Movement Therapies
A broad range of Eastern and Western complementary health approaches use movement, including postural realignment, to increase physical, mental, and emotional well-being and reduce limitations in body functioning. Two commonly available approaches are as follows:

- The *Alexander technique* is a movement education method designed to release harmful tension in the body to improve ease of movement, balance, and coordination.
- The *Feldenkrais method* is a system of gentle movements and exercises designed to improve movement, flexibility, coordination, and overall functioning through techniques that enhance the client's awareness and retrain the nervous system.

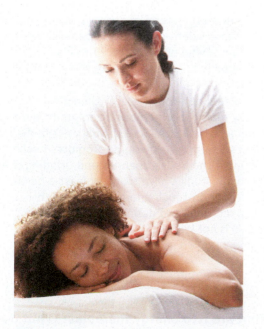

Oh, your aching back? Try massage!

Check Yourself

- What are manipulative therapies? What treatments do they involve?

15.8 Mind and Body Practices: Energy Therapies

Learning Outcome

15.8 Describe several mind and body practices involving energy therapies.

Some mind and body practices involve **energy therapies** that focus on energy fields thought to originate either within the body (biofields) or from other sources (electromagnetic fields). The existence of these fields has not been experimentally proven. Popular examples of energy therapy are acupuncture, acupressure, qigong, reiki, and therapeutic touch.

Acupuncture

One of the oldest and most popular TCM therapies, **acupuncture** is used to relieve a wide variety of health conditions, from musculoskeletal dysfunction to depression. The therapist stimulates various points on the body with a series of precisely placed and extremely fine needles. The stimulation of these acupuncture points is thought to increase the flow of *qi* through the *meridians*, or energy pathways, in the body.

Following acupuncture treatments, most participants in clinical studies report satisfaction with the treatment and improvement in their condition. However, there is significant controversy over whether or not such results are simply a placebo response.[36] A recent review study, for example, found acupuncture effective in achieving at least a 50 percent reduction in headache frequency; however, sham acupuncture achieved a 43 percent reduction.[37] Moreover, a 2017 clinical trial found sham acupuncture to be as effective as true acupuncture for the treatment of irritable bowel syndrome.[38] In contrast, a 2016 review study found acupuncture beneficial for back pain and knee pain.[39]

Acupuncture licensing requirements vary by state. Most states require a diploma from the National Certification Commission for Acupuncture and Oriental Medicine. In addition, many conventional physicians and dentists practice acupuncture.[40]

Acupressure

Like acupuncture, **acupressure** is based on the principles of energy flow as *qi*. Instead of inserting needles, however, the therapist applies pressure. The goal of acupressure is for *qi* to be evenly distributed and flow freely throughout the body. Practitioners typically have the same basic training and understanding of meridians and acupuncture points as do acupuncturists.

Other Forms of Energy Therapy

Qigong, a technique of TCM, brings together movement, meditation, and regulation of breathing to increase the flow of *qi*, enhance blood circulation, and improve immune function. A 2015 systematic review of meta-analyses found that the practice of qigong and other meditative movement therapies was associated

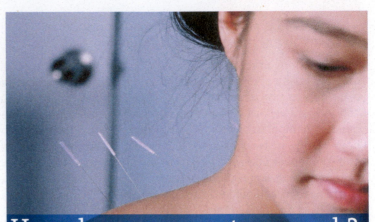

How does acupuncture work?

In acupuncture, long, thin needles are inserted into specific points along the body. This is thought to increase the flow of life-force energy, providing many physical and mental benefits.

with statistically significant improvements in pain management and other aspects of health-related quality of life for people recovering from breast cancer, as well as people with low back pain, heart failure, and other conditions.[41]

Reiki is a non-touch form of energy therapy that originated in Japan. The name is derived from the Japanese words representing "universal" and "vital energy," or *ki*. Reiki is based on the belief that by channeling *ki* to the patient, the practitioner facilitates healing.

In two related non-touch energy therapies, *therapeutic touch* and *healing touch*, the therapist attempts to perceive, through his or her hands held just above the patient's body, imbalances in the patient's energy. The therapist promotes healing by increasing the flow of the body's energies and bringing them into balance. Although studies have found at least a partial therapeutic response from non-touch energy therapies, the contribution of patient expectations and desires to the outcome (a form of placebo effect) is not known.[42]

Check Yourself

- What are two energy therapies? What do their treatments involve?

15.9 Mind and Body Practices: Mindfulness Meditation

Learning Outcome

15.9 **Summarize the benefits of mindfulness meditation.**

Another mind and body practice that is gaining wide attention is *mindfulness meditation*. It is relatively well known that the regular practice of mindfulness can reduce symptoms of stress, anxiety, and depression and improve physical conditions such as obesity, hypertension, and asthma. But the benefits of mindfulness go beyond your psychological and physical health to intellectual health and even academic success.

A growing body of research links the long-term practice of mindfulness meditation to improvements in both the structure and function of the brain. Over time, mindfulness meditation appears to preserve and even enhance the integrity and connectivity of nerve cells in the white matter of the brain, thereby helping to reduce the amount of age-related brain tissue degeneration that takes place.

In particular, through the practice of mindfulness meditation the prefrontal cortex—the part of the brain associated with decision making and concentration—enlarges and its connectivity to other parts of the brain increases. At the same time, the brain's fight-or-flight center, the amygdala, which is associated with fear and the stress response, appears to decrease in size, whereas its connectivity with other parts of the brain decreases. The same positive effect has been found for brain regions involved in the perception of pain.[43]

Even among novices, mindfulness meditation has been shown to boost cognitive skills, leading to better classroom performance. In one study, university students who participated in a one-semester mindfulness meditation course experienced significant improvements in both attention and memory, as well as the overall effectiveness of their learning.

But a full semester of mindfulness training isn't required. Another group of students who participated in a two-week mindfulness training program saw improvements in reading comprehension and working memory as well as less mind wandering.

Even a short period of mindfulness meditation has been shown to provide benefits in terms of academic performance and stress reduction. In another study, students who practiced just 6 minutes of meditation before a lecture scored higher on a quiz after the lecture than did students who did not meditate. The researchers speculated that meditation before class could be especially helpful to students who have trouble maintaining focus. A similar study found that students who engaged in a 5-minute instructor-led mindfulness meditation at the start of class reported feeling more grounded and focused on the class content.[44]

So instead of rushing into class at the last possible moment, get there 5 minutes early, close your eyes, breathe deeply, and tune in.

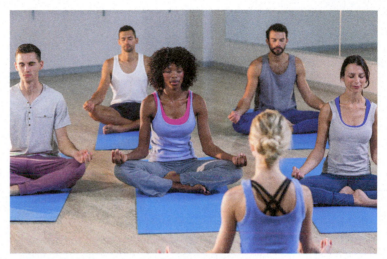

Research indicates that mindfulness meditation may be good for your brain—and for your academic performance!

You might find that you feel more focused and engaged in class, retain more afterward, and perform better on the next exam.

Several studies have shown that mindfulness may be beneficial in:

- Reducing anxiety
- Reducing age and race bias
- Preventing and treating depression
- Increasing body satisfaction and self compassion
- Improving cognition
- Helping the brain reduce distractions

See the *Forbes* article summarizing the research that appears to show that these six benefits may be a result of mindfulness meditation at this URL: https://www.forbes.com/sites/jeenacho/2016/07/14/10-scientifically-proven-benefits-of-mindfulness-and-meditation/#5167699f63ce

Check Yourself

- **What is mindfulness meditation? What do research studies say about it?**

- **Have you ever tried mindfulness meditation? Did you notice any effects from it?**

Natural Products and Dietary Supplements

15.10 Explain why caution is important in using natural products and dietary supplements.

Natural products include functional foods and dietary supplements. They are the most commonly used and perhaps the most controversial of complementary health approaches because of the sheer number of options available, the many claims that are made about their effects, and the fact that they do not undergo FDA approval.

The FDA has not developed a definition for the term *natural* and cautions consumers to avoid assuming that any food or dietary supplement claiming to be "natural" is safe.[45] In recent years, dietary supplements have caused a variety of health problems, such as liver damage, heart problems, and miscarriage, and some have been found to be contaminated with bacteria, toxic metals, hidden drug ingredients, and grass, gluten, or other potential allergens. When seeking out supplements, choose those labeled with the U.S. Pharmacopeia Verified Mark (**Figure 15.3**)—a label that means that what it says on the bottle is in the bottle, that the supplement doesn't contain unsafe levels of contaminants, and that the product was created with well-controlled, sanitary manufacturing processes.[46]

The NCCIH "Alerts and Advisories" web page frequently releases notifications of natural products that are contaminated or contain hidden drug ingredients. In 2017, for example, the FDA recalled three weight-loss supplements containing sibutramine, a controlled substance linked to life-threatening surges in blood pressure and pulse, and a fourth containing ephedra, an herb banned for its association with heart attack, stroke, and sudden death.[47] Moreover, the NCCIH warns that some natural products can be dangerous when combined with prescription or OTC drugs, can disrupt the normal action of the drugs, or can cause unusual side effects.[48]

In recent years, there have been increasing media claims about the health benefits of various hormones, enzymes, and other biological and synthetic compounds. Although a few products, such

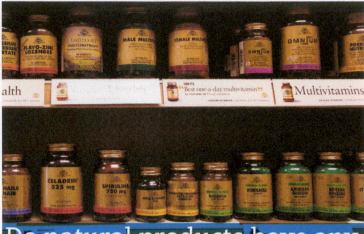

Do natural products have any risks or side effects?

Herbs and other natural products have the potential to cause negative side effects. St. John's wort, for example, has potentially dangerous interactions with some prescription antidepressants and should never be taken with them. Other herbs, such as kava, can have negative effects even when taken alone.

as melatonin (a hormone) or zinc lozenges (a mineral), have been widely studied, there is little high-quality research to support the claims of many others. **Table 15.1** gives an overview of some of the most popular natural products and dietary supplements on the market.

Always consult your primary health care provider before using dietary supplements. See the **Skills for Behavior Change** for tips on how to make smart decisions about integrating complementary therapies into your health care.

Skills for **Behavior Change**

Complementary Health Approaches and Self-Care

To help you make the best decisions about complementary health approaches, consider these pointers:

- **Research the safety and effectiveness of the product or treatment you're considering. Consult established journals and government resources such as the NCCIH, the National Library of Medicine's PubMed, and the FDA.**
- **Check the credentials of any complementary health practitioner you are considering using. Also check with your insurer to find out whether the services will be covered.**
- **Before using any complementary therapy, consult your primary health care provider. It is particularly important to talk with your provider if you are currently taking a prescription drug,**

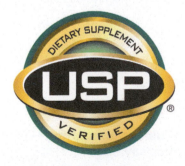

Figure 15.3 The U.S. Pharmacopeia Verified Mark

Source: Used with permission of The United States Pharmacopeial Convention, 12601 Twinbrook Parkway, Rockville, MD 20851.

Herb	Claims of Benefits	Research Findings	Potential Risks
Echinacea (purple coneflower, *Echinacea purpurea, E. angustifolia, E. pallida*)	Stimulates the immune system and helps fight infection. Used to both prevent and treat colds.	Some studies have provided evidence that taking Echinacea slightly reduces the risk for catching a cold but does not shorten duration or severity of colds.	Allergic reactions, including rashes and anaphylaxis (a life-threatening allergic reaction), increased asthma, nausea, stomach pain.
Flaxseed (*Linum usitatissimum*) and flaxseed oil	Used to treat constipation, diabetes, and hot flashes and to reduce cholesterol levels and risk of heart disease and cancer.	Flaxseed contains soluble fiber and may have a laxative effect. It has not been shown to be effective in decreasing hot flashes. Insufficient data are available on the effect of flaxseed on diabetes, cholesterol levels, heart disease, or cancer risks.	Flaxseed may have hormonal effects and should not be used during pregnancy or nursing. Can cause diarrhea. Few other side effects. Flaxseed should be taken with plenty of water.
Ginkgo (*Ginkgo biloba*)	Popularly used to prevent cognitive decline, dementia, vision and hearing problems, and vascular disease.	There is no conclusive evidence that ginkgo has any health benefits.	Headache, nausea, upset stomach, and allergic skin reactions. Ginkgo seeds are highly toxic; only products made from leaf extracts should be used.
Ginseng (*Panax ginseng*)	Claimed to increase resistance to stress, boost the immune system, slow aging, and relieve various physical and psychological disorders.	There is no conclusive evidence that ginseng has any health benefits.	Headaches, insomnia, and gastrointestinal problems are the most commonly reported adverse effects.
Green tea (*Camellia sinensis*)	Useful for reducing the risk for heart disease and some cancers, increasing mental alertness, and promoting weight loss.	Green tea contains caffeine and is thought to increase mental alertness; both green and black tea may reduce heart disease risk factors; studies of green tea and cancer are limited and results inconsistent; data suggest that green tea is not effective for weight loss.	Insomnia, anxiety, irritability, headaches, liver problems, abdominal pain.
Zinc (mineral)	Supports the immune system; lozenges, syrup, and nasal sprays are used to lessen duration and severity of cold symptoms; slows the progression of age-related macular degeneration (AMD).	Some research suggests that zinc lozenges or syrup can reduce the severity and duration of a cold if taken within 24 hours of onset of symptoms. Zinc may help to slow the progression of AMD.	Use of zinc lozenges or syrup can cause nausea. Use of nasal sprays can results in loss of sense of smell, which can be permanent. Prolonged excessive use can reduce immune function and levels of copper and HDL cholesterol.

Sources: National Center for Complementary and Integrative Health, "Herbs at a Glance," November 2016, https://nccih.nih.gov/health/herbsataglance.htm; Office of Dietary Supplements, National Institutes of Health, "Zinc: Fact Sheet for Consumers," February 2016, https://ods.od.nih.gov/factsheets/Zinc-Consumer.

have a chronic medical condition, are planning to have surgery, or are pregnant or nursing.

■ **Get your primary health care provider's approval before you combine supplements.** Also avoid combining supplements with either prescription or OTC drugs. Seek help if you notice any unusual side effects.

15.10

Check Yourself

■ **What factors should you consider when evaluating natural products, herbs, and supplements?**

■ **Why is it important to discuss any supplements you are taking with your health care provider?**

Health Insurance

15.11 Outline the structure of the U.S. health insurance system.

No matter how you're treated, chances are that you'll use some form of health insurance to pay for your care. The fundamental principle of insurance underwriting is that the cost of health care can be predicted for large populations. This is how health care **premiums** are determined. Policyholders pay premiums into a pool from which insurance companies pay claims. When you are sick or injured, the insurance company pays your care provider out of the pool regardless of your total contribution. Depending on your health and circumstances, you might never pay anything close to the actual cost of your care, or you might end up paying much more. In profit-oriented systems, insurers prefer to have healthy people in their plans who pour money into risk pools without requiring much money to be spent on their care.

Private Health Insurance

Originally, health insurance consisted solely of coverage for hospital costs (it was called *major medical*), but it was gradually extended to cover routine physicians' treatment and other services, such as dental care, vision care, and pharmaceuticals. These payment mechanisms laid the groundwork for today's steadily rising health care costs as hospitals were reimbursed for the costs of providing care plus an amount for profit. Physicians were reimbursed on a fee-for-service (indemnity) basis determined by "usual, customary, and reasonable" fees. This system encouraged physicians to charge high fees, raise them often, and perform as many procedures as possible. Until the mid- to late-twentieth century, most insurance did not cover routine or preventive services, and consumers generally waited until illness developed to see a health care provider instead of seeking preventive care. Consumers were also free to choose any provider or service they wished, including even inappropriate—and often expensive—levels of care.

To limit potential losses, private insurance companies began increasingly employing the following cost-sharing mechanisms and coverage limits:

See It! Videos

Need ideas for finding the best prices for dental care? Watch **Real Money: Saving Big on Dental Bills** in the Study Area of Mastering Health.

- *Deductibles* are payments (which can range from about $500 to $5,000 annually) you make for health care before insurance coverage kicks in to pay for eligible services.
- *Co-payments* are set amounts that you pay per service or product received, regardless of the total cost (e.g., $20 per doctor visit or per prescription filled).
- *Coinsurance* is the percentage of costs that you must pay based on the terms of the policy (e.g., 20 percent of the total bill).
- Some group plans specify a *waiting period* that cannot exceed 90 days before they will provide coverage.

- All insurers set some limits on the types of *covered services* (e.g., most exclude cosmetic surgery, private rooms, and experimental procedures).
- *Preexisting condition clauses* once limited the insurance company's liability for medical conditions that a consumer had before obtaining coverage. Under the 2010 Patient Protection and Affordable Care Act (ACA), no one can be discriminated against because of a preexisting condition.
- Some plans imposed an *annual upper limit* or *lifetime limit*, on coverage. The ACA makes this practice illegal.

Managed Care

Managed care describes a health care delivery system consisting of the following:

- A network of physicians, hospitals, and other providers and facilities linked contractually to deliver comprehensive health benefits within a predetermined budget and sharing economic risk for any budget deficit or surplus
- A budget based on an estimate of the annual cost of delivering health care for a given population
- An established set of administrative rules regarding how services are to be obtained from participating health care providers under the terms of the health plan

Many managed care plans pay their contracted health care providers a fixed monthly amount for each enrolled patient regardless

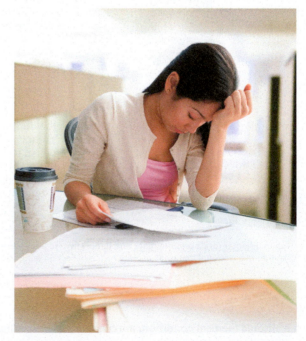

Choosing a health insurance plan can be confusing. Some things to think about include how comprehensive your coverage needs to be, how convenient your care must be, how much you are willing to spend on premiums and co-payments, what the overall cost will be, and whether the services of the plan meet your needs.

of services provided. Some plans pay health care providers a salary, and some are still fee-for-service plans. Doctors participating in managed care networks are motivated (and sometimes given incentives) to keep their patient pool healthy and avoid preventable catastrophic ailments through prevention and early intervention.

There are three common types of managed care plans in the United States:[49]

- *Health maintenance organizations (HMOs)* provide a wide range of covered health benefits (e.g., physician visits, lab tests, surgery) for a fixed amount prepaid by the patient, the employer, Medicaid, or Medicare. HMO premiums are typically the least expensive form of managed care but also the most restrictive (offering more limited choices of staff and health care facilities). Patients are required to use the plan's doctors and hospitals. Concerns have arisen about care allocation and access to services, profit-motivated medical decision making, and the degree of focus on prevention and intervention.
- *Preferred provider organizations (PPOs)* are networks of independent doctors and hospitals that contract to provide care at discounted rates. Although they often offer more provider choices than HMOs do, they are less likely to coordinate a patient's care. Members may choose to see doctors who are not on the preferred list at higher out-of-pocket costs.
- *Point of service (POS)*—a hybrid of HMO and PPO plans—provides a more familiar form of managed care for people who are used to traditional indemnity insurance, in which services are directly reimbursed. This might explain why it is among the fastest-growing of managed care plans. Under POS plans, members select an in-network PCP, but they can go to non-network providers for care without a referral and must pay the extra cost.

Other Types of Managed Care Other types of managed care include *independent practice associations (IPAs)*, in which independent physicians maintain their own offices but enroll patients from an insurer for a fee, and *exclusive provider organizations (EPOs)*, which do not cover services received outside of the EPO.

Government-Funded Programs

The federal government currently funds about 45 percent of the total U.S. health care spending, mainly through Medicare and Medicaid.[50] **Medicare** is a federal insurance program that employees and employers pay into over the course of a person's working life, a form of long-term savings plan for health insurance and care. The funds are used to cover a broad range of services, except long-term care. Medicare covers citizens or permanent residents of the United States who are 65 or older, have certain disabilities, or have permanent end-stage kidney damage. Currently, 55.3 million people receive Medicare (46.3 million people age 65 or older and 9 million disabled people).[51] As the costs of medical care have continued to increase, Medicare has placed limits on the amount of reimbursement to providers.[52] As a result, some providers no longer accept Medicare patients, and patients must pay increasing levels of out-of-pocket expenses.

Currently, Medicare is divided into two major parts. Part A helps to pay for care while in hospitals, skilled nursing facilities, hospice care, and limited home health care. Part B requires monthly payments; people with a higher income pay more than lower-income individuals. Typically, Part B covers most of your care as long as your provider or facility agrees to charge only what Medicare reimburses.

If providers charge more than Medicare allows, either the individual or a so-called *Medigap* plan must make up the difference. Consumers may purchase additional plans that offer varying degrees of dental, vision, or medication coverage.

A federal–state matching funds program, **Medicaid** provides health insurance for approximately 74 million low-income Americans, including children, pregnant women, seniors, and people with disabilities who meet eligibility requirements, based on income.[53] There are vast differences in the way Medicaid operates from state to state. The ACA provides generous federal subsidies to states that expand Medicaid coverage to all Americans with incomes up to about 133 percent of the federal poverty threshold (about $24,300 for a four-person household).[54] State compliance with the Medicaid expansion brought insurance coverage to 12.3 million previously uninsured low-income Americans between 2013 and 2015.[55]

The Children's Health Insurance Program (CHIP) provides health insurance coverage to more than 8 million uninsured children whose family income is too high to qualify for Medicaid.[56] Like Medicaid, CHIP is jointly funded by federal and state funds and is administered by state governments.

Insurance Coverage by the Numbers

For 2016, the average family's annual health insurance premium was estimated to exceed $18,142.[57] For workers employed in organizations that offer health care insurance, most of this cost is hidden: The worker pays 15 to 25 percent of the full premium, usually as a deduction from his or her paycheck, and earns lower wages in return for the remaining cost of the coverage. People who are self-employed or work in companies that do not provide group health insurance must pay their premiums independently, often at extremely high rates.

Although the vast majority of uninsured Americans are employed or are dependents of people who are employed, 28.2 million uninsured Americans (over 9 percent of Americans) do not find health insurance affordable, even with implementation of the ACA.[58] These numbers could increase significantly if the ACA is changed during this presidential term. Lack of health insurance has been associated with delayed health care and increased mortality. *Underinsurance* (i.e., the inability to pay out-of-pocket expenses despite having insurance) also may result in adverse health consequences. Among young adults age 18 to 24, nearly 15 percent lack health insurance coverage; among those age 25 to 34, nearly 16 percent lack coverage.[59]

Check Yourself

- **What are four common barriers to adequate health insurance?**

Issues Facing the Health Care System

15.12 Discuss the major challenges facing the U.S. health care system.

In 2010, Congress passed the *Patient Protection and Affordable Care Act (ACA)* to provide a means for all Americans to obtain affordable health care. In addition to increasing access to care, the ACA is addressing the high cost of care and improving the overall quality of care.

Access

The most significant factors in determining access to health care are the supply and proximity of providers and facilities and the availability of insurance coverage.

Access to Providers, Facilities, and Treatments
In 2016, there were more than 926,000 physicians in the United States.[60] However, there is an oversupply of higher-paid specialists and a shortage of lower-paid primary care physicians (family practitioners, internists, pediatricians, etc.). Moreover, most nongovernment hospitals in the United States are located in urban areas, leaving many rural communities with a lack of facilities.[61]

Managed care health plans determine access on the basis of participating providers, health plan benefits, and administrative rules, which means that consumers have little say in who treats them or what facility they can use.

The ACA and other government investments have helped in the training of many new health care providers, as well as encouraged primary care providers to set up their practices in high-need areas. Some of these efforts are as follows:

- Investing in new primary care training programs such as the National Health Service Corps and the Graduate Medical Education program
- Training new primary care providers through increased funding of medical training programs
- Supporting mental and behavioral health training to boost numbers of those practicing in mental and behavioral health

Access to High-Quality Health Insurance
Key provisions in the ACA aim to increase access to high-quality health insurance among Americans. These include the following:

- Insurers are now required to cover 15 preventive services (22 for women), such as health screenings for breast, cervical, and colorectal cancer; blood glucose and cholesterol screenings for patients of certain ages or with certain health risks; immunizations; contraception; and counseling on topics such as losing weight, quitting smoking, treating depression, and reducing alcohol use.

- Insurers are required to cover young adults on a parent's plan through age 26.
- Coverage is in place for prescription medications, including psychotropic medications.
- Americans with preexisting conditions cannot be denied coverage.
- No annual and lifetime limits on benefits are allowed.
- An online insurance marketplace helps consumers shop for and enroll in plans and to apply for federal subsidies that lower the cost of premiums for many Americans.
- Small businesses, which typically paid as much as 18 percent more than large businesses, now qualify for special tax credits to help fund insurance plans.

Even before passage of the ACA, Congress provided assistance with insurance coverage for employees who change jobs. Under the Consolidated Omnibus Budget Reconciliation Act (COBRA), former employees, retirees, spouses, and dependents have the option to continue their insurance for up to 18 months at group rates. People who enroll in COBRA do pay a higher amount than they did when they were employed because they are covering both the personal premium and the amount previously covered by the employer.

Cost

Both per capita and as a percentage of gross domestic product (GDP), the United States spends more on health care than

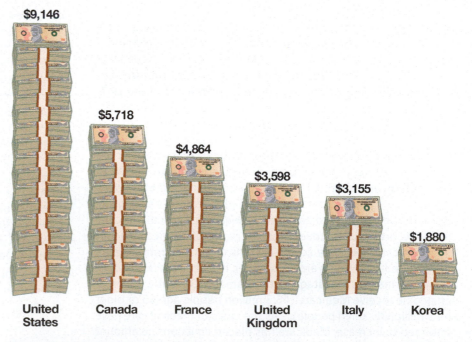

$9,146

$5,718

$4,864

$3,598

$3,155

$1,880

| United States | Canada | France | United Kingdom | Italy | Korea |

Figure 15.4 Health Care Spending per Person, 2014

Source: The World Bank, "Health Care Expenditure per Capita," 2016, http://data.worldbank.org/indicator/SH.XPD.PCAP.

Mastering Health & Nutrition Being a Good Health Care Consumer

any other nation (Figure 15.4). In 2015, our national health expenditures were estimated to exceed $3.2 trillion, about $9,990 for every man, woman, and child.[62] Health care expenditures are projected to grow by 5.6 percent each year and to climb to over 20 percent of our projected GDP by 2025.[63]

Why are U.S. health care costs so high? Many factors are involved: duplication of services; an aging population; growing rates of obesity, inactivity, and related health problems; demand for new diagnostic and treatment technologies; an emphasis on crisis-oriented care instead of prevention; physician over-treatment; and inappropriate use of services.

Our insurance system is also to blame. Currently, more than 2,000 companies provide health insurance in the United States, each with different coverage structures and administrative requirements. This lack of uniformity prevents our system from achieving the *economies of scale* (bulk purchasing at a reduced cost) and administrative efficiency realized in countries with a single-payer delivery system. On average, America's commercial insurance companies commonly spend about 16 percent of their total premiums on administrative costs.[64] These expenses contribute to the high cost of health care. See Figure 15.5 for a breakdown of how health care dollars are spent.

The ACA's 80/20 rule mandates that insurance companies that spend less than 80 percent of premium dollars on medical care in a given year now must send enrollees a rebate. Also, insurance companies now have to publicly justify their actions if they plan to raise rates by 10 percent or more.

Another way our insurance system contributes to America's high health care costs is through increasing consolidation. Excluding HMOs and other forms of managed care, just four companies dominate 83 percent of the private health insurance market, a market share that expanded from 74 percent a decade ago.[65] Since affordable insurance depends on rivalry within the market, reduced competition promotes higher premiums. Moreover, despite the fact that these large companies serve more patients within a geographic area and thus have been able to negotiate lower charges from hospitals and physicians, they have not passed this savings along to their policyholders in the form of lower premiums.[66]

Quality

The United States has several mechanisms for ensuring high-quality services. Providers are assessed according to education, licensure, certification/registration, accreditation, peer review, and the legal system of malpractice litigation. OTC and prescription medications, as well as medical devices, must be approved by the FDA. Insurance companies and the U.S. Centers for Medicare and Medicaid Services may also require a higher level of quality by linking payment to whether a practitioner is board certified, a facility is accredited, or a treatment is an approved therapy. In addition, most insurance plans now require prior authorization

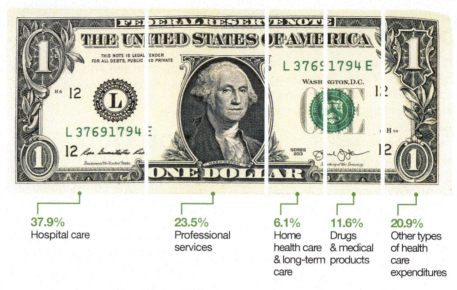

| 37.9% Hospital care | 23.5% Professional services | 6.1% Home health care & long-term care | 11.6% Drugs & medical products | 20.9% Other types of health care expenditures |

Figure 15.5 Where Do We Spend Our Health Care Dollars?

Source: U.S. Department of Health and Human Services, "Health, United States, 2015," National Center for Health Statistics, May 2016, www.cdc.gov/nchs/data/hus/hus14.pdf.

and/or second opinions, not only to reduce costs, but also to improve quality of care.

Although our health care spending far exceeds that of any other nation, we rank far below many other nations in key indicators of quality. For example, in 2017, the Central Intelligence Agency ranked the United States 42nd in life expectancy among 224 nations.[67] At a projected 79.8 years, U.S. life expectancy was a decade below that of the top-ranked country, Monaco.[68] And our *infant mortality rate*, at 5.8 deaths per every 1,000 live births, is higher than that of 56 other nations.[69]

The ACA is intended to improve the quality of health care in the United States. As a first step, in 2011, the Department of Health and Human Services released to Congress a National Strategy for Quality Improvement in Health Care. Updated annually, the National Quality Strategy emphasizes promoting the safest, most preventive, and most effective care; making care affordable for individuals, families, employers, and governments; increasing communication and coordination among providers; and ensuring that patients and families are engaged as partners in their care.[70]

Still, many health experts believe that our health care system has failed and should be replaced. As a consumer, your best strategy is to read the accumulated evidence on what is and is not working in the system and base your decisions on a rational, unbiased approach as we work to improve health care delivery in the United States.

Check Yourself

- What are three challenges faced by the U.S. health care system?

- What is the Patient Protection and Affordable Care Act (ACA)? Has it affected you personally? If so, how?

Summary

LO 15.1 Self-care and individual responsibility are key factors in reducing rising health care costs and improving health status. Planning can help you navigate health care treatment in unfamiliar situations or emergencies.

LO 15.2 Evaluate health professionals by considering their qualifications, their record of treating similar problems, and their ability to work with you.

LO 15.3 Conventional Western (allopathic) medicine is based on scientifically validated methods and procedures. Medical doctors, specialists of various kinds, nurses, and physician assistants practice allopathic medicine.

LO 15.4 Consumers need to understand the risks and benefits of prescription drugs and over-the-counter (OTC) medications. Regulations governing drug labels help to ensure that information about these products is available.

LO 15.5 People are using complementary health approaches and integrative medicine in increasing numbers.

LO 15.6 Complementary medical systems include traditional Chinese medicine (TCM), Ayurveda, homeopathy, and naturopathy.

LO 15.7–LO 15.9 Mind and body practices include manipulative therapies, energy therapies, and mindfulness meditation.

LO 15.10 The FDA does not study and approve dietary supplements or so-called natural products before they are brought to market, so there is no guarantee of their safety or effectiveness. However, the USP Verified Mark indicates that a supplement has met certain criteria for product purity and manufacturing standards.

LO 15.11 Health insurance is based on the concept of spreading risk. Insurance is provided by private insurance companies (which charge premiums) and government Medicare and Medicaid programs (which are funded by taxes). Managed care attempts to control costs by streamlining administration and stressing preventive care.

LO 15.12 Concerns about the U.S. health care system are related to access, cost, and quality. Congress passed the Patient Protection and Affordable Care Act (ACA) to address these issues.

Pop Quiz

Visit Mastering Health to personalize your study plan with Chapter Review Quizzes and Dynamic Study Modules.

LO 15.1 **1.** Which of the following conditions would be appropriately managed by self-care?
a. A persistent temperature of 104°F or higher
b. Sudden weight loss of more than a few pounds without changes in diet or exercise patterns
c. A sore throat, runny nose, and cough that persist for a few days
d. Yellowing of the skin or the whites of the eyes

LO 15.3 **2.** What medical practice is based on procedures whose objective is to heal by countering the patient's symptoms?
a. Allopathic medicine
b. Nonallopathic medicine
c. Osteopathic medicine
d. Chiropractic medicine

LO 15.5 **3.** Complementary health approaches focus on treating both the mind and the whole body, which makes them part of a
a. natural approach.
b. psychological approach.
c. holistic approach.
d. gentle approach.

LO 15.6 **4.** What type of medicine addresses imbalances of *qi*?
a. Chiropractic medicine
b. Naturopathic medicine
c. Traditional Chinese medicine
d. Homeopathic medicine

LO 15.6 **5.** The system of medicine based on the principle that "like cures like" is
a. naturopathic medicine.
b. homeopathic medicine.
c. Ayurvedic medicine.
d. chiropractic medicine.

LO 15.6 **6.** What system places equal emphasis on body, mind, and spirit and strives to restore the innate harmony of the individual?
a. Ayurvedic medicine
b. Homeopathic medicine
c. Naturopathic medicine
d. Traditional Chinese medicine

LO 15.7–15.9 **7.** Massage therapy, reiki, and mindfulness are all examples of
a. acupressure.
b. mind and body practices.
c. naturopathic medicine.
d. meditation.

LO 15.10 **8.** The USP Dietary Supplement Verified seal indicates that a supplement is
a. safe and pure.
b. effective.
c. low cost.
d. child safe.

LO 15.11 **9.** What mechanism used by private insurance companies requires that the subscriber pay a certain amount directly to the provider before the insurance company will begin paying for services?
a. Coinsurance
b. Cost sharing
c. Co-payments
d. Deductibles

LO 15.11 **10.** Andrea, 28, is a single parent on welfare. Her medical bills are paid by a federal health insurance program for the poor. This program is
a. an HMO.
b. Social Security.
c. Medicaid.
d. Medicare.

Answers to these questions can be found on page A-1. If you answered a question incorrectly, review the module identified by the Learning Outcome. For even more study tools, visit Mastering Health.

Answers to Pop Quiz Questions

Chapter 1

1. b; 2. a; 3. b; 4. a; 5. c; 6. d; 7. a; 8. c; 9. a; 10. a

Chapter 2

1. c; 2. a; 3. b; 4. a; 5. b; 6. b; 7. b; 8. b; 9. c; 10. c

Chapter 3

1. c; 2. c; 3. d; 4. b; 5. c; 6. d; 7. c; 8. c; 9. d; 10. c

Chapter 4

1. b; 2. c; 3. c; 4. d; 5. d; 6. c; 7. c; 8. a; 9. b; 10. b

Chapter 5

1. b; 2. c; 3. b; 4. b; 5. c; 6. a; 7. b; 8. d; 9. a; 10. a

Chapter 6

1. b; 2. d; 3. a; 4. c; 5. c; 6. c; 7. a; 8. c; 9. b; 10. c

Chapter 7

1. d; 2. d; 3. c; 4. a; 5. b; 6. c; 7. d; 8. c; 9. b; 10. c

Chapter 8

1. a; 2. b; 3. b; 4. a; 5. d; 6. c; 7. b; 8. d; 9. a; 10. d

Chapter 9

1. a; 2. c; 3. b; 4. b; 5. c; 6. b; 7. a; 8. a; 9. b; 10. b

Chapter 10

1. c; 2. b; 3. d; 4. c; 5. a; 6. a; 7. b; 8. a; 9. d; 10. a

Chapter 11

1. c; 2. c; 3. b; 4. a; 5. b; 6. d; 7. a; 8. c; 9. b; 10. a

Chapter 12

1. c; 2. a; 3. c; 4. a; 5. c; 6. c; 7. a; 8. c; 9. b; 10. d

Chapter 13

1. b; 2. c; 3. a; 4. b; 5. c; 6. c; 7. b; 8. b; 9. a

Chapter 14

1. d; 2. b; 3. d; 4. d; 5. a; 6. c; 7. a; 8. a; 9. b; 10. a

Chapter 15

1. c; 2. a; 3. c; 4. c; 5. b; 6. b; 7. a; 8. a; 9. d; 10. c

Glossary

abortion The termination of a pregnancy by expulsion or removal of an embryo or fetus from the uterus.

abstinence Refraining from a behavior.

accountability Accepting responsibility for personal decisions, choices, and actions.

acid deposition The acidification process that occurs when pollutants are deposited by precipitation, clouds, or directly on the land.

acquaintance rape A rape in which the rapist is known to the victim (replaces the formerly used term *date rape*).

acquired immunodeficiency syndrome (AIDS) A disease caused by a retrovirus, the human immunodeficiency virus (HIV), that attacks the immune system, reducing the number of helper T cells and leaving the victim vulnerable to infections, malignancies, and neurological disorders.

acupressure Technique of traditional Chinese medicine related to acupuncture that uses the application of pressure to selected points along the meridians to balance energy.

acupuncture Branch of traditional Chinese medicine that uses the insertion of long, thin needles to affect flow of energy (*qi*) along energy pathways (meridians) within the body.

acute stress The short-term physiological response to an immediate perceived threat.

adaptive response Form of adjustment in which the body attempts to restore homeostasis.

adaptive thermogenesis Theoretical mechanism by which the brain regulates metabolic activity according to caloric intake.

addiction Persistent, compulsive dependence on a behavior or substance, including mood-altering behaviors or activities, despite ongoing negative consequences.

aerobic capacity (or power) The functional status of the cardiorespiratory system; refers specifically to the volume of oxygen the muscles consume during exercise.

aerobic exercise Any type of exercise that requires oxygen to make energy for activity.

aggravated rape Rape that involves one or multiple attackers, strangers, weapons, or physical beating.

alcohol abuse Use of alcohol that interferes with work, school, or personal relationships or that entails violations of the law.

alcohol poisoning A potentially lethal blood alcohol concentration that inhibits the brain's ability to control consciousness, respiration, and heart rate; usually occurs as a result of drinking a large amount of alcohol in a short period of time. Also known as *acute alcohol intoxication*.

alcoholic hepatitis A condition resulting from prolonged use of alcohol in which the liver is inflamed; can be fatal.

Alcoholics Anonymous (AA) An organization whose goal is to help alcoholics stop drinking; includes auxiliary branches such as Al-Anon and Alateen.

alcoholism (alcohol dependency) Condition in which personal and health problems related to alcohol use are severe and stopping alcohol use results in withdrawal symptoms.

allopathic medicine Conventional, Western medical practice; in theory, based on scientifically validated methods and procedures.

allostatic load Wear and tear on the body caused by prolonged or excessive stress responses.

alternative (whole) medical systems Specific theories of health and balance that have developed outside the influence of conventional medicine.

alternative insemination A fertilization procedure accomplished by depositing semen from a partner or donor into a woman's vagina via a thin tube.

alternative medicine Treatment used in place of conventional medicine.

altruism The giving of oneself out of genuine concern for others.

Alzheimer's disease (AD) A chronic condition involving changes in nerve fibers of the brain that results in mental deterioration.

amino acids The nitrogen-containing building blocks of protein.

amniocentesis A medical test in which a small amount of fluid is drawn from the amniotic sac to test for Down syndrome and other genetic diseases.

amniotic sac The protective pouch surrounding the fetus.

amphetamines A large and varied group of synthetic agents that stimulate the central nervous system.

anabolic steroids Artificial forms of the hormone testosterone that promote muscle growth and strength.

anal intercourse The insertion of the penis into the anus.

androgyny High levels of traditional masculine and feminine traits in a single person.

aneurysm A weakened blood vessel that may bulge under pressure and, in severe cases, burst.

angina pectoris Chest pain occurring as a result of reduced oxygen flow to the heart.

angiography A technique for examining blockages in heart arteries.

angioplasty A technique in which a catheter with a balloon at the tip is inserted into a clogged artery; the balloon is inflated to flatten fatty deposits against artery walls and a stent is typically inserted to keep the artery open.

anorexia nervosa An eating disorder characterized by deliberate food restriction, self-starvation or extreme exercising to achieve weight loss, and an extremely distorted body image.

antagonism A drug interaction in which two drugs compete for the same available receptors, potentially blocking each other's actions.

antibiotic resistance The ability of bacteria or other microbes to withstand the effects of an antibiotic.

antibiotics Medicines used to kill microorganisms, such as bacteria.

antibodies Substances produced by the body that are individually matched to specific antigens.

antigen Substance capable of triggering an immune response.

antioxidants Substances believed to protect against oxidative stress and resultant tissue damage at the cellular level.

anxiety disorders Mental illnesses characterized by persistent feelings of threat and worry in coping with everyday problems.

appetite The desire to eat; normally accompanies hunger but is more psychological than physiological.

appraisal The interpretation and evaluation of information provided to the brain by the senses.

arrhythmia An irregularity in heartbeat.

arteries Vessels that carry blood away from the heart to other regions of the body.

arterioles Branches of the arteries.

asbestos A mineral compound that separates into stringy fibers and lodges in the lungs, where it can cause various diseases.

asthma A long-term, chronic inflammatory disorder that causes tiny airways in the lung to spasm in response to triggers. Many cases of asthma are triggered by environmental pollutants.

atherosclerosis Condition characterized by deposits of fatty substances (plaque) on the inner lining of an artery.

atria (singular: *atrium*) The heart's two upper chambers, which receive blood.

attention-deficit/hyperactivity disorder (ADHD) A learning disability characterized by hyperactivity and distraction.

autism spectrum disorder (ASD) A neurodevelopmental disorder characterized by difficulty mastering communication and social behavior skills.

autoerotic behaviors Sexual self-stimulation.

autoimmune disease Disease caused by an overactive immune response against the body's own cells.

autoinoculate Transmission of a pathogen from one part of your body to another part.

autonomic nervous system (ANS) The portion of the central nervous system regulating body functions that a person does not normally consciously control.

Ayurveda (Ayurvedic medicine) A comprehensive system of medicine, derived largely from ancient India, that places equal emphasis on the body, mind, and spirit, and strives to restore the body's innate harmony through diet, exercise, meditation, herbs, massage, exposure to sunlight, and controlled breathing.

background distressors Environmental stressors of which people are often unaware.

bacteria (singular: *bacterium*) Simple, single-celled microscopic organisms; about 100 known species of bacteria cause disease in humans.

barbiturates Drugs that depress the central nervous system and have sedating, hypnotic, and anesthetic effects.

barrier methods Contraceptive methods that block the meeting of egg and sperm by means of a physical barrier (such as condom, diaphragm, or cervical cap), a chemical barrier (such as spermicide), or both.

basal metabolic rate (BMR) The rate of energy expenditure by a body at complete rest in a neutral environment.

belief Appraisal of the relationship between some object, action, or idea and some attribute of that object, action, or idea.

benign Harmless; refers to a noncancerous tumor.

benzodiazepines A class of central nervous system depressant drugs with sedative, hypnotic, and muscle relaxant effects.

bereavement The loss or deprivation experienced by a survivor when a loved one dies.

bidis Hand-rolled flavored cigarettes.

binge drinking A *binge* is a pattern of drinking alcohol that brings blood alcohol concentration (BAC) to 0.08 gram-percent or above; for a typical adult, this pattern corresponds to consuming five or more drinks (male) or four or more drinks (female) in about 2 hours.

binge-eating disorder A type of eating disorder characterized by gorging on food once a week or more, but not typically followed by a purge.

biofeedback A technique using a machine to self-monitor physical responses to stress.

biopsy Removal and examination of a tissue sample to determine if a cancer is present.

biopsychosocial model of addiction Theory of the relationship between an addict's biological (genetic) nature and psychological and environmental influences.

bipolar disorder A form of mood disorder characterized by alternating mania and depression; also called *manic depression*.

bisexual Experiencing attraction to and preference for sexual activity with people of both sexes.

blood alcohol concentration (BAC) The ratio of alcohol to total blood volume; the factor used to measure the physiological and behavioral effects of alcohol.

body composition Describes the relative proportions of fat and fat-free (muscle, bone, water, organs) tissues in the body.

body dysmorphic disorder (BDD) A psychological disorder characterized by an obsession with one's appearance and a distorted view of one's body or with a minor or imagined flaw in appearance.

body image How you see yourself in your mind, what you believe about your appearance, and how you feel about your body.

body mass index (BMI) A number calculated from a person's weight and height that is used to assess risk for possible present or future health problems.

bulimia nervosa An eating disorder characterized by binge eating followed by inappropriate purging measures or compensatory behavior, such as vomiting or excessive exercise, to prevent weight gain.

caffeine A stimulant drug that is legal in the United States and found in many coffees, teas, chocolates, energy drinks, and certain medication.

calorie A unit of measure that indicates the amount of energy obtained from a particular food.

cancer A large group of diseases characterized by the uncontrolled growth and spread of abnormal cells.

candidiasis Yeast-like fungal infection often transmitted sexually; also called moniliasis or yeast infection.

capillaries Minute blood vessels that branch out from the arterioles and venules; their thin walls permit exchange of oxygen, carbon dioxide, nutrients, and waste products among body cells.

carbohydrates Basic nutrients that supply the body with glucose, the energy form most commonly used to sustain normal activity.

carbon dioxide (CO₂) Gas created by the combustion of fossil fuels, exhaled by animals, and used by plants for photosynthesis; the primary greenhouse gas in Earth's atmosphere.

carbon footprint The amount of greenhouse gases produced by an individual, nation, or other entity, usually expressed in equivalent tons of carbon dioxide emissions.

carbon monoxide A gas found in cigarette smoke that binds at oxygen receptor sites in the blood.

carcinogens Cancer-causing agents.

cardiometabolic risks Physical and biochemical changes that are risk factors for the development of cardiovascular disease and type 2 diabetes.

cardiorespiratory fitness The ability of the heart, lungs, and blood vessels to supply oxygen to skeletal muscles during sustained physical activity.

cardiovascular disease (CVD) Diseases of the heart and blood vessels.

cardiovascular system Organ system, consisting of the heart and blood vessels, that transports nutrients, oxygen, hormones, metabolic wastes, and enzymes throughout the body.

carotenoids Fat-soluble plant pigments with antioxidant properties.

carpal tunnel syndrome (CTS) A common occupational injury in which the median nerve in the wrist becomes irritated, causing numbness, tingling, and pain in the fingers and hands.

carrying capacity of the earth The largest population that can be supported indefinitely given the resources available in the environment.

celiac disease An inherited autoimmune disorder affecting the digestive process of the small intestine and triggered by the consumption of gluten.

celibacy State of abstaining from sexual activity.

cell-mediated immunity Aspect of immunity that is mediated by specialized white blood cells that attack pathogens and antigens directly.

cervical cap A small cup made of latex or silicone that is designed to fit snugly over the entire cervix.

cervix Lower end of the uterus that opens into the vagina.

cesarean section (C-section) Surgical birthing procedure in which a baby is removed through an incision made in the mother's abdominal wall and uterus.

chancre Sore often found at the site of syphilis infection.

chemotherapy The use of drugs to kill cancerous cells.

chewing tobacco A stringy type of tobacco that is placed in the mouth and then sucked or chewed.

chickenpox A highly infectious disease caused by the herpes varicella zoster virus.

child abuse Deliberate, intentional words or actions that cause harm, potential for harm, or threat of harm to a child.

child maltreatment Any act or series of acts of commission or omission by a parent or caregiver that results in harm, potential for harm, or threat of harm to a child.

chiropractic medicine Manipulation of the spine and neuromuscular structure to promote proper energy flow.

chlamydia Bacterially caused STI of the urogenital tract; most commonly reported STI in the United States.

chlorofluorocarbons (CFCs) Chemicals that contribute to the depletion of the atmospheric ozone layer.

cholesterol A form of fat circulating in the blood that can accumulate on the inner walls of arteries, causing a narrowing of the channel through which blood flows.

chorionic villus sampling (CVS) A prenatal test that involves snipping tissue from the fetal sac to be analyzed for genetic defects.

chronic disease A disease that typically begins slowly, progresses, and persists, with a variety of signs and symptoms that can be treated but not cured by medication.

chronic mood disorder Experience of persistent emotional states, such as sadness, despair, and hopelessness.

chronic stress An ongoing state of physiological arousal in response to ongoing or numerous perceived threats.

cirrhosis The last stage of liver disease associated with chronic heavy alcohol use, during which liver cells die and damage becomes permanent.

climate change A shift in typical weather patterns that includes fluctuations in seasonal temperatures, rain or snowfall amounts, and the occurrence of catastrophic storms.

clitoris A pea-sized nodule of tissue located at the top of the labia minora; central to sexual arousal in women.

club drugs Synthetic analogs (drugs that produce similar effects) of existing illicit drugs.

codependence A self-defeating relationship pattern in which a person is controlled by an addict's addictive behavior.

cognitive restructuring The modification of thoughts, ideas, and beliefs that contribute to stress.

cohabitation Living together without being married.

collateral circulation Adaptation of the heart to partial damage accomplished by rerouting needed blood through unused or underused blood vessels while the damaged heart muscle heals.

collective violence Violence perpetrated by groups against other groups.

common-law marriage Cohabitation lasting a designated period of time (usually 7 years) that is considered legally binding in some states.

comorbidities The presence of one or more diseases at the same time.

complementary medicine Treatment used in conjunction with conventional medicine.

complete (high-quality) proteins Proteins that contain all nine of the essential amino acids.

complex carbohydrates A major type of carbohydrate that provides sustained energy.

compulsion Preoccupation with a behavior and an overwhelming need to perform it.

compulsive buying disorder People who are preoccupied with shopping and spending.

compulsive exercise Disorder characterized by a compulsion to engage in excessive amounts of exercise and feelings of guilt and anxiety if the level of exercise is perceived as inadequate.

compulsive shoppers People who are preoccupied with shopping and spending.

computerized axial tomography (CAT) scan A scan by a machine that uses radiation to view internal organs not normally visible in X-rays.

conception The fertilization of an ovum by a sperm.

conflict An emotional state that arises when the behavior of one person interferes with the behavior of another.

conflict resolution A concerted effort by all parties to constructively resolve points of contention.

congeners Forms of alcohol that are metabolized more slowly than ethanol and produce toxic by-products.

congenital cardiovascular defect Cardiovascular problem that is present at birth.

congestive heart failure (CHF) or heart failure (HF) An abnormal cardiovascular condition that reflects impaired cardiac pumping and blood flow; pooling blood leads to congestion in body tissues.

consummate love A relationship that combines intimacy, compassion, and commitment.

contemplation A practice of concentrating the mind on a spiritual or ethical question or subject, a view of the natural world, or an icon or other image representative of divinity.

contraception (birth control) Methods of preventing conception.

contraceptive sponge Contraceptive device, made of polyurethane foam and containing nonoxynol-9, that fits over the cervix to create a barrier against sperm.

coping Managing events or conditions to lessen the physical or psychological effects of excess stress.

core strength Strength in the body's core muscles, including deep back and abdominal muscles that attach to the spine and pelvis.

coronary artery disease (CAD) A narrowing or blockage of coronary arteries, usually caused by atherosclerotic plaque buildup.

coronary bypass surgery A surgical technique whereby a blood vessel taken from another part of the body is implanted to bypass a clogged coronary artery.

coronary heart disease (CHD) A narrowing of the small blood vessels that supply blood to the heart.

coronary thrombosis A blood clot occurring in a coronary artery.

corpus luteum A body of cells that forms from the remains of the graafian follicle following ovulation; it secretes estrogen and progesterone during the second half of the menstrual cycle.

cortisol Hormone released by the adrenal glands that makes stored nutrients more readily available to meet energy demands.

countering Substituting a desired behavior for an undesirable one.

Cowper's glands Glands that secrete a fluid that lubricates the urethra and neutralizes any acid remaining in the urethra after urination.

cross-tolerance Development of a physiological tolerance to one drug that reduces the effects of another, similar drug.

cunnilingus Oral stimulation of a woman's genitals.

Daily Values (DVs) Percentages listed as "% DV" on food and supplement labels; made up of the RDIs and DRVs together.

defensive medicine The use of medical practices designed to avert the possibility of malpractice suits in the future.

dehydration Abnormal depletion of body fluids; a result of lack of water.

delirium tremens (DTs) A state of confusion brought on by withdrawal from alcohol; symptoms include hallucinations, anxiety, and trembling.

dementias Progressive brain impairments that interfere with memory and normal intellectual functioning.

denial Inability to perceive or accurately interpret the self-destructive effects of the addictive behavior.

dentist Specialist who diagnoses and treats diseases of the teeth, gums, and oral cavity.

Depo-Provera, Depo-subQ Provera Injectable method of birth control that lasts for 3 months.

depressants Drugs that slow down the activity of the central nervous and muscular systems and cause sleepiness or calmness.

determinants of health The range of personal, social, economic, and environmental factors that influence health status.

detoxification The early abstinence period during which an addict adjusts physically and cognitively to being free from the influences of the addiction.

diabetes mellitus A group of diseases characterized by elevated blood glucose levels.

diaphragm A latex, cup-shaped device designed to cover the cervix and block access to the uterus; should always be used with spermicide.

diastolic blood pressure The lower number in the fraction that measures blood pressure, indicating pressure on arterial walls during the relaxation phase of heart activity.

dietary supplements Vitamins and minerals taken by mouth that are intended to supplement existing diets.

digestive process The process by which the body breaks down foods and either absorbs or excretes them.

dilation and evacuation (D&E) An abortion technique that uses a combination of instruments and vacuum aspiration.

dioxins Highly toxic chlorinated hydrocarbons found in herbicides and produced during certain industrial processes.

dipping Placing a small amount of chewing tobacco between the front lip and teeth for rapid nicotine absorption.

disaccharides Combinations of two monosaccharides.

discrimination Actions that deny equal treatment or opportunities to a group, often based on prejudice.

disease prevention Actions or behaviors designed to keep people from getting sick.

disordered eating A pattern of atypical eating behaviors that is used to achieve or maintain a lower body weight.

gambling disorder Compulsive gambling that cannot be controlled.

distillation The process whereby mash is subjected to high temperatures to release alcohol vapors, which are then condensed and mixed with water to make the final product.

distress Stress that can have a detrimental effect on health; negative stress.

domestic violence The use of force to control and maintain power over another person in the home environment, including both actual harm and the threat of harm.

downshifting Taking a step back and simplifying a lifestyle that has become focused on trying to keep up, is hectic, and is packed with pressure and stress; also known as voluntary simplicity.

drug abuse Excessive use of a drug.

drug misuse Use of a drug for a purpose for which it was not intended.

drug resistance That which occurs when microbes, such as bacteria, viruses, or other pathogens, grow and proliferate in the presence of chemicals that would normally kill them or slow their growth.

dysfunctional families Families in which there is violence; physical, emotional, or sexual abuse; parental discord; or other negative family interactions.

dysmenorrhea Condition of pain or discomfort in the lower abdomen just before or after menstruation.

dyslexia A language-based learning disorder characterized by reading, writing, and spelling problems.

dyspareunia Pain experienced by women during intercourse.

dysthymic disorder (dysthymia) A type of depression that is milder and harder to recognize than major depression; chronic and often characterized by fatigue, pessimism, or a short temper.

eating disorder A psychiatric disorder characterized by severe disturbances in body image and eating behaviors.

ecological or public health model A view of health in which diseases and other negative health events are seen as the result of an individual's interaction with his or her social and physical environment.

ecosystem The collection of physical (nonliving) and biological (living) components of an environment and the relationships between them.

ectopic pregnancy Dangerous condition that results from the implantation of a fertilized egg outside the uterus, usually in a fallopian tube.

ejaculation The propulsion of semen from the penis.

ejaculatory duct Tube formed by the junction of the seminal vesicle and the vas deferens that carries semen to the urethra.

electrocardiogram (ECG) A record of the electrical activity of the heart; may be measured during a stress test.

embolus A blood clot that becomes dislodged from a blood vessel wall and moves through the circulatory system.

embryo The fertilized egg from conception through the eighth week of development.

emergency contraceptive pills (ECPs) Drugs taken within 3 to 5 days after unprotected intercourse to prevent fertilization or implantation.

emotional health The feeling part of psychosocial health; includes your emotional reactions to life.

emotional intelligence A person's ability to identify, understand, use, and manage emotional states effectively and interact positively with others in relationships.

emotions Intensified feelings or complex patterns of feelings.

emphysema A chronic lung disease in which the tiny air sacs in the lungs are destroyed, making breathing difficult.

enablers People who knowingly or unknowingly protect addicts from the natural consequences of their behavior.

endemic Describing a disease that is always present to some degree.

endometriosis Disorder in which endometrial tissue establishes itself outside the uterus.

endometrium Soft, spongy matter that makes up the uterine lining.

endorphins Opioid-like hormones that are manufactured in the human body and contribute to natural feelings of well-being.

energy medicine Therapies using energy fields, such as magnetic fields or biofields.

enhanced greenhouse effect The warming of Earth's surface as a direct result of human activities that release greenhouse gases into the atmosphere, trapping more of the sun's radiation than is normal.

environmental stewardship A responsibility for environmental quality shared by all those whose actions affect the environment.

environmental tobacco smoke (ETS) Smoke from tobacco products, including sidestream and mainstream smoke; commonly called *secondhand smoke*.

epidemic Disease outbreak that affects many people in a community or region at the same time.

epididymis The duct system atop the testis where sperm mature.

epinephrine Also called *adrenaline*, a hormone that stimulates body systems in response to stress.

episodic acute stress The state of regularly reacting with wild, acute stress about one thing or another.

erectile dysfunction (ED) Difficulty in achieving or maintaining a penile erection sufficient for intercourse.

ergogenic drug Substance believed to enhance athletic performance.

erogenous zones Areas of the body that, when touched, lead to sexual arousal.

essential amino acids Nine of the basic nitrogen-containing building blocks of protein, which must be obtained from foods to ensure health.

estrogens Hormones secreted by the ovaries that control the menstrual cycle.

ethnoviolence Violence directed at persons affiliated with a particular ethnic group.

ethyl alcohol (ethanol) An addictive drug produced by fermentation and found in many beverages.

eustress Stress that presents opportunities for personal growth; positive stress.

evidence-based medicine Decisions regarding patient care based on clinical expertise, patient values, and current best scientific evidence.

exercise Planned, structured, and repetitive bodily movement done to improve or maintain one or more components of physical fitness.

exercise addicts People who exercise compulsively to try to meet needs of nurturance, intimacy, self-esteem, and self-competency.

exercise metabolic rate (EMR) The energy expenditure that occurs during exercise.

extensively drug-resistant TB (XDR-TB) Form of TB that is resistant to nearly all existing antibiotics.

fallopian tubes (oviducts) Tubes that extend from near the ovaries to the uterus; site of fertilization and passageway for fertilized eggs.

family of origin People present in the household during a child's first years of life—usually parents and siblings.

fats Basic nutrients composed of carbon and hydrogen atoms; needed for the proper functioning of cells, insulation of body organs against shock, maintenance of body temperature, and healthy skin and hair.

fellatio Oral stimulation of a man's genitals.

female athlete triad A syndrome of three interrelated health problems seen in some female athletes: disordered eating, amenorrhea, and poor bone density.

female condom A single-use polyurethane sheath for internal use during vaginal or anal intercourse to catch semen on ejaculation.

female orgasmic disorder A woman's inability to achieve orgasm.

fermentation The process whereby yeast organisms break down plant sugars to yield ethanol.

fertility A person's ability to reproduce.

fertility awareness methods (FAMs) Several types of birth control that require alteration of sexual behavior rather than chemical or physical intervention in the reproductive process.

fertility rate Average number of births a female in a certain population has during her reproductive years.

fetal alcohol syndrome (FAS) A pattern of birth defects, learning, and behavioral problems in a child caused by the mother's alcohol consumption during pregnancy.

fetus A developing human from the ninth week until birth.

fiber The indigestible portion of plant foods that helps move food through the digestive system and softens stools by absorbing water.

fibrillation A sporadic, quivering pattern of heartbeat that results in extreme inefficiency in moving blood through the cardiovascular system.

fight-or-flight response Physiological arousal response in which the body prepares to combat or escape a real or perceived threat.

FITT Acronym for Frequency, Intensity, Time, and Type; the terms that describe the essential components of a program or plan to improve a health-related component of physical fitness.

flexibility The range of motion, or the amount of movement possible, at a particular joint or series of joints.

foams Spermicide packaged in aerosol cans and inserted into the vagina with an applicator.

food allergy Overreaction by the body to normally harmless proteins, which are perceived as allergens. In response, the body produces antibodies, triggering allergic symptoms.

food intolerance Adverse effects resulting when people who lack the digestive chemicals needed to break down certain substances eat those substances.

food irradiation Treating foods with gamma radiation from radioactive cobalt, cesium, or other sources of X-rays to kill microorganisms.

formaldehyde A colorless, strong-smelling gas released through off-gassing; causes respiratory and other health problems.

fossil fuels Carbon-based material used for energy; includes oil, coal, and natural gas.

frequency As part of the FITT prescription, refers to how many days per week a person should exercise to improve a component of physical fitness.

functional foods Foods believed to have specific health benefits and/or to prevent disease.

fungi A group of multicellular and unicellular organisms that obtain their food by infiltrating the bodies of other organisms, both living and dead; several microscopic varieties are pathogenic.

gay Sexual orientation involving primary attraction to people of the same sex.

gender The psychological condition of being feminine or masculine as defined by the society in which one lives.

gender identity Personal sense or awareness of being masculine or feminine, a male or a female.

gender roles Expressions of maleness or femaleness in everyday life.

gender-role stereotypes Generalizations concerning how men and women should express themselves and the characteristics each possesses.

gene Discrete segment of DNA in a chromosome that stores the code for assembling a particular body protein.

general adaptation syndrome (GAS) The pattern followed in the physiological response to stress, consisting of the alarm, resistance, and exhaustion phases.

generalized anxiety disorder (GAD) A constant sense of worry that may cause restlessness, difficulty in concentrating, tension, and other symptoms.

generic drugs Medications sold under chemical names rather than brand names.

genetically modified (GM) foods Foods derived from organisms whose DNA has been altered using genetic engineering techniques.

genital herpes STI caused by the herpes simplex virus.

genital warts Warts that appear in the genital area or the anus; caused by the human papillomavirus (HPV).

gestational diabetes Form of diabetes mellitus in which women who have never had diabetes before have high blood sugar (glucose) levels during pregnancy.

global warming A type of climate change in which average temperatures increase.

globesity High number of countries and large percentages of populations within countries who are classified as obese.

glycemic index (GI) Compares foods with the same amount of carbohydrates and determines how much each raises blood glucose levels.

glycemic load (GL) A food's glycemic index (potential to raise blood glucose) multiplied by the grams of carbohydrates it provides, divided by 100.

glycogen The polysaccharide form in which glucose is stored in the liver and, to a lesser extent, in muscles.

gonads The reproductive organs in a male (testes) or female (ovaries) that produce sperm (male), eggs (female), and sex hormones.

gonorrhea Second most common bacterial STI in the United States; if untreated, may cause sterility.

graafian follicle Mature ovarian follicle that contains a fully developed ovum, or egg.

greenhouse gases Gases that accumulate in the atmosphere, where they contribute to global warming by trapping heat near Earth's surface.

grief An individual's reaction to significant loss, including one's own impending death, the death of a loved one, or a quasi-death experience; grief can involve mental, physical, social, or emotional responses.

habit A repeated behavior in which the repetition may be unconscious.

hallucinogens Substances capable of creating auditory or visual distortions and unusual changes in mood, thoughts, and feelings.

hangover The physiological reaction to excessive drinking, including headache, upset stomach, anxiety, depression, diarrhea, and thirst.

hate crime A crime targeted against a particular societal group and motivated by bias against that group.

hazardous waste Waste that, due to its toxic properties, poses a hazard to humans or to the environment.

health The ever-changing process of achieving individual potential in the physical, social, emotional, mental, spiritual, and environmental dimensions.

health belief model (HBM) Model for explaining how beliefs may influence behaviors.

health disparities Differences in the incidence, prevalence, mortality, and burden of diseases and other health conditions among specific population groups.

health promotion The combined educational, organizational, procedural, environmental, social, and financial supports that help individuals and groups reduce negative health behaviors and promote positive change.

healthy life expectancy Expected number of years of full health remaining at a given age, such as at birth.

healthy weight Having a BMI of 18.5 to 24.9, the range of lowest statistical health risk.

heat cramps Involuntary and forcible muscle contractions that occur during or following exercise in hot and/or humid weather.

heat exhaustion A heat stress illness caused by significant dehydration resulting from exercise in hot and/or humid conditions.

heatstroke A deadly heat stress illness resulting from dehydration and overexertion in hot and/or humid conditions.

hepatitis A viral disease in which the liver becomes inflamed, producing symptoms such as fever, headache, and possibly jaundice.

herpes A general term for infections characterized by sores or eruptions on the skin caused by the herpes simplex virus.

herpes gladiatorum A skin infection caused by the herpes simplex type 1 virus and seen among athletes participating in contact sports.

heterosexual Experiencing primary attraction to and preference for sexual activity with people of the opposite sex.

high-density lipoproteins (HDLs) Compounds that facilitate the transport of cholesterol in the blood to the liver for metabolism and elimination from the body.

holistic Relating to or concerned with the whole body and the interactions of systems, rather than treatment of individual parts.

homeopathic medicine Unconventional Western system of medicine based on the principle that "like cures like."

homeostasis A balanced physiological state in which all the body's systems function smoothly.

homicide Death that results from intent to injure or kill.

homosexual Experiencing primary attraction to and preference for sexual activity with people of the same sex.

hormonal contraception Contraceptive methods that introduce synthetic hormones into the woman's system to prevent ovulation, thicken cervical mucus, or prevent a fertilized egg from implanting.

hormone replacement therapy or menopausal hormone therapy Use of synthetic or animal estrogens and progesterone to compensate for decreases in estrogens in a woman's body during menopause.

hostility Cognitive, affective, and behavioral tendencies toward anger and cynicism.

human chorionic gonadotropin (HCG) Hormone detectable in blood or urine samples of a mother within the first few weeks of pregnancy.

human immunodeficiency virus (HIV) The virus that causes AIDS by infecting helper T cells.

human papillomavirus (HPV) A group of viruses, many of which are transmitted sexually; some types of HPV can cause genital warts or cervical cancer.

humoral immunity Aspect of immunity that is mediated by antibodies secreted by white blood cells.

hunger The physiological impulse to seek food, prompted by the lack or shortage of basic foods needed to provide the energy and nutrients that support health.

hymen Thin tissue covering the vaginal opening in some women.

hyperglycemia Elevated blood glucose level.

hyperplasia A condition characterized by an excessive number of fat cells.

hypertension Sustained elevated blood pressure.

hypertrophy The act of swelling or increasing in size, as with cells.

hypnosis A trancelike state that allows people to become unusually responsive to suggestion.

hyponatremia or water intoxication The overconsumption of water, which leads to a dilution of sodium concentration in the blood with potentially fatal results.

hypothalamus An area of the brain located near the pituitary gland; works in conjunction with the pituitary gland to control reproductive functions. It also controls the sympathetic nervous system and directs the stress response.

hypothermia Potentially fatal condition caused by abnormally low body core temperature.

hysterectomy Surgical removal of the uterus.

hysterotomy The surgical removal of the fetus from the uterus.

imagined rehearsal Practicing, through mental imagery, to become better able to perform an event in actuality.

immunocompetence The ability of the immune system to respond to attack.

immunocompromised Having an immune system that is impaired.

Nexplanon (Implanon) A plastic capsule inserted in a woman's upper arm that releases a low dose of progestin to prevent pregnancy.

in vitro fertilization Fertilization of an egg in a nutrient medium and subsequent transfer back to the mother's body.

incomplete proteins Proteins that lack one or more of the essential amino acids.

incubation period The time between exposure to a disease and the appearance of symptoms.

induction abortion An abortion technique in which chemicals are injected into the uterus through the uterine wall; labor begins, and the woman delivers a dead fetus.

infection The state of pathogens being established in or on a host and causing disease.

infertility Inability to conceive after a year or more of trying.

influenza A common viral disease of the respiratory tract.

inhalants Products that are sniffed or inhaled in order to produce highs.

inhalation The introduction of drugs through the respiratory tract via sniffing, smoking, or inhaling.

inhibited sexual desire Lack of sexual appetite or lack of interest and pleasure in sexual activity.

inhibition A drug interaction in which the effects of one drug are eliminated or reduced by the presence of another drug at the same receptor site.

injection The introduction of drugs into the body via a hypodermic needle.

insulin Hormone secreted by the pancreas and required by body cells for the uptake and storage of glucose.

insulin resistance State in which body cells fail to respond to the effects of insulin; obesity increases the risk that cells will become insulin resistant.

intact dilation and extraction (D&X) A late-term abortion procedure in which the body of the fetus is extracted up to the head and then the contents of the cranium are aspirated.

intensity As part of the FITT prescription, refers to how hard or how much effort is needed when a person exercises to improve a component of physical fitness.

intentional injuries Injury, death, or psychological harm inflicted with the intent to harm.

Internet addiction The compulsive use of the computer, personal digital device, cell phone, or other forms of technology to access the Internet for activities such as e-mail, games, shopping, social networking, or blogging.

interpersonal violence Violence inflicted against one individual by another, or by a small group of others.

intersex General term for a variety of conditions in which a person is born with reproductive or sexual anatomy that doesn't seem to fit the typical definitions of female or male. Also termed disorders of sexual development (DSDs).

intervention A planned process of confronting an addict carried out by close family, friends, and a professional counselor.

intimate partner violence (IPV) Violent behavior, including physical violence, sexual violence, threats, and emotional abuse, occurring between current or former spouses or dating partners.

intimate relationships Relationships with family members, friends, and romantic partners, characterized by behavioral interdependence, need fulfillment, emotional attachment, and emotional availability.

intolerance A drug interaction in which the combination of two or more drugs in the body produces extremely uncomfortable reactions.

intrauterine device (IUD) A device, often T-shaped, that is implanted in the uterus to prevent pregnancy.

ionizing radiation Electromagnetic waves and particles having short wavelengths and energy high enough to ionize atoms.

ischemia Reduced oxygen supply to a body part or organ.

jealousy An aversive reaction evoked by a real or imagined relationship involving a person's partner and a third person.

jellies and creams Spermicide packaged in tubes and inserted into the vagina with an applicator.

labia majora "Outer lips," or folds of tissue covering the female sexual organs.

labia minora "Inner lips," or folds of tissue just inside the labia majora.

leach To dissolve and filter through soil.

lead A highly toxic metal found in emissions from lead smelters and processing plants; also sometimes found in pipes or paint in older houses.

learned helplessness Pattern of responding to situations by giving up because of repeated failure in the past.

learned optimism Teaching oneself to think positively.

lesbian Sexual orientation involving attraction of women to other women.

leukoplakia A condition characterized by leathery white patches inside the mouth; produced by contact with irritants in tobacco juice.

libido Sexual drive or desire.

life expectancy Expected number of years of life remaining at a given age, such as at birth.

locavore A person who primarily eats food grown or produced locally.

locus of control The location, *external* (outside oneself) or *internal* (within oneself), that an individual perceives as the source and underlying cause of events in his or her life.

loss of control Inability to reliably predict whether a particular instance of involvement with the addictive substance or behavior will be healthy or damaging.

low-density lipoproteins (LDLs) Compounds that facilitate the transport of cholesterol in the blood to the body's cells and cause the cholesterol to build up on artery walls.

low sperm count A sperm count below 20 million sperm per milliliter of semen.

lymphocyte A type of white blood cell involved in the immune response.

macrominerals Minerals that the body needs in fairly large amounts.

macrophage A type of white blood cell that ingests foreign material.

magnetic resonance imaging (MRI) A device that uses magnetic fields, radio waves, and computers to generate an image of internal tissues of the body for diagnostic purposes without the use of radiation.

mainstream smoke Smoke that is drawn through tobacco while inhaling.

major depression Severe depressive disorder that entails chronic mood disorder, physical effects such as sleep disturbance and exhaustion, and mental effects such as the inability to concentrate; also called *clinical depression*.

male condom A single-use sheath of thin latex or other material designed to fit over an erect penis and to catch semen upon ejaculation.

malignant Very dangerous or harmful; refers to a cancerous tumor.

malignant melanoma A virulent cancer of the melanocytes (pigment-producing cells) of the skin.

managed care Cost-control procedures used by health insurers to coordinate treatment.

manipulative and body-based practices Treatments involving manipulation or movement of one or more body parts.

marijuana Chopped leaves and flowers of *Cannabis indica* or *Cannabis sativa* (hemp); a psychoactive stimulant.

marital rape Any unwanted intercourse or penetration obtained by force, threat of force, or when the spouse is unable to consent.

massage therapy Soft tissue manipulation by trained therapists for relaxation and healing.

masturbation Self-stimulation of genitals.

measles A viral disease that produces symptoms such as an itchy rash and a high fever.

Medicaid A federal-state matching funds program that provides health insurance to low-income people.

Medicare A federal health insurance program that covers people age 65 and older, the permanently disabled, and people with end-stage kidney disease.

medical abortion The termination of a pregnancy during its first 9 weeks using hormonal medications that cause the embryo to be expelled from the uterus.

medical model A view of health in which health status focuses primarily on the individual and a biological or diseased organ perspective.

meditation A relaxation technique that involves concentrated focus to quiet the mind and increase awareness of the present moment.

menarche The first menstrual period.

meningitis An infection of the meninges, the membranes that surround the brain and spinal cord.

menopause The permanent cessation of menstruation, generally between the ages of 40 and 60.

mental health The thinking part of psychosocial health; includes your values, attitudes, and beliefs.

mental illnesses Disorders that disrupt thinking, feeling, moods, and behaviors, and that impair daily functioning.

metabolic syndrome (MetS) A group of metabolic conditions occurring together that increase a person's risk of heart disease, stroke, and diabetes.

metastasis Process by which cancer spreads from one area to different areas of the body.

methicillin-resistant *Staphylococcus aureus* (MRSA) Highly resistant form of staph infection that is growing in international prevalence.

migraine A condition characterized by localized headaches that possibly result from alternating dilation and constriction of blood vessels.

mind-body medicine Techniques designed to enhance the mind's ability to affect bodily functions and symptoms.

mindfulness A practice of purposeful, nonjudgmental observation in which we are fully present in the moment.

minerals Inorganic, indestructible elements that aid physiological processes.

miscarriage Loss of the fetus before it is viable; also called *spontaneous abortion*.

modeling Learning specific behaviors by watching others perform them.

monogamy Exclusive sexual involvement with one partner.

mononucleosis A viral disease that causes pervasive fatigue and other long-lasting symptoms.

monosaccharides Simple sugars that contain only one molecule of sugar.

mons pubis Fatty tissue covering the pubic bone in females; in physically mature women, the mons is covered with coarse hair.

morbidly obese Having a body weight 100 percent or more above healthy recommended levels; in an adult, having a BMI of 40 or more.

mortality The proportion of deaths to the total population, within a given period of time.

motivation A social, cognitive, and emotional force that directs human behavior.

multidrug-resistant TB (MDR-TB) Form of TB that is resistant to at least two of the best antibiotics available.

multifactorial disease Disease caused by interactions of several factors.

mumps A once common viral disease that is controllable by vaccination.

municipal solid waste (MSW) Solid wastes such as durable goods; nondurable goods; containers and packaging; food waste; yard waste; and miscellaneous wastes from residential, commercial, institutional, and industrial sources.

muscle dysmorphia Body image disorder in which men believe that their body is insufficiently lean or muscular.

muscular endurance A muscle's ability to exert force repeatedly without fatiguing or the ability to sustain a muscular contraction for a length of time.

muscular strength The amount of force that a muscle is capable of exerting in one contraction.

mutant cells Cells that differ in form, quality, or function from normal cells.

myocardial infarction (MI) or heart attack A blockage of normal blood supply to an area in the heart.

natural products Treatments using substances found in nature, such as herbs, special diets, or vitamin megadoses.

naturopathy (naturopathic medicine) System of medicine in which practitioners work with nature to restore people's health.

negative consequences Severe problems associated with addiction, such as physical damage, legal trouble, financial problems, academic failure, or family dissolution.

neglect Failure to provide for a child's basic needs such as food, shelter, medical care, and clothing.

neoplasm A new growth of tissue that results from uncontrolled, abnormal cellular development and serves no physiological function.

neurotransmitters Chemicals that relay messages between nerve cells or from nerve cells to other body cells.

nicotine The primary stimulant chemical in tobacco products; nicotine is highly addictive.

nicotine poisoning Symptoms often experienced by beginning smokers, including dizziness, diarrhea, lightheadedness, rapid and erratic pulse, clammy skin, nausea, and vomiting.

nicotine withdrawal Symptoms, including nausea, headaches, irritability, and intense tobacco cravings, suffered by addicted smokers who stop using tobacco.

nonionizing radiation Electromagnetic waves having relatively long wavelengths and enough energy to move atoms around or cause them to vibrate.

nonpoint source pollutants Pollutants that run off or seep into waterways from broad areas of land.

nonverbal communication All unwritten and unspoken messages, both intentional and unintentional.

nuclear meltdown An accident that results when the temperature in the core of a nuclear reactor increases enough to melt the nuclear fuel and the containment vessel housing it.

nurse Health professional who provides many services for patients and who may work in a variety of settings.

nurse practitioner (NP) Professional nurse with advanced training obtained through either a master's degree program or a specialized nurse practitioner program.

nutraceuticals Food or food-based supplements that have combined nutritional and pharmaceutical benefits; used interchangeably with the term *functional foods*.

nutrients The constituents of food that sustain humans physiologically: proteins, carbohydrates, fats, vitamins, minerals, and water.

nutrition The science that investigates the relationship between physiological function and the essential elements of foods eaten.

NuvaRing A soft, flexible ring inserted into the vagina that releases hormones, preventing pregnancy.

obesity A body weight more than 20 percent above healthy recommended levels; in an adult, a BMI of 30 or more.

obesogenic Characterized by environments that promote increased food intake, nonhealthful foods, and physical inactivity; refers to conditions that lead people to become excessively fat.

obsession Excessive preoccupation with an addictive object or behavior.

obsessive-compulsive disorder (OCD) A form of anxiety disorder characterized by recurrent, unwanted thoughts and repetitive behaviors.

oncogenes Suspected cancer-causing genes present on chromosomes.

one repetition maximum (1 RM) The amount of weight or resistance that can be lifted or moved only once.

open relationship A relationship in which partners agree that sexual involvement can occur outside the relationship.

ophthalmologist Physician who specializes in the medical and surgical care of the eyes, including prescriptions for glasses.

opioids Drugs that induce sleep and relieve pain; includes derivatives of opium and synthetics with similar chemical properties; also called *narcotics*.

opium The parent drug of the opioids; made from the seedpod resin of the opium poppy.

opportunistic infections Infections that occur when the immune system is weakened or compromised.

optometrist Eye specialist whose practice is limited to prescribing and fitting lenses.

oral contraceptives Pills containing synthetic hormones that prevent ovulation by regulating hormones.

oral ingestion Intake of drugs through the mouth.

organic Grown without use of pesticides, chemicals, or hormones.

Ortho Evra A patch that releases hormones similar to those in oral contraceptives; each patch is worn for 1 week.

osteopath General practitioner who receives training similar to a medical doctor's but with an emphasis on the skeletal and muscular systems; often uses spinal manipulation as part of treatment.

other specified feeding or eating disorder (OSFED) Eating disorders that are a true psychiatric illness but that do not fit the strict diagnostic criteria for anorexia nervosa, bulimia nervosa, or binge-eating disorder.

ovarian follicles Areas within the ovary in which individual eggs develop.

ovaries Almond-sized organs that house developing eggs and produce hormones.

overload A condition in which a person feels overly pressured by demands.

overuse injuries Injuries that result from the cumulative effects of day-after-day stresses placed on tendons, muscles, and joints.

overweight Having a body weight more than 10 percent above healthy recommended levels; in an adult, having a BMI of 25 to 29.

ovulation The point of the menstrual cycle at which a mature egg ruptures through the ovarian wall.

ovum A single mature egg cell.

pancreas Organ that secretes digestive enzymes into the small intestine, and hormones, including insulin, into the bloodstream.

pandemic Global epidemic of a disease that occurs in several countries at the same time.

panic attack Severe anxiety reaction in which a particular situation, often for unknown reasons, causes terror.

Pap test A procedure in which cells taken from the cervical region are examined for abnormal cellular activity.

parasitic worms The largest of the pathogens, most of which are more a nuisance than they are a threat.

parasympathetic nervous system Branch of the autonomic nervous system responsible for slowing systems stimulated by the stress response.

pathogen A disease-causing agent.

pelvic inflammatory disease (PID) Term used to describe various infections of the female reproductive tract; can be caused by chlamydia or gonorrhea.

penis Male sexual organ that releases sperm.

peptic ulcer Damage to the stomach or intestinal lining, usually caused by digestive juices; most ulcers result from infection by the bacterium *Helicobacter pylori.*

perfect-use failure rate The number of pregnancies (per 100 users) that are likely to occur in the first year of use of a particular birth control method if the method is used consistently and correctly.

perineum Tissue that forms the "floor" of the pelvic region in both men and women.

peripheral artery disease (PAD) Atherosclerosis occurring in the lower extremities, such as in the feet, calves, or legs, or in the arms.

personal flotation device A device worn to provide buoyancy and keep the wearer, conscious or unconscious, afloat with the nose and mouth out of the water; also known as a life jacket.

personality disorders A class of mental disorders that are characterized by inflexible patterns of thought and beliefs that lead to socially distressing behavior.

pesticides Chemicals that kill pests such as insects, weeds, and rodents.

phobia A deep and persistent fear of a specific object, activity, or situation that results in a compelling desire to avoid the source of the fear.

smog Brownish haze that is a form of pollution produced by the photochemical reaction of sunlight with hydrocarbons, nitrogen compounds, and other gases in vehicle exhaust.

physical activity Refers to all body movements produced by skeletal muscles resulting in substantial increases in energy expenditure, but generally refers to movement of the large muscle groups.

physical fitness Refers to a set of attributes that allow you to perform moderate- to vigorous-intensity physical activities on a regular basis without getting too tired and with energy left over to handle physical or mental emergencies.

physician assistant (PA) A midlevel practitioner trained to handle most standard cases of care under the supervision of a physician.

physiological dependence The adaptive state that occurs with regular addictive behavior and results in withdrawal syndrome.

pituitary gland The endocrine gland that controls the release of hormones from the gonads.

placenta The network of blood vessels connected to the umbilical cord that transports oxygen and nutrients to a developing fetus and carries away fetal wastes.

plant sterols Essential components of plant membranes that, when consumed in the diet, appear to help lower cholesterol levels.

plaque Buildup of deposits in the arteries.

platelet adhesiveness Stickiness of red blood cells associated with blood clots.

pneumonia Inflammatory disease of the lungs characterized by chronic cough, chest pain, chills, high fever, and fluid accumulation; may be caused by bacteria, viruses, fungi, chemicals, or other substances.

point source pollutants Pollutants that enter waterways at a specific location.

poison Any substance harmful to the body when ingested, inhaled, injected, or absorbed through the skin.

pollutant A substance that contaminates some aspect of the environment and causes potential harm to living organisms.

polychlorinated biphenyls (PCBs) Toxic chemicals that were once used as insulating materials in high-voltage electrical equipment.

polydrug use Taking several medications, vitamins, recreational drugs, or illegal drugs simultaneously.

polysaccharides Complex carbohydrates formed by the combination of long chains of monosaccharides.

positive reinforcement Presenting something positive following a behavior that is being reinforced.

positron emission tomography (PET) scan Method for measuring heart activity by injecting a patient with a radioactive tracer that is scanned electronically to produce a three-dimensional image of the heart and arteries.

postpartum depression A mood disorder experienced by women who have given birth; involves depression, fatigue, and other symptoms and may last for weeks or months.

post-traumatic stress disorder (PTSD) A collection of symptoms that may occur as a delayed response to a serious trauma.

power The ability to make and implement decisions.

prayer Communication with a transcendent Presence.

preconception care Medical care received prior to becoming pregnant that helps a woman assess and address potential maternal health issues.

prediabetes Condition in which blood glucose levels are higher than normal, but not high enough to be classified as diabetes.

preeclampsia A pregnancy complication characterized by high blood pressure, protein in the urine, and edema.

pre-gaming A strategy of drinking heavily at home before going out to an event or other location.

prehypertensive Blood pressure is above normal, but not yet in the hypertensive range.

prejudice A negative evaluation of an entire group of people that is typically based on unfavorable and often wrong ideas about the group.

premature ejaculation Ejaculation that occurs prior to or almost immediately following penile penetration of the vagina.

premenstrual dysphoric disorder (PMDD) Collective name for a group of negative symptoms similar to but more severe than PMS, including severe mood disturbances.

premenstrual syndrome (PMS) Comprises the mood changes and physical symptoms that occur in some women during the 1 or 2 weeks prior to menstruation.

premium Payment made to an insurance carrier, usually in monthly installments, that covers the cost of an insurance policy.

primary aggression Goal-directed, hostile self-assertion that is destructive in character.

primary care practitioner (PCP) A medical practitioner who treats routine ailments, advises on preventive care, gives general medical advice, and makes appropriate referrals when necessary.

prion A recently identified self-replicating, protein-based pathogen.

process addictions Behaviors such as disordered gambling, compulsive buying, compulsive Internet or technology use, work addiction, compulsive exercise, and sexual addiction that are known to be addictive because they are mood altering.

procrastinate To intentionally put off doing something.

progesterone Hormone secreted by the ovaries; helps the endometrium develop and helps maintain pregnancy.

proof A measure of the percentage of alcohol in a beverage.

prostate gland Gland that secretes nutrients and neutralizing fluids into the semen.

prostate-specific antigen (PSA) An antigen found in prostate cancer patients.

proteins The essential constituents of nearly all body cells; necessary for the development and repair of bone, muscle, skin, and blood; the key elements of antibodies, enzymes, and hormones.

protozoans Microscopic single-celled organisms that can be pathogenic.

psychoactive drugs Drugs that have the potential to alter mood or behavior.

psychological hardiness A personality trait characterized by control, commitment, and the embrace of challenge.

psychological resilience The process of adapting well in the face of adversity, trauma, tragedy, threats, or significant sources of stress, such as family and relationship problems, serious health problems, or workplace and financial stressors.

psychological health The mental, emotional, social, and spiritual dimensions of health.

psychoneuroimmunology (PNI) The study of the interrelationship between the mind and body on immune system functioning.

puberty The period of sexual maturation.

pubic lice Parasitic insects that can inhabit various body areas, especially the genitals.

qi Element of traditional Chinese medicine that refers to the vital energy force that courses through the body; when *qi* is in balance, health is restored.

radiation absorbed doses (rads) Units that measure exposure to radiation.

radiotherapy The use of radiation to kill cancerous cells.

radon A naturally occurring radioactive gas resulting from the decay of certain radioactive elements.

rape Sexual penetration without the victim's consent.

reactive aggression Hostile emotional reaction brought about by frustrating life experiences.

receptor sites Specialized areas of cells and organs where chemicals, enzymes, and other substances interact.

relapse The tendency to return to the addictive behavior after a period of abstinence.

religion A system of beliefs, practices, rituals, and symbols designed to facilitate closeness to the sacred or transcendent.

repetitive motion disorder (RMD) An injury to soft tissue, tendons, muscles, nerves, or joints due to the physical stress of repeated motions; sometimes called *overuse syndrome*, *cumulative trauma disorders*, or *repetitive stress injuries*.

resiliency The ability to adapt to change and stressful events in healthy and flexible ways.

resting metabolic rate (RMR) The energy expenditure of the body under BMR conditions plus other daily sedentary activities.

rheumatic heart disease A heart disease caused by untreated streptococcal infection of the throat.

RICE Acronym for the standard first aid treatment for virtually all traumatic and overuse injuries: **r**est, **i**ce, **c**ompression, and **e**levation.

rickettsia A small form of bacteria that live inside other living cells.

risk behaviors Actions that increase susceptibility to negative health outcomes.

rubella (German measles) A milder form of measles that causes a rash and mild fever in children and may damage a fetus or a newborn baby.

satiety The feeling of fullness or satisfaction at the end of a meal.

saturated fats Fats that are unable to hold any more hydrogen in their chemical structure; derived mostly from animal sources; solid at room temperature.

schizophrenia A mental illness with biological origins that is characterized by irrational behavior, severe alterations of the senses, and often an inability to function in society.

scrotum External sac of tissue that encloses the testes.

seasonal affective disorder (SAD) A type of depression that occurs in the winter months, when sunlight levels are low.

secondary sex characteristics Characteristics associated with sex but not directly related to reproduction, such as vocal pitch, degree of body hair, and location of fat deposits.

self-disclosure Sharing personal feelings or information with others.

self-efficacy Describes a person's belief about whether he or she can successfully engage in and execute a specific behavior.

self-esteem Refers to one's realistic sense of self-respect or self-worth.

self-injury Intentionally causing injury to one's own body in an attempt to cope with overwhelming negative emotions; also called *self-mutilation*, *self-harm*, or *nonsuicidal self-injury* (NSSI).

self-nurturance Developing individual potential through a balanced and realistic appreciation of self-worth and ability.

self-talk The customary manner of thinking and talking to yourself, which can affect your self-image.

semen Fluid containing sperm and nutrients that increase sperm viability and neutralize vaginal acid.

seminal vesicles Glandular ducts that secrete nutrients for the semen.

serial monogamy A series of monogamous sexual relationships.

set point theory Theory that a form of internal thermostat controls our weight and fights to maintain this weight around a narrowly set range.

sexual abuse of children Sexual interaction between a child and an adult or older child.

sexual addiction Compulsive involvement in sexual activity.

sexual assault Any act in which one person is sexually intimate with another without that person's consent.

sexual aversion disorder Desire dysfunction characterized by sexual phobias and anxiety about sexual contact.

sexual dysfunction Problems associated with achieving sexual satisfaction.

sexual fantasies Sexually arousing thoughts and dreams.

sexual harassment Any form of unwanted sexual attention related to any condition of employment, education, or performance evaluation.

sexual identity Recognition of oneself as a sexual being; a composite of biological sex characteristics, gender identity, gender roles, and sexual orientation.

sexual orientation A person's enduring emotional, romantic, sexual, or affectionate attraction to other persons.

sexual performance anxiety A condition of sexual difficulties caused by anticipating some sort of problem with the sex act.

sexual prejudice Negative attitudes and hostile actions directed at sexually identified social groups; also referred to as sexual bias.

sexuality All the thoughts, feelings, and behaviors associated with being male or female, experiencing attraction, being in love, and being in relationships that include sexual intimacy and activity.

sexually transmitted infections (STIs) Infectious diseases caused by pathogens transmitted through some form of intimate, usually sexual, contact.

shaping Using a series of small steps to gradually achieve a particular goal.

shift and persist A strategy of reframing appraisals of current stressors and focusing on a meaningful future that protects a person from the negative effects of too much stress.

shingles A disease characterized by a painful rash that occurs when the chickenpox virus is reactivated.

sick building syndrome (SBS) Occurs when occupants of a building experience acute health effects linked to time spent in a building, but no specific illness or cause can be identified; symptoms diminish when occupants are away from the building.

sidestream smoke The cigarette, pipe, or cigar smoke breathed by nonsmokers.

simple carbohydrates A major type of carbohydrate that provides short-term energy; also called *simple sugars*.

simple rape Rape by one person, usually known to the victim, that does not involve physical beating or use of a weapon.

sinoatrial node (SA node) Cluster of electric pulse-generating cells that serves as a natural pacemaker for the heart.

situational inducement Attempt to influence a behavior through situations and occasions that are structured to exert control over that behavior.

sleep debt The difference between the number of hours of sleep an individual needed in a given time period and the number of hours he or she actually slept.

snuff A powdered form of tobacco that is sniffed or absorbed through the mucous membranes in the nose or placed inside the cheek and sucked.

social bonds The level of closeness and attachment with other individuals.

social cognitive model (SCM) Model of behavior change emphasizing the role of social factors and thought processes (cognition) in behavior change.

social health Aspect of psychosocial health that includes interactions with others, ability to use social supports, and ability to adapt to various situations.

social learning theory Theory that people learn behaviors by watching role models—parents, caregivers, and significant others.

social phobia A phobia characterized by fear and avoidance of social situations; also called *social anxiety disorder*.

social physique anxiety (SPA) A desire to look good that has a destructive effect on a person's ability to function well in social interactions and relationships.

social support Network of people and services with whom you share ties and from whom you get support.

socialization Process by which a society communicates behavioral expectations to its individual members.

spermatogenesis The development of sperm.

spermicides Substances designed to kill sperm.

spiritual health The aspect of psychosocial health that relates to having a sense of meaning and purpose to one's life, as well as a feeling of connection with others and with nature.

spiritual intelligence (SI) The ability to access higher meanings, values, abiding purposes, and unconscious aspects of the self, a characteristic that helps us find a moral and ethical path to guide us through life.

spirituality An individual's sense of purpose and meaning in life, beyond material values.

stalking The willful, repeated, and malicious following, harassing, or threatening of another person.

standard drink The amount of any beverage that contains about 14 grams of pure alcohol (about 0.6 fluid ounce or 1.2 tablespoons).

staphylococci A group of round bacteria, usually found in clusters, that cause a variety of diseases in humans and other animals.

starch Polysaccharide that is the storage form of glucose in plants.

static stretching Stretching techniques that slowly and gradually lengthen a muscle or group of muscles and their tendons.

stent A stainless steel, mesh-like tube that is inserted to prop open the artery.

sterilization Permanent fertility control achieved through surgical procedures.

stereotactic radiosurgery A type of radiation therapy that can be used to zap tumors; also known as gamma knife surgery.

stillbirth A fetus that is dead at birth.

stimulants Drugs that increase activity of the central nervous system.

Streptococcus A round bacterium, usually found in chain formation.

stress A series of mental and physiological responses and adaptations to a real or perceived threat to one's well-being.

stress inoculation A stress-management technique in which a person consciously anticipates and prepares for potential stressors.

stressor A physical, social, or psychological event or condition that upsets homeostasis and produces a stress response.

stroke A condition occurring when the brain is damaged by disrupted blood supply; also called *cerebrovascular accident*.

subjective well-being An uplifting feeling of inner peace.

suction curettage An abortion technique that uses gentle suction to remove fetal tissue from the uterus.

sudden cardiac death Death that occurs as a result of abrupt, profound loss of heart function.

sudden infant death syndrome (SIDS) The sudden death of an infant under 1 year of age for no apparent reason.

suicidal ideation A desire to die and thoughts about suicide.

Superfund Fund established under the Comprehensive Environmental Response, Compensation, and Liability Act to be used for cleaning up toxic waste dumps.

suppositories Waxy capsules that are inserted deep into the vagina, where they melt and release a spermicide.

sustainable development Development that meets the needs of the present without compromising the ability of future generations to meet their own needs.

sympathetic nervous system Branch of the autonomic nervous system responsible for stress arousal.

sympathomimetics Food substances that can produce stresslike physiological responses.

synergism The interaction of two or more drugs that produce more profound effects than would be expected if the drugs were taken separately; also called *potentiation*.

syphilis One of the most widespread bacterial STIs; characterized by distinct phases and potentially serious results.

systolic blood pressure The upper number in the fraction that measures blood pressure, indicating pressure on the walls of the arteries when the heart contracts.

tar A thick, brownish substance condensed from particulate matter in smoked tobacco.

target heart rate The heart rate range of aerobic exercise that leads to improved cardiorespiratory fitness (i.e., 64% to 96% of maximal heart rate).

temperature inversion A weather condition occurring when a layer of cool air is trapped under a layer of warmer air, preventing the air from circulating.

teratogenic Causing birth defects; may refer to drugs, environmental chemicals, radiation, or diseases.

terrorism The unlawful use of force or violence against persons or property to intimidate or coerce a government, the civilian population, or any segment thereof in furtherance of political or social objectives.

testes Male sex organs that manufacture sperm and produce hormones.

testosterone The male sex hormone manufactured in the testes.

tetrahydrocannabinol (THC) The chemical name for the active ingredient in marijuana.

thrombolysis Injection of an agent to dissolve clots and restore some blood flow, thereby reducing the amount of tissue that dies from ischemia.

thrombus Blood clot attached to a blood vessel's wall.

time As part of the FITT prescription, refers to how long a person needs to exercise each time to improve a component of physical fitness.

tolerance Phenomenon in which progressively larger doses of a drug or more intense involvement in a behavior is needed to produce the desired effects.

toxic shock syndrome (TSS) A potentially life-threatening disease that occurs when specific bacterial toxins multiply and spread to the bloodstream, most commonly through improper use of tampons or diaphragms.

toxins Poisonous substances produced by certain microorganisms that cause various diseases.

toxoplasmosis A disease caused by an organism found in cat feces that, when contracted by a pregnant woman, may result in stillbirth or an infant with mental retardation or birth defects.

trace minerals Minerals that the body needs in only very small amounts.

traditional Chinese medicine (TCM) Ancient comprehensive system of healing that uses herbs, acupuncture, and massage to bring vital energy, *qi*, into balance and to remove blockages of qi that lead to disease.

***trans* fats (*trans* fatty acids)** Fatty acids that are produced when polyunsaturated oils are hydrogenated to make them more solid.

transdermal The introduction of drugs through the skin.

transgendered Having a gender identity that does not match one's biological sex.

transient ischemic attack (TIA) Brief interruption of the blood supply to the brain that causes only temporary impairment; often an indicator of impending major stroke.

transsexual A person who is psychologically of one sex but physically of the other.

transtheoretical model Model of behavior change that identifies six distinct stages people go through in altering behavior patterns; also called the *stages of change model*.

traumatic injuries Injuries that are accidental and occur suddenly and violently.

traumatic stress A physiological and mental response that occurs for a prolonged period of time after a major accident, war, assault, natural disaster, or an event in which one may be seriously hurt, or killed, or witness horrible things.

trichomoniasis Protozoan STI characterized by foamy, yellowish discharge and unpleasant odor.

triglycerides The most common form of fat in the body; excess calories consumed are converted into triglycerides and stored as body fat.

trimester A 3-month segment of pregnancy; used to describe specific developmental changes that occur in the embryo or fetus.

triple marker screen (TMS) A common maternal blood test that can be used to identify fetuses with certain birth defects and genetic abnormalities.

tubal ligation Sterilization of the woman that involves the cutting and tying off or cauterizing of the fallopian tubes.

tuberculosis (TB) A disease caused by bacterial infiltration of the respiratory system.

tumor A neoplasmic mass that grows more rapidly than surrounding tissue.

type As part of the FITT prescription, refers to what kind of exercises a person needs to do to improve a component of physical fitness.

type 1 diabetes Form of diabetes mellitus in which the pancreas is not able to make insulin and therefore blood glucose cannot enter the cells to be used for energy.

type 2 diabetes Form of diabetes mellitus in which the pancreas does not make enough insulin or the body is unable to use insulin correctly.

typical-use failure rate The number of pregnancies (per 100 users) that are likely to occur in the first year of use of a particular birth control method if the method's use is not consistent or always correct.

ultrasonography (ultrasound) A common prenatal test that uses high-frequency sound waves to create a visual image of the fetus.

underweight Having a body weight more than 10 percent below healthy recommended levels; in an adult, having a BMI below 18.5.

unintentional injuries Injury, death, or psychological harm caused unintentionally or without premeditation.

unsaturated fats Fats that have room for more hydrogen in their chemical structure; derived mostly from plants; liquid at room temperature.

urethral opening The opening through which urine is expelled.

urinary tract infection (UTI) Infection, more common among women than men, of the urinary tract; causes include untreated STIs.

uterus (womb) Hollow, pear-shaped muscular organ whose function is to contain the developing fetus.

vaccination Inoculation with killed or weakened pathogens or similar, less dangerous antigens in order to prevent or lessen the effects of a disease.

vagina The passage in females leading from the vulva into the uterus.

vaginal intercourse The insertion of the penis into the vagina.

vaginismus A state in which the vaginal muscles contract so forcefully that penetration cannot occur.

values Principles that influence our thoughts and emotions and guide the choices we make in our lives.

variant sexual behavior A sexual behavior that is not practiced by most people.

vas deferens Tube that transports sperm from the epididymis to the ejaculatory duct.

vasectomy Sterilization of the man that involves the cutting and tying off of both vasa deferentia.

vasocongestion The engorgement of the genital organs with blood.

vegetarian A person who follows a diet that excludes some or all animal products.

veins Vessels that transport waste and carry blood back to the heart from other regions of the body.

ventricles The heart's two lower chambers, which pump blood through the blood vessels.

venules Branches of the veins.

very-low-calorie diets (VLCDs) Diets with a daily caloric value of 400 to 700 calories.

violence Aggressive behaviors that produce injuries and can result in death.

virulent Strong enough to overcome host resistance and cause disease.

viruses Pathogens that invade and inject their own DNA or RNA into a host cell, take it over, and force it to make copies of the pathogen.

visualization The creation of mental images to promote relaxation.

vitamins Essential organic compounds that promote growth and reproduction and help maintain life and health.

vulva Collective term for the external female genitalia.

waist-to-hip ratio Waist circumference divided by hip circumference; a high ratio indicates increased health risks due to unhealthy fat distribution.

wellness The achievement of the highest level of health possible in each of several dimensions.

whole grains Grains that are milled in their complete form, and thus include the bran, germ, and endosperm, with only the husk removed.

withdrawal

1. A method of contraception that involves withdrawing the penis from the vagina before ejaculation; also called coitus interruptus.

2. A series of temporary physical and biopsychosocial symptoms that occurs when an addict abruptly abstains from an addictive chemical or behavior.

work addiction The compulsive use of work and the work persona to fulfill needs for intimacy, power, and success.

yoga A system of physical and mental training involving controlled breathing, physical postures (*asanas*), meditation, chanting, and other practices that are believed to cultivate unity with the *Atman*, or spiritual life principle of the universe.

yo-yo diets Cycles in which people diet and regain weight.

zoonotic diseases Diseases of animals that may be transmitted to humans.

References

Chapter 1

1. World Health Organization, "Constitution of the World Health Organization," *Chronicles of the World Health Organization*, Available at www.who.int/governance/eb/constitution/en/index.html.
2. R. Dubos, *So Human an Animal: How We Are Shaped by Surroundings and Events* (New York: Scribner, 1968), 15.
3. J. Xu et al., "Mortality in the United States, 2015," *NCHS Data Brief*, no. 267 (December 2016), Available at https://www.cdc.gov/nchs/products/databriefs/db267.htm.
4. R.A. Rudd et al., "Increases in Drug and Opioid-Involved Overdose Deaths—United States, 2010–2015," *Morbidity and Mortality Weekly Report* 65 (2016): 1445–52, doi:http://dx.doi.org/10.15585/mmwr.mm655051e1.
5. Organization for Economic Cooperation and Development, *Health at a Glance 2015: OECD Indicators, 2015, Key Findings: United States*, http://www.oecd.org/unitedstates/Health-at-a-Glance-2015-Key-Findings-UNITED-STATES.pdf.
6. M. Heron, "Deaths: Leading Causes for 2014, Table 1," *National Vital Statistics Reports* 65, no. 5, June 2016, www.cdc.gov/nchs/data/nvsr/nvsr65/nvsr65_05.pdf.
7. Office of Disease Prevention and Health Promotion (ODPHP). *Healthy People 2020*, Accessed August,2016. https://www.healthypeople.gov/
8. Ibid.
9. Ibid.
10. Ibid.
11. Ibid.
12. Centers for Disease Control and Prevention, "Chronic Disease Overview: Prevention and Health Promotion: Chronic Disease Overview," February 2016, www.cdc.gov/chronicdisease/overview/index/htm.
13. Ibid.
14. J.F. Sallis and J.A. Carlson, "Physical Activity: Numerous Benefits and Effective Interventions," July 2015, Agency for Healthcare Research and Quality, http://www.ahrq.gov/professionals/education/curriculum-tools/population-health/sallis.html.
15. X. Wang et al., "Fruit and Vegetable Consumption and Mortality from All Causes, Cardiovascular Disease, and Cancer: Systematic Review and Dose-Response Meta-analysis of Prospective Cohort Studies," *British Medical Journal* 349 (2014): g4490, doi:10.1136/bmj.g4490.
16. Centers for Disease Control and Prevention, "Alcohol Use and Health Fact Sheets: Chronic Disease Overview," 2016. https://www.cdc.gov/alcohol/fact-sheets/alcohol-use.htm
17. Centers for Disease Control and Prevention, "Smoking and Tobacco Use Fast Facts," December 2016, www.cdc.gov/tobacco/data_statistics/fact_sheets/fast_facts/index.htm#toll.
18. Centers for Disease Control and Prevention, "Wide-ranging Online Data for Epidemiologic Research (WONDER)," 2016, Available at http://wonder.cdc.gov.
19. U.S. Department of Health and Human Services, *Healthy People 2020*, 2016. https://www.healthypeople.gov/
20. P. Pilkington et al., "Evidence-Based Decision Making When Designing Environments for Physical Activity: The Role of Public Health," *Sports Medicine* 46 (2016): 997–1002.
21. U.S. Department of Health and Human Services, "New Report Details Impact of the Affordable Care Act," January 2017, https://www.hhs.gov/healthcare/facts-and-features/fact-sheets/new-report-details-impact-affordable-care-act.html#.
22. J. Donald, et al. "Daily Stress and the Benefits of Mindfulness: Examining the Daily and Longitudinal Relations between Present-Moment Awareness and Stress Responses." *Journal of Research in Personality*. 65: 30–37. 2016.
23. T. Hendriks, et al. "The Effect of Yoga on Positive Mental Health Among Healthy Adults: A Systematic Review and Meta-Analysis." *The Journal of Alternative and Complementary Medicine*. Jul 2017: 505–517.
24. S. Bowen, et al. "Mindfulness-Based Relapse Prevention for Methadone Maintenance: A Feasibility Trial." *The Journal of Alternative and Complementary Medicine*. Jul 2017: 541–544.
25. P. M. Herman, et al. "Cost-Effectiveness of Mindfulness-Based Stress Reduction vs. Cognitive Behavioral Therapy or Usual Care among Adults with Chronic Low-Back Pain." *Spine*. July 24, 2017. Epub ahead of print.
26. M. Blake. "Systematic Review and Meta-Analysis of Adolescent Cognitive-Behavioral Sleep Interventions." *Clinical Child and Family Psychology Review*. Sep 2017: 227–249.
27. J. Kabat-Zinn, *Wherever You Go, There You Are* (New York: Hachette Books, 2014).
28. I. Rosenstock, "Historical Origins of the Health Belief Model," *Health Education Monographs* 2, no. 4 (1974): 328–35.
29. J.J. Annesi et al., "Effects of the Youth Fit 4 Life Physical Activity/Nutrition Protocol on Body Mass Index, Fitness and Targeted Social Cognitive Theory Variables in 9- to 12-Year-Olds during After-school Care," *Journal of Paediatrics and Child Health* January 4, 2017, doi:10.1111/jpc.13447.
30. J.O. Prochaska and C.C. DiClemente, "Stages and Processes of Self-Change of Smoking: Toward an Integrative Model of Change," *Journal of Consulting and Clinical Psychology* 51 (1983): 390–95.
31. M. Jung, "Implications of Graphic Cigarette Warning Labels on Smoking Behavior: An International Perspective," *Journal of Cancer Prevention* 21, no. 1 (2016): 21–5, doi:10.15430/JCP.2016.21.1.21.
32. Y. Kang, et al, "Dispositional Mindfulness Predicts Adaptive Affective Responses to Health Messages and Increased Exercise Motivation," *Mindfulness* 8, no. 2 (2017): 387–97, doi:10.1007/s12671-016-0608-7.
33. G. Goldzweig et al., "Perceived Threat and Depression among Patients with Cancer: The Moderating Role of Health Locus of Control," *Psychology, Health, and Medicine* 21, no. 5 (2016): 601–7.
34. Ibid.
35. A. Ellis and M. Benard, *Clinical Application of Rational Emotive Therapy* (New York: Plenum, 1985).
36. K. Davis et al., "Mirror, Mirror on the Wall: How the Performance of the U.S. Health Care System Compares Internationally," 2014 Update, Commonwealth Fund, Available at www.commonwealthfund.org/publications/fund-reports/2014/jun/mirror-mirror.
37. World Health Organization, "Health Systems: Equity," 2017, Available at www.who.int/healthsystems/topics/equity/en.
38. M.C. Arcaya et al., "Inequalities in Health: Definitions, Concepts, and Theories," *Global Health Action* 8, no. 10 (2015), doi:10.3402/gha.v8.27106, Available at www.ncbi.nlm.nih.gov/pmc/articles/PMC4481045.
39. S.L. Colby and J. M. Ortman, "Projections of the Size and Composition of the U.S. Population: 2014-2060, U.S. Census Bureau, March, 2015. https://www.census.gov/content/dam/Census/library/publications/2015/demo/p25-1143.pdf
40. G. Goldzweig et al., "Perceived Threat and Depression among Patients with Cancer: The Moderating Role of Health Locus of Control," *Psychology, Health, and Medicine* 21, no. 5 (2016): 601–7.
41. Harris Interactive, "The GLBT Market Research Leaders—Hands Down," 2013, Available at http://www.witeck.com/wp-content/uploads/2013/03/partnership-with-harris-interactive.pdf.
42. G.J. Gates, "In U.S., More Adults Identifying as LGBT," Gallup, January 11, 2017, Available at www.gallup.com/poll/201731/lgbt-identification-rises.aspx.
43. Pew Research Center, "Nones on the Rise," October 9, 2012, Available at http://www.pewforum.org/2012/10/09/nones-on-the-rise.
44. Pew Research Center, "America's Changing Religious Landscape," May 12, 2015. http://www.pewforum.org/2015/05/12/americas-changing-religious-landscape/
45. Ibid.
46. J.Z. Ayanian, "The Costs of Racial Disparities in Health Care," *Harvard Business Review*, October 1, 2015, Available at https://hbr.org/2015/10/the-costs-of-racial-disparities-in-health-care
47. U.S. Department of Health and Human Services, *Healthy People 2020*, "Disparities," 2017. https://www.healthypeople.gov/2020/about/foundation-health-measures/Disparities
48. C. Stone et al., "A Guide to Statistics on Historical Trends in Income Inequality," Center on Budget and Policy Priorities, November 7, 2016, Available at http://www.cbpp.org/research/poverty-and-inequality/a-guide-to-statistics-on-historical-trends-in-income-inequality.
49. B.D. Proctor et al., "Income and Poverty in the United States: 2015," U.S. Census Bureau, Report Number P60-256, September 26, 2016, Available at https://www.census.gov/library/publications/2016/demo/p60-256.html.
50. K.L. Walters et al., "Health Equity: Eradicating Health Inequalities for Future Generations," American Academy of Social Work and Social Welfare. 2016. http://aaswsw.org/wp-content/uploads/2016/01/WP19-with-cover2.pdf
51. B.P. Bosworth et al, "What Growing Life Expectancy Gaps Mean for the Promise of Social Security," Brookings Institution, February 12, 2016, Available at https://www.brookings.edu/research/what-growing-life-expectancy-gaps-mean-for-the-promise-of-social-security/#recent.

52. P. Bravemen et al., "The Social Determinants of Health: Coming of Age," *Annual Review of Public Health* 32 (2011): 381–98, doi:10.1146/annurev-publhealth-031210-101218.

53. American Psychological Association, "Stress in America: Impact of Discrimination," March 10, 2016, Available at www.stressinamerica.org.

54. Ibid.

55. Ibid.

56. National Library of Medicine, "Health Literacy: Definition," 2017, Available at https://nnlm.gov/professional-development/topics/health-literacy.

57. Ibid.

58. J.J. Wing et al., "Change in Neighborhood Characteristics and Change in Coronary Artery Calcium," *Circulation*, 134 (2016): 504–13, doi:https://doi.org/10.1161/CIRCULATIONAHA.115.020534.

59. A.J. Cohen et al., "Estimates and 25-year Trends of the Global Burden of Disease Attributable to Ambient Air Pollution: An Analysis of Data from the Global Burden of Diseases Study 2015," *Lancet*, 389, no. 10082 (2017): 1907–18, doi:10.1016/S0140-6736(17)30505-6.

60. Centers for Disease Control and Prevention, "Lead: Data, Statistics, and Surveillance," February 9, 2017, Available at www.cdc.gov/nceh/lead/default.htm.

61. K.P. Theall et al., "Association between Neighborhood Violence and Biological Stress in Children," *JAMA Pediatrics* 171, no. 1 (2017): 53–60, doi:10.1001/jamapediatrics.2016.2321.

62. J. Nothling et al., "Differences in Abuse, Neglect, and Exposure to Community Violence in Adolescents with and without PTSD and Depression," *Journal of Interpersonal Violence* (2016): pii: 0886260516674944.

63. S.A. Sumner et al., "Violence in the United States: Status, Challenges, and Opportunities," *Journal of the American Medical Association* 31, no. 5 (2015): 478–88, doi:10.1001/jama.2015.8371.

64. K. Eldeirawi et al., "Association of Neighborhood Crime with Asthma and Asthma Morbidity among Mexican American Children in Chicago, Illinois," *Annals of Allergy and Asthma Immunology* 117, no. 5 (2016): 502–7, doi:10.1016/j.anal.2016.09.429.

65. S.A. Sumner et al., "Violence in the United States: Status, Challenges, and Opportunities," *Journal of the American Medical Association* 31, no. 5 (2015): 478–88, doi:10.1001/jama.2015.8371.

66. J. Pykett et al., "Mindfulness, Behaviour Change and Decision Making: An Experimental Trial," Economic and Social Research Council, January 2016, Available at http://www.sps.ed.ac.uk/staff/sociology/rachel_howell/Mindfulness_Behaviour_Change_and_Decision_Making_Final_Report.pdf.

67. A. Lueke and B. Gibson, "Mindfulness Meditation Reduces Implicit Age and Race Bias," *Social Psychology and Personality Science* 6, no. 3 (2015): 284–91, doi:10.1177/1948550614559651.

68. N. Torres, "Mindfulness Mitigates Biases You May Not Know You Have," *Harvard Business Review*, December 24, 2014, Available at https://hbr.org/2014/12/mindfulness-mitigates-biases-you-may-not-know-you-have.

69. A. Thompson and J.B. Cuseo, *Diversity and the College Experience: Research-Based Strategies for Appreciating Human Differences*, 2nd ed. (Dubuque, Iowa: Kendall Hunt, 2014).

70. A.S. Noonan et al., "Improving the Health of African Americans in the USA: An Overdue Opportunity for Social Justice," *Public Health Reviews* 37, not. 12 (2016), doi:10.1186/s40985-016-0025-4.

71. Department of Health and Human Services, "National Prevention Strategy: Elimination of Health Disparities—A Report of the Surgeon General," May 2014. https://www.surgeon-general.gov/priorities/prevention/strategy/elimination-of-health-disparities.html

72. Ibid.

73. S. Artiga, "Disparities in Health and Health Care: Five Key Questions and Answers," Henry J. Kaiser Family Foundation.

74. Ibid.

75. Department of Health and Human Services, "National Prevention Strategy: Elimination of Health Disparities—A Report of the Surgeon General," May 2014.

Chapter 2

1. A.H. Maslow, *Motivation and Personality*, 2nd ed. (New York: Harper and Row, 1970).

2. D.J. Anspaugh and G. Ezell, *Teaching Today's Health*, 10th ed. (Boston: Pearson, 2013).

3. D. Goleman et al., *Primal Leadership: Unleashing the Power of Emotional Intelligence* (Boston: Harvard Business Review Press, 2013); I. Tuhovsky, *Emotional Intelligence: A Practical Guide to Making Friends with Your Emotions and Raising Your EQ* (Ian Tuhovsky, 2015).

4. Y. Yang et al., "Social Relationships and Physiological Determinants of Longevity across the Lifespan," *Proceedings of the National Academy of Sciences of the United States of America* 113, no. 3 (2016): 578–83; M. Ramsey and A. Gentzler, "An Upward Spiral: Bidirectional Associations between Positive Affect and Positive Aspects of Close Relationships across the Life Span," *Developmental Review* 36, (2015): 58–104.

5. S. Levens et al., "The Role of Family Support and Perceived Stress Reactivity in Predicting Depression in College Freshman," *Journal of Social and Clinical Psychology* 35, no. 4 (2016): 342–55; D. Lamis et al., "Depressive Symptoms and Suicidal Ideation in College Students: The Mediating and Moderating Roles of Hopelessness, Alcohol Problems, and Social Support," *Journal of Clinical Psychology* 72, no. 9 (2016): 919–32.

6. National Cancer Institute, "Spirituality in Cancer Care," May 18, 2015, www.cancer.gov/cancertopics/pdq/supportivecare/spirituality/patient.

7. D. *Melkasha*. *Friendship and Happiness across the Lifespan* (New York: Springer, 2015).

8. S. Straussner and C. Fewel. "Children of Parents Who Abuse Alcohol and Drugs," in *Parental Psychiatric Disorder: Distressed Parents and Their Children*, edited by A. Reupert, D. Mayberry, and J. Licholson (Cambridge, UK: Cambridge University Press, 20XX), xxx–xxx.

9. M. Seligman, *Helplessness: On Depression, Development, and Death* (New York: W. H. Freeman, 1975).

10. P.L. Hill et al., "Examining Concurrent and Longitudinal Relations between Personality Traits and Social Well-Being in Adulthood," *Social Psychological and Personality Science* 3 (2012): 698–705.

11. K. Huffman and C.A. Sanderson, *Real World Psychology* (Hoboken, NJ: Wiley, 2014).

12. M. Seligman et al., "White Paper: Positive Health and Heath Assets: Re-analysis of Longitudinal Datasets." *U Penn Positive Health* (2015), Available at https://ppc.sas.upenn.edu/sites/ppc.sas.upenn.edu/files/positivehealthassetspub.pdf.

13. Ibid.

14. M. Seligman, *Flourish: A Visionary New Understanding of Happiness and Well-Being* (New York: Free Press, 2011).

15. S. Donaldson et al., "Happiness, Excellence, and Optimal Human Functioning Revisited: Examining the Peer Reviewed Literature Linked to Positive Psychology," *Journal of Positive Psychology* 10, no. 3 (2015): 185–95.

16. M. Garaigordobil, "Predictor Variables of Happiness and Its Connection with Risk and Protective Factors for Health," *Frontiers in Psychology* 6 (2015): 1176.

17. Ibid.

18. P. de Souto Barreto and Y. Rolland, "Happiness and Unhappiness Have No Direct Effect on Mortality," *Lancet* XX (2015): xx–xx.

19. K. Eagan et al., *The American Freshman: National Norms Fall 2015* (Los Angeles: Higher Education Research Institute, UCLA, 2015), Available at https://www.heri.ucla.edu/monographs/TheAmericanFreshman2015-Expanded.pdf.

20. Ibid.

21. H.G. Koenig, "Religion, Spirituality and Health: A Review and Update," *Advances in Mind–Body Medicine* 29, no. 3 (2015): 19–26.

22. Pew Research Center, *The Global Religious Landscape* (Washington, DC: Pew Research Center's Forum on Religion and Public Life, 2012), Available at http://www.pewforum.org/2012/12/18/global-religious-landscape-exec.

23. Ibid.

24. B.A. Alper, "Millennials Are Less Religious Than Older Americans, but Just as Spiritual," Pew Research Center, November 23, 2015, www.pewresearch.org/fact-tank/2015/11/23/millennials-are-less-religious-than-older-americans-but-just-as-spiritual.

25. D. Maschi. "Why Millenials Are Less Religious than Older Americans," Pew Research FactTank, January 8, 2016. http://www.pewresearch.org/fact-tank/2016/01/08/qa-why-millennials-are-less-religious-than-older-americans.

26. B.L. Seaward, *Managing Stress: Principles and Strategies for Health and Well Being*, 7th ed. (Sudbury, MA: Jones and Bartlett, 2012).

27. DanahZohar.com, "Learn the Qs," Accessed July, 2017., http://dzohar.com/?page_id=622.

28. National Institutes of Health, National Center for Complementary and Integrative Health, *2016 Strategic Plan*, accessed March 2017, https://nccih.nih.gov/about/strategic-plans/2016.

29. D. Fishbein et al., "Behavioral and Psychophysiological Effects of a Yoga Intervention on High-Risk Adolescents: A Randomized Control Trial," *Journal of Child and Family Studies* 25, no. 2 (2016): 518–29; H. Lu et al., "The Brain Structure Correlates of Individual Differences in Trait Mindfulness: A Voxel-Based Morphometry Study," *Neuroscience* 272 (2014): 21–8; H. Huang et al., "A Meta-Analysis of the Benefits of Mindfulness-Based Stress Reduction (MBSR) on Psychological Function among Breast Cancer (BC) Survivors," *Breast Cancer*, Published online March 28, 2015 at http://link.springer.com/article/10.1007/s12282-015-0604-0#page-1 E. Hoge et al., "Effects of Mindfulness Meditation on Occupational Functioning and Health Care Utilization in Individuals with Anxiety," *Journal of Psychosomatic Research* 95 (2017): 7–11.

30. National Cancer Institute, "Spirituality in Cancer Care," July 17, 2015, www.cancer.gov/cancertopics/pdq/supportivecare/-spirituality/HealthProfessional/page1.

31. M. Mollica et al., "Spirituality Is Associated with Better Prostate Cancer Treatment Decision Making Experiences," *Journal of Behavioral Medicine* 39, no. 1 (2016): 161–69.

32. P. Rajguru et al., "Use of Mindfulness Meditation in the Management of Chronic Pain: A Systematic Review of Randomized Controlled Trials,"

American Journal of Lifestyle Medicine 9, no 3 (2015): 176–84.

33. E. Singer, R. McElroy, and P. Muennig, "Social Capital and the Paradox of Poor but Healthy Groups in the United States," *Journal of Immigrant and Minority Health*, Published online 23 March 2016, doi:10.1007/s10903-016-0396-0.

34. C. Aldwin et al., "Differing Pathways between Religiousness, Spirituality, and Health: A Self-Regulation Perspective," *Psychology of Religion and Spirituality* 6, no. 1 (2014): 9–21.

35. H. Jim et al., "Religion, Spirituality, and Physical Health in Cancer Patients: A Meta-Analysis," *Cancer* 121, no. 21 (2015): 3760–68.

36. S. Hooker, K. Masters, and K. Carey, "Multidimensional Assessment of Religiousness/Spirituality and Health Behaviors in College Students," *International Journal for the Psychology of Religion* 24, no. 3 (2014): 228–40; V. Kress et al., "Spirituality/Religiosity, Life Satisfaction, and Life Meaning as Protective Factors for Nonsuicidal Self-Injury in College Students," *Journal of College Counseling* 18, no. 2 (2015): 160–74.

37. National Cancer Institute, "Spirituality in Cancer Care," July 17, 2015, www.cancer.gov/cancertopics/pdq/supportivecare/-spirituality/HealthProfessional/page1.

38. L. Waters, A. Barsky, A. Ridd, and K. Allen, "Contemplative Education: A Systematic, Evidence-Based Review of the Effect of Meditation Interventions in Schools," *Educational Psychology Review* 27, no. 1 (2015): 103–34, doi:10.1007/s10648-014-9258-2.

39. National Center for PTSD, "Spirituality and Trauma: Professionals Working Together," February 23, 2016, www.ptsd.va.gov/-professional/provider-type/community/fs-spirituality.asp.

40. Ibid.; National Center for Complementary and Alternative Medicine, "Prayer and Spirituality in Health: Ancient Practices, Modern Science," *CAM at the NIH: Focus on Complementary and Alternative Medicine* 12, no. 1 (2005), www.jpsych.com/pdfs/NCCAM%20-%20Prayer%20and%20Spirituality%20in%20Health.pdf; National Cancer Institute, "Spirituality in Cancer Care," July 17, 2015, www.cancer.gov/cancertopics/pdq/supportivecare/-spirituality/HealthProfessional/page1.

41. G.G. Ano and E.B. Vasconcelles, "Religious Coping and Psychological Adjustment to Stress: A Meta-Analysis," *Journal of Clinical Psychology* 61, no. 4 (2005): 461–80; U. Winter et al., "The Psychological Outcome of Religious Coping with Stressful Life Events in a Swiss Sample of Church Attendees," *Psychotherapy and Psychosomatics* 78, no. 4 (2009): 240–44; G. Lucchetti, "Impact of Spirituality/Religiosity," 2011; Y. Matchim, "Breast Cancer Survivors Benefit," 2011.

42. A. Chiesa and A. Serretti, "Mindfulness-based Stress Reduction for Stress Management in Healthy People: A Review and Meta-Analysis," *Journal of Alternative and Complementary Medicine* 15, no. (2009): 593–600. G. Lucchetti, "Impact of Spirituality/Religiosity," 2011; Y. Matchim, "Breast Cancer Survivors Benefit," 2011.

43. D.R. Vago and D.A. Silbersweig, "Self-awareness, Self-regulation, and Self-transcendence (S-ART): A Framework for Understanding the Neurobiological Mechanisms of Mindfulness," *Human Neuroscience* 6, no. 269 (2012), Available at www.ncbi.nlm.nih.gov/pmc/articles/PMC3480633.

44. G. Desbordes et al., "Effects of Mindful-Attention and Compassion Meditation Training on Amygdala Response to Emotional Stimuli in an Ordinary, Non-meditative State," *Frontiers in Human Neuroscience* 6, no. 292 (2012), doi:10.3389/fnhum.2012.00292.

45. D. Desteno, "The Kindness Cure," *Atlantic*, July 21, 2015, https://www.theatlantic.com/health/archive/2015/07/mindfulness-meditation-empathy-compassion/398867.

46. F. Zeidan et al., "Neural Correlates of Mindfulness Meditation-Related Anxiety Relief," *Social Cognitive and Affective Neuroscience* 9, no. 6 (2014): 751–59, doi:10.1093/scan/nst041; G. Desbordes et al, "Effects of Mindful-Attention and Compassion Meditation Training on Amygdala Response to Emotional Stimuli in an Ordinary, Non-meditative State," *Frontiers in Human Neuroscience* 6, no. 292 (2012), doi:10.3389/fnhum.2012.00292; J.C. Ong et al., "A Randomized Controlled Trial of Mindfulness Meditation for Chronic Insomnia," *Sleep* 37, no. 9 (2013): 1553–63; National Center for Complementary and Integrative Health, "Research Spotlight," 2014.

47. W. Marchand, "Neural Mechanisms of Mindfulness and Meditation: Evidence from Neuroimaging Studies," *World Journal of Radiology* 6, no. 7 (2014): 471–70, doi:10.4329/wjr.v6.i7.471.

48. S. Keng et al., "Effects of Mindfulness on Psychological Health," *Clinical Psychology Review* 31, no. 6 (2011); 1041–56; M. Spijkerman, W. Pots, and E. Bohlmeijer, "Effectiveness of Online Mindfulness-Based Interventions in Improving Mental Health: A Review and Meta-analysis of Randomised Controlled Trials," *Clinical Psychology Review* 45 (2016): 102–14.

49. W. Marchand, "Neural Mechanisms of Mindfulness and Meditation: Evidence from Neuroimaging Studies," *World Journal of Radiology* 6, no. 7 (2014): 471–70, doi:10.4329/wjr.v6.i7.471; B. Holzel et al., "Neural Mechanisms of Symptom Improvements in Generalized Anxiety Disorder Following Mindfulness Training," *Neuroimage: Clinical* 2 (2013): 448–58; A. Taren et al., "Mindfulness Meditation Training Alters Stress-Related Amygdala Resting State Functional Connectivity: A Randomized Controlled Trial," *Social Cognitive and Affective Neuroscience* 10, no. 12 (2015): 1758–68.

50. A. Lucette et al., "Spirituality and Religiousness Are Associated with Fewer Depressive Symptoms in Individuals with Medical Conditions," *Psychosomatics* (2016), doi:10.1016/j.psym.2016.03.005; University of Minnesota Center for Spirituality and Healing, "What Is Prayer?," August 2013, www.takingcharge.csh.umn.edu/explore-healing-practices/prayer.

51. L. Larkey et al., "Randomized Controlled Trial of Qigong/Tai Chi Easy on Cancer-Related Fatigue in Breast Cancer Survivors," *Annals of Behavioral Medicine* 49, no. 2 (2015): 165–76; American Tai Chi Association, "Psychiatric Expert: Tai Chi and Qigong Can Improve Mood in Older Adults," September 6, 2013, www.americantaichi.net/TaiChiQigongForHealthArticle.asp?cID=2'sID=10'article=chi_201309_1'subject=Mental Health.

52. M. Rudd and J. Aakers, "How to Be Happy by Giving to Others," *Scientific American*, July 8, 2014, www.scientificamerican.com/article/how-to-be-happy-by-giving-to-others.

53. K. Azzarelli, "Rethinking Happiness: Using Your Power for Purpose," *Annals of the New York Academy of Sciences* 1384 (2016): 32–5, doi:10.1111/nyas.13149.

54. Mayo Clinic Staff, "Mental Illness: Causes," October 2015, www.mayoclinic.org/diseases-conditions/mental-illness/basics/causes/con-20033813.

55. Ibid.

56. Substance Abuse and Mental Health Services Administration, "Key Substance Use and Mental Health Indicators in the United States: Results from the 2015 National Survey on Drug Use and Health," September 2016, Available at https://www.samhsa.gov/data/sites/default/files/NSDUH-FFR1-2015/NSDUH-FFR1-2015/NSDUH-FFR1-2015.htm.

57. Ibid.

58. L. Szabo, "Cost of Not Caring: Nowhere to Go," *USA Today*, May 5, 2014, www.usatoday.com/story/news/nation/2014/05/12/mental-health-system-crisis/7746535; T. Insel, "Director's Blog: Mental Health Awareness Month: By the Numbers," *National Institute of Mental Health*, May 15, 2015, http://www.nimh.nih.gov/about/director/2015/mental-health-awareness-month-by-the-numbers.shtml.

59. R.P. Gallagher, "*National Survey of College Counseling 2014*," *International Association of Counseling Services, Inc. Monograph Series* 9V (2014), Available at http://0201.nccdn.net/1_2/000/000/088/0b2/NCCCS2014_v2.pdf.

60. American College Health Association, *American College Health Association–National College Health Assessment II (ACHA–NCHA II): Reference Group Data Report Fall 2016* (Baltimore: American College Health Association, 2017), Available at http://www.acha-ncha.org/docs/NCHA-II%20SPRING%202016%20US%20REFERENCE%20GROUP%20EXECUTIVE%20SUMMARY.pdf.

61. Ibid.

62. Ibid.

63. Substance Abuse and Mental Health Services Administration, "Mental Disorders: Anxiety Disorders," October 27, 2015, www.samhsa.gov/disorders/mental; R. Karg et al., "Past Year Mental Health Disorders among Adults in the U.S." 2014 K.R. Merikangas et al., "Lifetime Prevalence of Mental Disorders in U.S. Adolescents: Results from the National Comorbidity Survey Replication—Adolescent Supplement (NCS-A)," *Journal of the American Academy of Child and Adolescent Psychiatry* 49, no. 10 (2010): 980–89, doi:10.1016/j.jaac.2010.05.017.

64. American College Health Association, *American College Health Association–National College Health Assessment II (ACHA–NCHA II): Reference Group Data Report Fall 2016* (Baltimore: American College Health Association, 2017), Available at http://www.acha-ncha.org/docs/NCHA-II%20SPRING%202016%20US%20REFERENCE%20GROUP%20EXECUTIVE%20SUMMARY.pdf

65. National Institute of Mental Health, "Generalized Anxiety Disorder, GAD," Accessed April 2017, www.nimh.nih.gov/health/publications/anxiety-disorders/generalized-anxiety-disorder-gad.shtml.

66. American College Health Association, *American College Health Association–National College Health Assessment II (ACHA–NCHA II): Reference Group Data Report Fall 2016* (Baltimore: American College Health Association, 2017), Available at http://www.acha-ncha.org/docs/NCHA-II%20SPRING%202016%20US%20REFERENCE%20GROUP%20EXECUTIVE%20SUMMARY.pdf.

67. Mayo Clinic Staff, "Panic Attacks and Panic Disorder: Symptoms," May 2015, www.mayoclinic.org/diseases-conditions/panic-attacks/basics/symptoms/con-20020825.

68. WebMD, "Anxiety and Panic Disorders Health Center: Specific Phobias," February 24, 2016, www.webmd.com/anxiety-panic/specific-phobias

69. Ibid.

70. National Institute of Mental Health, "Obsessive Compulsive Disorder: Prevalence," Accessed February 23, 2015, www.nimh.nih.gov/health/statistics/prevalence/obsessive-compulsive-disorder-among-adults.shtml.

71. National Institute of Mental Health, "Obsessive Compulsive Disorder," January 2016, http://

www.nimh.nih.gov/health/topics/obsessive-compulsive-disorder-ocd/index.shtml.

72. Ibid; J. Gradus, "Epidemiology of PTSD," PTSD: National Center for PTSD, *U.S. Department of Veterans Affairs, National Center for PTSD,* February 23, 2016, http://www.ptsd.va.gov/professional/PTSD-overview/epidemiological-facts-ptsd.asp.

73. U.S. Department of Veterans Affairs, "PTSD: National Center for PTSD," October 3, 2016, www.ptsd.va.gov/public/PTSD-overview/basics/how-common-is-ptsd.asp.

74. National Institute of Mental Health, "Post-Traumatic Stress Disorder," February 2016, www.nimh.nih.gov/health/topics/post-traumatic-stress-disorder-ptsd/index.shtml#part4.

75. J. Gradus, "Epidemiology of PTSD," *U.S. Department of Veterans Affairs, National Center for PTSD,* February 23, 2016, www.ptsd.va.gov/professional/PTSD-overview/epidemiological-facts-ptsd.asp; S. Staggs, "Myths and Facts about PTSD," *PsychCentral,* February 2014, http://psychcentral.com/lib/myths-and-facts-about-ptsd.

76. National Institute of Mental Health, "Anxiety Disorders," March 2016 https://www.nimh.nih.gov/health/topics/anxiety-disorders/index.shtml.

77. U.S. National Library of Medicine, "Medline Plus: Mood Disorders," December 27, 2016, https://medlineplus.gov/mooddisorders.html.

78. National Institute of Mental Health, "Major Depression Among Adults," Accessed April 2017, https://www.nimh.nih.gov/health/statistics/prevalence/major-depression-among-adults.shtml.

79. Ibid.

80. Ibid.

81. American College Health Association, *American College Health Association–National College Health Assessment II (ACHA–NCHA II): Reference Group Data Report Fall, 2016.* (Baltimore: American College Health Association, 2017), Available at http://www.acha-ncha.org/docs/NCHA-II%20FALLI%202016%20US%20REFERENCE%20GROUP%20EXECUTIVE%20SUMMARY.pdf.

82. National Institute of Mental Health, "Dysthymic Disorder among Adults," Accessed April 2017, https://www.nimh.nih.gov/health/statistics/prevalence/dysthymic-disorder-among-adults.shtml.

83. Substance Abuse and Mental Health Services Administration, "Mental Disorders: Bipolar and Related Disorders," October 27, 2015, www.samhsa.gov/disorders/mental.

84. WebMD, "Seasonal Depression (Seasonal Affective Disorder)," Accessed February 23, 2015, www.webmd.com/depression/guide/seasonal-affective-disorder.

85. Cleveland Clinic, "Seasonal Depression," Accessed February 2016, https://my.clevelandclinic.org/services/neurological_institute/center-for-behavioral-health/-disease-conditions/hic-seasonal-depression.

86. Mayo Clinic Staff, "Depression: Causes," 2015, www.mayoclinic.org/diseases-conditions/depression/basics/causes/con-20032977.

87. Mayo Clinic, "Depression in Women: Understanding the Gender Gap," January 2016, www.mayoclinic.org/diseases-conditions/depression/in-depth/depression/art-20047725.

88. HelpGuide.org, "Depression in Men," April 2017, www.helpguide.org/mental/depression_men_male.htm.

89. NIH. "Major Depression among Adolescents Aged 12–17." Accessed June, 2017, https://www.nimh.nih.gov/health/statistics/prevalence/major-depression-among-adolescents; American Psychological Association, "Mental Health: Children," Accessed June, 2017, http://www.apa.org/pi/families/children-mental-health.aspx.

90. WebMD, "Depression in the Elderly," Accessed June 2017, http://www.webmd.com/depression/guide/depression-elderly#1; American Psychological Association, "Mental and Behavioral Health of Older Americans: Depression and Anxiety," Accessed June 2017, http://www.apa.org/about/gr/issues/aging/mental-health.

91. Centers for Disease Control and Prevention, "Faststats: Depression." October 2016, https://www.cdc.gov/nchs/fastats/depression.htm.

92. American Psychiatric Association, *Diagnostic and Statistical Manual of Mental Disorders,* 5th ed. (Washington, DC: American Psychiatric Association, 2013).

93. National Institute of Mental Health, "Any Personality Disorder," Accessed February 2016, www.nimh.nih.gov/health/statistics/prevalence/any-personality-disorder.shtml; P. Tyrer, F. Reed, and M. Crawford, "Classification, Assessment Prevalence, and Effect of Personality Disorder," *Lancet* 385, no. 9969 (2015): 717–26.

94. PubMed Health, "Antisocial Personality Disorder," *A.D.A.M. Medical Encyclopedia* (Bethesda, MD: U.S. National Library of Medicine, 2016).

95. Mayo Clinic Staff, "Borderline Personality Disorder," July 2015, http://www.mayoclinic.org/diseases-conditions/borderline-personality-disorder/basics/-symptoms/con-20023204.

96. Ibid.

97. National Institute of Mental Health, "Borderline Personality Disorder," Accessed February 2016, http://www.nimh.nih.gov/health/topics/borderline-personality-disorder/index.shtml.

98. S. Stines. "The Psychology of Cutting: The Reasoning behind self-mutilation." Psych Central. 2016. https://pro.psychcentral.com/recovery-expert/2016/03/the-psychology-of-cutting-the-reasoning-behind-self-mutilation/.

99. American College Health Association, *American College Health Association–National College Health Assessment II (ACHA–NCHA II): Reference Group Data Report, Fall 2016* (Baltimore: American College Health Association, 2017), Available at http://www.acha-ncha.org/docs/NCHA-II%20FALLI%202016%20US%20REFERENCE%20GROUP%20EXECUTIVE%20SUMMARY.pdf.; M. DeRiggi et al., "Non-suicidal Self-injury in Our Schools: A Review and Research-Informed Guidelines for School Mental Health Professionals," *Canadian Journal of School Psychology* 32, no. 2 (2017)122–43; M. Smith and J. Segal, "Cutting and Self-Harm," Updated February 2014, www.helpguide.org/mental/self_injury.htm.

100. National Institute of Mental Health, "Schizophrenia," February 2016, www.nimh.nih.gov/health/topics/schizophrenia/index.shtml.

101. Ibid.

102. Ibid.

103. Alzheimer's Association, "Quick Facts: Prevalence," 2017, http://www.alz.org/facts/#prevalence.

104. Ibid.

105. M. Heron, "Deaths: Leading Causes for 2014," *National Vital Statistics Reports* 65, no. 5 (2016), Available at https://www.cdc.gov/nchs/data/nvsr/nvsr65/nvsr65_05.pdf.

106. American College Health Association, *American College Health Association–National College Health Assessment II (ACHA–NCHA II): Reference Group Data Report Fall 2016* (Baltimore: American College Health Association, 2017), Available at http://www.acha-ncha.org/docs/NCHA-II%20SPRING%202016%20US%20REFERENCE%20GROUP%20EXECUTIVE%20SUMMARY.pdf.

107. Ibid.; Centers for Disease Control and Prevention, "Suicide Facts at a Glance 2015," Accessed February 2016, http://www.cdc.gov/violenceprevention/pdf/suicide-datasheet-a.pdf.

108. A. Haas et al., "Suicide Attempts among Transgender and Gender Non-conforming Adults: Findings of the National Transgender Discrimination Survey," American Foundation for Suicide Prevention, January 2014.

109. Centers for Disease Control and Prevention, "Suicide Facts at a Glance 2015," Accessed February 2016, http://www.cdc.gov/violenceprevention/pdf/suicide-datasheet-a.pdf.

110. Ibid.

111. American Foundation for Suicide Prevention, "Warning Signs of Suicide," Accessed February 2016, www.afsp.org/preventing-suicide/risk-factors-and-warning-signs.

112. Ibid.

113. Befrienders Worldwide, "Helping a Suicidal Friend or Relative," Accessed February 2016, http://www.befrienders.org/helping-a-friend; Befrienders Worldwide, "Suicidal Feelings," Accessed February 2016, http://www.befrienders.org/suicidal-feelings.

114. National Institute of Mental Health, "Use of Mental Health Services and Treatment among Adults," Accessed April 2017, https://www.nimh.nih.gov/health/statistics/prevalence/use-of-mental-health-services-and-treatment-among-adults.shtml.

115. S. Clement et al., "What Is the Impact of Mental Health-Related Stigma on Help-seeking? A Systematic Review of Quantitative and Qualitative Studies," *Psychological Medicine* 45, no. 1 (2015): 11–27.

116. K. Huffman and C. A. Sanderson, *Real World Psychology* (Hoboken, NJ: Wiley, 2014).

117. Ibid.

118. Mayo Clinic, "Cognitive Behavioral Therapy," February 2016, http://www.mayoclinic.org/tests-procedures/cognitive-behavioral–therapy/home/ovc-20186868.

119. National Institute of Mental Health, "Major Depression among Adults," Accessed April 2017, https://www.nimh.nih.gov/health/statistics/prevalence/major-depression-among-adults.shtml; National Institute of Mental Health, "Any Anxiety Disorder among Adults," Accessed April 2017, https://www.nimh.nih.gov/health/statistics/prevalence/any-anxiety-disorder-among-adults.shtml; National Institute of Mental Health, "Any Anxiety Disorder among Children," Accessed April 2017, https://www.nimh.nih.gov/health/statistics/prevalence/any-anxiety-disorder-among-children.shtml; N. Farm et al., "The Mindful Brain and Emotion Regulation in Mood Disorders," *Canadian Journal of Psychiatry* 57, no. 2 (2012): 70–7; J. Vøllestad et al., "Mindfulness and Acceptance based Interventions for Anxiety Disorders: A Systematic Review and Metaanalysis," *British Journal of Clinical Psychology* 51, no. 3 (2012): 239–60; J. Sundquist et al., "Mindfulness Group Therapy in Primary Care Patients with Depression, Anxiety and Stress and Adjustment Disorders: Randomised Controlled Trial," *British Journal of Psychiatry* 206, no. 2 (2015): 128–35.

120. Drug Watch, "FDA Warnings for Antidepressants," October 12, 2015, http://www.drugwatch.com/ssri/fda-warnings; R. Friedman, "Antidepressants' Black-Box Warning—10 Years Later," *New England Journal of Medicine* 371, no. 18 (2014): 1666–68.

Chapter 3

1. American Psychological Association, "Stress in America, Coping with Change," 2017.; https://www.apa.org/news/press/releases/stress/2016/coping-with-change.pdf; American Psychological Association, "Stress in America Annual Survey: Are Teens Adopting Adults' Stress Habits?" February 11, 2014, Accessed July 2017, Available at www.apa.org/news/press/releases/stress/2013/stress-report.pdf; American Psychological Association, "Stress in America: The Impact of Discrimination," March 2016, http://www.apa.org/news/press/releases/stress/2015/impact-of-discrimination.pdf.

2. American Psychological Association, "A Stress Snapshot: Women Continue to Face an Uphill Battle with Stress," Accessed January 30, 2015, http://apa.org/news/press/releases/stress/2013/snapshot.aspx: American Psychological Association, "Stress in America, Coping with Change," 2017.; https://www.apa.org/news/press/releases/stress/2016/coping-with-change.pdf

3. American Psychological Association, "Stress in America: Coping with Change," 2017. https://www.apa.org/news/press/releases/stress/2016/coping-with-change.pdf;.

4. American Psychological Association, "A Stress Snapshot: Women Continue to Face an Uphill Battle with Stress," Accessed January 30, 2015, http://apa.org/news/press/releases/stress/2013/snapshot.aspx.

5. B.L. Seaward, *Managing Stress: Principles and Strategies for Health and Well-Being*, 9th ed. (Sudbury, MA: Jones and Bartlett, 2015), ; National Institute of Mental Health (NIMH), "Fact Sheet on Stress," Accessed January 2017, www.nimh.nih.gov/health/publications/stress/index.shtml/index.shtml.

6. American Psychological Association, "Stress in America: The Impact of Discrimination," March 2016, http://www.apa.org/news/press/releases/stress/2015/impact-of-discrimination.pdf; American Psychological Association, "Stress in America: Paying with Our Health," 2015, Accessed April 2015, http://www.apa.org/news/press/releases/stress/2014/stress-report.pdf.

7. American Psychological Association, "Stress in America: Coping with Change." 2017.

8. Ibid.

9. H. Selye, *Stress without Distress* (New York: Lippincott Williams ' Wilkins, 1974), 28–9.

10. W.B. Cannon, *The Wisdom of the Body* (New York: Norton, 1932).

11. C. Fagundes and B. Way, "Early-Life Stress and Adult Inflammation," *Current Directions in Psychological Science* 23, no. 4 (2014): 277–83; J. Morey et al., "Current Directions in Stress and Human Immune Function," *Current Opinion in Psychology* 5 (2015): 13–7; Mayo Clinic, "Chronic Stress Puts Your Health at Risk," April 21, 2016, http://www.mayoclinic.org/healthy-lifestyle/stress-management/in-depth/stress/art-20046037; A. Marsland et al., "The Effects of Acute Psychological Stress on Circulating and Stimulated Inflammatory Markers: A Systematic Review and Meta-analysis," *Brain, Behavior and Immunity* 64 (2017): 208–19.

12. C. Cardoso and M.A. Ellenbogen, "Tend-and-Befriend Is a Beacon for Change in Stress Research: A Reply to Tops," *Psychoneuroendocrinology* 45 (2014): 212–13; J. Berger et al., "Cortisol Modulates Men's Affiliative Responses to Acute Social Stress," *Psychoneuroendocrinology* 63 (2016): 1–9.

13. N.K. Dess, "Tend and Befriend: Women Tend to Nurture and Men to Withdraw When Life Gets Hard," June 9, 2016, *Psychology Today*, https://www.psychologytoday.com/articles/200009/tend-and-befriend.

14. N. Rohleder, "Chronic Stress and Disease" in *Insights to Neuroimmune Biology*, 2nd ed., edited by I. Berci (Amsterdam: Elsevier Publishing, 2016); E. Dalton et al., "Pathways Maintaining Physical Health Problems from Childhood to Young Adulthood: The Role of Stress and Mood." *Psychology ' Health* 31, no. 11 (2016): 1255–71; P. Gianaros and T. Wager, "Brain–Body Pathways Linking Psychological Stress and Physical Health," *Current Directions in Psychological Science* 24, no. 4 (2015): 313–21; K.

15. J. Sumner et al., "Associations of Trauma Exposure and Posttraumatic Stress Symptoms with Venous Thromboembolism over 22 Years in Women." *Journal of the American Heart Association* 5, no. 5 (2016): e003197; H.M. Lagraauw et al., "Acute and Chronic Psychological Stress as Risk Factors for Cardiovascular Disease: Insights Gained from Epidemiological, Clinical, and Experimental Studies," *Brain, Behavior, and Immunity* 50 (2015): 18–30; A. Marsland et al., "The Effects of Acute Psychological Stress on Circulating and Stimulated Inflammatory Markers: A Systematic Review and Meta-analysis," *Brain, Behavior and Immunity* 64 (2017): 208–19; J. Holt-Lunstad and T. Smith, "Loneliness and Social Isolation as Risk Factors for CVD: Implications for Evidence-Based Patient Care and Scientific Inquiry," *Heart* 102, no. 13 (2016): 967–89.

16. I. Bot, et al, "Stressed brain, stressed heart?" The Lancet. Volume 389, No 10071, p770–771, (2017), DOI: http://dx.doi.org/10.1016/S0140-6736(17)30044-2M. Kivimäki and I. Kawachi, "Work Stress as a Risk Factor for Cardiovascular Disease," *Current Cardiology Reports* 17, no. 9 (2015): 1–9; M. Skogstad et al., "Systematic Review of the Cardiovascular Effects of Occupational Noise," *Occupational Medicine* 66, no. 1 (2016): 10–16.

17. H. Kim, et al. "Interaction between the *RGS6* gene and psychosocial stress on obesity-related traits." *Endocrine Journal.* Vol. 64 (2017) No. 3 p. 357-362 Doi: http://doi.org/10.1507/endocrj.EJ16-0438; S. Garbarino and N. Magnavita, "Work Stress and Metabolic Syndrome in Police Officers: A Prospective Study," *PLoS ONE* 10, no. 12 (2015): e0144318; F. Bartoli et al., "Posttraumatic Stress Disorder and Risk of Obesity: Systematic Review and Meta-analysis," *Journal of Clinical Psychiatry* 76, no. 10 (2015): e1253–61.

18. National Headache Foundation, "Fact Sheets." Accessed July, 2017. http://www.headaches.org/headache-fact-sheets/

19. Mayo Clinic, " Overview: Tension Headache: Symptoms," June, 2016. http://www.mayoclinic.org/diseases-conditions/tension-headache/home/ovc-20211413.

20. National Headache Foundation, "Fact Sheets: Migraine," Accessed July, 2017.

21. R. Lin et al., "Systemic Causes of Hair Loss," *Annals of Medicine* 48, no. 6 (2016): 393–402; A. Skrok and L. Rudnicka, "Stress-Related Hair Disorders," in *Stress and Skin Disorders: Basic and Clinical Aspects*, edited by K. França and M. Jafferany (New York: Springer International, 2017), 155–64.

22. S.H. Ley et al., "Contribution of the Nurses' Health Studies to Uncovering Risk Factors for Type 2 Diabetes: Diet, Lifestyle, Biomarkers, and Genetics," *American Journal of Public Health* 106, no. 9(2016): 1624– 30.

23. M. Virtanen et al., "Psychological Distress and Incidence of Type 2 Diabetes in High Risk and Low Risk Populations: The Whitehall II Cohort Study," *Diabetes Care* 37, no. 8 (2014): 2091–97; C. Crump et al., "Stress Resilience and Subsequent Risk of Type 2 Diabetes in 1.5 Million Young Men." *Diabetologia* 59, no. 4 (2016): 728–33.

24. National Digestive Diseases Information Clearinghouse (NDDIC), "Irritable Bowel Syndrome: How Does Stress Affect IBS?" Accessed January 2017, http://digestive.niddk.nih.gov/ddiseases/pubs/ibs/#stress.

25. B. Bartosz et al., "Mechanisms by Which Stress Affects the Experimental and Clinical Inflammatory Bowel Disease (IBD): Role of Brain-Gut Axis," *Current Neuropharmacology* 14, no. 8 (2016): 892–900; H. F. Herlong, "Digestive Disorders White Paper—2013," *Johns Hopkins Health Alerts*, 2013, www.johnshopkinshealthalerts.com.

26. E. Carlsson et al., "Psychological Stress in Children May Alter the Immune Response," *Journal of Immunology* 192, no. 5 (2014): 2071–81; J. Morey et al., "Current Directions in Stress and Human Immune Function," *Current Opinion in Psychology* 5 (2015): 13–7.

27. K. Murphy, et al. "Stress, cortisol, and B lymphocytes: a novel approach to understanding academic stress and immune function." *Stress*. 2016. 19(2). Stress Vol. 19 , Iss. 2,2016. https://doi.org/10.3109/10253890.2015.1127913; J. Morey et al., "Current Directions in Stress and Human Immune Function," *Current Opinion in Psychology* 5 (2015): 13–7.

28. American College Health Association, *American College Health Association–National College Health Assessment II (ACHA-NCHA II): Reference Group Data Report Fall, 2016* (Hanover, MD: American College Health Association, 2017).

29. O.T. Wolf et al., "Stress and Memory: A Selective Review on Recent Developments in the Understanding of Stress Hormone Effects on Memory and Their Clinical Relevance," *Journal of Neuroendocrinology* 28, no. 8 (2016); G. Shields et al., "The Effects of Acute Stress on Core Executive Functions: A Meta-analysis and Comparison with Cortisol," *Neuroscience ' Biobehavioral Reviews* 68 (2016): 651–68.

30. J. Oliver et al., "Impairments of the Spatial Working Memory and Attention Following Acute Psychosocial Stress," *Stress and Health* 31, no. 2 (2015): 115–23; G. Shields et al., "The Effects of Acute Stress on Core Executive Functions: A Meta-analysis and Comparison with Cortisol," *Neuroscience ' Biobehavioral Reviews* 68 (2016): 651–68.

31. D. Baglietto-Vargas et al., "Short-Term Modern Life-like Stress Exacerbates Ab-Pathology and Synapse Loss in 3xTg-AD Mice," *Journal of Neurochemistry* 134, no. 5 (2015): 915–26; E. Marcello, "Alzheimer's Disease and Modern Lifestyle: What Is the Role of Stress?," *Journal of Neurochemistry* 134, no. 5 (2015): 795–98.

32. L. Mah, C. Szabuniewicz, and Alexandra J. Fiocco, "Can Anxiety Damage the Brain?" *Current Opinion in Psychiatry* 29, no. 1 (2016): 56–62; D. Toral-Rios, "Oxidative Stress, Metabolic Syndrome and Alzheimer's Disease," *Biochemistry of Oxidative Stress* 16 (2016): 361–74; A. Pole et al., "Oxidative Stress, Cellular Senescence and Ageing," *AIMS Molecular Science/* 3, no. 3 (2016).

33. *American College Health Association, American College Health Association–National College Health Assessment II (ACHA–NCHA II): Reference Group Data Report Fall 2016* (Hanover, MD: American College Health Association, 2017), Available at www.achancha.org/reports_ACHA-NCHAII.html.

34. Ibid.

35. A. Prather et al., "Association of Insufficient Sleep with Respiratory Infections among Adults in the United States," *JAMA Internal Medicine* 176, no. 6 (2016): 850–52, doi:10.1001/jamainternmed.2016.0787; A. Prather et al., "Behaviorally Assessed Sleep and Susceptibility to the Common Cold," *Sleep* 38, no. 9 (2015): 1353–59.

36. V. Aho et al., "Prolonged Sleep Restriction Induces Changes in Pathways Involved in Cholesterol Metabolism and Inflammatory Responses," *Scientific Reports* 6 (2016): doi:10.1038/srep24828 M. Irwin et al., "Sleep Disturbance, Sleep Duration, and Inflammation: A Systematic Review and Meta-Analysis of Cohort Studies and Experimental Sleep Deprivation," *Biological Psychiatry* 80, no. 1 (2016): 40–52.

37. M. Irwin et al., "Sleep Disturbance, Sleep Duration, and Inflammation: A Systematic Review and Meta-Analysis of Cohort Studies and Experimental Sleep Deprivation," *Biological Psychiatry* 80, no. 1 (2016): 40–52; R. Yuan et al., "The Effect of Sleep Deprivation on Coronary Heart Disease," *Chinese Medical Sciences Journal* 31, no. 4 (2016): 247–53.

38. A. Cooper et al., "Sleep Duration and Cardio-metabolic Risk Factors among Individuals with Type 2 Diabetes," *Sleep Medicine* 16, no. 1 (2015): 119–25; M.A. Miller et al., "Sustained Short Sleep and Risk of Obesity: Evidence in Children and Adults," in *Handbook of Obesity*, vol. 1, 3rd ed., edited by G.A. Bray and C. Bouchard (Boca Raton, FL: CRC Press, 2014), 397–41.

39. M. Nagayoshi et al., "Obstructive Sleep Apnea and Incident Type 2 Diabetes," *Sleep Medicine* 25 (2016): 156–61; A. Cooper et al., "Sleep Duration and Cardio-metabolic Risk Factors among Individuals with Type 2 Diabetes," *Sleep Medicine* 16, no. 1 (2015): 119–25; M. Kohasieh and A. Makaryrus, "Sleep Deficiency and Deprivation Leading to Cardiovascular Disease," *International Journal of Hypertension* 2015 (2015); Z. Shan et al., "Sleep Duration and Risk of Type 2 Diabetes: A Meta-analysis of Prospective Studies," *Diabetes Care* 38, no. 3 (2015): 529–37; J. Ferrie et al., "Change in Sleep Duration and Type 2 Diabetes: The Whitehall II Study," *Diabetes Care* 38, no. 8 (2015): 1467–72.

40. L. Wise et al., "Sleep and Male Fecundity in a North American Preconception Cohort Study," *Fertility and Sterility* 106, no. 3 (2016): e79; N. White, "Influence of Sleep on Fertility in Women," *American Journal of Lifestyle Medicine* 10, no. 4 (2016): 239–41.

41. National Institutes of Health, "Information about Sleep," Accessed February 2016, http://science.education.nih.gov/supplements/nih3/sleep/guide/info-sleep.html; C. Peri, "What Lack of Sleep Does to Your Mind," WebMD, Accessed February 2017, www.webmd.com/sleep-disorders/excessive-sleepiness-10/emotions-cognitive.

42. A. Chatburn et al., "Complex Associative Memory Processing and Sleep: A Systematic Review and Meta-Analysis of Behavioural Evidence and Underlying EEG Mechanisms." *Neuroscience and Biobehavioral Reviews* 47 (2014): 645–55; S. Hershner and R. Chervin, "Causes and Consequences of Sleepiness among College Students," 2014.

43. H. Fullagar et al., "Sleep and Athletic Performance: The Effects of Sleep Loss on Exercise Performance, and Physiological and Cognitive Responses to Exercise," *Sports Medicine* 45, no. 2 (2015): 161–86.

44. AAA Foundation for Traffic Safety, "Acute Sleep Deprivation and Crash Risk," Accessed February 2017, https://www.aaafoundation.org/acute-sleep-deprivation-and-crash-risk.

45. National Sleep Foundation, "Depression and Sleep," Accessed February 2016, https://sleepfoundation.org/sleep-disorders-problems/depression-and-sleep.

46. A. Ramkisoengsing and J. Meijer, "Synchronization of Biological Clock Neurons by Light and Peripheral Feedback Systems Promotes Circadian Rhythms and Health," *Frontiers in Neurology* 6, no. 128 (2015): 128; M. Vitaterna, J. Takahashi, and F. Turek, "Overview of Circadian Rhythms," National Institute on Alcohol Abuse and Alcoholism, Accessed July 2017, http://pubs.niaaa.nih.gov/publications/arh25-2/85-93.htm.

47. B. Rasch and J. Born, "About Sleep's Role in Memory," *Physiological Reviews* 93, no. 2 (2013): 681–766; R. Boyce and A. Adamantidis, "REM: Sleep on It!" *Neuropsychopharmacology* 42, no. 1 (2017): 375.

48. N. Watson et al., "Joint Consensus Statement of the American Academy of Sleep Medicine and Sleep Research Society on the Recommended Amount of Sleep for a Healthy Adult: Methodology and Discussion," *Journal of Clinical Sleep Medicine* 11, no. 8 (2015): 931–52; N.F. Watson et al., "Recommended Amount of Sleep for a Healthy Adult: A Joint Consensus Statement of the American Academy of Sleep Medicine and Sleep Research Society," *Sleep 38, no. 6 (2015):* 843–44.

49. National Sleep Foundation, "Recommendations: Sleep Hygiene," April, 2016. https://com-jax-emergency-pami.sites.medinfo.ufl.edu/files/2016/08/Sleep-Hygiene.pdf

50. K. Donahue, "Daily Hassles, Mental Health Outcome and Dispositional Mindfulness in Student Registered Nurse Anesthetists," Doctoral Dissertation, Oregon Health and Science University, OHSU Digital Commons, 2016; Y. Jeong et al., "Do Hassles and Uplifts Trajectories Predict Mortality? Longitudinal Findings from the VA Normative Aging Study," *Journal of Behavioral Medicine* 39, no. 3 (2016): 408–19; C. Aldwin et al., "Do Hassles Mediate between Life Events and Mortality in Older Men? Longitudinal Findings from the VA Normative Aging Study," *Experimental Gerontology* 59 (2014): 74–80.

51. Y. Jeong et al., "Do Hassles and Uplifts Trajectories Predict Mortality? Longitudinal Findings from the VA Normative Aging Study," *Journal of Behavioral Medicine* 39, no. 3 (2016): 408–19; C. Aldwin et al., "Do Hassles Mediate between Life Events and Mortality in Older Men? Longitudinal Findings from the VA Normative Aging Study," *Experimental Gerontology* 59 (2014): 74–80.

52. APA. Stress in America: Technology and Social Media. 2017. https://www.apa.org/news/press/releases/stress/2017/technology-social-media.PDF; S. Deatherage, H. Servaty-Seib, and I. Aksoz, "Stress, Coping and the Internet Use of College Students," *Journal of American Health* 62, no. 1 (2014): 40–6; Y. Lee et al., "The Dark Side of Smartphone Usage: Psychological Traits, Compulsive Behavior and Technostress," *Computers in Human Behavior* 31 (2014): 373–81; A. Lepp, J. Barkley, and A. Karpinski, "The Relationship between Cell Phone Use, Academic Performance, Anxiety, and Satisfaction with Life in College Students," *Computers in Human Behavior* 31 (2014):1.

53. American Psychological Association, "Stress in America, The Impact of Discrimination," March 2016, Accessed July 2017, http://www.apa.org/news/press/releases/stress/2015/impact-of-discrimination.pdf.

54. Ibid.

55. Ibid.

56. Ibid.

57. A. Gold, "Why Self Esteem Is Important for Mental Health," NAMI, July 12, 2016, http://www.nami.org/Blogs/NAMI-Blog/July-2016/Why-Self-Esteem-Is-Important-for-Mental-Health; K.N. Mossakowski, "Disadvantaged Family Background and Depression among Young Adults in the United States: The Roles of Chronic Stress and Self-esteem," *Stress and Health* 31, no. 1 (2015): 52–62; K.R. Conner et al., "Posttraumatic Stress Disorder and Suicide in 5.9 Million Individuals Receiving Care in the Veterans Health Administration Health System," *Journal of Affective Disorders* 166 (2014): 1–5.

58. J. Twenge, *Generation Me—Revised and Updated: Why Today's Young Americans Are More Confident, Assertive, Entitled and More Miserable Than Ever* (New York: Simon and Schuster, 2014).

59. E. Anderson, (2016) "Giving Negative Feedback to Millennials: How Can Managers Criticize the 'Most Praised' Generation," *Management Research Review* 39, no. 6 (2016): 692–705.

60. P. Schonfeld et al., "The Effects of Daily Stress on Positive and Negative Mental Health: Mediation through Self-efficacy," *International Journal of Clinical and Health Psychology* 6, no. 1 (2016): 692–705.

61. A. Peng and J. Schaubroeck, "When Confidence Comes and Goes: How Variation in Self-efficacy Moderates Stressor-Strain Relationships," *Journal of Occupational Health Psychology* 20, no. 3 (2015): 359–76; M. Komarraju and D. Nadler, "Self Efficacy and Academic Achievement: Who Do Implicit Beliefs, Goals and Effort Regulation Matter?" *Learning and Individual Differences* 25 (2013): 67–72.

62. T. Honicke and J. Broadbent, "The Influence of Academic Self-efficacy on Academic Performance: A Systematic Review," *Educational Research Review* 17 (2016): 63–84; P.N. von der Embse and S. Witmer, "High-Stakes Accountability: Student Anxiety and Large-Scale Testing," *Journal of Applied School Psychology* 30, no. 2 (2014): 132–56, doi:10.1080/15377903.2014.888529.

63. T. Honicke and J. Broadbent, "The Influence of Academic Self-efficacy on Academic Performance: A Systematic Review," *Educational Research Review* 17 (2016): 63–84.

64. M. Friedman and R.H. Rosenman, *Type A Behavior and Your Heart* (New York: Knopf, 1974).

65. P. Pimple et al., "Association between Anger and Mental Stress–Induced Myocardial Ischemia," *American Heart Journal* 169, no. 1 (2015): 115–21.

66. G. Mate, *When the Body Says No: Understanding the Stress-Disease Connection,* (Hoboken, NJ: John Wiley ' Sons, 2011).

67. J. Thayer et al., "Potential Biological Pathways Linking Type-D Personality and Poor Health: A Cross-Sectional Investigation," *Psychotherapy and Psychosomatics* 84 (2015); R. Garcia-Retamero et al., "On the Relationship between Type-D Personality and Cardiovascular Health," *European Health Psychologist* 17, Supplement (2015): 707.

68. S.C. Kobasa, "Stressful Life Events, Personality, and Health: An Inquiry into Hardiness," *Journal of Personality and Social Psychology* 37, no. 1 (1979): 1–11.

69. R. Graber, F. Pichon, and E. Carubine, "Psychological Resilience: State of Knowledge and Future Research Agendas: Working Paper 425," October 2015, Available at http://www.odi.org/sites/odi.org.uk/files/odi-assets/publications-opinion-files/9872.pdf.

70. E. Chen, K.C. McLean, and G. E. Miller, "Shift-and-Persist Strategies: Associations with Socioeconomic Status and the Regulation of Inflammation among Adolescents and Their Parents," *Psychosomatic Medicine* 77, no. 4 (2015): 371–82.

71. M.E.P. Seligman, *Flourishing: A Visionary New Understanding of Happiness and Well-Being* (New York: Free Press/Simon and Schuster, 2011); M. Seligman. "The New Era of Positive Psychology: TED TALK." Accessed July, 2017. http://www .nationalwellbeingservice.com/wellbeing-videos/ martin-seligman-flourishing-a-new-under- standing-of-wellbeing-at-happiness-its-causes- 2012/M.E.P. Seligman, *Authentic Happiness: Using the New Positive Psychology to Realize Your Potential for Lasting Fulfillment* (New York: Free Press/Simon and Schuster, 2002).

72. B.L. Seaward, *Managing Stress: Principles and Strategies for Health and Well-Being,*" 8th ed. (Sudbury, MA: Jones and Bartlett, 2015).

73. Action for Happiness, "10 Keys To Happier Living," Accessed January 30, 2015, www.action- forhappiness.org/10-keys-to-happier-living.

74. W. Lovallo, *Stress and Health: Biological and Psychological Interactions*, 3rd ed. (Thousand Oaks, CA: Sage, 2016); D.A. Girdano, D.E. Dusek, and G.S. Everly, *Controlling Stress and Tension,* 9th ed. (San Francisco: Benjamin Cummings, 2013), 375.

75. W. Lovallo, *Stress and Health: Biological and Psychological Interactions*, 3rd ed. (Thousand Oaks, CA: Sage, 2016); A. Lurie and K. Monahan, "Humor, Aging, and Life Review: Survival through the Use of Humor," *Social Work in Mental Health* 13, no. 1 (2015): 82–91; C. Dormann, "Laughter as the Best Medicine: Exploring Humour-Mediated Health Applications," in *Distributed, Ambient, and Pervasive Interactions*, edited by N. Streitz (New York: Springer, 2015), 639–50.

76. B.L. Seaward, *Managing Stress Principles and Strategies for Health and Well-Being*, 8th ed. (Sudbury, MA: Jones and Bartlett, 2015).

77. P. Norman and A. Wrona-Clarke, "Combining Self-affirmation and Implementation Intentions to Reduce Heavy Episodic Drinking in University Students," *Psychology of Addictive Behaviors*, 30, no. 4 (2016): 434–41; A. Toli, T. Webb, and G.E. Hardy, "Does Forming Implementation Intentions Help People with Mental Health Problems to Achieve Goals? A Meta-analysis of Experimental Studies with Clinical and Analogue Samples," *British Journal of Clinical Psychology* 55, no. 1 (2016): 69–90.

78. American College Health Association, *National College Health Assessment II: Reference Group Data Report, Fall 2016* (Hanover, MD: American College Health Association, 2017).

79. Yoga Journal and Yoga Alliance, "Yoga in America Study," January 2016, Available at https://www. yogaalliance.org/Home/Media_Inquiries/2016_ Yoga_in_America_Study_Conducted_by_Yoga_ Journal_and_Yoga_Alliance_Reveals_Growth_ and_Benefits_of_the_Practice.

80. C. Lau, R. Yu, and J. Woo, "Effects of a 12-Week Hatha Yoga Intervention on Cardiorespiratory Endurance, Muscular Strength and Endurance, and Flexibility in Hong Kong Chinese Adults: A Controlled Clinical Trial," *Evidence-Based Complementary and Alternative Medicine* 2015 (2015); M.E. Papp et al., "Effects of High-Intensity Hatha Yoga on Cardiovascular Fitness, Adipocytokines, and Apolipoproteins in Healthy Students: A Randomized Controlled Study," *Journal of Alternative and Complementary Medicine* 22, no. 1 (2016): 81–7.

81. S. Lu et al., "Meditation and Blood Pressure: A Meta-analysis of Randomized Clinical Trials," *Journal of Hypertension* (2016); S.R. Steinhubl et al., "Cardiovascular and Nervous System Changes during Meditation," *Frontiers in Human Neuroscience* 9 (2015): 145; R.D. Brook et al., "Beyond Medications and Diet: Alternative Approaches to Lowering Blood Pressure," *Hypertension* 61, no. 6 (2013): 1360–83.

82. K. Eagan et. al., "The American Freshman: Fifty-Year Trends, 1966–2015," Los Angeles Higher Education Research Institute, UCLA (2016), Available at https://www.heri.ucla.edu/monogra phs/50YearTrendsMonograph2016.pdf.

83. Higher Education Research Institute, "A Year of Change: First Year," Accessed January 31, 2015, www.heri.ucla.edu/infographics/YFCY-2014-In- fographic.pdf; J.K. Eagen et al., *The American Freshman: National Norms Fall 2014—Expanded Edition* (Los Angeles: Higher Education Research Institute, 2015), www.heri.ucla.edu/monographs/ TheAmericanFreshman2014-Expanded.pdf.

84. Ibid.

85. K. Donahue, "Daily Hassles, Mental Health Outcomes, and Dispositional Mindfulness in Student Registered Nurse Anesthetists," Doctoral Dissertation, Oregon Health and Science University, OSU Digital Commons, http://digitalcommons. ohsu.edu/cgi/viewcontent.cgi?article=16915'co ntext=etd.

86. J. Gu et al., "How Do Mindfulness-based Cognitive Therapy and Mindfulness-based Stress Reduction Improve Mental Health and Well Being? A Systematic Review and Meta-analysis of Mediation Studies," *Clinical Psychology Review* 37 (2015):1–12; A. Rosenberg et al., "Promoting Resilience in Stress Management: A Pilot Study of a Novel Resilience-Promoting Intervention for Adolescents and Young Adults with Serious Illness," *Journal of Pediatric Psychology* 40, no. 9 (2015): 992–99; J. Donald et al., "Daily Stress and the Benefits of Mindfulness: Examining the Daily and Longitudinal Relations between Present Moment Awareness and Stress Responses," *Journal of Research in Personality* 65 (2016): 30–47.

Chapter 4

1. J. Holt-Lunstad et al., "Loneliness and Social Isolation as Risk Factors for Mortality," *Perspectives on Psychological Science* 10, no. 2 (2015): 227-237.

2. H. C. Espeleta et al., "The Impact of Child Abuse Severity on Adult Attachment Anxiety and Avoidance in College Women: The Role of Emotion Dysregulation," *Journal of Family Violence* (2016): 1-9.

3. R. Sternberg, "A Triangular Theory of Love," *Psychological Review* 93 (1986): 119–35.

4. H. Fisher, *Anatomy of Love: A Natural History of Mating, Marriage, and Why We Stray* (New York: W. W. Norton, 2016).

5. H. Fisher, *Anatomy of Love: A Natural History of Mating, Marriage, and Why We Stray* (New York: W. W. Norton, 2016).

6. R. L. Crooks and K. Baur, *Our Sexuality*, 2016.

7. Sources: M. A. Monto and A. G. Carey, "A New Standard of Sexual Behavior? Are Claims Associated with the "Hookup Culture" Supported by General Social Survey Data?," *Journal of Sex Research* 56, no. 6 (2014): 605–15; P. N. E. Roberson et al., "Hooking Up During College Years: Is There a Pattern?," *Culture, Health & Sexuality* 17, no. 5 (2015): 576-591; J. M. Bearak, "Casual Contraception in Casual Sex: Life-Cycle Change in Undergraduates' Sexual Behavior in Hookups,"

Social Forces 93, no. 2 (2014): 483–513.

8. T. Worley, "Exploring the Association between Relational Uncertainty, Jealousy About Partner's Friendships, and Jealousy Expression in Dating Relationships," *Communication Studies* 65, no. 4 (2014): 370–88; B. D. L. Zandbergen and S. G. Brown, "Culture and Gender Differences in Romantic Jealousy," *Personality and Individual Differences* 72 (2015): 122–7.

9. United States Department of Labor, Bureau of Labor Statistics, "American Time Use Survey Summary–2015 Results," June 24, 2016, http:// www.bls.gov/news.release/atus.pdf

10. N. Baym, *Personal Connections in the Digital Age* (Cambridge: Polity, 2015).

11. p. 227, A. Smith, "15% of American Adults Have Used Online Dating Sites or Mobile Dating Apps," Pew Research, 2016, www.pewinternet. org/2016/02/11/15-percent-of-american-adults- have-used-online-dating-sites-or-mobile-dating- apps/.

12. C. Finkenauer and A. Buyukcan-Tetik, "To Know You Is to Feel Intimate with You: Felt Knowledge is Rooted in Disclosure, Solicitation, and Intimacy," *Family Science* 6, no. 1 (2015): 109–18; C. R. Rogers, "Interpersonal Relationship: The Core of Guidance," in *Person to Person: The Problem of Being Human,* eds. C. R. Rogers and B. Stevens (Lafayette, CA: Real People Press, 1967).

13. K. Stolz, *Unfriending My Ex: Confessions of a Social Media Addict* (New York: Scribner, 2015); N. Baym, *Personal Connections in the Digital Age* (Cambridge: Polity, 2015); CareerBuilder.com, "Number of Employers Using Social Media to Screen Candidates Has Increased 500 Percent over the Last Decade," April 28, 2016, http:// www.careerbuilder.com/share/aboutus/press- releasesdetail.aspx?ed=12%2F31%2F2016&id=p r945&sd=4%2F28%2F2016.

14. B. Johnson, "Privacy No Longer a Social Norm, Says Facebook Founder," *The Guardian*, January 10, 2010, www.guardian.co.uk

15. D. Worthington and M. Fitch-Hauser, *Listening: Processes, Functions, and Competency* (London: Routledge, 2016).

16. J. Wood, *Interpersonal Communication: Everyday Encounters, 8th ed.* (Boston, MA: Woodsworth Publishing, 2015).

17. Ibid.

18. F. Newport and J. Wilke, "Most in U.S. Want Marriage, but Its Importance Has Dropped," Gallup, August 2, 2013, www.gallup.com/poll/163802/ marriage-importance-dropped.aspx

19. G. Livingston and A. Caumont. "5 Facts on Love and Marriage in America." Pew Research Center. February, 2017. http://www.pewresearch.org/ fact-tank/2017/02/13/5-facts-about-love-and- marriage/.

20. U.S. Census Bureau, "Families and Living Arrangements: 2016, Table MS-2 Estimated Median Age at First Marriage, by Sex: 1890 to the Present," www.census.gov/hhes/families/ data/marital.html.

21. P. N. E. Roberson, et al. "Do Differences Matter? A Typology of Emerging Adult Romantic Relationship." *Journal of Social and Personal Relationships* (2016): doi:0265407516661589.

22. R. G. Watt et al., "Social Relationships and Health Related Behaviors Among Older US Adults," *BMC Public Health* 14, no. 1 (2014): 533; G. E. Miller and Y. Pylypchuk, "Marital Status, Spousal Characteristics, and the Use of Preventive Care," *Journal of Family and Economic Issues* 35, no. 3 (2014): 323–38.

23. C. C. Miller, "Study Finds More Reasons to Get and Stay Married," *New York Times*, January 8,

2015, www.nytimes.com/2015/01/08/upshot/study-finds-more-reasons-to-get-and-stay-married.html?rref=upshot&abt=0002&abg=0&_r=2.

24. R. G. Watt et al., "Social Relationships and Health Related Behaviors Among Older US Adults," *BMC Public Health* 14, no. 1 (2014); G. E. Miller and Y. Pylypchuk, "Marital Status, Spousal Characteristics, and the Use of Preventive Care," *Journal of Family and Economic Issues* 35, no. 3 (2014): 323–38.

25. Ibid.

26. U.S. Census Bureau, "Table C2. Household Relationship And Living Arrangements Of Children Under 18 Years, By Age And Sex: 2012," *America's Families and Living Arrangements: 2012*, November 2013, www.census.gov/hhes/families/data/cps2012.html

27. M. Lino, *Expenditures on Children by Families, 2012* (Alexandria, VA: U.S. Department of Agriculture, Center for Nutrition Policy and Promotion, 2013), www.cnpp.usda.gov/Publications/CRC/crc2012.pdf

28. U.S. Census Bureau, "America's Families and Living Arrangements: 2016: Adults, Table AD-3" https://www.census.gov/hhes/families/data/adults.html.

29. U.S. Department of Health and Human Services, Division of Vital Statistics, "First Premarital Cohabitation in the United States: 2006–2010 National Survey of Family Growth," *National Health Statistics Report* 64 (2013), Available at www.cdc.gov/nchs/data/nhsr/nhsr064.pdf; U.S. Department of Health and Human Services, Center for Health Statistics, "Key Statistics from the National Survey of Family Growth," April 20, 2015, www.cdc.gov/nchs/nsfg/key_statistics/c.htm.

30. A. Kuperberg, "Age at Co-Residence, Premarital Cohabitation and Marriage Dissolution: 1985–2009," *Journal of Marriage and Family* 76, no. 2 (2014): DOI: 10.1111/jomf.12092.

31. U.S. Census Bureau, "Characteristics of Same-Sex Households: 2014," Accessed February 2017, www.census.gov/hhes/samesex/data/acs.html.

32. Obergefell v. Hodges, 576 U.S. (2015).

33. Ibid.

34. U.S. Census Bureau, "Marital Status: 2007–2011 American Community Survey, 5-Year Estimates, Table S1201," http://factfinder2.census; U.S. Census Bureau. "Marital Status of the Population 15 Years Old and Over, by Sex, Race and Hispanic Origin: 1950 to Present, Table MS-1", Accessed February 2017, https://www.census.gov/hhes/families/data/marital.html.

35. U.S. Census Bureau, "Marital Status: 2007–2011 American Community Survey, 5-Year Estimates, Table S1201," http://factfinder2.census; U.S. Census Bureau. "Marital Status of the Population 15 Years Old and Over, by Sex, Race and Hispanic Origin: 1950 to Present, Table MS-1", Accessed February 2017, https://www.census.gov/hhes/families/data/marital.html.

36. S. Kennedy and S. Ruggles, "Breaking Up Is Hard to Count: The Rise of Divorce in the United States, 1980–2010," *Demography* 51, no. 2 (2014): 587–98.

37. K. Heller, "The Myth of the High Rate of Divorce," *Psych Central*, 2016, http://psychcentral.com/lib/the-myth-of-the-high-rate-of-divorce

38. C. C. Miller, "The Divorce Surge Is Over, but the Myth Lives On," *New York Times*, December 2, 2014, www.nytimes.com/2014/12/02/upshot/the-divorce-surge-is-over-but-the-myth-lives-on.html.

39. Ibid.

40. The Gottman Institute, "Research FAQs," Accessed February 3, 2017, https://www.gottman.com/about/research/faq/.

41. J. S. Greenberg, C. E. Bruess, and S. B. Oswalt, *Ex-

42. W. J. Chambliss and D. S. Eglitis, *Discover Sociology*, 2nd ed. (Los Angeles: Sage Publications, 2015).

43. Ibid.

44. Ibid.

45. GLAAD, "GLAAD Media Reference Guide—Terms to Avoid," Accessed March 2017, http://www.glaad.org/reference/offensive.

46. Federal Bureau of Investigation, "Bias Breakdown," November 16, 2015, https://www.fbi.gov/news/stories/2015/november/latest-hate-crime-statistics-available.

47. Intersex Society of North America, "How Common Is Intersex?," Accessed March 2017, www.isna.org faq/frequency.

48. J. S. Greenberg, C. E. Bruess, and S. B. Oswalt, *Exploring the Dimensions of Human Sexuality*, 6th ed. (Burlington, MA: Jones and Bartlett, 2016).

49. Womenshealth.gov, "Premenstrual Symptoms Fact Sheet," January 4, 2017, https://www.womenshealth.gov/a-z-topics/premenstrual-syndrome\#e.

50. E.W. Freeman, "Epidemiology and Etiology of Premenstrual Syndromes," March 3, 2017, http://www.medscape.org/viewarticle/553603.

51. Ibid.

52. Womenshealth.gov, "Menstruation and the Menstrual Cycle," January 4, 2017, https://www.womenshealth.gov/a-z-topics/menstruation-and-menstrual-cycle.

53. Ibid.

54. MedlinePlus, "Menopause," February 17, 2017, https://www.nlm.nih.gov/medlineplus/menopause.html.

55. Ibid.

56. Ibid.

57. Ibid.; H. Levine, "Is Hormone Replacement Therapy Making a Comeback?," *Consumer Reports*, May 15, 2016, http://www.consumerreports.org/women-s-health/is-hormone-replacement-therapy-making-a-comeback/.

58. Division of STD Prevention-Centers for Disease Control and Prevention, "2015 Sexually Transmitted Diseases Treatment Guidelines," June 4, 2015, https://www.cdc.gov/std/tg2015/clinical.htm; M. Owings, S. Uddin, and S. Williams, "Trends in Circumcision for Male Newborns in U.S. Hospitals: 1979–2010," August 2013, www.cdc.gov/nchs/data/hestat/circumcision_2013/circumcision_2013.pdf.

59. Mayo Clinic Staff, "Male Menopause: Myth or Reality?," 2011, Available at www.mayoclinic.com/health/male-menopause/MC00058

60. Ibid.

61. F. Kelly, *Sexuality Today*, 11th ed. (New York: McGraw-Hill, 2014).

62. Ibid.

63. American College Health Association, *American College Health Association–National College Health Assessment II (ACHA-NCHA II) Reference Group Data Report, Fall 2016* (Hanover, MD: American College Health Association, 2017), Available at http://www.acha-ncha.org/docs/NCHA-II%20SPRING%202016%20UNDERGRADUATE%20REFERENCE%20GROUP%20DATA%20REPORT.pdf.

64. Ibid.

65. Ibid.

66. Mayo Clinic Staff, "Antidepressants: Get Tips to Cope with Side Effects," July 2013, http://www.mayoclinic.org/diseases-conditions/depression/in-depth/antidepressants/art-20049305.

67. Mayo Clinic Staff, "Erectile Dysfunction," February 2012, Available at www.mayoclinic.com/

health/erectile-dysfunction/DS00162

68. National Kidney and Urological Diseases Information Clearinghouse, "Erectile Dysfunction," 2012, Available at http://kidney.niddk.nih.gov/KUDiseases/pubs/ED/index.aspx

69. S. G. Deem et al., "Premature Ejaculation," (2013), http://emedicine.medscape.com/article/435884-overview

70. Medline Plus, "Sexual Problems Overview: Medline PlusMen's Health: Sexual Problems," Updated May January 2011, http://womenshealth.gov/mens-health/sexual-health-for-men/sexual-problems.html; J. A. Simon, "Problems of Sexual Function in Menopausal Women," *Menopausal Medicine* 20, no. 4 (2012): S1–S6.

71. D. G. Duryea, N. G. Calleja, and D. A. MacDonald, "Nonmedical Use of Prescription Drugs by College Students with Minority Sexual Orientations," *Journal of College Student Psychotherapy* 29, no. 2 (2015): 147–59.

72. T. M. Hall, S. Shoptaw, and C. J. Reback, "Sometimes Poppers Are Not Poppers: Huffing as an Emergent Health Concern Among MSM Substance Users," *Journal of Gay and Lesbian Mental Health* 19, no. 1 (2015): 118–21; T. Kofler, et al. "Use of Poppers (Amyl Nitrite): Unpleasant Side Effects in a Brothel," *European Journal of Case Reports in Internal Medicine* 1, no. 1 (2014): doi: 10.12890/2014_000139.

73. Rape, Abuse, and Incest National Network, "Drug-Facilitated Sexual Assault," Accessed February 2017, https://rainn.org/get-information/types-of-sexual-assault/drug-facilitated-assault.

74. SIECUS, "Life Behaviors of a Sexually Healthy Adult," Accessed May 2016, www.siecus.org.

Chapter 5

1. American College Health Association, *National College Health Assessment II: Reference Group Data Report Fall, 2016* (Hanover, MD: American College Health Association, 2017).

2. Adapted from R. Hatcher et al., *Contraceptive Technology*, 20th rev. ed. (New York: Ardent Media, 2011); Planned Parenthood, "Birth Control," Accessed March 2017, www.plannedparenthood.org.

3. Ibid.

4. Ibid.

5. Ibid.

6. Ibid.

7. World Health Organization, "Nonoxynol-9 Ineffective in Preventing HIV Infection," Accessed March 2017, www.who.int/mediacentre/news/notes/release55/en.

8. R. Hatcher et al., *Contraceptive Technology*, 20th rev. ed. (New York: Ardent Media, 2011); Planned Parenthood, "Birth Control," Accessed March 2017, www.plannedparenthood.org.

9. Ibid.

10. HPSRx Enterprises, "Caya: For Patients," Accessed March 2017, http://caya.us.com/services/for-patients.

11. R. Hatcher et al., *Contraceptive Technology*, 20th rev. ed. (New York: Ardent Media, 2011); Planned Parenthood, "Birth Control," Accessed March 2017, www.plannedparenthood.org.

12. Ibid.

13. Ibid.

14. Data from American College Health Association, *American College Health Association—National College Health Assessment II: Reference Group Data, Fall 2016* (Hanover, MD: American College Health Association, 2017).

15. R. Hatcher et al., *Contraceptive Technology*, 20th rev. ed. (New York: Ardent Media, 2011); Planned Parenthood, "Birth Control," Accessed March 2017, www.plannedparenthood.org.

16. J. Trussell, "Contraceptive Efficacy,". Contraception. 2011 May; 83(5): 397–404. doi: 10.1016/j.contraception.2011.01.021 https://www.ncbi.nlm.nih.gov/pmc/articles/PMC3638209/

17. O. Lidegaard, "The Risk of Arterial Thrombosis Increases with the Use of Combined Oral Contraceptives," *Evidence Based Medicine* 21, no. 1 (2016): 38; A. Weill et al., "Low Dose Oestrogen Combined Oral Contraception and Risk of Pulmonary Embolism, Stroke, and Myocardial Infarction in Five Million French Women: Cohort Study," *British Medical Journal* 353, (2016): i2002.

18. R. Hatcher et al., *Contraceptive Technology*, 20th rev. ed. (New York: Ardent Media, 2011); Planned Parenthood, "Birth Control," Accessed March 2017, www.plannedparenthood.org.

19. Mylan Pharmaceuticals, "Xulane," Accessed March 2017, www.xulane.com; Drugs.com, "Xulane," March 2017, www.drugs.com/mtm/xulane_transdermal.html.

20. R. Hatcher et al., *Contraceptive Technology*, 20th rev. ed. (New York: Ardent Media, 2011); Planned Parenthood, "Birth Control," Accessed March 2017, www.plannedparenthood.org.

21. Drugs.com, "Xulane," March 2017, http://www.drugs.com/pro/xulane.html.

22. Drugs.com, "Xulane," March 2017, http://www.drugs.com/pro/xulane.html.

23. R. Hatcher et al., *Contraceptive Technology*, 20th rev. ed. (New York: Ardent Media, 2011); Planned Parenthood, "Birth Control," Accessed March 2017, www.plannedparenthood.org.

24. Ibid.

25. Pfizer, "Depo-subQ Provera U.S. Patient Product Information," Accessed March 2017, http://www.pfizer.com/products/product-detail/depo_subq_provera_104.

26. R. Hatcher et al., *Contraceptive Technology*, 20th rev. ed. (New York: Ardent Media, 2011); Planned Parenthood, "Birth Control," Accessed March 2017, www.plannedparenthood.org.

27. K. Daniels et al., "Current Contraceptive Use and Variation by Selected Characteristics Among Women Aged 15–44: United States, 2011–2013," *National Health Statistics Reports* 86 (2015): 1–15.

28. R. Hatcher et al., *Contraceptive Technology*, 20th rev. ed. (New York: Ardent Media, 2011); Planned Parenthood, "Birth Control," Accessed March 2017, www.plannedparenthood.org.

29. Office of Population Research & Association of Reproductive Health Professionals, The Emergency Contraception Website, "Answers to Frequently Asked Questions about Effectiveness," Updated January 2017, http://ec.princeton.edu/questions/eceffect.html.

30. American College Health Association, *National College Health Assessment II (ACHA-NCHA II): Undergraduate Students Reference Group Data Fall 2016,* (Hanover, MD: American College Health Association, 2017).

31. American College Health Association, *National College Health Assessment II (ACHA-NCHA III): Reference Group Data Report Fall 2016,* (Hanover, MD: American College Health Association, 2017), Available at http://www.acha-ncha.org/reports_ACHA-NCHAIIc.html.

32. J. Trussell, "Contraceptive Efficacy,". Contraception. 2011 May; 83(5): 397–404. doi: 10.1016/j.contraception.2011.01.021 https://www.ncbi.

33. American College Health Association, *National College Health Assessment III (ACHA-NCHA II): Reference Group Data Report Fall, 2016* (Hanover, MD: American College Health Association, 2017).

34. J. Trussell, "Contraceptive Efficacy,". Contraception. 2011 May; 83(5): 397–404. doi: 10.1016/j.contraception.2011.01.021 https://www.ncbi.nlm.nih.gov/pmc/articles/PMC3638209/J.

35. A.R.A. Aiken et al., "Similarities and Differences in Contraceptive Use Reported by Women and Men in the National Survey of Family Growth," *Contraception*, 2016, http://dx.doi.org/10.1016/j.contraception.2016.10.008.

36. U.S. Food and Drug Administration, "Medical Devices, FDA Activities," November 16, 2016, https://www.fda.gov/MedicalDevices/ProductsandMedicalProcedures/ImplantsandProsthetics/EssurePermanentBirthControl/ucm452254.htm.

37. J. Trussell, "Contraceptive Efficacy,". Contraception. 2011 May; 83(5): 397–404. doi: 10.1016/j.contraception.2011.01.021https://www.ncbi.nlm.nih.gov/pmc/articles/PMC3638209/JJ.

38. Ibid.

39. Guttmacher Institute, "Fact Sheet: Induced Abortion in the United States," January 2017, www.guttmacher.org/fact-sheet/induced-abortion-united-states.

40. Ibid.

41. *Roe v. Wade*, 410 U.S. 113 (1973).

42. L. Saad, "Americans' Attitudes Toward Abortion Unchanged," *Gallup Social Issues*, May 25, 2016, http://www.gallup.com/poll/191834/americans-attitudes-toward-abortion-unchanged.aspx.

43. Center for Reproductive Rights, "Standing Up for Our Reproductive Rights: A Look Back at the 114th Congress," Report, 2017, Available at:https://www.reproductiverights.org/sites/crr.civicactions.net/files/documents/Standing-Up-for-Reproductive-Rights-A%20-Look-Back-at-the-114th-Congress.pdf.

44. Guttmacher Institute, "Induced Abortions Worldwide: Global Incidence and Trends—Fact Sheet." May 2016, https://www.guttmacher.org/fact-sheet/unduced abortion-worldwide.

45. Ibid.

46. M.A. Biggs et al., "Mental Health Diagnoses 3 Years after Receiving or Being Denied an Abortion in the United States," *American Journal of Public Health* 105, no. 12 (2015): 2557–63; J.R. Steinberg et al., "Abortion and Mental Health: Findings from the National Comorbidity Survey-Replication," *Obstetrics & Gynecology* 123, no. 2 (2014): 263–70.

47. Ibid.

48. Ibid.

49. Guttmacher Institute, "Fact Sheet: Induced Abortion in the United States," 2017, https://www.guttmacher.org/fact-sheet/induced-abortion-united-states?gclid=CNKFrYXc79ICFc-6wAodb1wKcQ.

50. Ibid.

51. Guttmacher Institute, "Bans on Specific Abortion Methods Used after the First Trimester," March 2017, https://www.guttmacher.org/state-policy/explore/bans-specific-abortion-methods-used-after-first-trimester.

52. Ibid.

53. Ibid.

54. A. Norton. "U.S. Maternal Death Rate Is Rising." Health Day, August 2016, https://consumer.healthday.com/pregnancy-information-29/pregnancy-risks-news-546/u-s-maternal-death-rate-is-rising-713685.html.

55. Planned Parenthood, "The Abortion Pill," Accessed March 2017, https://www.plannedparenthood.org/learn/abortion/the-abortion-pill.

56. M.J. Chen and M.D. Creinin, "Mifepristone with Buccal Misoprostol for Medical Abortion: A Systematic Review," *Obstetrics & Gynecology* 126, no. 1 (2015): 12–21.

57. Ibid.

58. Ibid.

59. Centers for Disease Control and Prevention, "Preconception Health and Health Care: Women," September 2016, www.cdc.gov/preconception/women.html.

60. T.J. Mathews and B.E. Hamilton, "*Mean Age of Mothers in on the Rise,*" *NCHS Data Brief* 232 (2016): 1–7, https://www.cdc.gov/nchs/data/databriefs/db232.pdf.

61. B.E. Hamilton et al., "Births: Preliminary Data for 2015," *National Vital Statistics Report* 65, no. 13 (2016), Available at https://www.cdc.gov/nchs/data/nvsr/nvsr65/nvsr65_03.pdf.

62. American Pregnancy Association, "Miscarriage," Updated August 2016, http://american pregnancy.org/pregnancycomplications/miscarriage.html.

63. J.P. Bonde et al., "The Epidemiologic Evidence Linking Prenatal and Postnatal Exposure to Endocrine Disrupting Chemicals with Male Reproductive Disorders: A Systematic Review and Meta-analysis," *Human Reproduction Update* 23, no. 1 (2016): 104–25; G.C. Di Renzo et al., "International Federation of Gynecology and Obstetrics Opinion on Reproductive Health Impacts of Exposure to Toxic Environmental Chemicals," *International Journal of Gynecology & Obstetrics* 131, no. 3 (2015): 219–25; Centers for Disease Control and Prevention, "Preconception Health and Healthcare," September 2016, www.cdc.gov/preconception/careformen/exposures.html.

64. D. Malaspina et al., "Paternal Age and Mental Health of Offspring," *Fertility and Sterility* 103, no. 6 (2015): 1392–96.

65. M. Lino et al., "Expenditures on Children by Families, 2015," *U.S. Department of Agriculture, Center for Nutrition Policy and Promotion, Miscellaneous Publication No. 1528-2015. (2017),* Available at https://www.cnpp.usda.gov/sites/default/files/crc2015_March2017_0.pdf.

66. Castlight Health, "New Study Shows Huge Cost Differences for Having a Baby, Often in Same City," June 2016, http://www.castlighthealth.com/press-releases/new-study-shows-huge-cost-differences-for-having-a-baby-often-in-the-same-city.

67. Planned Parenthood, "Pregnancy Tests," Accessed March 2017, https://www.planned parenthood.org/learn/pregnancy/pregnancy-test.

68. American Congress of Obstetricians and Gynecologists, "ACOG Committee Opinion no. 548: Weight Gain During Pregnancy," *Obstetrics and Gynecology* 121, no. 1 (2013): 210–2, doi:10.1097/01.AOG.0000425668.87506.4c.

69. Ibid.

70. Ibid.

71. American Congress of Obstetricians and Gynecologists, "Tobacco, Alcohol, Drugs, and Pregnancy," December 2013, www.acog.org/~/media/For%20Patients/faq170.pdf?dmc=1&ts=20140516T2242271513.

72. National Center for Chronic Disease Prevention and Health Promotion, "Tobacco Use and Pregnancy," *Reproductive Health*, Updated July 2016, https://www.cdc.gov/reproductivehealth/maternalinfanthealth/tobaccousepregnancy/index.htm; American Congress of Obstetricians and Gynecologists, "Tobacco, Alcohol, Drugs, and

References

Pregnancy," December 2013, www.acog.org/~/media/For%20Patients/faq170.pdf?dmc=1 & ts=20140516T2242271513.

73. Centers for Disease Control and Prevention, "Facts about Cleft Lip and Cleft Palate," 2015, www.cdc.gov/ncbddd/birthdefects/cleftlip.html.

74. B.E. Hamilton et al., "Births: Preliminary Data for 2015," *National Vital Statistics Report* 65, no. 13 (2016), Available at https://www.cdc.gov/nchs/data/nvsr/nvsr65/nvsr65_03.pdf.

75. M. Thielking, *Stat News*, "Sky-high C-section Rates in the US Don't Translate into Better Birth Outcomes," December 1, 2015, https://www.statnews.com/2015/12/01/cesarean-section-childbirth.

76. American Pregnancy Association, "Preeclampsia," Updated August 2015, http://americanpregnancy.org/pregnancy-complications/preeclampsia.

77. V.P. Sepilian et al., "Ectopic Pregnancy," *Medscape Reference*, Updated November 2015, http://emedicine.medscape.com/article/2041923-overview.

78. American Pregnancy Association, "Miscarriage," Updated August 2016, http://americanpregnancy.org/pregnancy-complications/miscarriage.

79. What to Expect, "Stillbirth," Accessed March 2017, www.whattoexpect.com/pregnancy/pregnancy-health/complications/stillbirth.aspx.

80. American Psychological Association, "What Is Postpartum Depression and Anxiety?," Accessed March 2017, http://www.apa.org/pi/women/resources/reports/postpartum-depression.aspx.

81. Ibid.

82. American Academy of Pediatrics, "Policy Statement: Breastfeeding and the Use of Human Milk," *Pediatrics* 129, no. 3 (2012): 496.

83. National Institute of Child Health and Human Development, "What Are the Benefits of Breastfeeding?," Accessed March 2017, https://www.nichd.nih.gov/health/topics/breastfeeding/conditioninfo/Pages/benefits.aspx.

84. Centers for Disease Control and Prevention, "Sudden Unexpected Infant Death and Sudden Infant Death Syndrome," February 2017, www.cdc.gov/sids/aboutsuidandsids.htm.

85. Ibid.

86. Ibid.

87. Centers for Disease Control and Prevention, "Infertility FAQs," Reproductive Health, February 2017, www.cdc.gov/reproductivehealth/Infertility.

88. Mayo Clinic, "Infertility Symptoms and Causes," August, 2016. http://www.mayoclinic.org/diseases-conditions/infertility/symptoms-causes/dxc-20228738.

89. U.S. Department of Health and Human Services, "Polycystic Ovary Syndrome (PCOS) Fact Sheet," June 2016, www.womenshealth.gov/publications/our-publications/fact-sheet/polycystic-ovary-syndrome.html.

90. A. Talmor and B. Dunphy, "Female Obesity and Infertility," *Best Practice & Research Clinical Obstetrics & Gynaecology* 29, no. 4 (2015): 498–506.

91. Centers for Disease Control and Prevention, "Pelvic Inflammatory Disease CDC Fact Sheet," Sexually Transmitted Diseases, May 2016, www.cdc.gov/std/PID/STDFact-PID.htm.

92. Centers for Disease Control and Prevention, "Infertility: FAQs," February 2017, www.cdc.gov/reproductivehealth/Infertility/index.htm#4.

93. National Infertility Association, "The Semen Analysis," Accessed March 2017, http://www.resolve.org/about-infertility/male-workup/the-semen-analysis.html.

94. National Infertility Association, "The Semen Analysis," Accessed March 2017, http://www.resolve.org/about-infertility/male-workup/the-semen-analysis.html; Mayo Clinic Staff, "Low Sperm Count," July 2015, www.mayoclinic.org/diseases-conditions/low-sperm-count/basics/causes/con-20033441.

95. Centers for Disease Control and Prevention, "Infertility: FAQs," February 2017, www.cdc.gov/reproductivehealth/Infertility/index.htm#4.

96. Ibid.

97. WebMD, "Fertility Drugs," June 2015, www.webmd.com/infertility-and-reproduction/guide/fertility-drugs.

98. American Society for Reproductive Medicine, "Fertility Drugs and the Risk for Multiple Births," Accessed March 2017, www.asrm.org/uploadedFiles/ASRM_Content/Resources/Patient_Resources/Fact_Sheets_and_Info_Booklets/fertilitydrugs_multiple births.pdf.

99. WebMD, "Using a Surrogate Mother, What You Need to Know," September 2015, www.webmd.com/infertility-and-reproduction/guide/using-surrogate-mother.

100. R.M. Kreider and D.A. Loftquist, *Adopted Children and Stepchildren: 2010*, U.S. Census Bureau, April 2014, www.census.gov/content/dam/Census/library/publications/2014/demo/p20-572.pdf.

Chapter 6

1. U.S. Department of Health and Human Services, Office of the Surgeon General, *Facing Addiction in America: The Surgeon General's Report on Alcohol, Drugs, and Health* (Washington, DC: HHS, 2016).

2. S. Williams. "Behavioral Addiction vs Substance Addiction: Are they the Same?" MentalHelp.net. March, 2016.

3. N. Volkow et al., "Neurobiologic Advances from the Brain Disease Model of Addiction," *New England Journal of Medicine* 374, no. 4 (2016): 363–71.

4. American Society of Addiction Medicine, "Definition of Addiction," Accessed May, 2017, www.asam.org/for-the-public/definition-of-addiction.

5. L. Wu et al., "Association Study of Gene Polymorphisms in GABA, Serotonin, Dopamine, and Alcohol Metabolism Pathways with Alcohol Dependence in Taiwanese Han Men," *Alcoholism: Clinical and Experimental Research* 40 (2016): 284–90. doi:10.1111/acer.12963.

6. R. Rakerd et al., "Age at First Use and Later Substance Use Disorder: Shared Genetic and Environmental Pathways for Nicotine, Alcohol, and Cannabis," *Journal of Abnormal Psychology* 125, No. 7 (2016): 946–959. doi:10.1037/abn0000191; G. Saunders, "Parent Offspring Resemblance for Drinking Behaviors in a Longitudinal Twin Sample," *Journal of Studies on Alcohol and Drugs* 78, no. 1 (2017): 49–58.

7. J. Kinney, *Loosening the Grip: A Handbook of Alcohol Information*, 11th ed. (Boston: McGraw-Hill, 2014).

8. G. Hanson and P. Venturelli, *Drugs and Society*, 12th ed. (Sudbury, MA: Jones and Bartlett, 2014).

9. Ibid.

10. National Institute on Drug Abuse, National Institutes of Health, U.S. Department of Health and Human Services, *Drugs, Brains, and Behavior: The Science of Addiction*, NIH Publication No. 07-5605 (Bethesda, MD: National Institute on Drug Abuse, Revised 2014), Available at www.nida.nih.gov/-scienceofaddiction.

11. National Council on Problem Gambling, "March Madness and Gambling: Have the Conversation," March 9, 2016, Available at https://images.production.membersuite.com/7339289f-0004-c76f-a8b9-0b3842784d72/20987/7339289f-001c-c537-bd2e-0b3b1 fb1a928; American Psychiatric Association, *Diagnostic and Statistical Manual of Mental Disorders*, 5th ed. (Arlington, VA: American Psychiatric Publishing, 2013), 585.

12. American Psychiatric Association, *Diagnostic and Statistical Manual of Mental Disorders*, 5th ed. (Arlington, VA: American Psychiatric Publishing, 2013), 585.

13. D. Nutt et al., "The Dopamine Theory of Addiction: 40 Years of Highs and Lows," *Nature Reviews Neuroscience* 16, no. 5 (2015): 305–12.

14. D.V. Rinker et al., "Racial and Ethnic Differences in Problem Gambling among College Students," *Journal of Gambling Studies* 32, no. 2 (2015): 581–90; National Center for Responsible Gambling, "Fact Sheet: Gambling on College Campuses," Accessed February 2016, http://www.collegegambling.org/just-facts/gambling-college-campuses.

15. A. Muller et al., "Compulsive Buying," *American Journal on Addictions* 24, no. 2 (2015): 132–37.

16. A. Weinstein et al., "Compulsive Buying-Features and Characteristics of Addiction," *Neuropathology of Drug Addictions and Substance Misuse* 3 (2016): http://dx.doi.org/10.1016/B978-0-12-800634-4.00098-6; A. Muller et al., "Compulsive Buying," *American Journal on Addictions* 24, no. 2 (2015): 132–37.

17. Net Addiction, "FAQs," Accessed March 2016, http://netaddiction.com/faqs; H. Pontes, D. Kuss, and M. Griffiths, "Clinical Psychology of Internet Addiction: A Review of Its Conceptualization, Prevalence, Neuronal Processes, and Implications for Treatment," *Neuroscience and Neuroeconomics* 4 (2015): 11–23.

18. American College Health Association, *American College Health Association—National College Health Assessment II: Reference Group Data Report Fall 2016* (Baltimore. MD: American College Health Association, 2017).

19. Ibid.

20. Ibid.

21. M. Clark et al., "All Work and No Play?: A Meta-analytic Examination of the Correlates and Outcomes of Workaholism," *Journal of Management* 42, no. 7 (2016): 1836–73.

22. A. Szabo et al., "Methodological and Conceptual Limitations in Exercise Addiction Research," *Yale Journal of Biology and Medicine* 88, no. 3 (2015): 303–8; A .Muller, et al. "OP-76: Risk for exercise dependence, eating disorder pathology, alcohol use disorder and addictive behaviors among clients of fitness centers." *Journal of Behavioral Addictions*, vol. 6, no. S1, 2017, p. 36+. *Academic OneFile*, Accessed 14 July; H. Hausenblas, et al. "Addiction to Exercise." BMJ 2017;357:j1745, doi: https://doi.org/10.1136/bmj.j1745.

23. R. Weiss, "Hypersexuality: Symptoms of Sexual Addiction," *Psych Central*, March 2016, http://psychcentral.com/lib/hypersexuality-symptoms-of-sexual-addiction.

24. Substance Abuse and Mental Health Services Administration, Center for Behavioral Health Statistics and Quality, *Treatment Episode Data Set (TEDS): 2000–2010; National Admissions to Substance Abuse Treatment Services*, 2012, DASIS Series S-61, HHS Publication No. (SMA) 12-4701 (Rockville, MD: Substance Abuse and Mental Health Services Administration), Available at www.samhsa.gov/data/2k12/TEDS2010N/TEDS2010NWeb.pdf.

25. Centers for Disease Control and Prevention, "Therapeutic Drug Use," January 19, 2017, https://www.cdc.gov/nchs/fastats/drug-use-therapeutic.htm.

26. Consumer Health Care Products Association, "Statistics on OTC Use," Accessed May 2016, http://www.chpa.org/MarketStats.aspx.

27. U.S. National Library of Medicine, "Over-the-Counter Medicines," February 8, 2017, https://www.nlm.nih.gov/medlineplus/overthe counter-medicines.html.

28. L.D. Johnston et al., *Monitoring the Future National Results on Drug Use* (Ann Arbor, MI: Institute for Social Research, University of Michigan, 2016.)

29. Erowid, The DXM Vault, Accessed June 2016, www.erowid.org.

30. Center for Behavioral Health Statistics and Quality, "Behavioral Health Trends in the United States: Results from the 2015 National Survey on Drug Use and Health," 2016. ttps://www.samhsa.gov/data/sites/default/files/NSDUH-DetTabs-2015/NSDUH-DetTabs-2015/NSDUH-DetTabs-2015.pdfR. Miech et al. "The Influence of College Attendance on Risk for Marijuana Initiation in the United States: 1977–2015," *American Journal of Public Health*, Posted online on April 20, 2017.

31. Ibid.

32. Ibid.

33. L.D. Johnston et al., *Monitoring the Future National Results on Drug Use* (Ann Arbor, MI: Institute for Social Research, University of Michigan, 2016).

34. American College Health Association, *American College Health Association–National College Health Assessment Fall 2016 Reference Group Executive Summary*, 2017, Available at http://www.acha-ncha.org/docs/NCHA-II_WEB_Fall,2016_REFERENCE_GROUP_EXECUTIVE_SUMMARY.2017. pdf.

35. American College Health Association, *American College Health Association—National College Health Assessment* Fall *Reference Group Data Report*, 2017, Available at http://www.acha-ncha.org/docs/NCHA-II%20SPRING%20 2016%20REFERENCE%20GROUP%20DATA%20 REPORT.pdf.

36. Ibid.

37. Ibid.

38. Center for Behavioral Health Statistics and Quality, "Behavioral Health Trends in the United States: Results from the 2015 National Survey on Drug Use and Health," 2016; ttps://www.samhsa.gov/data/sites/default/files/NSDUH-DetTabs-2015/NSDUH-DetTabs-2015/NSDUH-DetTabs-2015.pdfR. Miech et al. "The Influence of College Attendance on Risk for Marijuana Initiation in the United States: 1977–2015," *American Journal of Public Health*, Posted online on April 20, 2017.

39. Ibid.

40. Ibid.

41. Ibid.

42. A. Arria et al., "Drug Use Patterns and Continuous Enrollment in College: Results from a Longitudinal Study," *Journal of Studies on Alcohol and Drugs* 74, no. 1 (2013): 71–83.

43. Ibid.

44. Higher Education Center for Alcohol and Drug Misuse Prevention and Recovery, "College Prescription Drug Study," Accessed June 2016, Available at http://hecaod.osu.edu/wp-content/uploads/2015/10/CPDS-Key-Findings-Report-1.pdf.

45. Center for Behavioral Health Statistics and Quality, "Behavioral Health Trends in the United States: Results from the 2015 National Survey on Drug Use and Health," 2016.

46. American College Health Association, *American College Health Association–National College Health Assessment Spring 2016 Reference Group Executive Summary*, 2016, Available at http://www.acha-ncha.org/docs/NCHA-II_WEB_SPRING_2016_REFERENCE_GROUP_EXECUTIVE_SUMMARY.pdf.

47. Addiction Center, "Drinking and Drug Abuse Is Higher among Greeks," February 15, 2015, www.addictioncenter.com/college/drinking-drug-abuse-greek-life.

48. Ibid.

49. Center for Behavioral Health Statistics and Quality, "Behavioral Health Trends in the United States: Results from the 2015 National Survey on Drug Use and Health," 2016. ttps://www.samhsa.gov/data/sites/default/files/NSDUH-DetTabs-2015/NSDUH-DetTabs-2015/NSDUH-DetTabs-2015.pdf

50. L.D. Johnston et al., *Monitoring the Future National Results on Drug Use* (Ann Arbor, MI: Institute for Social Research, University of Michigan, 2016).

51. National Institutes of Health, National Institute on Drug Abuse, "What Is Methamphetamine?," February 2017, https://www.drugabuse.gov/publications/drugfacts/methamphetamine; Medscape, "Methamphetamine Use Triples Parkinson's Risk," *Multispecialty*, 2014, http://www.medscape.com/viewarticle/837025.

52. National Institutes of Health, National Institute on Drug Abuse, "What Is Methamphetamine?," February 2017, https://www.drugabuse.gov/publications/drugfacts/methamphetamine.

53. National Institutes of Health, National Institute on Drug Abuse, "What Are Synthetic Cathinones?," January 2016, https://www.drugabuse.gov/publications/drugfacts/synthetic-cathinones-bath-salts.

54. Ibid.

55. Ibid.

56. D.C. Mitchell et al., "Beverage Caffeine Intakes in the U.S.," *Food and Chemical Toxicology* 63 (2014): 136–42.

57. Caffeineinformer, "20 Harmful Effects of Caffeine," February 1, 2017, http://www.caffeineinformer.com/harmful-effects-of-caffeine.

58. Caffeineinformer, "Top 24 Caffeine Health Benefits" January 19, 2017, https://www.caffeineinformer.com/top-10-caffeine-health-benefits.

59. Center for Behavioral Health Statistics and Quality, " " Results from the 2015 National Survey on Drug Use and Health, Detailed Tables" 2016. www.samhsa.gov/data/sites/default/files/NSDUH-DetTabs-2015/NSDUH-DetTabs-2015/NSDUH-DetTabs-2015.pdf

60. L.D. Johnston et al., *Monitoring the Future National Results on Drug Use* (Ann Arbor, MI: Institute for Social Research, University of Michigan, 2016).

61. National Institute on Drug Abuse, "Drug Facts: Marijuana," 2016. https://www.drugabuse.gov/publications/drugfacts/marijuana

62. National Institutes of Health, "Marijuana," March 2016, https://www.drugabuse.gov/sites/default/files/marijuanadrugfacts_march_2016.pdf.

63. AAA Foundation, "Impaired Driving and Cannabis," May 2016, https://www.aaafoundation.org/impaired-driving-and-cannabis.

64. T. Johnson, "Fatal Road Crashes Involving Marijuana Double after State Legalizes Drugs," AAA, May 10, 2016, http://newsroom.aaa.com/2016/05/fatal-road-crashes-involving-marijuana-double-state-legalizes-drug.

65. American Lung Association, "Marijuana and Lung Health," March 23, 2015, http://www.lung.org/stop-smoking/smoking-facts/marijuana-and-lung-health.html.

66. National Institute on Drug Abuse, "Drug Facts: Marijuana," 2016. https://www.drugabuse.gov/publications/drugfacts/marijuana

67. D. Tashkin, "How Beneficial Is Vaping Cannabis to Respiratory Health Compared to Smoking?," *Addiction* 110, no. 11 (2015): 1706–7.

68. National Institute on Drug Abuse, "Drug Facts: Marijuana," 2016. https://www.drugabuse.gov/publications/drugfacts/marijuana

69. C. Blanco et al., "Cannabis Use and Risk of Psychiatric Disorders," *JAMA Psychiatry* 73, no. 4 (2016): 388–95.

70. Ibid.

71. American Academy of Pediatrics, "Marijuana Legalization," March 2016, https://www.aap.org/en-us/advocacy-and-policy/state-advocacy/Documents/Marijuana%20Legalization.pdf.

72. Ibid.

73. Ibid.

74. National Institute on Drug Abuse, "Marijuana: Facts for Teens," May 2015, www.drugabuse.gov/publications/marijuana-facts-teens; Science Daily, "Marijuana Use Prior to Pregnancy Doubles Risk of Premature Birth," July 17, 2012, www.sciencedaily.com.

75. National Institute on Drug Abuse, "Drug Facts: Is Marijuana Medicine?," July 2015, www.drugabuse.gov; DrugRehab.us, "Pros and Cons of Legalizing Recreational Marijuana," 2016, www.drugrehab.us/news/pros-cons-legalizing-recreational-marijuana; N. Volkow et al., "Adverse Health Effects of Marijuana Use," *New England Journal of Medicine* 370 (2014): 2219–27.

76. Ibid.

77. National Institute on Drug Abuse, "Drug Facts: Synthetic Cannabinoids," November 2015, https://www.drugabuse.gov/publications/drug-facts/synthetic-cannabinoids.

78. L.D. Johnston et al., *Monitoring the Future National Survey Results on Drug Use* (Ann Arbor, MI: Institute for Social Research, University of Michigan, 2016).

79. K.L. Egan et al., "K2 and Spice Use among a Cohort of College Students in the Southeast Region of the USA," *American Journal of Drug and Alcohol Abuse* 41 no. 4 (2015): 317–22.

80. L.D. Johnston et al., *Monitoring the Future National Survey Results on Drug Use* (Ann Arbor, MI: Institute for Social Research, University of Michigan, 2016).

81. National Institute on Drug Abuse, "Drug Facts: Synthetic Cannabinoids," November 2015, https://www.drugabuse.gov/publications/drug-facts/synthetic-cannabinoids.

82. Substance Abuse and Mental Health Services Administration, "Not for Human Consumption: Spice and Bath Salts," March 3, 2015, http://newsletter.samhsa.gov/2015/03/03/not-for-human-consumption-spice-and-bath-salts.

83. National Institute on Drug Abuse, "What Are CNS Depressants?," 2016, https://www.drugabuse.gov/publications/research-reports/prescription-drugs/cns-depressants/what-are-cns-depressants.

84. WebMD, "Barbiturate Abuse: Overview, 2016, http://www.webmd.com/mental-health/addiction/barbiturate-abuse.

85. Partnership for Drug-Free Kids, "GHB," Accessed June 2016, www.drugfree.org/drug-guide/ghb.

86. National Institute on Drug Abuse, "Drug Facts: What Is Heroin?," January 2017, https://www.drugabuse.gov/publications/drugfacts/heroin.

87. Ibid.

88. Center for Behavioral Health Statistics and Quality, "Behavioral Health Trends in the United States: Results from the 2015 National Survey on Drug Use and Health," 2016 (HHS Publication No. SMA 16-4984, NSDUH Series H-51); Healthline, "Prescription Drugs are Leading to Heroin Addiction," February, 2016. http://www.health-line.com/health-news/prescription-drugs-lead-to-addiction.

89. Centers for Disease Control and Prevention, "Vital Signs: Demographic and Substance Use Trends among Heroin Users—United States 2002–2013," *Morbidity and Mortality Weekly* 64, no. 26 (2015): 719–25; T. Cicero, "The Changing Face of Heroin Use in the United States: A Retrospective Analysis of the Past 50 Years," *Journal of the American Medical Association* 71, no. 7 (2014): 821–26.

90. National Institute on Drug Abuse, "Drug Facts: What Is Heroin?," January 2017, https://www.drugabuse.gov/publications/drugfacts/heroin.

91. Center for Behavioral Health Statistics and Quality, "Behavioral Health Trends in the United States: Results from the 2015 National Survey on Drug Use and Health," 2016.

92. L.D. Johnston et al., *Monitoring the Future National Survey Results on Drug Use* (Ann Arbor, MI: Institute for Social Research, University of Michigan, 2016).

93. National Institute on Drug Abuse, "Hallucinogens," 2016, https://www.drugabuse.gov/publications/drugfacts/hallucinogens.

94. Ibid.

95. National Institute on Drug Abuse, "What Is MDMA?," 2016, https://www.drugabuse.gov/publications/drugfacts/mdma-ecstasymolly.

96. Ibid.

97. Partnership at DrugFree.org, "Experts: People Who Think They Are Taking 'Molly' Don't Know What They Are Getting," June 24, 2013, www.drugfree.org/join-together/drugs/experts-people-who-think-they-are-taking-molly-dont-know-what-theyre-getting.

98. Drugs.com, "Mescaline," 2016, http://www.drugs.com/illicit/mescaline.html.

99. National Institute on Drug Abuse "Hallucinogens," 2016, https://www.drugabuse.gov/publications/drugfacts/hallucinogens.

100. Drugs.com, "PCP (Phencyclidine)," http://www.drugs.com/illicit/pcp.html.

101. Ibid.

102. National Institute on Drug Abuse, "Commonly Used Club Drugs," 2016, https://www.drugabuse.gov/drugs-abuse/commonly-abused-drugs-charts#ketamine; Drugs.com, "Ketamine," 2016, http://www.drugs.com/cdi/ketamine.html.

103. National Institute on Drug Abuse, "Hallucinogens," January 2016, www.drugabuse.gov/publications/drugfacts/hallucinogens.

104. Ibid.

105. Ibid.

106. Ibid.

107. Partnership for Drug-Free Kids, "Inhalants," 2016, http://www.drugfree.org/drug-guide/inhalants.

108. Ibid.

109. National Collegiate Athletic Association, "NCAA National Study of Substance Use Habits of College Student Athletes—Final Report 2014," August 2014, www.ncaa.org/sites/default/files/Substance%20Use%20Final%20Report_FINAL.pdf.

110. National Collegiate Athletic Association, "Substance Use: National Study of Substance Use Trends among NCAA College Student-Athletes," 2012, www.ncaapublications.com/product-downloads/SAHS09.pdf.

111. H.G. Pope et al., "The Lifetime Prevalence of Anabolic-Androgenic Steroid Use and Dependence in Americans: Current Best Estimates," *American Journal on Addictions* 23, no. 4 (2014): 371–77.

112. American College Health Association, *American College Health Association, National College Health Assessment, Reference Group, Spring 2016*, 2016, http://www.acha-ncha.org/docs/NCHA-II%20SPRING%202016%20REFER-ENCE%20GROUP%20DATA%20REPORT.pdf.

113. National Institute on Drug Abuse, "What Are Anabolic Steroids?," 2016, https://www.drugabuse.gov/publications/drugfacts/anabolic-steroids.

114. Ibid.

115. Association Against Steroid Use, "Legal Ramifications of Steroid Use," http://www.steroida-buse.com/legal-ramifications-of-steroid-abuse.html.

116. Substance Abuse and Mental Health Services Administration, "Results from the 2015 National Survey," 2016; U.S. Department of Health and Human Services, Office of the Surgeon General, *Facing Addiction in America: The Surgeon General's Report on Alcohol, Drugs, and Health* (Washington, DC: HHS, 2016).

117. U.S. Department of Health and Human Services, Office of the Surgeon General, *Facing Addiction in America: The Surgeon General's Report on Alcohol, Drugs, and Health* (Washington, DC: HHS, 2016).

118. Alcoholic Anonymous, "Over 80 Years of Growth," 2016, http://www.aa.org/pages/en_US/aa-timeline/to/1; Rehabs.com, "AA Success Rates," 2016, http://luxury.rehabs.com/12-step-programs/aa-success-rates.

119. U.S. Department of Health and Human Services, Office of the Surgeon General, *Facing Addiction in America: The Surgeon General's Report on Alcohol, Drugs, and Health* (Washington, DC: HHS, 2016).

120. M.L. Dennis et al., "A Pilot Study to Examine the Feasibility and Potential Effectiveness of Using Smartphones to Provide Recovery Support for Adolescents," *Substance Abuse* 36, no. 4 (2015): 486–92.

121. S. Gaidos, "Vaccines Could Counter Addictive Opioids," *Science News*, June 28, 2016, https://www.sciencenews.org/article/vaccines-could-counter-addictive-opioids.

122. S. Gaidos, "Vaccines Could Counter Addictive Opioids," *Science News*, June 28, 2016, https://www.sciencenews.org/article/vaccines-could-counter-addictive-opioids; National Institute on Drug Abuse, "Dr. Thomas Kosten Q & A: Vaccines to Treat Addiction," 2015, https://www.druga-buse.gov/news-events/nida-notes/2015/06/dr-thomas-kosten-q-vaccines-to-treat-addiction.

123. Office of National Drug Control Policy, "How Illicit Drug Use Affects Business and the Economy," Executive Office of the President, Accessed June 2016, www.whitehouse.gov/ondcp/ondcp-fact-sheets/how-illicit-drug-use-affects-business-and-the-economy.

124. Ibid.

125. Pew Research Center, "America's New Drug Policy Landscape," April 2, 2014, http://www.people-press.org/2014/04/02/americas-new-drug-policy-landscape; SAMSHA, "Prevention of Substance Abuse and Mental Illness," 2016, http://www.samhsa.gov/prevention.

Chapter 7

1. Center for Behavioral Health Statistics and Quality, "Key Substance Use and Mental Health Indicators in the United States: Results from the 2015 National Survey on Drug Use and Health, 2016, (HHS Publication No. SMA 16-4984, NA-SUH Series H-51), http://www.samhsa.gov/data.

2. Ibid.

3. Centers for Disease Control and Prevention, "Current Cigarette Smoking among Adults—United States, 2005–2015," *Morbidity and Mortality Weekly Report* 64, no. 44 (2016): 1205–11.

4. U.S. Department of Health and Human Services, *The Health Consequences of Smoking—50 Years of Progress*, 2014.

5. Centers for Disease Control and Prevention, "Fast Facts and Fact Sheets: Smoking and Tobacco Use," December 2016, www.cdc.gov/tobacco/data_statistics/fact_sheets/fast_facts/index.htm

6. American College Health Association, *National College Health Assessment II: Reference Group Executive Summary Fall 2016* (Hanover, MD: American College Health Association, *2017*), http://www.acha-ncha.org/docs/NCHA-II%20FALL%202016%20REFERENCE%20GROUP%20EXECUTIVE%20SUMMARY.pdf.

7. Ibid.

8. U.S. Department of Health and Human Services, National Institute on Alcohol Abuse and Alcoholism, "Moderate and Binge Drinking," Accessed May 2016, http://www.niaaa.nih.gov/alcohol-health/overview-alcohol-consumption/moderate-binge-drinking.

9. Ibid.

10. A. White and R. Hingson, "The Burden of Alcohol Use: Excessive Alcohol Consumption and Related Consequences among College Students," *Alcohol Research: Current Reviews* 35, no. 2 (2014): 201.

11. Ibid.

12. American College Health Association, *National College Health Assessment II: Reference Group Executive Summary Fall2016* (Hanover, MD: American College Health Association, 2017), http://www.acha-ncha.org/docs/NCHA-

13. L. Fucito et al., "Perceptions of Heavy Drinking College Students about a Sleep and Alcohol Health Intervention," *Behavioral Sleep Medicine* 13, no. 5 (2016): 395–411 doi:10.1080/15402002.2014.919919.

14. Ibid.

15. J. Merrill et al., "The Effect of Descriptive Norms on Pre-gaming Frequency: Tests of Five Moderators," *Substance Use & Misuse* 51, no. 8 (2016): 1002–12 .

16. J. Merrill and K. Carey, "Drinking over the Lifespan: A Focus on College Ages," *Alcohol Research* 38, no. 1 (2016): 103–14.

17. B. Zamboanga and P. Peake, "Moving House Parties to the Lab: A Call for Experimental Studies on Drinking Games" *Addictive Behaviors* 67 (2017): 18–19.

18. Ibid.

19. B. Zamboanga et al., "Drinking Game Participation among High School and Incoming Students: A Narrative Review," *Journal of Addictions Nursing* 24, no. 1 (2016): 24–31.

20. R. Martin et al., "Hazardous Drinking and Weight-Conscious Drinking Behaviors in a Sample of College Students and College Student Athletes," *Substance Abuse* (2016). doi:10.1080/08897077.2016.1142922.

21. "Poll: One in Five Women Say They Have Been Sexually Assaulted in College," *Washington Post*, June 12, 2015, https://www.washingtonpost.com/graphics/local/sexual-assault-poll.

22. Ibid.

23. National Institute on Alcohol Abuse and Alcoholism, "Planning Alcohol Interventions Using

NIAAA's College AIM: Alcohol Intervention Matrix," September 2015, NIH Publication No. 15-AA-8017.

24. Ibid.

25. Centers for Disease Control and Prevention, "Alcohol and Public Health: Fact Sheets—Caffeine and Alcohol," 2015, https://www.cdc.gov/alcohol/fact-sheets/caffeine-and-alcohol.htm; M. Patrick et al., "Who Uses Alcohol Mixed with Energy Drinks? Characteristics of College Student Users," *Journal of American College Health* 64, no. 1 (2016): 74–7; A. Haas et al., "Proportion as a Metric of Problematic Alcohol-Energy Drink Consumption in College Students," *Journal of Substance Abuse* doi:10.1080/14659891.2016.1271037; Verster et al., "Motives for Mixing Alcohol with Energy Drinks and Other Nonalcoholic Beverages and Consequences for Overall Alcohol Consumption," *International Journal of Internal Medicine* 7 (2014): 285–93.

26. National Institute on Alcohol Abuse and Alcoholism, "Beyond Hangovers: Understanding Alcohol's Impact on Your Health," October 2015, https://pubs.niaaa.nih.gov/publications/Hangovers/beyondHangovers.pdf; National Institute on Alcohol Abuse and Alcoholism, "Alcohol's Effects on the Body," Accessed May 4, 2016, http://niaaa.nih.gov/alcohol-health/alcohols-effects-body.

27. "Blowfish for Hangovers," Accessed May 2016, http://forhangovers.com.

28. Centers for Disease Control and Prevention, "Unintentional Drowning: Get the Facts," April 28, 2016, http://www.cdc.gov/HomeandRecreationalSafety/Water-Safety/waterinjuries-factsheet.html.

29. Ibid.

30. Mental Health America, "Suicide," June 18, 2016, http://www.mentalhealthamerica.net/suicide.

31. K. Conner et al., "Alcohol and Suicidal Behavior: What Is Known and What Can Be Done," *American Journal of Preventive Medicine* 47, no. 3 (2014): S204–8.

32. American College Health Association, *American College Health Association—National College Health Assessment II: Reference Group Executive Summary Fall 2016* (Hanover, MD: American College Health Association, 2017).

33. K. Bountress, et al. "Reducing sexual risk behaviors: secondary analyses from a randomized controlled trial of a brief web-based alcohol intervention for underage, heavy episodic drinking college women." Addiction Research & Theory. Vol. 25 , Iss. 4, 2017; T. Kilwein et al. "Predicting risky Sexual behaviors among college student drinkers as a function of event-level drinking motives and alcohol use." 2018. 76:100-104. https://doi.org/10.1016/j.addbeh.2017.07.032

34. Bureau of Justice Statistics, "Criminal Victimization in the United States, 2008 Table 32, Percent Distribution of Victimizations by Perceived Drug or Alcohol Use by Offender, 2008," May 2011, www.bjs.gov/content/pub/pdf/cvus0802.pdf.

35. "Poll: One in Five Women Say They Have Been Sexually Assaulted in College," Washington Post, June 12, 2015, https://www.washingtonpost.com/graphics/local/sexual-assault-poll.

36. Ibid.

37. R. Rettner, "Cheers?: Counting the Calories in Alcoholic Drinks," *Livescience,* December 7, 2015, http://www.livescience.com/52990-alcohol-calories-weight-loss-be-healthy.html.

38. L. Squeglia et al., "Brain Development in Heavy Drinking Adolescents," *American Journal of Psychiatry* 172, no. 6 (2015): 531–42.

39. I. Romieu et al., "Alcohol Intake and Breast Cancer in the European Prospective Investigation into Cancer and Nutrition,"

40. *International Journal of Cancer* 137, no. 8 (2015): 1921–30.

40. Ibid.

41. Y. Cao et al., "Light to Moderate Intake of Alcohol, Drinking Patterns, and Risk of Cancer: Results from Two Prospective US Cohort Studies," *British Medical Journal* 351 (2015): h4238.

42. I. Romieu et al., "Alcohol Intake and Breast Cancer in the European Prospective Investigation into Cancer and Nutrition," *International Journal of Cancer* 137, no. 8 (2015): 1921–30.

43. Ibid.

44. Substance Abuse and Mental Health Services Administration, "Protect Your Unborn Baby," Accessed January 2016, http://www.samhsa.gov/sites/default/files/programs_campaigns/fasd/fasd-infographic.pdf.

45. Centers for Disease Control and Prevention, "Fetal Alcohol Spectrum Disorders (FASDs): Data and Statistics," March 13, 2017, www.cdc.gov/ncbddd/fasd/data.html/

46. Ibid.

47. Centers for Disease Control and Prevention, "Ten Leading Causes of Death by Age Group," February 2016, www.cdc.gov/injury/wisqars/leadingcauses.html.

48. Centers for Disease Control and Prevention, "Impaired Driving: Get the Facts," January 26, 2017, http://www.cdc.gov/motorvehiclesafety/impaired_driving/impaired-drv_factsheet.html.

49. Ibid.

50. American College Health Association, *National College Health Assessment II: Reference Group Data Report, Fall 2016* (Hanover, MD: American College Health Association, 2017) , Available from www.achancha.org/reports_ACHA-NCHAII.html.

51. Insurance Institute for Highway Safety, "Alcohol-Impaired Driving 2015," November 2016, http://www.iihs.org/iihs/topics/t/alcohol-impaired-driving/fatalityfacts/alcohol-impaired-driving/2015.

52. Ibid.

53. Ibid.

54. Ibid.

55. Medline Plus, "Alcoholism and Alcohol Abuse," March 2015, www.nlm.nih.gov/medlineplus/ency/article/000944.htm.

56. National Institute on Alcohol Abuse and Alcoholism, "College Drinking," December 2015, http://pubs.niaaa.nih.gov/publications/CollegeFactSheet/CollegeFactSheet.pdf.

57. A. Arria, "College Student Success: The Impact of Health Concerns and Substance Abuse," Lecture presented at NASPA Alcohol and Mental Health Conference (Fort Worth, TX: January 19, 2013).

58. M. Waldron et al., "Parental Separation and Early Substance Involvement: Results from Children of Alcoholic and Cannabis Twins," *Drug and Alcohol Dependence* 134 (2014): 78–84.

59. M. Schuckit, "A Brief History of Research on the Genetics of Alcohol and Other Drug Use Disorders," *Journal of Studies on Alcohol and Drugs* 75, Suppl. 17 (2014): 59–67.

60. Ibid.

61. B. Taub, "Here's What Happens to Alcoholics' Brains When They Quit Drinking," *IFLScience,* March 3, 2016, http://www.iflscience.com/brain/what-happens-alcoholics-brains-when-they-quit-drinking.

62. Centers for Disease Control and Prevention, Fact Sheet, "Excessive Alcohol Use and Risks to Women's Health," March 7, 2016, www.cdc.gov/alcohol/fact-sheets/womens-health.htm.

63. W. Jacobs. "Hispanic/Latino Adolescents' Alcohol Use: Influence of Family Structure, Perceived Peer Norms, and Family Members' Alcohol Use,"

American Journal of Health Education 47, no. 4 (2016): 253–61;AKUA Mind and Body, "Addiction as A Family Disease," 2016, https://akuatreatmentprograms.com/addiction-family-disease; M. Haverfield et al. "Characteristics of Communication in Families of Alcoholics," Journal of Family Communication 2016. 16, no. 2 (2016): 111–27.

64. Centers for Disease Control and Prevention, "Excessive Drinking Is Draining the U.S. Economy," January 12, 2016, www.cdc.gov/features/CostsOfDrinking.

65. Ibid.

66. Ibid.

67. Ibid.

68. World Health Organization, "Global Status Report on Alcohol and Health," 2014, www.who.int/substance_abuse/publications/global_alcohol_report/en; World Health Organization, "Alcohol Fact Sheet," 2015, www.who.int/mediacenter/News/en.

69. Ibid.

70. S. Finn, "Alcohol Consumption, Dependence, and Treatment Barriers: Perceptions among Nontreatment Seekers with Alcohol Dependence," *Substance Use and Misuse* 49, no. 6 (2014): 762–69.

71. A. Laudet et al., "Collegiate Recovery Community Programs: What Do We Know and What Do We Need to Know?," *Journal of Social Work Practice in the Addictions* 14 (2014): 84–100; A. Laudet, et al., "Characteristics of Students Participating in Collegiate Recovery Programs: A National Survey," *Journal of Substance Abuse Treatment* 51 (2014): 38–46.

72. O. Manejwala, "How Often Do Long-Term Sober Alcoholics and Addicts Relapse?" *Psychology Today,* February 13, 2014, https://www.psychologytoday.com/blog/craving/201402/how-often-do-long-term-sober-alcoholics-and-addicts-relapse.

73. Centers for Disease Control and Prevention, "Current Cigarette Smoking Among Adults—United States, 2005–2015," *Morbidity and Mortality Weekly Report* 64, no. 44 (2016): 1205–11.

74. Ibid.

75. J. Suckling and L. Nestor, "The Neurobiology of addiction: The Perspective from Magnetic Resonance Imaging Present and Future," *Addiction* 112, no. 2 (2017): 360–69; M. Sutherland et al. "Chronic Cigarette Smoking Is Linked with Structural Alterations in Brain Regions Showing Acute Nicotinic Drug-induced Functional Modulations." *Behavioral and Brain Functions* 12 (2016):16. doi:10.1186/s12993-016-0100-5; M. Spitz and P. Cinciripini, "Chipping Away at the Genetics of Smoking Behavior," *Nature Genetics* 42, no. 5 (2010): 366–68.

76. Campaign for Tobacco-Free Kids, "Toll of Tobacco in the United States of America," April 3, 2017, www.tobaccofreekids.org/research/factsheets/pdf/0072.pdf?utm_source=factsheets_finder'utm_medium=link'utm_campaign=analytics.

77. Ibid.

78. Ibid.

79. American Cancer Society, "Cancer Facts & Figures 2017," Accessed March 2017, www.cancer.org/research/cancerfactsstatistics/cancerfactsfigures2017.

80. U.S. Department of Health and Human Services, *The Health Consequences of Smoking—50 Years of Progress*, 2014.

81. Centers for Disease Control and Prevention, "Fast Facts and Fact Sheets: Smoking and Tobacco Use," December 2016, www.cdc.gov/tobacco/data_statistics/fact_sheets/fast_facts/index.htm.

82. Campaign for Tobacco-Free Kids, "Toll of Tobacco in the United States of America," 2017.

83. U.S. Department of Health and Human Services, *The Health Consequences of Smoking—50 Years of Progress*, 2014.
84. Campaign for Tobacco-Free Kids, "Toll of Tobacco in the United States of America," 2017.
85. American College Health Association, *American College Health Association–National College Health Assessment II: Reference Group Data Report, Fall2016* (Hanover, MD: American College Health Association, 2017), Available from www.achancha.org/reports_ACHA-NCHAII.html.
86. Ibid.
87. Ibid.
88. J. Rosa and P. Aloise-Young, "A Qualitative Study of Smoker Identity among College Student Smokers," *Substance Use & Misuse* 50, no. 12 (2015): 1510–17.
89. American Cancer Society, "Light Smoking as Risky as a Pack a Day?," January 2013, http://blogs.cancer.org/expertvoices/2013/01/02/light-smoking-as-risky-as-a-pack-a-day.
90. U.S. Department of Health and Human Services, *The Health Consequences of Smoking—50 Years of Progress*, 2014; U.S. Department of Health and Human Services, "How Tobacco Smoke Causes Disease: The Biology and Behavioral Basis for Smoking Attributable Disease: A Report of the Surgeon General," 2010, Available at www.ncbi.nlm.nih.gov.
91. American Cancer Society, "Cancer Facts & Figures 2016," 2016, https://www.cancer.org/research/cancer-facts-statistics/all-cancer-facts-figures/cancer-facts-figures-2016.html.
92. National Cancer Institute, "Cigar Smoking and Cancer," Accessed March 13, 2016, http://www.cancer.gov/about-cancer/causes-prevention/risk/tobacco/cigars-fact-sheet.
93. American Cancer Society, "Cancer Facts & Figures 2016," 2016, https://www.cancer.org/research/cancer-facts-statistics/all-cancer-facts-figures/cancer-facts-figures-2016.html.
94. National Cancer Institute, "Cigar Smoking and Cancer," Accessed March 13, 2016, http://www.cancer.gov/about-cancer/causes-prevention/risk/tobacco/cigars-fact-sheet.
95. Centers for Disease Control and Prevention, "Smoking ' Tobacco Use: Hookahs," December 1, 2016, https://www.cdc.gov/tobacco/data_statistics/fact_sheets/tobacco_industry/hookahs/; Centers for Disease Control and Prevention, "CDC Features: Dangers of Hookah," November 9, 2015, https://www.cdc.gov/features/hookahsmoking.
96. Centers for Disease Control and Prevention, "Smoking & Tobacco Use: Bidis and Kreteks," December 1, 2016, www.cdc.gov/tobacco/data_statistics/fact_sheets/tobacco_industry/bidis_kreteks.
97. Campaign for Tobacco Free Kids, "Smokeless Tobacco in the United States," 2016.
98. U.S. Department of Health and Human Services, *E-Cigarette Use among Youth and Young Adults: A Report of the Surgeon General—Executive Summary* (Atlanta, GA: U.S. Department of Health and Human Services, Centers for Disease Control and Prevention, National Center for Chronic Disease Prevention and Health Promotion, Office on Smoking and Health, 2016).
99. American College Health Association, *American College Health Association–National College Health Assessment II: Reference Group Data Report, Fall2016* (Hanover, MD: American College Health Association, 2017), Available from www.achancha.org/reports_ACHA-NCHAII.html.
100. A. Littlefield et al., "Electronic Cigarette Use among College Students: Links to Gender, Race/Ethnicity, Smoking and Heavy Drinking," *Journal of American College Health* 63, no. 8 (2015): 523–29.
101. Campaign for Tobacco Free Kids, "Toll of Tobacco in the United States of America," 2017.
102. National Cancer Institute, "Lung Cancer Prevention," February 2016, www.cancer.gov/cancertopics/pdq/prevention/lung/HealthProfessional/page2.
103. American Cancer Society, "Cancer Facts & Figures 2017," Accessed March 2017, www.cancer.org/research/cancerfactsstatistics/cancerfactsfigures2017.
104. American Cancer Society, "What Are Oral Cavity and Oropharyngeal Cancers?," January 2016, www.cancer.org/cancer/oralcavityandoropharyngealcancer/detailed guide/oral-cavity-and-oropharyngeal-cancer-what-is-oral-cavity-cancer.
105. American Cancer Society, "Cancer Facts & Figures 2017," Accessed March 2017, www.cancer.org/research/cancerfactsstatistics/cancerfactsfigures2017.
106. American Heart Association, *Heart Disease and Stroke Statistics—2017 Update: A Report from the American Heart Association* (Dallas, TX: American Heart Association, 2016), Available at http://circ.ahajournals.org/content/early/2017/01/25/CIR.0000000000000485.
107. Ibid.
108. Ibid.
109. Ibid
110. U.S. Department of Health and Human Services, *The Health Consequences of Smoking—50 Years of Progress: A Report of the Surgeon General*, 2014.
111. American Lung Association, "Lung Health Diseases: What Causes COPD," November 1, 2016, http://www.lung.org/lung-health-and-diseases/lung-disease-lookup/copd/symptoms-causes-risk-factors/what-causes-copd.html.
112. C.B. Harte et al., "Association between Cigarette Smoking and Erectile Tumescence: The Mediating Role of Heart Rate Variability," *International Journal of Impotence Research* (2013): doi:10.1038/ijir.2012.43.
113. Centers for Disease Control and Prevention, "Tobacco Use and Pregnancy," September 2016, www.cdc.gov/reproductivehealth/TobaccoUsePregnancy.
114. Ibid.
115. American Academy of Periodontology, "Gum Disease Risk Factors," Accessed March 2017, www.perio.org/consumer/risk-factors; Centers for Disease Control and Prevention, "Smoking, Gum Disease, and Tooth Loss," September 2015, http://www.cdc.gov/tobacco/campaign/tips/diseases/periodontal-gum-disease.html.
116. S. Karama et al., "Cigarette Smoking and Thinning of the Brain's Cortex," *Molecular Psychiatry* 20 (2015): 778–85; I. Moreno-Gonzalez et al., "Smoking Exacerbates Amyloid Pathology in a Mouse Model of Alzheimer's Disease," *Nature Communications* 4 (2013), www.nature.com/ncomms/journal/v4/n2/abs/ncomms2494.html.
117. Centers for Disease Control and Prevention, "Secondhand Smoke (SHS) Facts," February 21, 2017, https://www.cdc.gov/tobacco/data_statistics/fact_sheets/secondhand_smoke/general_facts/index.htm.
118. American Lung Association, "Health Effects of Secondhand Smoke," Accessed April 2016, http://www.lung.org/stop-smoking/smoking-facts/health-effects-of-secondhand-smoke.html.
119. American Nonsmokers' Rights Foundation, "Overview List—How Many Smoke-Free Laws," 2016.
120. Centers for Disease Control and Prevention, "Secondhand Smoke (SHS) Facts," February 21, 2017, https://www.cdc.gov/tobacco/data_statistics/fact_sheets/secondhand_smoke/general_facts/index.htm.
121. Centers for Disease Control and Prevention, "Health Effects of Secondhand Smoke Fact Sheet," February 2016, http://www.cdc.gov/tobacco/data_statistics/fact_sheets/secondhand_smoke/health_effects/index.htm.
122. Centers for Disease Control and Prevention, "Smoking and Tobacco Use: Secondhand Smoke Facts," 2014.
123. Ibid.
124. U.S. Department of Health and Human Services, *The Health Consequences of Involuntary Exposure to Tobacco Smoke*, 2011.
125. Z. Kabir, G. Connolly, and H. Alpert, "Secondhand Smoke Exposure and Neurobehavioral Disorders among Children in the United States," *Pediatrics* (2011), doi:10.1542/peds.2011-00232011-0023.
126. Ibid.
127. O. Shafey, M. Eriksen, H. Ross, and J. Mackay, "Secondhand Smoking," in *The Tobacco Atlas*, 3d ed. (Atlanta, GA: American Cancer Society, 2009), Available at www.cancer.org/aboutus/GlobalHealth/CancerandTobaccoControlResources/the-tobacco-atlas-3rd-edition.
128. U.S. Department of Health and Human Services, *The Health Consequences of Smoking—50 Years of Progress*, 2014.
129. Tobacco-Free Kids, "1998 State Tobacco Settlement 17 Years Later," December 2015, http://www.tobaccofreekids.org/microsites/statereport2016.
130. U.S. Food and Drug Administration Press Release. "FDA announces comprehensive regulatory plan to shift trajectory of tobacco-related disease, death." July 28, 2017. https://www.fda.gov/NewsEvents/Newsroom/PressAnnouncements/ucm568923.htm.
131. 111th Congress of the United States of America, *Family Smoking Prevention and Tobacco Control Act of 2009*, HR 1256, www.govtrack.us.
132. L. Weber et al., "E-Cigarette Rise Poses Quandary for Employers," *Wall Street Journal*, January 16, 2014, 41–42.
133. Centers for Disease Control and Prevention, "Quitting Smoking among Adults—United States 2000–2015," *Morbidity and Mortality Weekly* 65 no. 52 (2017):1457–64; Centers for Disease Control and Prevention, "Tobacco Use: Smoking Cessation," February 2016, www.cdc.gov/tobacco/data_statistics/fact_sheets/cessation/quitting/index.htm#quitting.
134. American Lung Association, "Benefits of Quitting," Accessed March 2017, www.lung.org/stop-smoking/i-want-to-quit/benefits-of-quitting.html; Centers for Disease Control and Prevention, "Smoking and Tobacco Use: Quitting Smoking," February 2017, https://www.cdc.gov/tobacco/data_statistics/fact_sheets/cessation/quitting.
135. Ibid.
136. Ibid.
137. Ibid.
138. H. Holmes, "What a Pack of Cigarettes Costs Now, State by State," *The Awl*, July 6, 2016, https://theawl.com/what-a-pack-of-cigarettes-costs-in-every-state-266d285b8a68#.xhj2e7evz.
139. Drugs.com, "Nicotine Patch," Accessed March 2016, http://www.drugs.com/price-guide/nicotine.

140. Ibid.

141. U.S. Food and Drug Administration, "FDA 101: Smoking Cessation Products," February 2016, http://www.fda.gov/ForConsumers/ConsumerUpdates/ucm198176.htm.

142. J. Brewer, "A Randomized Controlled Trial of Smartphone-Based Mindfulness Training for Smoking Cessation: A Study Protocol," *BMC Psychiatry* 15, no. 83 (2015): 2–7; J. Brewer, "A Simple Way to Break a Habit," TED TalkMED, November, 2015; Centers for Disease Control and Prevention, "Smoking & Tobacco Use: Quitting Smoking," February 1, 2017, https://www.cdc.gov/tobacco/data_statistics/fact_sheets/cessation/quitting; L. Peltz, "Practicing Mindfulness to Help You Break the Habit of Smoking," *Expert Beacon*, 2016, https://expertbeacon.com/practicing-mindfulness-help-you-break-habit-smoking/#.WM2YbhAfSPV; A. Ruscio et al., "Effect of Brief Mindfulness Practice on Self-Reported Affect, Craving and Smoking: A Pilot Randomized Controlled Trial Using Ecological Momentary Assessment," *Nicotine Tobacco Research* 18, no. 1 (2016): 64–73.

143. Ibid.

Chapter 8

1. Institute of Medicine, "Dietary Reference Intakes: Applications in Dietary Planning," 2003, Updated 2013, Accessed February 2017, Available at http://fnic.nal.usda.gov.

2. U.S. Department of Agriculture, "Food Availability (per Capita) Data System," Accessed March 2017, https://www.ers.usda.gov/data-products/food-availability-per-capita-data-system.

3. U.S. Department of Agriculture, "Part D: Section 6: Sodium, Potassium, and Water," *Report of the Dietary Guidelines Advisory Committee on the Dietary Guidelines for Americans, 2010* (Washington, DC.: U.S. Department of Agriculture, Agricultural Research Service, 2010).

4. A.E. Carroll, "No, You Do Not Have to Drink 8 Glasses of Water a Day," *New York Times,* August 24, 2015, www.nytimes.com/2015/08/25/upshot/no-you-do-not-have-to-drink-8-glasses-of-water-a-day.html?_r=0.

5. S.C. Killer, A.K. Blannin, and A.E. Jeukendrup, "No Evidence of Dehydration with Moderate Daily Coffee Intake: A Counterbalanced Cross-over Study in a Free-living Population," *PLoS ONE* 9, no. 1 (2014): e84154, doi:10.1371/journal.pone.0084154; R. Maugham et al., "A Randomized Trial to Assess the Potential of Different Beverages to Affect Hydration Status: Development of a Beverage Hydration Index," *American Journal of Clinical Nutrition*, 2015, doi:10.3945/ajcn.115.114769.

6. American College of Sports Medicine, "Selecting and Effectively Using Hydration for Fitness," 2011, www.acsm.org/docs/brochures/selecting-and-effectively-using-hydration-for-fitness.pdf.

7. U.S. Department of Agriculture, "*What We Eat in America,*" NHANES 2011–2012, February 11, 2015, www.ars.usda.gov/SP2UserFiles/Place/80400530/pdf/1112/Table_1_NIN_GEN_11.pdf.

8. Food and Nutrition Board, Institute of Medicine, *Dietary Reference Intakes for Energy, Carbohydrate, Fiber, Fat, Fatty Acids, Cholesterol, Protein, and Amino Acids (Macronutrients)* (Washington, DC: National Academies Press, 2005), Available at www.nap.edu/openbook.php?isbn=0309085373; R. Wolf et al., "Optimizing Protein Intake in Adults: Interpretation and Application of the Recommended Dietary Allowance Compared with the Acceptable Macronutrient Distribution Range." *Advances in Nutrition* 8 (2017): 266–75, doi:10.3945/an.116.013821.

9. Dietitians of Canada, the Academy of Nutrition and Dietetics, and the American College of Sports Medicine, "Nutrition and Athletic Performance: Position of Dietitians of Canada, the Academy of Nutrition and Dietetics, and the American College of Sports Medicine," February 2016, Accessed March 2017, Available at https://www.dietitians.ca/Downloads/Public/noap-position-paper.aspx.

10. Institute of Medicine of the National Academies, "Dietary, Functional, and Total Fiber," *Dietary Reference Intakes for Energy, Carbohydrate, Fiber, Fat, Fatty Acids, Cholesterol, Protein, and Amino Acids* (Washington, DC: The National Academies Press, 2005), 339–421, Available at www.nap.edu/openbook.php?isbn=0309085373.

11. Ibid.

12. U.S. Department of Health and Human Services and U.S. Department of Agriculture. *2015–2020 Dietary Guidelines for Americans*, 8th ed., December 2015, Available at http://health.gov/dietaryguidelines/2015/guidelines.

13. C.E. Ramsden et al., "Use of Dietary Linoleic Acid for Secondary Prevention of Coronary Heart Disease and Death: Evaluation of Recovered Data from the Sydney Diet Heart Study and Updated Meta-Analysis," *British Medical Journal* 346 (2013): e8707; M.A. Leslie et al., "A Review of the Effect of Omega-3 Polyunsaturated Fatty Acids on Blood Triacylglycerol Levels in Normolipidemic and Borderline Hyperlipidemic Individuals," *Lipids in Health and Disease* 14, no. 1 (2015): 1.

14. W. Willet, "Dietary Fats and Coronary Heart Disease," *Journal of Internal Medicine* 272, no. 1 (2012): 13–24; R. Micha et al., "Etiologic Effects and Optimal Intakes of Foods and Nutrients for Risk of Cardiovascular Diseases and Diabetes: Systematic Reviews and Meta-analyses from the Nutrition and Chronic Diseases Expert Group (NutriCoDE)," *PLoS ONE* 12, no. 4 (2017): e0175149. https://doi.org/10.1371/journal.pone.0175149.

15. U.S. Food and Drug Administration, "FDA Targets Trans Fats in Processed Foods," FDA Consumer Updates, March 17, 2017, www.fda.gov/ForConsumers/ConsumerUpdates/ucm372915.htm.

16. U.S. Food and Drug Administration, "FDA Targets Trans Fats in Processed Foods," *FDA Consumer Updates*, December 2013, www.fda.gov/ForConsumers/ConsumerUpdates/ucm372915.htm.

17. Ibid.

18. Ibid.

19. U.S. Department of Health and Human Services and U.S. Department of Agriculture. *2015–2020 Dietary Guidelines for Americans*, 8th ed., December 2015, Available at http://health.gov/dietaryguidelines/2015/guidelines; A. Trichpoulou et al., "Definitions and Potential Health Benefits of the Mediterranean Diet: Views from Experts Around the World," *BMC Medicine* 12, no. 1 (2014): 112.

20. National Institutes of Health Office of Dietary Supplements, "Dietary Supplement Fact Sheet: Vitamin D," March, 2017, http://ods.od.nih.gov/factsheets/VitaminD-HealthProfessional.

21. U.S. Department of Agriculture, *What We Eat in America*, 2010.

22. U.S. Department of Health and Human Services and U.S. Department of Agriculture, *2015–2020 Dietary Guidelines for Americans*, 8th ed., December 2015, Available at http://health.gov/dietaryguidelines/2015/guidelines.

23. Ibid.

24. Academy of Nutrition and Dietetics, "Position of the Academy of Nutrition and Dietetics: Functional Foods," *Journal of the Academy of Nutrition and Dietetics* 113 no. 8 (2013): 1096–103.

25. Ibid.

26. J. Harasym and R. Oledzki, "Effect of Fruit and Vegetable Antioxidants on Total Antioxidant Capacity of Blood Plasma," *Nutrition* 30, no. 5 (2014): 511–17.

27. M.E. Obrenovich et al., "Antioxidants in Health, Disease, and Aging," *CNS' Neurological Disorders Drug Targets* 10, no. 2 (2011): 192–207; V. Ergin et al., "Carbonyl Stress in Aging Process: Role of Vitamins and Phytochemicals as Redox Regulators," *Aging and Disease* 4, no. 5 (2013): 276–94.

28. H. Stutz et al., "Analytical Tools for the Analysis of Beta-Carotene and Its Degradation Products," *Free Radical Research* 49, no. 4 (2015): 650–80; M.J. Gostner et al., "The Good and Bad of Antioxidant Foods: An Immunological Perspective," *Food and Chemical Toxicology* 80 (2015): 72–79.

29. Academy of Nutrition and Dietetics, "Position of the Academy of Nutrition and Dietetics: Functional Foods," *Journal of the Academy of Nutrition and Dietetics* 113 (2013): 1096–1103; S.C. Dyall, "Long-chain Omega-3 Fatty Acids and the Brain: A Review of the Independent and Shared Effects of EPA, DPA, and DHA," *Frontiers in Aging Neuroscience* 7 (2015): 52; A.P.S. Hungin et al., "Systematic Review: Probiotics in the Management of Lower Gastrointestinal Symptoms in Clinical Practice: An Evidence-Based International Guide," *Alimentary Pharmacology and Therapeutics* 38, no. 8 (2013): 864–86; N. Khan et al., "Cocoa Polyphenols and Inflammatory Markers of Cardiovascular Disease," *Nutrients* 6, no. 2 (2014): 844–80.

30. Ibid.

31. Ibid.

32. U.S. Department of Agriculture, "Empty Calories: How Do I Count the Empty Calories I Eat?" September 30, 2015, Accessed April 2017, http://archive.rhizome.org/artbase/53981/www.choosemyplate.gov/food-groups/emptycalories_count_table.html.

33. E. Forman et al., "Mindful Decision Making and Inhibitory Control Training as Complementary Means to Decrease Snack Consumption," *Appetite* 103 (2016): 176–83; M. Mantzios and J.C. Wilson, "Mindfulness, Eating Behaviours, and Obesity: A Review and Reflection on Current Findings," *Current Obesity Reports* 4, no. 1 (2015): 141–46; S. Katteman et al., "Mindfulness Meditation as an Intervention for Binge Eating, Emotional Eating, and Weight Loss: A Systematic Review," *Eating Behaviors* 15, no. 2 (2014): 197–204; C. Dawn et al., "Impact of Non-diet Approaches on Attitudes, Behaviors, and Health Outcomes: A Systematic Review," *Journal of Nutrition Education and Behavior* 47, no. 2 (2015): 143–55; M. Mantzios and J.C. Wilson, "Making Concrete Construals Mindful: A Novel Approach for Developing Mindfulness and Self-Compassion to Assist Weight Loss," *Psychology and Health* 29, no. 4 (2014): 422–41, doi:10.1080/08870446.2013.863883.

34. Vegetarian Resource Group, "How Many Adults in the U.S. Are Vegetarian or Vegan: Results of a 2016 National Harris Poll," 2017, http://www.vrg.org/nutshell/Polls/2016_adults_veg.htm.

35. Ibid.

36. Y. Yokoyama et al., "Vegetarian Diets and Blood Pressure: A Meta-Analysis," *Journal of the Ameri-*

can *Medical Association Internal Medicine* 174, no. 4 (2014): 577–87.

37. M. Dinu et al., "Vegetarian, Vegan Diets and Multiple Health Outcomes: A Systematic Review with Meta-analysis of Observational Studies," *Critical Reviews in Food Science and Nutrition* 57, no. 17 (2017): 3640–49, doi:10.1080/10408 398.2016.1138447.

38. Council for Responsible Nutrition, "2015 CRN Consumer Survey on Dietary Supplements," October 23, 2015, www.crnusa.org/CRNPR15-CCSurvey102315.html.

39. Ibid.

40. Office of Dietary Supplements, "Frequently Asked Questions," July 2013, http://ods.od.nih.gov/Health_Information/ODS_Frequently_Asked_Questions.aspx#; V.A. Moyer, "Vitamin, Mineral, and Multi-vitamin Supplements for the Primary Prevention of Cardiovascular Disease and Cancer: U.S. Preventive Services Task Force Recommendation Statement," *Annals of Internal Medicine* 160, no. 8 (2014): 558–64.

41. M.J. Krantz et al., "Effects of Omega-3 Fatty Acids on Arterial Stiffness in Patients with Hypertension: A Randomized Pilot Study," *Journal of Negative Results in Biomedicine* 14, no. 1 (2015): 21; D. Siscovick et al., "Omega-3 Polyunsaturated Fatty Acid (Fish Oil) Supplementation and the Prevention of Clinical Cardiovascular Disease: A Science Advisory from the American Heart Association," *Circulation* 135, no. 24 (2017), http://circ.ahajournals.org/content/early/2017/03/13/CIR.0000000000000482; P. Ridker, "Fish Consumption, Fish Oils, and Cardiovascular Events: Still Waiting for Definitive Evidence," *American Journal of Clinical Nutrition* 104, no. 4 (2016):951–52.

42. New York State Office of the Attorney General, "Attorney General Schneiderman Asks Major Retailers to Halt Sales of Certain Herbal Supplements as DNA Tests Fail to Detect Plant Materials Listed on Majority of Products Tested," February 3, 2015, Accessed March 2017, www .ag.ny.gov/press-release/ag-schneiderman-asks-major-retailers-halt-sales-certain-herbal-supplements-dna-tests.

43. FDA, "'Natural' on Food Labeling," December 24, 2015, Accessed March 2017, www.fda.gov/Food/Guidance-Regulation/GuidanceDocumentsRegulatoryInformation/LabelingNutrition/ucm456090.htm.

44. Organic Trade Association, "Market Analysis: U.S. Organic Industry Survey, 2015," Accessed March 2017, https://www.ota.com/resources/market-analysis.

45. T. Burfield. "Organic Produce Sales up Significantly in 2016Q3," *The Packer*, January 6, 2017, www.thepaanic-produce-sales-significantly-2016-q3cker.com/news/org.

46. U.S. Environmental Protection Agency, "Food and Pesticides," December 2015, Accessed March 2017, www.epa.gov/safepestcontrol/food-and-pesticides.

47. F. Galgano et al., "Conventional and Organic Foods: A Comparison Focused on Animal Products." *Cogent Food 'Agriculture* 2, no. 1 (2016), http://www.tandfonline.com/doi/full/10.1080/23311932.2016.1142818?scroll=top' needAccess=tru'.

48. J. Miquel, " Organic versus Conventional Food: A Comparison Regarding Food Safety," *Food Reviews International* 33, no. 4 (2017): 424–46, doi:10.1080/87559129.2016.1196490.

49. J.L. Wood et al., "Microbiological Survey of Locally Grown Lettuce Sold at Farmers' Markets in Vancouver, British Columbia," *Journal of Food Protection* 78, no. 1 (2015): 203–8.

50. U.S. Food and Drug Administration, "Food Irradiation: What You Need to Know," June 2016, www.fda.gov/Food/ResourcesForYou/Consumers/ucm261680.htm.

51. W. Klumper and M. Qaim, "A Meta-Analysis of the Impacts of Genetically Modified Crops," *PLoS ONE* 9, no. 11 (2014): e111629.

52. Center for Food Safety, "About Genetically Engineered Foods," Accessed March 2014, www.centerforfoodsafety.org/issues/311/ge-foods/about-ge-foods.

53. Union of Concerned Scientists, "Genetic Engineering Risks and Impacts," November 2013, www.ucsusa.org/food_and_agriculture/our-failing-food-system/genetic-engineering/risks-of-genetic-engineering.html.

54. L.P. Brower et al., "Decline of Monarch Butterflies Overwintering in Mexico: Is the Migratory Phenomenon at Risk?" *Insect Conservation and Diversity* 5, no. 2 (2012): 95–100.

55. American Association for the Advancement of Science, "Statement by the AAAS Board of Directors on Labeling of Genetically Modified Foods," March 31, 2014, www.aaas.org/news/statement-aaas-board-directors-labeling-genetically-modified-foods. World Health Organization, "Frequently Asked Questions on Genetically Modified Foods," May 2014, http://www.who.int/foodsafety/areas_work/food-technology/faq-genetically-modified-food/en.

56. National Institute of Allergy and Infectious Diseases, "Food Allergy," January 2016, www.niaid.nih.gov/topics/foodallergy/Pages/default.aspx.

57. National Institute of Allergy and Infectious Diseases, "Guidelines for the Diagnosis and Management of Food Allergy: What's in It for Patients?" October 2016, Accessed April 2017, https://www.niaid.nih.gov/diseases-conditions/food-allergy-guidelines-patients.

58. U.S. Food and Drug Administration, "Food Allergies: What You Need to Know," April 5, 2017, www.fda.gov/food/resourcesforyou/consumers/ucm079311.htm.

59. National Institute of Child Health and Human Development, "Lactose Intolerance," Accessed March 2017, https://www.nichd.nih.gov/health/topics/lactose/Pages/default.aspx.

60. National Institute of Diabetes and Digestive and Kidney Diseases, "Celiac Disease," Accessed March 2017, www.niddk.nih.gov/health-information/health-topics/digestive-diseases/celiac-disease/Pages/facts.aspx.

61. U.S. Department of Health and Human Services, "Food Safety Modernization Act (FSMA)," November 2013, Accessed March 2017, www.fda.gov/Food/GuidanceRegulation/FSMA/ucm304045.htm.

62. Centers for Disease Control and Prevention, "Burden of Food-Borne Illness: Findings," January 2016, Accessed March 2017, www.cdc.gov/foodborneburden/index.html.

63. Centers for Disease Control and Prevention. *Foodborne Diseases Active Surveillance Network (FoodNet): FoodNet 2015 Surveillance Report (Final Data)* (Atlanta, GA: Centers for Disease Control and Prevention, 2017).

64. Centers for Disease Control and Prevention, "Estimates of Foodborne Illness in the United States, CDC 2011 Estimates: Findings," Updated January 8, 2014, www.cdc.gov/foodborneburden/2011-foodborne-estimates.html.

65. Centers for Disease Control and Prevention, "Botulism," May 3, 2016, Accessed March 2017, Available at https://www.cdc.gov/botulism.

66. U.S. Government Accountability Office, "Progress on Many High-Risk Areas, While Substantial Efforts Needed on Others," February 15, 2017, Available at http://www.gao.gov/products/GAO-17-317.

67. M. Jay-Russell et al., "Exploration of the Impact of Application Intervals for the Use of Raw Animal Manure as a Soil Amendment, on Tomato Contamination," Accessed March 2017, Available at www.wifss.ucdavis.edu/wp-content/uploads/2015/pdfs/OryangJayRussellPosterOFVM-ScienceaResearchConference_08_14.pdf.

68. Centers for Disease Control and Prevention, "Surveillance for Foodborne Disease Outbreaks—United States, 1998–2008," *Morbidity and Mortality Weekly Report* 62, no. SS2 (2013), www.cdc.gov/foodsafety/fdoss/data/annual-summaries/mmwr-questions-and-answers-1998-2008.html.

Chapter 9

1. S. Higgs and J. Thomas, "Social Influences on Eating," *Current Opinion in Behavioral Sciences* 9 (2016): 1–6; M. Gurnani, C. Birken, and J. Hamilton, "Childhood Obesity: Causes, Consequences, and Management," *Pediatric Clinics of North America* 62, no. 4 (2015): 821–40; J. Woo Baidal et al., "Risk Factors for Childhood Obesity in the First 1,000 Days: A Systematic Review," *American Journal of Preventive Medicine* 50, no. 6 (2016): 761–79, doi:10.1016/j.amepre.2016.11.012.

2. M. Ng et al., "Global, Regional, and National Prevalence of Overweight and Obesity in Children and Adults during 1980–2013: A Systematic Analysis for the Global Burden of Disease Study 2013," *Lancet* 384, no. 9945 (2014): 766–81.

3. C.L. Ogden et al., "Trends in Obesity Prevalence among Children and Adolescents in the United States: 1988 through 2013–2014," *JAMA* 315, no. 21 (2016): 2292–99, doi:10.1001/jama.2016.636; K. Flegal et al., "Trends in Obesity among Adults in the United States, 2005–2014, *JAMA* 315, no. 21 (2016): 2284–91.

4. K. Flegal et al., "Trends in Obesity among Adults in the United States, 2005–2014, *JAMA* 315, no. 21 (2016): 2284–91.

5. C.L. Ogden et al., "Trends in Obesity Prevalence among Children and Adolescents in the United States: 1988 through 2013–2014," *JAMA* 315, no. 21 (2016): 2292–99, doi:10.1001/jama.2016.636; E.J. Benjamin et al., "Heart Disease and Stroke Statistics—2017 Update: A Report from the American Heart Association," *Circulation* 135, no. 10 (2017): e146–e603.

6. E.J. Benjamin et al. "Heart Disease and Stroke Statistics—2017 Update: A Report from the American Heart Association," *Circulation* 135, no. 10 (2017): e146–e603.

7. Ibid.

8. Ibid.

9. Ibid.

10. World Health Organization, "Obesity and Overweight Fact Sheet," January 2015, www.who.int/mediacentre/factsheets/fs311/en.

11. World Health Organization, "Obesity and Overweight Fact Sheet," January 2015, www.who.int/mediacentre/factsheets/fs311/en; S. Blumenthal and S. Levin, "Global Obesity: A Growing Epidemic," February 2017, *Huffington Post*, http://www.huffingtonpost.com/susan-blumenthal/global-obesity-a-growing-_b_9139554.html.

12. S. Vandevijvere et al., "Increased Food Energy Supply as a Major Driver of the Obesity

Epidemic: A Global Analysis," *Bulletin of the World Health Organization* 93, no. 7(2015): 446–56.

13. L. Ferrucci et al., "Age-Related Change in Mobility: Perspectives from Life Course Epidemiology and Geroscience," *Journals of Gerontology Series A: Biological Sciences and Medical Sciences* 71, no. 9 (2016): 1184–94.

14. Robert Wood Johnson Foundation, "The Healthcare Costs of Obesity," 2016, stateofobesity.org/healthcare-costs-obesity; A. Dee et al., "The Direct and Indirect Costs of Both Overweight and Obesity: A Systematic Review," *BMC Research Notes* 7, no. 1 (2014): 242; T.C. Roberts et al., "Patchy Progress on Obesity Prevention: Emerging Examples, Entrenched Barriers and New Thinking," *Lancet* 385, no. 9985 (2015): 2400–9; McKinsey & Company, "How the World Could Better Fight Obesity," November 2014, www.mckinsey.com/insights/economic_studies/how_the_world_could_better_fight_obesity.

15. Ibid.

16. Robert Wood Johnson Foundation, "The Healthcare Costs of Obesity," 2016, stateofobesity.org/healthcare-costs-obesity; A. Dee et al., "The Direct and Indirect Costs of Both Overweight and Obesity: A Systematic Review," *BMC Research Notes* 7, no. 1 (2014): 242; T.C. Roberts et al., "Patchy Progress on Obesity Prevention: Emerging Examples, Entrenched Barriers and New Thinking," *Lancet* 385, no. 9985 (2015): 2400–9; McKinsey & Company, "How the World Could Better Fight Obesity," November 2014, www.mckinsey.com/insights/economic_studies/how_the_world_could_better_fight_obesity; L. Quan et al., "Association of Fat-Mass and Obesity-Associated Gene FTO rs9939609 Polymorphism with the Risk of Obesity among Children and Adolescents: A Meta-Analysis," *European Review for Medical and Pharmacological Sciences* 19, no. 4 (2015): 614–23.

17. E. Horn et al., "Behavioral and Environmental Modification of the Genetic Influence on BMI: A Twin Study," *Behavior Genetics* 45, no. 4 (2015): 409–26.

18. O. Al Massadi et al., "Current Understanding of the Hypothalamic Ghrelin Pathways Inducing Appetite and Adiposity," *Trends in Neurosciences* 40, no. 3 (2017): 167–80; HealthyChildren.org, "Organic Causes of Weight Gain and Obesity," November 21, 2015, https://www.healthychildren.org/English/health-issues/conditions/obesity/Pages/Organic-Causes-of-Weight-Gain-and-Obesity.aspx.

19. H. Feng et al., "Review: The Role of Leptin in Obesity and the Potential for Leptin Replacement Therapy," *Endocrine* 44, no. 1 (2013): 33–9; C. Llewelyn and J. Wardle, "Behavioral Susceptibility to Obesity: Gene-Environment Interplay in the Development of Weight," *Physiology & Behavior* 152, Part B (2015): 494–501.

20. C. Llewelyn and J. Wardle, "Behavioral Susceptibility to Obesity: Gene-Environment Interplay in the Development of Weight," *Physiology & Behavior* 152, Part B (2015): 494–501.

21. L.K. Mahan and J. Raymond, *Krause's Food and Nutrition Care Processes*, 14th ed. (St. Louis, MO: Elsevier, 2017).

22. M. Reinhart et al., "A Human Thrifty Phenotype Associated with Less Weight Loss during Caloric Restriction," *Diabetes* 64, no. 8 (2015): 2859–67.

23. M. Simmonds et al., "Predicting Adult Obesity from Childhood Obesity: A Systematic Review and Meta-analysis," *Obesity Reviews* 17, no. 2 (2016): 95–107; A. Llewellyn et al., "Childhood Obesity as a Predictor of Morbidity in Adult-

hood: A Systematic Review and Meta-analysis," *Obesity Reviews* 17, no. 1 (2016): 56–7.

24. S. Higgs and J. Thomas, "Social Influences on Eating," *Current Opinion in Behavioral Sciences* 9 (2016): 1–6; W. Willett et al., *Thinfluence: The Powerful and Surprising Effect Friends, Family, Work and Environment Have on Weight* (Emmaus, PA: Rodale Press: 2014).

25. J. Kolodziejczyk et al., "Influence of Specific Individual and Environmental Variables on the Relationship between Body Mass Index and Health-Related Quality of Life in Overweight and Obese Adolescents," *Quality of Life Research* 24, no. 1 (2015): 251–61.

26. Centers for Disease Control and Prevention, "Early Release of Selected Estimates Based on Data from the National Health Interview Survey," January–September 2016, Available at https://www.cdc.gov/nchs/data/nhis/earlyrelease/earlyrelease201702_06.pdf.

27. Ibid.

28. A. Tambo et al., "The Microbial Hypothesis: Contributions of Adenovirus Infection and Metabolic Endotoxaemia to the Pathogenesis of Obesity," *International Journal of Chronic Diseases*, 2016 (2016): 703–95, doi:10.1155/2016/7030795.

29. H. Lawman et al., "The Role of Prescription Medications in the Association of Self-reported Sleep Duration and Obesity in U.S. Adults 2007–2012," *Obesity* 24, no. 10 (2016): 2210–16; V. Medici et al., "Common Medications Which Lead to Unintended Alterations in Weight Gain or Organ Lipotoxicity," *Current Gastroenterology Reports* 18, no. 1 (2016): 1.

30. A.W. McHill and K.P. Wright, "Role of Sleep and Circadian Disruption on Energy Expenditure and in Metabolic Predisposition to Human Obesity and Metabolic Disease," *Obesity Reviews* 18, Suppl. 1 (2017): 15–24.

31. CDC, "Defining Overweight and Obesity," June 16, 2016, https://www.cdc.gov/obesity/adult/defining.html.

32. Ibid.

33. Ibid.

34. Ibid.

35. K.M. Flegal, "Trends in Obesity among Adults in the United States, 2005–2016," *Journal of the American Medical Association* 315, no. 21 (2016): 2284–91; Centers for Disease Control and Prevention, "Obesity Prevalence Maps," September 11, 2015, www.cdc.gov/obesity/data/prevalence-maps.html.

36. B. Major et al., **"The Ironic Effects of Weight Stigma,"** *Journal of Experimental Social Psychology* 51 (2014): 74–80; S.A. Mustillo et al., "Obesity, Labeling, and Psychological Distress in Late-Childhood and Adolescent Black and White Girls: The Distal Effects of Stigma," *Social Psychology Quarterly* 76, no. 3 (2013): 268–89.

37. National Heart, Lung, and Blood Institute, "Classification of Overweight and Obesity by BMI, Waist Circumference and Associated Disease Risks," Accessed March 2017, www.nhlbi.nih.gov/health/public/heart/obesity/lose_wt/bmi_dis.htm.

38. F. Ortega et al., "Obesity and Cardiovascular Disease," *Circulation* 118 (2016): 1752–70.

39. University of Maryland Medical Center, Rush University, "Waist to Hip Ratio," February 7, 2016, http://umm.edu/health/medical/reports/images/waisttohip-ratio.

40. P. Brambilla et al., "Waist Circumference-to-Height Ratio Predicts Adiposity Better Than Body Mass Index in Children and Adolescents," *International Journal of Obesity* 37, no. 7 (2013): 943–46.

41. S. Vangsness, "Mastering the Mindful Meal," Brigham Health Nutrition and Wellness Hub, April 13, 2016, http://www.brighamandwomens.org/Patients_Visitors/pcs/nutrition/services/healtheweightforwomen/special_topics/intelihealth0405.aspx.

42. S.N. Bleich et al., "Diet-Beverage Consumption and Caloric Intake among US Adults, Overall and by Body Weight," *American Journal of Public Health* 104, no. 3 (2014): e72–78; B.M. Popkin and C. Hawkes, "Sweetening of the Global Diet, Particularly Beverages: Patterns, Trends, and Policy Responses," *Lancet Diabetes ' Endocrinology* 4, no. 2 (2016): 174–86; "The Awful Truth about Diet Soda and Weight Gain, According to Science," *Forbes*, September 8, 2016, https://www.forbes.com/sites/quora/#2b99a7244a0d.

43. A. Saltiel, "New Therapeutic Approaches for the Treatment of Obesity," *Science Translational Medicine* 8, no. 323 (2016): 323rv2; J. Domecq et al., "Drugs Commonly Associated with Weight Change: A Systematic Review and Meta-analysis," *Journal of Clinical Endocrinology and Metabolism* 100, no. 2 (2015): 363–70.

44. Drugs.com, "Medications for Obesity," Accessed March 2017, https://www.drugs.com/condition/obesity.html.

45. Mayo Clinic, "Gastric Bypass Surgery: Risks," Accessed March, 2017, www.mayoclinic.org/tests-procedures/bariatric-surgery/basics/risks/prc-20019138.

46. Johns Hopkins Health Library, "BPD/DS Weight-Loss Surgery," Accessed March 2017, http://www.hopkinsmedicine.org/healthlibrary/test_procedures/gastroenterology/bpdds_weight-loss_surgery_135,64.

47. I. Lanza, "Enhancing the Metabolic Benefits of Bariatric Surgery: Tipping the Scales with Exercise," *Diabetes* 64, no. 11 (2015): 3656–58. J. Yu et al., "The Long Term Effects of Bariatric Surgery for Type 2 Diabetes: Systematic Review and Meta-analysis of Randomized and Non-randomized Evidence," *Obesity Surgery* 25, no. 1 (2015): 143–58.

48. M. Dahl, "Stop Obsessing: Women Spend 2 Weeks a Year on Their Appearance, TODAY Survey Shows," *Today*, February 24, 2014, http://www.today.com/health/stop-obsessing-women-spend-2-weeks-year-their-appearance-today-2D12104866.

49. A. Conason, "Is Facebook Making Us Hate Our Bodies?," *Psychology Today*, June 9, 2015, https://www.psychologytoday.com/blog/eating-mindfully/201506/is-facebook–making-us-hate-our-bodies.

50. K. Schreiber, "Promoting a Thin and Ultra-athletic Physique Has Unforeseen Consequences," *Psychology Today*, September 1, 2015, https://www.psychologytoday.com/articles/201509/mind-your-body-body-conscious.

51. Centers for Disease Control and Prevention, "FASTSTATS: Obesity and Overweight," February 25, 2016, www.cdc.gov/nchs/fastats/obesity-overweight.htm.

52. L. Choate, "Dads: What's Your Impact on Your Daughter's Body Image?," *Psychology Today*, July 3, 2015, https://www.psychologytoday.com/blog/girls-women-and-wellness/201507/dads-whats-your-impact-your-daughters-body-image; L. Choate, "Moms: What Will Your Body Image Legacy Be?," *Psychology Today*, June 29, 2015, https://www.psychologytoday.com/blog/girls-women-and-wellness/201506/moms-what-will-your-body-image-legacy-be?collection=1076687.

53. R. Puhl et al., "Cross-national Perspectives about Weight-based Bullying in Youth: Nature, Extent and Remedies," *Pediatric Obesity* 11, no. 4 (2015): 241–50, doi:10.1111/ijpo.12051.

54. L. Rakhkovskaya et al., "Sociocultural and Identity Predictors of Body Dissatisfaction in Ethnically Diverse College Women," *Body Image* 16 (2016): 32–40.

55. Mayo Clinic Staff, "Body Dysmorphic Disorder," April 2016, http://www.mayoclinic.org/diseases-conditions/body-dysmorphic-disorder/home/ovc-20200935w.

56. S. Rossell et al., "Can Understanding the Neurobiology of Body Dysmorphic Disorder (BDD) Inform Treatment?," *Australasian Psychiatry* 23, no. 4 (2015), doi:10.1177/1039856215591327.

57. Body Image Health, "The Model for Healthy Body Image and Weight," Accessed February 2016, http://bodyimagehealth.org/model-for-healthy-body-image.

58. I. Ahmed et al., "Body Dysmorphic Disorder," *Medscape Reference*, August 2014, http://emedicine.medscape.com/article/291182-overview.

59. Mayo Clinic Staff, "Body Dysmorphic Disorder," April 2016, http://www.mayoclinic.org/diseases-conditions/body-dysmorphic-disorder/home/ovc-20200935w; KidsHealth, "Body Dysmorphic Disorder," February 2016, http://kidshealth.org/parent/emotions/feelings/bdd.html.

60. I. Ahmed et al., "Body Dysmorphic Disorder," *Medscape Reference*, August 2014, http://emedicine.medscape.com/article/291182-overview.

61. American Psychiatric Association, *Diagnostic and Statistical Manual of Mental Disorders*, 5th ed. (Washington, DC: American Psychiatric Association, 2013).

62. National Eating Disorders Association, "Get the Facts on Eating Disorders," Accessed February 2016, www.nationaleatingdisorders.org/get-facts-eating-disorders.

63. American College Health Association, *National College Health Assessment II: Undergraduates Reference Group Executive Summary Fall, 2016* (Hanover, MD: American College Health Association, 2017), Available at www.acha-ncha.org/reports_ACHA-NCHAII.html.

64. Alliance for Eating Disorder Awareness, "What Are Eating Disorders?," Accessed February 2017, http://www.allianceforeatingdisorders.com/portal/what-are-eating-disorders#.VrKm-r5MrKRt.

65. Ibid.

66. National Eating Disorders Association, "Anorexia: Overview and Statistics," Accessed April 2017, https://www.nationaleatingdisorders.org/anorexia-nervosa.

67. American Psychiatric Association, *Diagnostic and Statistical Manual of Mental Disorders*, 5th ed. (Washington, DC: American Psychiatric Association, 2013).

68. National Eating Disorders Association, "Anorexia Nervosa," Accessed February 2017, www.nationaleatingdisorders.org/anorexia-nervosa.

69. C.M. Pearson et al., "Stability and Change in Patterns of Eating Disorder Symptoms from Adolescence to Young Adulthood," *International Journal of Eating Disorders* 50, no. 7 (2017): 748–57, doi:10.1002/eat.22692.

70. U.S. National Library of Medicine, "Anorexia Nervosa," *A.D.A.M. Medical Encyclopedia*, March 10, 2014, https://www.nlm.nih.gov/medlineplus/ency/article/000362.htm; B. Suchan et al., "Reduced Connectivity between the Left Fusiform Body Area and the Extrastriate Body Area in Anorexia Nervosa Is Associated with Body Image Distortion," *Behavioural Brain Research* 241 (2013): 80–5.

71. T. Insel, "Director's Blog: Spotlight on Eating Disorders," National Institute of Mental Health, February 24, 2012, http://www.nimh.nih.gov/about/director/2012/spotlight-on-eating-disorders.shtml#i; Mirasol Eating Disorder Recovery Centers, "Eating Disorder Statistics," Accessed March 2016, http://www.mirasol.net/learning-center/eating-disorder-statistics.php.

72. R. Kessler et al., "The Prevalence and Correlates of Binge Eating Disorder in the World Health Organization World Mental Health Surveys," *Biological Psychiatry* 73, no. 9 (2013): 904–14, doi:10.1016/j.biopsych.2012.11.020.

73. American Psychiatric Association, "DSM-5 Feeding and Eating Disorders," 2013, www.dsm5.org/documents/eating%20disorders%20fact%20sheet.pdf.

74. National Institute of Mental Health, "Eating Disorders," February 2016, www.nimh.nih.gov/health/topics/eating-disorders/index.shtml.

75. M. Skunde et al., "Neural Signature of Behavioural Inhibition in Women with Bulimia Nervosa," *Journal of Psychiatry 'Neuroscience*, 41, no. 5 (2016), E69–E78, doi:10.1503/jpn.150335.

76. Mayo Clinic, "Binge-Eating Disorder," February 9, 2016, http://www.mayoclinic.org/diseases-conditions/binge-eating-disorder/basics/definition/con-20033155.

77. R. Kessler et al., "The Prevalence and Correlates of Binge Eating Disorder in the World Health Organization World Mental Health Surveys," 2013.

78. American Psychiatric Association. "Diagnosis and Statistical Manual of Mental Disorders, Update (Supplement)," September 2016, http://psychiatryonline.org/pb-assets/dsm/update/DSM5Update2016.pdf..

79. T. Insel, "Director's Blog: Spotlight on Eating Disorders," National Institute of Mental Health, February 24, 2012, http://www.nimh.nih.gov/about/director/2012/spotlight-on-eating-disorders.shtml#i; Mirasol Eating Disorder Recovery Centers, "Eating Disorder Statistics," Accessed July 2017, http://www.mirasol.net/learning-center/eating-disorder-statistics.php.

80. B. Cook, "Exercise Addiction and Compulsive Exercising: Relationship to Eating Disorders, Substance Use Disorders, and Addictive Disorders," in *Eating Disorders, Addictions and Substance Use Disorders, eds. T. Brewer and A. Baker Dennis* (New York: Springer, 2014), 127–44.

81. J.J. Waldron, "When Building Muscle Turns into Muscle Dysmorphia," Association for Sport Applied Psychology, Accessed February 2016, www.appliedsportpsych.org/resource-center/health-fitness-resources/when-building-muscle-turns-into-muscle-dysmorphia.

82. T. David et al., "Muscle Dysmorphia: Current Insights," *Psychology Research and Behavior Management* 9 (2016): 179–88; M. Silverman, "What Is Muscle Dysmorphia?" Massachusetts General Hospital, February 18, 2011, https://mghocd.org/what-is-muscle-dysmorphia; J.J. Waldron, "When Building Muscle Turns into Muscle Dysmorphia," 2014.

83. Committee on Adolescent Healthcare. "Female Athlete Triad," American Congress of Obstetrics and Gynecology. June 2017, https://www.acog.org/Resources-And-Publications/Committee-Opinions/Committee-on-Adolescent-Health-Care/Female-Athlete-Triad.

Chapter 10

1. Centers for Disease Control and Prevention, "Data, Trend and Maps," Accessed May 8, 2017, https://www.cdc.gov/nccdphp/dnpao/data-trends-maps/index.html.

2. C. Bouchard et al., "Less Sitting, More Physical Activity, or Higher Fitness?," *Mayo Clinic Proceedings* 90, no. 11 (2015): 1–8; A. Biswas et al., "Sedentary Time and Its Association with Risk for Disease Incidence, Mortality, and Hospitalization in Adults," *Annals of Internal Medicine* 162, no. 2 (2015): 123–32.

3. American College Health Association, *American College Health Association–National College Health Assessment II (ACHA-NCHA II): Reference Group Executive Summary, Fall 2016* (Hanover, MD: American College Health Association, 2017), Available at http://www.acha-ncha.org/docs/NCHA-II_FALL_2016_REFERENCE_GROUP_EXECUTIVE_SUMMARY.pdf.

4. National Heart, Lung, and Blood Institute, U.S. Department of Health and Human Services, National Institutes of Health, "What Is Physical Activity," Updated September 2011, www.nhlbi.nih.gov/health/health-topics/topics/phys; Office of Disease Prevention and Health Promotion, *2008 Physical Activity Guidelines for Americans, 2008*, Available at www.health.gov/paguidelines.

5. C. Bouchard et al., "Less Sitting, More Physical Activity, or Higher Fitness?," *Mayo Clinic Proceedings* 90, no. 11 (2015): 1–8.

6. C. Bouchard et al., "Less Sitting, More Physical Activity, or Higher Fitness?," *Mayo Clinic Proceedings* 90, no. 11 (2015): 1–8; A. Biswas et al., "Sedentary Time and Its Association with Risk for Disease Incidence, Mortality, and Hospitalization in Adults," *Annals of Internal Medicine* 162, no. 2 (2015): 123–32; S. Biddle et al., "Too Much Sitting and All-cause Mortality: Is There a Causal Link?" *BMC Public Health* 16 (2016): 635, doi:1186/s12889-016-3307-3.

7. S. Biddle et al., "Too Much Sitting and All-cause Mortality: Is There a Causal Link?" *BMC Public Health* 16:635. doi:1186/s12889-016-3307-3; A. Biswas et al., "Sedentary Time and Its Association with Risk for Disease Incidence, Mortality, and Hospitalization in Adults," *Annals of Internal Medicine* 162, no. 2 (2015): 123–32.

8. Ibid.

9. S. Plowman and D. Smith, *Exercise Physiology for Health, Fitness, and Performance*, 5th ed. (Philadelphia, PA: Wolters Kluwer, 2017).

10. M. Böejesson et al., "Physical Activity and Exercise Lower Blood Pressure in Individuals with Hypertension: Narrative Review of 27 RTCs," *British Journal of Sports Medicine* 50, no. 6 (2016): 356–61.

11. D.J. Elmer et al., "Inflammatory, Lipid and Body Composition Response to Interval Training or Moderate Aerobic Training," *European Journal of Applied Physiology* 116 (2016): 601–9; B.B. Gibbs et al., "Six-Month Changes in Ideal Cardiovascular Health vs. Framingham 10-Year Coronary Heart Disease Risk among Adults Enrolled in a Weight Loss Intervention," *Preventive Medicine* 86 (2016): 123–9.

12. Ibid.

13. D.T. Lackland and J.H. Voeks, "Metabolic Syndrome and Hypertension: Regular Exercise as Part of Lifestyle Management," *Current Hypertension Reports* 16, no. 11 (2014): 1–7; P.R.P. Nunes et al., "Effects of Resistance Training on Muscular Strength and Indicators of Abdominal Adiposity, Metabolic Risk, and Inflammation in Postmenopausal: Controlled and Randomized

Clinical Trial of Efficacy or Training Volume," *Age* 38, no. 2 (2016): 1–13.

14. Ibid.

15. M. Santama et al., "Exercise Intensity and Incidence of Metabolic Syndrome: The SUN Project," *American Journal of Preventive Medicine* 52, no. 4 (2017): e95–e101; D.T. Lackland and J.H. Voeks, "Metabolic Syndrome and Hypertension: Regular Exercise as Part of Lifestyle Management," *Current Hypertension Reports* 16, no. 11 (2014): 1–7.

16. J. Henson et al., "Sedentary Behavior as a New Behavioural Target in the Prevention and Treatment of Type 2 Diabetes," *Diabetes Metabolism Research and Reviews* 32, suppl. 1 (2016): 213–20; L. Pai et al., "The Effectiveness of Regular Leisure-time Physical Activities on Long-Term Glycemic Control in People with Type 2 Diabetes: A Systemic Review and Meta-Analysis," *Diabetes Research and Clinical Practice* 113 (2016): 77–85.

17. E.M. Balk et al., "Combined Diet and Physical Activity Promotion Programs to Prevent Type 2 Diabetes among Persons at Increased Risk: A Systematic Review for the Community Preventive Task Force," *Annals of Internal Medicine* 163, no. 6 (2015): 437–51; M.J. Armstrong and R.J. Sigal, "Exercise Is Medicine: Key Concepts in Discussing Physical Activity with Patients Who Have Type 2 Diabetes," *Canadian Journal of Diabetes* 39 (2015): s129–s133.

18. J. Erdrich et al., "Proportion of Colon Cancer Attributable to Lifestyle in a Cohort of US Women," *Cancer, Causes and Control* 26, no. 9 (2015): 1271–79, doi:10.1007/s10552-015-0619-z; M. Harvie et al., "Can Diet and Lifestyle Prevent Breast Cancer: What Is the Evidence?" *ASCO Educational Book* 35 (2015): e66–e73, doi:10.14694/EdBook_AM.2015.35.e66.

19. L.F.M. Rezende et al., "All-cause Mortality Attributable Risk to Sitting Time Analysis of 54 Countries Worldwide," *American Journal of Preventive Medicine* 51, no. 2 (2016): 253–63; A. Biswas et al., "Sedentary Time and Its Association with Risk for Disease Incidence, Mortality, and Hospitalization in Adults," *Annals of Internal Medicine* 162, no. 2 (2015): 123–32.

20. American Cancer Society, "Diet and Physical Activity: What's the Cancer Connection?," April 2017, www.cancer.org/cancer/cancercauses/dietandphysicalactivity/diet-and-physical-activity.

21. J. Xu et al., "Effects of Exercise on Bone Status in Female Subjects, from Young Girls to Postmenopausal Women: An Overview of Systematic Reviews and Meta-analyses." *Sports Medicine* 46, no. 8 (2016): 1165–82; R. Rizzoli et al., "Nutrition and Bone Health: Turning Knowledge and Beliefs in Healthy Behavior," *Current Medical Research & Opinion* 30, no. 1 (2014): 131–41.

22. B.K. Greer et al., "EPOC Comparison between Isocaloric Bouts of Steady-State Aerobic, Intermittent Aerobic, and Resistance Training," *Research Quarterly for Exercise and Sport* 86, no. 2 (2015): 190–95.

23. J.E. Turner, "Is Immunosenescence Influenced by Our Lifetime 'Dose' of Exercise?," *Biogerontology* 17, no. 3 (2016): 581–602.

24. G.J. Koelwyn et al., "Exercise in Regulation of Inflammation-Immune Axis Function in Cancer Initiation and Progression," *Oncology*, December 15, 2015, www.cancernetwork.com/oncology-journal/exercise-regulation-inflammation-immune-axis-function-cancer-initiation-and-progression; N. Sallam and I. Laher, "Exercise Modulates Oxidative Stress and Inflammation in Aging and Cardiovascular Disease," *Oxidative Medicine and Cellular Longevity* 2016 (2016): 7239639, doi:10.1155/2016/7239639.

25. P. Zimmer et al., "Exercise Induced Alterations in NK-cell Cytotoxicity: Methodological Issues and Future Perspectives," *Exercise Immunology Review* 23 (2017): 66–81, http://eir-isei.de/2017/eir-2017-066-article.pdf; M. Cook et al., "Exercise and Gut Immune Function: Evidence of Alternations in Colon Immune Cell Homeostasis and Microbiome Characteristics with Exercise Training," *Immunology and Cell Biology* 94, no. 2 (2016): 158–63.

26. C. Jin et al., "Exhaustive Submaximal Endurance and Resistance Exercises Induce Temporary Immunosuppression via Physical and Oxidative Stress," *Journal of Exercise Rehabilitation* 11, no. 4 (2015): 198–203.

27. J. Richards et al., "Don't Worry, Be Happy: Cross-Sectional Associations between Physical Activity and Happiness in 15 European Countries," *BMC Public Health* 15, no. 1 (2015): 1.

28. H. Hausenblas and R.E. Rhodes, *Exercise Psychology, Physical Activity and Sedentary Behavior*, 2017.

29. Ibid.

30. J.W. de Greeff et al., "Physical Fitness and Academic Performance in Primary School Children with and without a Social Disadvantage," *Health Education Research* 29, no. 5 (2014): 853–60.

31. J.D. de Vries et al., "Exercise as an Intervention to Reduce Study-related Fatigue among University Students," *PLOS One* 11, no. 3 (2016): e0152137, doi:10.1371/journal.pone.0152137.

32. A.N. Slade and S.M. Kies, "The Relationship between Academic Performance and Recreation Use among First-Year Medical Students," *Medical Education Online* 20 (2015), doi:10.3404/meo.v20.25105.

33. Ibid.

34. M. Beckett et al., "A Meta-analysis of Prospective Studies on the Role of Physical Activity and the Prevention of Alzheimer's Disease in Older Adults," *BMC Geriatrics* 15, no. 9 (2015), doi:10.10.1186/s12877-015-0007-2.

35. C. Bouchard et al., "Less Sitting, More Physical Activity, or Higher Fitness?," *Mayo Clinic Proceedings* 90, no. 11 (2015): 1–8.

36. C. Bouchard et al., "Less Sitting, More Physical Activity, or Higher Fitness?," *Mayo Clinic Proceedings* 90, no. 11 (2015): 1–8; L.F.M. Rezende et al., "All-cause Mortality Attributable Risk to Sitting Time Analysis of 54 Countries Worldwide," *American Journal of Preventive Medicine* 51, no. 2 (2016): 253–63.

37. D. Dunlop et al., "Sedentary Time in US Older Adults Associated with Disability in Activities of Daily Living Independent of Physical Activity," *Journal of Physical Activity and Health* 12, no. 1 (2015): 93–101.

38. K. Brown and D. Stanforth, "Go Green with Outdoor Activity," *ACSM's Health & Fitness Journal* 21, no. 1 (2017): 10-15.

39. Ibid.

40. Ibid.

41. C.A. Celis-Morales et al., "Association between Active Commuting and Incident Cardiovascular Disease, Cancer, and Mortality: Prospective Cohort Study," *BMJ* 357 (2017): j1456; "The Top 10 Reasons Everyone Should Bike to Work," Momentum, https://momentummag.com/top-10-reasons-you-should-bike-to-work, June 1, 2015; Rails-to-Trails Conservancy, "Investing in Trails: Cost-Effective Improvements—for Everyone," 2013, www.railstotrails.org /resourcehandler.ashx?id=3629; U.S. Environmental Protection Agency, "Climate Change: What You Can Do: On the Road," Updated April 2014, www.epa.gov/climatechange/wycd/road.html; B. McKenzie, "Modes Less Traveled—Bicycling and Walking to Work in the United States: 2008–2012," U.S. Department of Commerce, May 2014, www.census.gov/prod/2014pubs/acs-25.pdf.

42. American College of Sports Medicine, *ACSM's Guidelines for Exercise Testing and Prescription*, 9th ed. (Philadelphia, PA: Lippincott Williams & Wilkins, 2014).

43. American College of Sports Medicine, *ACSM's Resource Manual for Guidelines for Exercise Testing and Prescription*, 7th ed. (Philadelphia, PA: Lippincott Williams & Wilkins, 2014).

44. D.G. Behm et al., "Acute Effects of Muscle Stretching on Physical Performance, Range of Motion, and Injury Incidence in Healthy Active Individuals: A Systematic Review," *Applied Journal of Nutrition and Metabolism* 41 (2016): 1–11; S.G. Sadler et al., "Restriction in Lateral Bending Range of Motion, Lumbar Lordosis, and Hamstring Flexibility Predicts the Development of Low Back Pain: A Systematic Review of Prospective Cohort Studies," *BMC Musculoskeletal Disorders* 18 (2017): 179, doi:10.1186/s12891-1534-0.

45. American College of Sports Medicine, *ACSM's Guidelines for Exercise Testing and Prescription*, 10th ed. (Philadelphia, PA: Lippincott Williams & Wilkins, 2018).

46. Ibid.

47. D.G. Behm et al., "Acute Effects of Muscle Stretching on Physical Performance, Range of Motion, and Injury Incidence in Healthy Active Individuals: A Systematic Review," *Applied Journal of Nutrition and Metabolism* 41 (2016): 1–11.

48. Ibid.

49. J. Calstayud et al., "Core Muscle Activity in a Series of Balance Exercises with Different Stability Conditions," *Gait ' Posture* 42, no. 2 (2015): 186–92.

50. D.G. Behm et al., "Acute Effects of Muscle Stretching on Physical Performance, Range of Motion, and Injury Incidence in Healthy Active Individuals: A Systematic Review," *Applied Journal of Nutrition and Metabolism* 41 (2016): 1–11.

51. C. Winn et al., "Effect of High-intensity Exercise on Aerobic Performance and Airway Inflammation in Asthma," *European Respiratory Journal* 48 (2016): OA4804; doi:10.1183/13993003.congress-2016.OA4804; "Exercise and Asthma," WebMD, Accessed July 2017, http://www.webmd.com/asthma/guide/exercising-asthma#.

52. C. Winn et al., "Effect of High-intensity Exercise on Aerobic Performance and Airway Inflammation in Asthma," *European Respiratory Journal* 48 (2016): OA4804; doi:10.1183/13993003.congress-2016.OA4804; "Exercise and Asthma," WebMD, Accessed July, 2017, http://www.webmd.com/asthma/guide/exercising-asthma#; A. Bauman et al., "Updating the Evidence for Physical Activity: Summative Reviews of the Epidemiological Evidence, Prevalence, and Interventions to Promote 'Active Aging,'" *Gerontologist* 56, suppl. 2 (2016): S268–S280, doi:10.1093/geront/gnw031.

53. Ibid.

54. Ibid.

55. W.J. Chodzko-Zajko et al., "American College of Sports Medicine Position Stand: Exercise and Physical Activity for Older Adults," *Medicine and Science in Sports and Exercise* 41, no. 7 (2009): 1510–30. A. Bauman et al., "Updating

the Evidence for Physical Activity: Summative Reviews of the Epidemiological Evidence, Prevalence, and Interventions to Promote 'Active Aging,'" *Gerontologist* 56, suppl. 2 (2016): S268–S280, doi:10.1093/geront/gnw031.

56. D. McCartney et al., "The Effect of Fluid Intake Following Dehydration on Subsequent Athletic and Cognitive Performance: A Systematic Review and Meta-analysis," *Sports Medicine—Open* 3 (2017): 13, doi:10.1186/s40798-017-0079-y.

57. Ibid.

58. S. Cutts et al., "Plantar Fasciitis," *Annals of the Royal College of Surgeons of England* 94, no. 8 (2012): 539–42.

59. J.A. Rixe et al., "A Review of the Management of Patellofemoral Pain Syndrome," *Physician and Sports Medicine* 41, no. 3 (2013): 19–28.

60. J. Kraschnewski et al., "Is Strength Training Associated with Mortality Benefits? A 15year Cohort Study of US Older Adults," *Preventive Medicine* 87 (2016): 121, doi:10.1016/j.ypmed.2016.02.038.

61. American Academy of Ophthalmology, "Eye Health in Sports and Recreation," March 2016, www.aao.org/eye-health/tips-prevention/injuries-sports.

62. Ibid.

63. Bicycle Helmet Safety Institute, "Helmet-Related Statistics from Many Sources," January 2016, www.helmets.org/stats.htm.

64. American College Health Association, *National College Health Assessment II: Reference Group Data Report, Fall 2016* (Hanover, MD: American College Health Association, 2017).

65. Bicycle Helmet Safety Institute, "Helmet-Related Statistics from Many Sources," January 2016, www.helmets.org/stats.htm.

66. American College of Sports Medicine, *ACSM's Guidelines for Exercise Testing and Prescription*, 7th ed. (Philadelphia, PA: Lippincott Williams & Wilkins, 2014).

67. Mayo Clinic, "Hypothermia: Definition," May 11, 2017, www.mayoclinic.org/diseases-conditions/hypothermia/basics/definition/con-20020453.

68. American College of Sports Medicine, *ACSM's Guidelines for Exercise Testing and Prescription*, 9th ed. (Philadelphia, PA: Lippincott Williams & Wilkins, 2014).

Chapter 11

1. E. Benjamin et al., "Heart Disease and Stroke Statistics—2017 Update: A Report from the American Heart Association," *Circulation* 135, no. 10 (2017): e146–3603.

2. C. Bommer et al., "The Global Economic Burden of Diabetes in Adults Aged 20–79 Years: A Cost of Illness Study," *Lancet Diabetes & Endocrinology* 5, no. 6 (2017): 423–30; NCD Risk Factor Collaboration, "Worldwide Trends in Diabetes since 1980: A Pooled Analysis of 751 Population-based Studies with 4.4 Million Participants," *Lancet* 387, no. 10027 (2016): 1513–30.

3. Centers for Disease Control and Prevention, "Deaths: Final Data for 2014," *National Vital Statistics Reports* 65, no. 4, June 30, 2016.

4. E. Benjamin et al., "Heart Disease and Stroke Statistics—2017 Update: A Report from the American Heart Association," *Circulation* 135, no. 10 (2017): e146–3603.

5. American Cancer Society, *"Cancer Facts ' Figures 2017,"* Available at https://www.cancer.org/content/dam/cancer-org/research/cancer-facts-and-statistics/annual-cancer-facts-and-figures/2017/cancer-facts-and-figures-2017.pdf.

6. E. Benjamin et al., "Heart Disease and Stroke Statistics—2017 Update: A Report from the American Heart Association," *Circulation* 135, no. 10 (2017): e146–3603.

7. World Health Organization, "Cardiovascular Diseases (CVDs): Fact Sheet," September 2016, http://www.who.int/mediacentre/factsheets/fs317/en; E. Benjamin et al., "Heart Disease and Stroke Statistics—2017 Update: A Report from the American Heart Association," *Circulation* 135, no. 10 (2017): e146–3603.

8. A.S. Go et al., "Heart Disease and Stroke Statistics—2014 Update, A Report from the American Heart Association," *Circulation* 129 (2014): e28–e292.

9. E. Benjamin et al., "Heart Disease and Stroke Statistics—2017 Update: A Report from the American Heart Association," *Circulation* 135, no. 10 (2017): e146–3603.

10. A.S. Go et al., "Heart Disease and Stroke Statistics—2014 Update, A Report from the American Heart Association," *Circulation* 129 (2014): e28–e292.

11. A.S. Go et al., "Heart Disease and Stroke Statistics—2014 Update, A Report from the American Heart Association," *Circulation* 129 (2014): e28–e292; E. Benjamin et al., Heart Disease and Stroke Statistics—2017 Update: A Report from the American Heart Association," *Circulation* 135, no. 10 (2017): e146–3603.

12. S. Go et al., Heart Disease and Stroke Statistics—2014 Update, A Report from the American Heart Association," *Circulation* 129 (2014): e28–e292.

13. Ibid.

14. Ibid.

15. Ibid.

16. Ibid.

17. Ibid.

18. Ibid.

19. World Health Organization, "Cardiovascular Diseases (CVDs): Fact Sheet," September 2016, http://www.who.int/mediacentre/factsheets/fs317/en; E. Benjamin et al., "Heart Disease and Stroke Statistics—2017 Update: A Report from the American Heart Association," *Circulation* 135, no. 10 (2017): e146–3603.

20. World Health Organization, "Cardiovascular Diseases (CVDs)—Key Facts," Updated May 2017, www.who.int/mediacentre/factsheets/fs317/en/#.

21. Ibid.

22. E. Benjamin et al., "Heart Disease and Stroke Statistics—2017 Update: A Report from the American Heart Association," *Circulation* 135, no. 10 (2017): e146–3603.

23. A.S. Go et al., "Heart Disease and Stroke Statistics—2014 Update, A Report from the American Heart Association," *Circulation* 129 (2014): e28–e292; ACC/AHA/AAPA/ABC/ACPM/AGS/APhA/ASH/ASPC/NMA/PCNA Guideline for the Prevention, Detection, Evaluation, and Management of High Blood Pressure in Adults. *Journal of the American College of Cardiology* 2017, doi: 10.1016/j.jacc.2017.11.006.

24. ACC/AHA/AAPA/ABC/ACPM/AGS/APhA/ASH/ASPC/NMA/PCNA Guideline for the Prevention, Detection, Evaluation, and Management of High Blood Pressure in Adults. *Journal of the American College of Cardiology* 2017, doi: 10.1016/j.jacc.2017.11.006.

25. E. Benjamin et al., "Heart Disease and Stroke Statistics—2017 Update: A Report from the American Heart Association," *Circulation* 135, no. 10 (2017): e146–3603.

26. Centers for Disease Control and Prevention, "Peripheral Arterial Disease (PAD) Fact Sheet," June 2016, https://www.cdc.gov/dhdsp/data_statistics/fact_sheets/fs_pad.htm; American Heart Association, "Understand Your Risk for PAD," February 17, 2017, https://www.heart.org/HEARTORG/Conditions/VascularHealth/PeripheralArteryDisease/Understand-Your-Risk-for-PAD_UCM_301304_Article.jsp.

27. American Heart Association, "About Peripheral Artery Disease," November 16, 2016, www.heart.org/HEARTORG/Conditions/More/PeripheralArteryDisease/About-Peripheral-Artery-Disease-PAD_UCM_301301_Article.jsp.

28. American Heart Association, "Understand Your Risk for PAD," February 17, 2017, https://www.heart.org/HEARTORG/Conditions/VascularHealth/PeripheralArteryDisease/Understand-Your-Risk-for-PAD_UCM_301304_Article.jsp.

29. E. Benjamin et al., "Heart Disease and Stroke Statistics—2017 Update: A Report from the American Heart Association," *Circulation* 135, no. 10 (2017): e146–3603.

30. Ibid.

31. Ibid.

32. Ibid.

33. U.K. Patel et al., "Trends in Acute Ischemic Stroke Hospitalizations and Risk Factors among Young Adults: 12 Years of Nationally Representative Data," *Stroke* 48, suppl. 1 (2017): AWP182; D. Ingram and J. Montresor-Lopez, "Differences in Stroke Mortality, Adults Aged 45 and Over: United States 2010–2013," *NCHS Data Brief* 207 (2015), Available at http://www.cdc.gov/nchs/data/databriefs/db207.pdf; E. Benjamin et al., "Heart Disease and Stroke Statistics—2017 Update: A Report from the American Heart Association," *Circulation* 135, no. 10 (2017): e146–3603

34. American Heart Association, "Angina (Chest Pain)," April 14, 2017, www.heart.org/HEARTORG/Conditions/HeartAttack/SymptomsDiagnosisofHeartAttack/Angina-Chest-Pain_UCM_450308_Article.jsp; American Heart Association, "Angina in Women Can Be Different Than Men," April 18, 2016, http://www.heart.org/HEARTORG/Conditions/HeartAttack/WarningSignsofaHeartAttack/Angina-in-Women-Can-Be-Different-Than-Men_UCM_448902_Article.jsp#.VzJHJmQrIfE.

35. WebMD, " Pre-Ventricular Contractions," Accessed April 2017, http://www.webmd.com/heart-disease/tc/premature-ventricular-contractions-pvcs-topic-overview.

36. E. Benjamin et al., "Heart Disease and Stroke Statistics—2017 Update: A Report from the American Heart Association," *Circulation* 135, no. 10 (2017): e146–3603.

37. American Heart Association, "Congenital Cardiovascular Defects—Statistical Fact Sheet," 2017 Update, https://www.heart.org/idc/groups/ahamah-public/@wcm/@sop/@smd/documents/downloadable/ucm_495091.pdf.

38. Ibid.

39. C.J.L. Murray et al., "The State of US Health, 1990–2010 Burden of Diseases, Injuries, and Risk Factors," *Journal of the American Medical Association* 310, no. 6 (2013): 591–608.

40. S. Gardener et al., "Dietary Patterns Associated with Alzheimer's Disease and Related Chronic Disease Risk: A Review," *Journal of Alzheimer's Disease and Parkinsonism* S10 (2013): 2161–460; S. Sharp et al., "Hypertension Is a Potential Risk Factor for Vascular Dementia: Systematic Review," *International Journal of Geriatric Psychiatry* 26, no. 7 (2011): 661–69 ; I. van de Vorst et al., "Effect of Vascular Risk Factors and Diseases on Mortality in Individuals with Dementia: A Systematic Review and Meta-Analysis."

Journal of the American Geriatrics Society 64, no. 1 (2016):37–46, doi:10.1111/jgs.13835.

41. E. Benjamin et al., "Heart Disease and Stroke Statistics—2017 Update: A Report from the American Heart Association," *Circulation* 135, no. 10 (2017): e146–3603; A. Noortie, "Ischaemic Stroke in Young Adults: Risk Factors and Long-term Consequences," *Nature Reviews Neurology* 10, no. 6 (2014): 315–25; Y. Yano et al., "Isolated Systolic Hypertension in Young and Middle-Aged Adults and 31-year Risk for Cardiovascular Mortality," *Journal of the American College of Cardiology* 65, no. 4 (2015): 327–33.

42. M. Aguilar et al., "Prevalence of the Metabolic Syndrome in the United States, 2003–2012," *Journal of the American Medical Association* 313, no. 19 (2015): 1973–74.

43. Ibid.

44. Centers for Disease Control and Prevention, "Health Effects of Cigarette Smoking," May 2017, https://www.cdc.gov/tobacco/data_statistics/fact_sheets/health_effects/effects_cig_smoking/index.htm.

45. Ibid.

46. L.K. Sustersic Gawlik et al., "An Epidemiological Study of Population Health Reveals Social Smoking as a Major Cardiovascular Risk Factor," *American Journal of Health Promotion*, 2017; 089011711770642, doi:10.1177/0890117117706420.

47. Ibid.

48. Centers for Disease Control and Prevention. "Health Effects of Cigarette Smoking." May 2017, https://www.cdc.gov/tobacco/data_statistics/fact_sheets/health_effects/effects_cig_smoking/index.htm Centers for Disease Control and Prevention," Quitting Smoking," February 2017, https://www.cdc.gov/tobacco/data_statistics/fact_sheets/cessation/quitting/index.htm.

49. U.S. Department of Health and Human Services and U.S. Department of Agriculture, *2015–2020 Dietary Guidelines for Americans*, 8th ed., December 2015, Available at http://health.gov/dietaryguidelines/2015/guidelines.

50. V. Papademetriou et al., "Effects of High Density Lipoprotein Raising Therapies on Cardiovascular Outcomes in Patients with Type 2 Diabetes Mellitus, with or without Renal Impairment: The Action to Control Cardiovascular Risk in Diabetes Study," *American Journal of Nephrology* 45, no. 2 (2017): 136–45; D. Keene et al., "Effect on Cardiovascular Risk of High Density Lipoprotein Targeted Drug Treatments Niacin, Fibrates, and CETP Inhibitors: Meta-analysis of Randomised Controlled Trials Including 117,411 Patients," *British Medical Journal* 349 (2014): g4379; T. Wood et al., "The Cardiovascular Risk Reduction Benefits of a Low-carbohydrate Diet Outweigh the Potential Increase in LDL-Cholesterol," *British Journal of Nutrition* 115, no. 6 (2016): 1126–28.

51. Y. Yang, "Serum Lipoprotein-associated Phospholipase A2 Predicts the Formation of Carotid Artery Plaque and Its Vulnerability in Anterior Circulation Cerebral Infarction," *Clinical Neurology and Neurosurgery* 160 (2017): 40–5, doi:10.1016/j.clineuro.2017.06.007; P. Grag et al., "Lipoprotein-associated Phospholipase A2 and Incident Peripheral Arterial Disease in Older Adults: The Cardiovascular Health Study."*Arteriosclerosis, Thrombosis and Vascular Biology* February 4, 2016, doi:10.1161/ATVBAHA.115.306647 ; K.M. Moon et al., "Lipoprotein-associated Phospholipase A2 Is Associated with Atherosclerotic Stroke Risk: The Northern Manhattan Study," *PLoS ONE* 9, no. 1 (2014): e83393, doi:10.1371/journal.pone.0083393.

52. B.M. Sondermeijer et al., "Non-HDL Cholesterol vs. Apo B for Risk of Coronary Heart Disease in Healthy Individuals: The EPIC-Norfolk Prospective Population Study," *European Journal of Clinical Investigation* 43, no. 10 (2013): 1009–15.

53. E. Benjamin et al., "Heart Disease and Stroke Statistics—2017 Update: A Report from the American Heart Association." *Circulation* 135, no. 10 (2017): e146–3603.

54. Z. Wang et al., "Black and Green Tea Consumption and the Risk of Coronary Artery Disease: A Meta Analysis," *American Journal of Clinical Nutrition* 93, no. 3 (2011): 506–15; L. Hooper et al., "Effects of Chocolate, Cocoa, and Flavan-3-ols on Cardiovascular Health: A Systematic Review and Meta-analysis of Randomized Trials," *American Journal of Clinical Nutrition* 95, no. 3 (2012): 740–51.

55. F. Magkos et al., "Effects of Moderate and Subsequent Progressive Weight Loss on Metabolic Function and Adipose Tissue Biology in Humans with Obesity," *Cell Metabolism*, 2016, doi:10.1016/j.cmet.2016.02.005.

56. E. Benjamin et al., "Heart Disease and Stroke Statistics—2017 Update: A Report from the American Heart Association," *Circulation* 135, no. 10 (2017): e146–3603.

57. S. Wood and R. Valentino, "The Brain Norepinephrine System, Stress and Cardiovascular Vulnerability," *Neuroscience and Biobehavioral Reviews* (2016), doi:10.1016/j.neurbiorev.2016.04.018; N. Batelaan et al., "Anxiety and New Onset of Cardiovascular Disease: Critical Review and Meta-Analysis," *British Journal of Psychiatry* 208, no. 3 (2016): 223–31.

58. Ibid.

59. E. Benjamin et al., "Heart Disease and Stroke Statistics—2017 Update: A Report from the American Heart Association," *Circulation* 135, no. 10 (2017): e146–3603.

60. E. Benjamin et al., "Heart Disease and Stroke Statistics—2017 Update: A Report from the American Heart Association," *Circulation* 135, no. 10 (2017): e146–3603; T. Huang and F. Hu, "Gene-Environmental Interactions and Obesity: Recent Developments and Future Directions," *BMC Medical Genomics* 8, suppl. 1 (2015): S2.

61. Ibid.

62. The Emerging Risk Factors Collaboration, "C-Reactive Protein, Fibrinogen and CVD Prediction," *New England Journal of Medicine* 367, no. 14 (2012): 1310–20.

63. P. Ridker, "A Test in Context: High Sensitivity C-Reactive Protein," *Journal of the American College of Cardiology* 67, no. 6 (2016): 712–23; M. Jimenez et al., "Association between High Sensitivity C-Reactive Protein and Total Stroke by Hypertensive Stroke among Men," *Journal of the American Heart Association* 4, no. 9 (2015): e002013.

64. "The PLAC Test: Predicting Heart Attack Risk in People with No Symptoms." *Scientific American—Health After 50* 27, no. 2 (2015): 1–2.

65. Heartsite, "Coronary Stents," Available at http://www.heartsite.com/html/stent.html.

66. U.S. Preventive Services Task Force, "Understanding Task Force Recommendations: Aspirin Use for the Primary Prevention of Cardiovascular Disease and Colorectal Cancer," April 2016, http://www.uspreventiveservicestaskforce.org/Home/GetFile/11/218/aspr-cvccrc-finalrsfact/pdf; U.S. Food and Drug Administration, "Can an Aspirin a Day Help Prevent a Heart Attack?," February 22, 2016, www.fda.gov/For-Consumers/ConsumerUpdates/ucm390539.htm.

67. American Heart Association, "Prevention and Treatment of Heart Attack," February 10, 2016, http://www.heart.org/HEARTORG/Conditions/HeartAttack/PreventionTreatmentofHeartAttack/Prevention-and-Treatment-of-Heart-Attack_UCM_002042_Article.jsp#.VzJaa2QrlfE.

68. American Cancer Society, "Cancer Statistics Center," Accessed April 2017, https://cancerstatisticscenter.cancer.org/#.

69. American Cancer Society, "Cancer Facts & Figures 2017," Available at https://www.cancer.org/content/dam/cancer-org/research/cancer-facts-and-statistics/annual-cancer-facts-and-figures/2017/cancer-facts-and-figures-2017.pdf.

70. Ibid.

71. E. Benjamin et al., "Heart Disease and Stroke Statistics—2017 Update: A Report from the American Heart Association," *Circulation* 135, no. 10 (2017): e146–3603; American Cancer Society, "Cancer Facts and Figures 2017," https://www.cancer.org/content/dam/cancer-org/research/cancer-facts-and-statistics/annual-cancer-facts-and-figures/2017/cancer-facts-and-figures-2017.pdf.

72. U.S. Surgeon General, "The Health Consequences of Smoking—50 Years of Progress: A Report of the Surgeon General, 2014," 2014, www.surgeongeneral.gov/library/reports/50-years-of-progress/index.html.

73. U.S. Surgeon General, "The Health Consequences of Smoking—50 Years of Progress: A Report of the Surgeon General, 2014," 2014, www.surgeongeneral.gov/library/reports/50-years-of-progress/index.html; American Cancer Society, "Cancer Facts and Figures 2017," www.cancer.org/research/cancerfactsstatistics/cancerfactsfigures2014/index; Centers for Disease Control and Prevention, "Tobacco Use: Targeting the Nation's Leading Killer—At-a-Glance 2011," Accessed May 2014, www.cdc.gov/chronicdisease/resources/publications/aag/pdf/2011/tobacco_aag_2011_508.pdf.

74. World Health Organization, "Report on the Global Tobacco Epidemic, 2015," July 7, 2015, Available at www.who.int/tobacco/global_report/2015/en.

75. Cancer Research UK, "Worldwide Cancer," May 2015, http://publications.cancerresearchuk.org/downloads/Product/CS_KF_WORLDWIDE.pdf.

76. V. Bagnardi et al., "Alcohol Consumption and Site-Specific Cancer Risk: A Comprehensive Dose-Response Meta-analysis," *British Journal of Cancer* 112, no. 3 (2015): 580–93.

77. Centers for Disease Control and Prevention, "Fact Sheet—Alcohol Use and Your Health," February 29, 2016, http://www.cdc.gov/alcohol/fact-sheets/alcohol-use.htm; Centers for Disease Control and Prevention, "Fact Sheets—Excessive Alcohol Use and Risks to Men's Health," March 7, 2016, http://www.cdc.gov/alcohol/fact-sheets/mens-health.htm; National Cancer Institute, "Alcohol and Cancer Risk Sheet," June 24, 2013, www.cancer.gov/cancertopics/factsheet/Risk/alcohol.

78. American Cancer Society, "Cancer Facts and Figures 2017," Available at https://www.cancer.org/content/dam/cancer-org/research/cancer-facts-and-statistics/annual-cancer-facts-and-figures/2017/cancer-facts-and-figures-2017.pdf.

79. American Cancer Society, "Cancer Facts and Figures 2017," Available at https://www.cancer.org/content/dam/cancer-org/research/cancer-facts-and-statistics/annual-cancer-facts-and-figures/2017/cancer-facts-and-figures-2017.pdf; D. Aune et al., "Anthropometric Factors and Endometrial Cancer Risk: A Systematic Review and Dose–Response Meta-Analysis of Prospective Studies," *Annals of Oncology* 26, no. 8 (2015): 1635–48.

80. Ibid.
81. Ibid.
82. A. Blanc-Lapierre, "Lifetime Report of Perceived Stress at Work and Cancer Among Men: A Case Control Study in Montreal, Canada," *Preventive Medicine* 96 (2017): 28–35; K. Heikkila et al., "Work Stress and Risk of Cancer: Meta-analysis of 5700 Incident Cancer Events in 116,000 European Men and Women," *British Medical Journal* 346 (2013): 1165.
83. Cancer.net, "Hereditary Cancer-Related Syndromes," Accessed April 2017, http://www.cancer.net/navigating-cancer-care/cancer-basics/genetics/hereditary-cancer-related-syndromes; American Cancer Society, "Family Cancer Syndromes," April 19, 2017, www.cancer.org/cancer/cancercauses/geneticsandcancer/heredity-and-cancer.
84. American Cancer Society, "Breast Cancer Overview: Do We Know What Causes Breast Cancer?," May 4, 2016, www.cancer.org/Cancer/BreastCancer/DetailedGuide/breast-cancer-what-causes; American Cancer -Society, "Cancer Facts and Figures," 2016.
85. American Cancer Society, "Cancer Facts and Figures for Hispanic/Latinos, 2012–2014," Accessed May 2014, www.cancer.org/acs/groups/content/@epidemiologysurveilance/documents/document/acspc-034778.pdf; M. Banegas et al., "The Risk of Developing Invasive Breast Cancer in Hispanic Women," *Cancer* 119, no. 7 (2013): 1373–80.
86. J. Godos, "Markers of Systemic Inflammation and Colorectal Adenoma Risk: Meta-Analysis of Observational Studies," *World Journal of Gastroenterology* 23, no. 10 (2017): 1909; R. Francescone et al., "Microbiome, Inflammation, and Cancer," *Cancer Journal* 20, no. 3 (2014): 181–89.
87. R. Francescone et al., "Microbiome, Inflammation, and Cancer," *Cancer Journal* 20, no. 3 (2014): 181–89; T. Deng, "Obesity, Inflammation and Cancer," *Annual Review of Pathology: Mechanisms of Disease* 11 (2016): 421–49.
88. Crohn's and Colitis Foundation of America, "Bringing to Light the Risk of Colorectal Cancer among Crohn's & Ulcerative Colitis Patients," Accessed June 2016, http://www.ccfa.org/resources/risk-of-colorectal-cancer.html; S. Sebastian et al., "Colorectal Cancer in Inflammatory Bowel Disease: Results of the 3rd ECCO Pathogenesis Scientific Workshop (I)," *Journal of Crohn's and Colitis* 8, no. 1 (2014): 5–18.
89. American Cancer Society, "Can Infections Cause Cancer?," July 11, 2016, https://www.cancer.org/cancer/cancer-causes/infectious-agents/infections-that-can-lead-to-cancer/intro.html.
90. Ibid.
91. D. Saslow et al., "Human Papillomavirus Vaccination Guideline Update: American Cancer Society Guideline Endorsement," *CA: A Cancer Journal for Clinicians* 66, no. 5 (2016): 375–85; Centers for Disease Control and Prevention, "Put Vaccination on Your Back to School List," August 5, 2015, https://www.cdc.gov/features/hpvvaccine.
92. American Cancer Society, "Cancer Facts and Figures 2017," Available at https://www.cancer.org/content/dam/cancer-org/research/cancer-facts-and-statistics/annual-cancer-facts-and-figures/2017/cancer-facts-and-figures-2017.pdf.
93. Ibid.
94. J. Manson, et al. "Menopausal Hormone Therapy and Long-term All-Cause and Cause-Specific Mortality: The Women's Health Initiative Randomized Trials." JAMA. 2017;318(10):927-938. doi:10.1001/jama.2017.11217.
95. American Cancer Society, "Cancer Facts and Figures 2017," Available at https://www.cancer.org/content/dam/cancer-org/research/cancer-facts-and-statistics/annual-cancer-facts-and-figures/2017/cancer-facts-and-figures-2017.pdf.
96. Ibid.
97. American Cancer Society, "Nonsmall Lung Cancer Survival Rates, by Stage," Revised: May 16, 2016, https://www.cancer.org/cancer/non-small-cell-lung-cancer/detection-diagnosis-staging/survival-rates.html.
98. Ibid.
99. American Cancer Society, "Benefits of Quitting over Time," September, 2016., http://www.cancer.org/healthy/stayawayfromtobacco/benefits-of-quitting-smoking-over-time.
100. S. Simon, "Why Non-smokers Sometimes Get Lung Cancer," November 2016, https://www.cancer.org/latest-news/why-lung-cancer-strikes-nonsmokers.html, www.cancer.org/cancer/news/why-lung-cancer-strikes-nonsmokers.
101. American Cancer Society, "Colorectal Cancer Facts and Figures, 2014–2016," Accessed June 2016, www.cancer.org/acs/groups/content/documents/document/acspc-042280.pdf; American Cancer Society, "Cancer Facts and Figures 2017," Available at https://www.cancer.org/content/dam/cancer-org/research/cancer-facts-and-statistics/annual-cancer-facts-and-figures/2017/cancer-facts-and-figures-2017.pdf.
102. American Cancer Society, "Colorectal Cancer Facts and Figures, 2014–2016," Accessed June 2016, www.cancer.org/acs/groups/content/documents/document/acspc-042280.pdf; American Cancer Society, "Cancer Facts and Figures 2017," Available at https://www.cancer.org/content/dam/cancer-org/research/cancer-facts-and-statistics/annual-cancer-facts-and-figures/2017/cancer-facts-and-figures-2017.pdf.
103. American Cancer Society, "Cancer Facts and Figures 2017," Available at https://www.cancer.org/content/dam/cancer-org/research/cancer-facts-and-statistics/annual-cancer-facts-and-figures/2017/cancer-facts-and-figures-2017.pdf.
104. Ibid.
105. Ibid.
106. American Cancer Society, "Colorectal Cancer Facts and Figures, 2017–2019," 2017, https://www.cancer.org/content/dam/cancer-org/research/cancer-facts-and-statistics/colorectal-cancer-facts-and-figures/colorectal-cancer-facts-and-figures-2017-2019.pdf.
107. Ibid.
108. American Cancer Society, "Can Colorectal Cancer Be Prevented?" March 1, 2017, https://www.cancer.org/cancer/colon-rectal-cancer/causes-risks-prevention/prevention.html.
109. Ibid.
110. Ibid.
111. American Cancer Society, "Cancer Facts and Figures 2017," 2017Available at https://www.cancer.org/content/dam/cancer-org/research/cancer-facts-and-statistics/annual-cancer-facts-and-figures/2017/cancer-facts-and-figures-2017.pdf.
112. Ibid.
113. Ibid.
114. American Cancer Society, "Magnetic Resonance Imaging," January 2014, www.cancer.org/cancer/breastcancer/moreinformation/breastcancerearlydetection/breast-cancer-early-detection-a-c-s-recs-m-r-i.
115. U.S. Preventative Services Task Force, "Breast Cancer: Screening," January 2016, https://www.uspreventiveservicestaskforce.org/Page/Document/UpdateSummaryFinal/breast-cancer-screening1?ds=1's=breast%20cancer%20screening.
116. American Cancer Society, "Cancer Facts and Figures 2017," 2017.Available at https://www.cancer.org/content/dam/cancer-org/research/cancer-facts-and-statistics/annual-cancer-facts-and-figures/2017/cancer-facts-and-figures-2017.pdf.
117. Ibid.
118. American Cancer Society, "Cancer Facts and Figures 2017," 2017Available at https://www.cancer.org/content/dam/cancer-org/research/cancer-facts-and-statistics/annual-cancer-facts-and-figures/2017/cancer-facts-and-figures-2017.pdf; M. Farvid, "Fruit and Vegetable Consumption in Adolescences and Early Adulthood and Risk of Breast Cancer: Population Based Cohort Study," *BMJ* 353 (2016): i2343.
119. S. Koman. "Genetics and Breast Cancer," http://ww5.komen.org/uploadedFiles/_Komen/Content/About_Breast_Cancer/Tools_and_Resources/Fact_Sheets_and_Breast_Self_Awareness_Cards/Genetics%20and%20Breast%20Cancer.pdf. 2015.
120. H. Kyu et al., "Physical Activity and Risk of Breast Cancer, Colon Cancer, Diabetes, Ischemic Heart Disease, and Ischemic Stroke Events: Systematic Review and Dose-Response Meta-analysis for the Global Burden of Disease Study 2013," *BMJ* 354 (2016): i3857; I. Lahart et al., "Physical Activity, Risk of Death and Recurrence in Breast Cancer Survivors: A Systematic Review and Meta-analysis of Epidemiological Studies," *Acta Oncologica* 54, no. 5 (2015): 635–54, doi:10.3109/0284186X.2014.998275.
121. American Cancer Society, "Cancer Facts and Figures 2017," Available at https://www.cancer.org/content/dam/cancer-org/research/cancer-facts-and-statistics/annual-cancer-facts-and-figures/2017/cancer-facts-and-figures-2017.pdf.
122. Ibid.
123. Ibid.
124. Ibid.
125. Ibid.
126. Ibid.
127. K. Zu et al., "Dietary Lycopene, Angiogenesis, and Prostate Cancer: A Prospective Study in the Prostate-Specific Antigen Era," *Journal of the National Cancer Institute* 106, no. 2 (2014): 1093–97.
128. American Cancer Society, "Cancer Facts and Figures 2017," 2017. https://www.cancer.org/content/dam/cancer-org/research/cancer-facts-and-statistics/annual-cancer-facts-and-figures/2017/cancer-facts-and-figures-2017.pdf.
129. American Cancer Society, "Cancer Facts and Figures 2017," Available at https://www.cancer.org/content/dam/cancer-org/research/cancer-facts-and-statistics/annual-cancer-facts-and-figures/2017/cancer-facts-and-figures-2017.pdf.
130. Ibid.
131. National Institute of Health, National Cancer Institute, "SEER Stat Fact Sheets: Testis Cancer," February 2016, http://seer.cancer.gov/statfacts/html/testis.html.
132. Ibid.
133. Skin Cancer Foundation, "Skin Cancer Facts," June 8, 2016, www.skincancer.org/skin-cancer-information/skin-cancer-facts.

134. American Cancer Society, "Cancer Facts and Figures 2017," Available at https://www.cancer.org/content/dam/cancer-org/research/cancer-facts-and-statistics/annual-cancer-facts-and-figures/2017/cancer-facts-and-figures-2017.pdf.
135. Ibid.
136. Ibid.
137. Ibid.
138. Ibid.
139. Ibid.
140. Ibid.
141. National Cancer Institute, "Endometrial Cancer," 2016, https://seer.cancer.gov/statfacts/html/corp.htm.
142. American Cancer Society, "Cancer Facts and Figures 2017," 2017. https://www.cancer.org/content/dam/cancer-org/research/cancer-facts-and-statistics/annual-cancer-facts-and-figures/2017/cancer-facts-and-figures-2017.pdf
143. Ibid.
144. L. Carlson, "Mindfulness-based Cancer Recovery: The Development of an Evidence-based psychosocial oncology intervention," Oncology Exchange 12, no. 2 (2013): 21–25; M. Zhang et al., "Effectiveness of Mindfulness-based Therapy for Reducing Anxiety and Depression in Patients with cancer: A Meta-Analysis," Medicine 94, no. 45 (2015): e0897; L. Carlson, Mindfulness-based Cancer Recovery: A Step-by-Step MBSR Approach to Help You Cope with Treatment and Reclaim Your Life (Oakland, CA: New Harbinger, 2011); J. Kabat-Zinn and Thich Nhat Hanh, Full Catastrophe Living: Using the Wisdom of Your Body and Mind to Face Stress, Pain, and Illness (New York: Bantam, 2013).
145. Centers for Disease Control and Prevention, "National Diabetes Statistics Report, 2017," Available at https://www.cdc.gov/diabetes/pdfs/data/statistics/national-diabetes-statistics-report.pdf.
146. World Health Organization, "Diabetes Fact Sheet," Updated July 2016; http://www.who.int/mediacentre/factsheets/fs312/en.
147. Ibid.
148. International Diabetes Federation, Diabetes Atlas, 6th ed., 2014, http://www.diabetesatlas.org/resources/previous-editions.html; Centers for Disease Control and Prevention, "National Diabetes Statistics Report," 2017, https://www.cdc.gov/diabetes/pdfs/data/statistics/national-diabetes-statistics-report.pdf.
149. C. Bommer et al., "The Global Economic Burden of Diabetes in Adults Aged 20–79 Years: A Cost of Illness Study," Lancet Diabetes 'Endocrinology 5, no. 6 (2017):423–30; NCD Risk Factor Collaboration, "Worldwide Trends in Diabetes since 1980: A Pooled Analysis of 751 Population-based Studies with 4.4 Million Participants," Lancet 387, no. 10027 (2016): 1513–30.
150. Centers for Disease Control and Prevention, "Press Release: Number of Americans with Diabetes Projected to Double or Triple by 2050," https://www.cdc.gov/media/pressrel/2010/r101022.html.
151. American Diabetes Association, "Economic Costs of Diabetes in the U.S. in 2012" Diabetes Care 36 no. 4 (2013): 1033–46.
152. Centers for Disease Control and Prevention, "At a Glance 2016 Diabetes," Accessed June 2017, www.cdc.gov/chronicdisease/resources/publications/aag/pdf/2016/diabetes-aag.pdf; American Diabetes Association, "Fast Facts," December 2015, http://professional.diabetes.org/sites/professional.diabetes.org/files/media/fast_facts_12-2015a.pdf.

153. Centers for Disease and Prevention. "Diabetes Surveillance Data," April, 2016, https://www.cdc.gov/diabetes/data/statistics/faqs.html.
154. E. Mayor-Davis et al., "Increasing Trends of Type 1 and Type 2 Diabetes among Youth, 2002–2012," New England Journal of Medicine 376(2017):1419–29.
155. F. He et al., "Abdominal Obesity and Metabolic Syndrome Burden in Adolescents—Penn State Children Cohort Study," Journal of Clinical Densitometry 18, no. 1 (2015): 30–6; T. Huang et al., "Genetic Predisposition to Central Obesity and Risk of Type 2 Diabetes: Two Independent Cohort Studies," Diabetes Care 38, no. 7 (2015): 1306–11.
156. F. He et al., "Abdominal Obesity and Metabolic Syndrome Burden in Adolescents—Penn State Children Cohort Study," Journal of Clinical Densitometry 18, no. 1 (2015): 30–6; T. Huang et al., "Genetic Predisposition to Central Obesity and Risk of Type 2 Diabetes: Two Independent Cohort Studies," Diabetes Care 38, no. 7 (2015): 1306–11; S. Millar et al., "General and Central Obesity Measurement Associations with Markers of Chronic Low-grade Inflammation and Type 2 Diabetes," Journal of Epidemiology and Community Health 69, suppl. 1 (2015): A54–A55.
157. P.L. Capers et al., "A Systematic Review and Meta-analysis of Randomized Controlled Trials of the Impact of Sleep Duration on Adiposity and Components of Energy Balance," Obesity Reviews 16, no. 9 (2015): 771–82; L. Bromley et al., "Sleep Restriction Decreases the Physical Activity of Adults at Risk for Type 2 Diabetes," Sleep 35, no. 7 (2012): 977–84.
158. Z. Shan et al., "Sleep Duration and Risk of Type 2 Diabetes: A Meta-analysis of Prospective Studies," Diabetes Care 38, no. 3 (2015): 529–37; H.C. Hung et al., "The Association between Self-Reported Sleep Quality and Metabolic Syndrome," PLoS ONE 8, no. 1 (2013): e54304, doi:10.1371/journal.pone.0054304.
159. T. Anothaisintawee et al., "Sleep Disturbances Compared to Traditional Risk Factors for Diabetes Development: Systematic Review and Meta-analysis," Sleep Medicine Reviews 30 (2016): 11–24; S. Kelly and M. Ismail, "Stress and Type 2 Diabetes: A Review of How Stress Contributes to the Development of Type 2 Diabetes," Annual Review of Public Health 36 (2015): 441–62.
160. Ibid.
161. L. Mongiello et al., "Many College Students Underestimate Diabetes Risk," Journal of Allied Health 45, no. 2 (2016): 81–6; N. Yahia et al., "Assessment of College Students' Awareness and Knowledge about Conditions Relevant to Metabolic Syndrome," Diabetology and Metabolic Syndrome 6, no. 1 (2014): 111; A. Lima et al., "Risk Factors for Type 2 Diabetes Mellitus in College Students: Association with Sociodemographic Variables," Revista Latino-Americana de Enfermagem 22, no. 3 (2014): 484–90.
162. M. Aguilar et al., "Prevalence of the Metabolic Syndrome in the United States, 2003–2012," Journal of the American Medical Association 313, no. 19 (2015): 1973–74.
163. American Diabetes Association, "What Is Gestational Diabetes?," November 21, 2016, www.diabetes.org/diabetes-basics/gestational/what-is-gestational-diabetes.html.
164. Ibid; E. Noctor and F. Dunne, "Type 2 Diabetes after Gestational Diabetes: The Influence of Changing Diagnostic Criteria," World Journal of Diabetes 6, no. 2 (2015): 234–44.
165. National Kidney Foundation, "Fast Facts," May 2016, www.kidney.org/news/newsroom/fact-

sheets/FastFacts.cfm; U.S. Renal Disease Data System, "Annual Data Report, 2015," Available at https://www.usrds.org/adr.aspx.
166. Centers for Disease Control and Prevention, "National Diabetes Statistics Report, 2014," May 2015.
167. Prevent Blindness America, "Diabetic Retinopathy Prevalence by Age," Accessed May 2017, www.visionproblemsus.org/diabetic-retinopathy/diabetic-retinopathy-by-age.html.
168. American Diabetes Association, "Standards of Medical Care in Diabetes—2016: Summary of Revisions," Diabetes Care/ 39, suppl. 1 (2016): S4–S5.
169. Ibid.
170. Diabetes Prevention Program Research Group, "Reduction in the Incidence of Type 2 Diabetes with Lifestyle Intervention or Metformin," New England Journal of Medicine 345 (2002): 393–403.
171. American Diabetes Association, "Diabetes Superfoods," Accessed May 2017, http://www.diabetes.org/food-and-fitness/food/what-can-i-eat/making-healthy-food-choices/diabetes-superfoods.html.
172. S. Bhupathiraju et al., "Glycemic Index, Glycemic Load and Risk of Type 2 Diabetes: Results from 3 Large US Cohorts and an Updated Meta-Analysis," Circulation 129, suppl. 1 (2014): AP140–AP140; American Diabetes Association, "Diabetes Superfoods," Accessed May 2017, http://www.diabetes.org/food-and-fitness/food/what-can-i-eat/making-healthy-food-choices/diabetes-superfoods.html.
173. A. Wallin et al., "Fish Consumption and Frying of Fish in Relation to Type 2 Diabetes Incidence: A Prospective Cohort Study of Swedish Men," European Journal of Nutrition (2015): 1–10; Y. Kim et al., "Fish Consumption, Long-Chain Omega-3 Polyunsaturated Fatty Acid Intake and Risk of Metabolic Syndrome: A Meta-analysis," Nutrients 7, no. 4 (2015): 2085–2100.
174. W. Cefalu et al., "Standards of Medical Care in Diabetes-2017," Diabetes Care 40, suppl. 1 (2017), Available at http://care.diabetesjournals.org/content/diacare/suppl/2016/12/15/40.Supplement_1.DC1/DC_40_S1_final.pdf.
175. O. Farr and C. Mantzorous, "Treatment Options to Prevent Diabetes in Subjects with Prediabetes: Efficacy, Cost Effectiveness, and Future Outlook," Metabolism 70, (2017); A. Anabtawj and J. Miles, "Metformin: Nonglycemic Effects and Potential Novel Indications," Endocrine Practice 22, no. 8 (2016): 999–1007; U. Hostalek et al., "Therapeutic Use of Metformin in Prediabetes and Diabetes Prevention," Drugs 75, no. 10 (2015): 1071–94.
176. F. Rubino et al., "Metabolic Surgery in the Treatment Algorithm for Type 2 Diabetes: A Joint Statement by International Diabetes Organizations," Surgery of Obesity and Related Diseases 12, no. 6 (2016): 1144–62; D.E. Cummings et al., "Gastric Bypass Surgery vs Intensive Lifestyle and Medical Intervention for Type 2 Diabetes: The CROSSROADS Randomised Controlled Trial," Diabetologia 59, no. 5 (2016): 945–53; J. Yu et al., "The Long Term Effects of Bariatric Surgery for Type 2 Diabetes: Systematic Review and Meta-analysis of Randomized and Non Randomized Evidence," Obesity Surgery 25, no. 1 (2015): 143–55.
177. Ibid.
178. M. Jenson et al., "2013 AHA/ACC/TOS Guideline for the Management of Overweight and Obesity in Adults: A Report of the American College of Cardiology/American Heart Association Task Force on Practice Guidelines and the Obesity Society," Circulation 25, suppl. 2 (2014): S139–40.

Chapter 12

1. X. Wu et al., "Impact of Climate Change on Human Infectious Diseases: Empirical Evidence and Human Adaptation," *Environment International* 86 (2016): 14–23; L. Liang and P. Gong, "Climate Change and Human Infectious Diseases: A Synthesis of Research Findings from Global and Spatio-temporal Perspectives," *Environment International* 103 (2017): 99–108; World Health Organization, "Climate Change and Infectious Disease," May 2015, www.who.int/global-change/publications/climatechangechap6.pdf; C. Heffernan, "Climate Change and Infectious Disease: Time for a New Normal?" *Lancet Infectious Diseases* 15, no. 2 (2015): 143–44.

2. D. Black and G. Slavich, "Mindfulness Meditation and the Immune System: A Systematic Review of Randomized Controlled Trials," *Annals of the New York Academy of Sciences* 1373 (2016): 13–24. doi:10.1111/nyas.1299.

3. M. Ewoenspoek, "The Effects of Early Life Adversity on the Immune System," *Psychoneuroendocrinology* 82 (2017): 140–54.

4. F. D'Acquisto, "Affective Immunology: Where Emotions and the Immune System Converge," *Dialogues in Clinical Neuroscience* 19, no. 1 (2017): 9–19.

5. National Institute of Allergy and Infectious Diseases, "Autoimmune Diseases," January 5, 2016, http://www.niaid.nih.gov/topics/autoimmune/Pages/default.aspx.

6. Centers for Disease Control and Prevention, 2017 Recommended Immunization for Adults: By Age," February 2017, https://www.cdc.gov/vaccines/schedules/downloads/adult/adult-schedule-easy-read.pdf;. Centers for Disease Control and Prevention, "Recommended Immunization Schedule for Adults Aged 19 Years or Older, United States, 2017," February 2017, https://www.cdc.gov/vaccines/schedules/downloads/adult/adult-combined-schedule.pdf.

7. Centers for Disease Control and Prevention, "Preventing Healthcare Associated Infections," Accessed May 2017, https://www.cdc.gov/washington/~cdcatWork/pdf/infections.pdf; Centers for Disease Control and Prevention, "HAI Data and Statistics," October 25, 2016, www.cdc.gov/HAI/surveillance; S. Magill et al., "Multistate Point-Prevalence Survey of Health Care–Associated Infections," *New England Journal of Medicine* 370, no. 13 (2014): 1198–208.

8. P. Span, "Doctors See Gains against 'an Urgent Threat,' C. Diff" *New York Times*, February 10, 2017, https://www.nytimes.com/2017/02/10/health/clostridium-difficile-c-diff.html.

9. Centers for Disease Control and Prevention, "Group B Strep (GBS)," May 23, 2016, https://www.cdc.gov/groupbstrep.

10. World Health Organization, "Global Health Observatory (GHO) Data: Meningococcal Meningitis," Accessed March 28, 2016, http://www.who.int/gho/epidemic_diseases/meningitis/en/; Centers for Disease Control and Prevention, "Meningococcal Disease: Surveillance," June 9, 2017, https://www.cdc.gov/meningococcal/surveillance.

11. Ibid.

12. Ibid.

13. World Health Organization, "Media Centre: Tuberculosis Fact Sheet," March 2017, www.who.int/mediacentre/factsheets/fs104/en.

14. K. Schmit et al., "Tuberculosis—United States, 2016," *Morbidity and Mortality Weekly Reports* 66, no. 11 (2017): 289–94.

15. Ibid.

16. World Health Organization, "Tuberculosis and Women," 2015, http://www.who.int/tb/publications/tb_women_factsheet_251013.pdf.

17. World Health Organization, "Tuberculosis and Women," 2015, http://www.who.int/tb/publications/tb_women_factsheet_251013.pdf; Centers for Disease Control and Prevention, "New Treatment Regimen for Latent Tuberculosis Infection," March 25, 2016, http://www.cdc.gov/tb/topic/treatment/12dose_video.htm; ScienceDaily, "Curcumin May Help Overcome Drug-Resistant Tuberculosis," March 25, 2016, www.sciencedaily.com/releases/2016/03/160325093704.htm.

18. Centers for Disease Control and Prevention, "TB-MultiDrug Resistant," May 11, 2016, https://www.cdc.gov/tb/publications/factsheets/drtb/mdrtb.htm.

19. Centers for Disease Control and Prevention. "Epstein-Barr Virus and Infectious Mononucleosis," September 2016, https://www.cdc.gov/epstein-barr/index.html.

20. Centers for Disease Control and Prevention, "Hepatitis A Questions and Answers for Public," October 2016, https://www.cdc.gov/hepatitis/hav/afaq.htm#statistics; T.V. Murphy, "Progress toward Eliminating Hepatitis A Disease in the United States," *Morbidity and Mortality Weekly Report Supplements* 65, no. 1 (2016): 29–41.

21. Centers for Disease Control and Prevention, "Viral Hepatitis Surveillance United States—2015, June 19, 2017, https://www.cdc.gov/hepatitis/statistics/2015surveillance/pdfs/2015HepSurveillanceRpt.pdf.html.

22. Ibid.

23. D. Lavanchy and M. Kane, *Hepatitis B Virus in Human Disease* (Switzerland: Springer Publishing, 2016), 187–202; World Health Organization, "Hepatitis B," October 2016, http://www.who.int/immunization/monitoring_surveillance/burden/vpd/surveillance_type/passive/hepatitis/en.

24. Centers for Disease Control and Prevention, "Viral Hepatitis Surveillance United States—2015," June 19, 2017, https://www.cdc.gov/hepatitis/statistics/2015surveillance/pdfs/2015HepSurveillanceRpt.pdf.html.

25. Centers for Disease Control and Prevention, "Viral Hepatitis Surveillance United States—2015," June 19, 2017, https://www.cdc.gov/hepatitis/statistics/2015surveillance/pdfs/2015HepSurveillanceRpt.pdf. html; Centers for Disease Control and Prevention, "Hepatitis C FAQs for the Public," October 2016, https://www.cdc.gov/hepatitis/hcv/cfaq.htm.

26. Ibid.

27. Ibid.

28. Ibid; J. Bastos, "Hepatitis C Virus: Promising discoveries and new Treatments." World J Gastroenterol. 2016 Jul 28; 22(28): 6393–6401.doi: 10.3748/wjg.v22.i28.6393

29. Centers for Disease Control and Prevention, "Shingles (Herpes Zoster)," August 2016, https://www.cdc.gov/shingles/index.htm.

30. Centers for Disease Control and Prevention, "Common Colds: Protect Yourself and Others," February 6, 2017, www.cdc.gov/features/rhinoviruses.

31. C. DerSarkissian, "What's Causing My Cold?," January 23, 2017, http://www.webmd.com/cold-and-flu/cold-guide/common_cold_causes.

32. Centers for Disease Control and Prevention, "Frequently Asked Flu Questions 2016–2017 Influenza Season," March 2017, https://www.cdc.gov/flu/about/season/flu-season-2016-2017.htm; Centers for Disease Control and Prevention, "Faststats: Leading Causes of Death, 2015," March 2017, https://www.cdc.gov/nchs/fastats/deaths.htm.

33. Centers for Disease Control and Prevention, "Selecting the Viruses in the Seasonal Influenza (Flu) Vaccine," October 20, 2015, www.cdc.gov/flu/about/season/vaccine-selection.htm.

34. Centers for Disease Control and Prevention, "ACIP Votes Down Use of LAIV for 2016–2017 Flu Season," June 2016, http://www.cdc.gov/media/releases/2016/s0622-laiv-flu.html.

35. Centers for Disease Control and Prevention, "Valley Fever (Coccidioidomycosis) Statistics," June 2017, https://www.cdc.gov/fungal/diseases/coccidioidomycosis/statistics.htm.

36. Ibid.

37. Centers for Disease Control and Prevention, "vCJD Factsheet (Variant Creutzfeldt-Jakob Disease)," February 2015, https://www.cdc.gov/prions/vcjd/index.html.

38. Ibid.

39. Ibid.

40. Centers for Disease Control and Prevention, "West Nile Virus Disease Cases and Presumptive Viremic Blood Donors by State—United States, 2016," January 17, 2017, http://www.cdc.gov/westnile/statsmaps/preliminarymapsdata/histatedate.html.

41. World Health Organization, "Cumulative Number of Confirmed Human Cases of Avian Influenza A (H5N1) Reported to WHO," January 2014, www.who.int/influenza/human_animal_interface/H5N1_cumulative_table_archives/en/index.html.

42. Pls. provide reference.

43. World Health Organization, "Factsheet on the World Malaria Report 2016," December 2013, www.who.int/malaria/media/world_malaria_report_2016/3n/3.

44. Ibid.

45. Ibid.

46. Centers for Disease Control and Prevention, "Fast Facts: Get Smart about Antibiotics," April 2017, www.cdc.gov/getsmart/community/about/index.html; World Health Organization, "Antimicrobial Resistance," May 2017, http://www.who.int/antimicrobial-resistance/en; Centers for Disease Control and Prevention, "Antibiotic-Antimicrobial Resistance—Biggest Threats," April, 14, 2017, https://www.cdc.gov/drugresistance.

47. Ibid.

48. Centers for Disease Control and Prevention, "Fact Sheet: Reported Cases of Sexually Transmitted Diseases in United States-2016: High Burden of STDs Threaten Millions of Americans," September 21, 2017. https://www.cdc.gov/nchhstp/newsroom/docs/factsheets/std-trends-508.pdf; Centers for Disease Control and Prevention. *Sexually Transmitted Disease Surveillance 2016.* Atlanta: U.S. Department of Health and Human Services; 2017.

49. IBID; 5.

50. Centers for Disease Control and Prevention, "STDs: Adolescents and Young Adults," December 2014, www.cdc.gov/std/stats13/adol.htm.

51. U.S. Department of Health and Human Services, Office of Adolescent Health, "Sexually Transmitted Diseases," May 2016, http://www.hhs.gov/ash/oah/adolescent-health-topics/reproductive-health/stds.html.

52. Centers for Disease Control and Prevention, "10 Ways STDs Impact Women Differently from Men," Accessed June 2017, https://www.cdc.gov/std/health-disparities/stds-women.pdf.

53. UNAIDS, "Fact Sheet," February 2017, http://www.unaids.org/en/resources/fact-sheet; AMFAR, "Statistics World Wide," February 2017, http://www.amfar.org/About-HIV-and-AIDS/Facts-and-Stats/Statistics—Worldwide.

54. UNAIDS "Fact Sheet: Latest Statistics on the Status of the AIDS Epidemic." ," February, 2017". http://www.unaids.org/en/resources/fact-sheet; AMFAR, "Statistics World Wide," February 2017, http://www.amfar.org/About-HIV-and-AIDS/Facts-and-Stats/Statistics–Worldwide/.

55. World Health Organization, "Mother to Child Transmission of HIV," July 2015, www.who.int/hiv/topics/mtct/en.

56. Ibid.

57. U.S. Food and Drug Administration, "Think Before You Ink: Are Tattoos Safe?" May 2017, https://www.fda.gov/ForConsumers/ConsumerUpdates/ucm048919.htm.

58. Centers for Disease Control and Prevention, "HIV Testing," September 21, 2017., www.cdc.gov/hiv/testing/index.html.

59. Pharmaceutical Research and Manufacturers of America, "Medicine in Development: 2014 Report," May 2015, www.phrma.org/sites/default/files/pdf/2014-meds-in-dev-hiv-aids.pdf.

60. U.S. Department of Health and Human Services, "Limitations to Treatment Safety and Efficacy: Cost Considerations and Antiretroviral Therapy," July 14, 2016, https://aidsinfo.nih.gov/guidelines/html/1/adult-and-adolescent-arv-guidelines/459/cost-considerations-and-antiretroviral-therapy.

61. Ibid.

62. Ibid.

63. Centers for Disease Control and Prevention, "CDC Fact Sheet: Chlamydia (Detailed)," October 17, 2016, http://www.cdc.gov/std/chlamydia/stdfact-chlamydia-detailed.htm.

64. Centers for Disease Control and Prevention, "CDC Fact Sheet: Gonorrhea (Detailed)," September 26, 2017. https://www.cdc.gov/std/gonorrhea/stdfact-gonorrhea-detailed.htm.

65. Ibid.

66. Ibid..

67. Ibid.

68. CDC. "Pelvic Inflammatory Disease (PID): Fact Sheet." July, 2017. https://www.cdc.gov/std/pid/stdfact-pid.htm.

69. J. Martel and A Gotter. "Epididymitis: Fast Facts." Healthline. 2016. https://www.healthline.com/health/epididymitis#overview1; CDC. "Epididymitis." June, 2015. https://www.cdc.gov/std/tg2015/epididymitis.htm Control and Prevention, "STD Treatment Guidelines 2010: Epididymitis," Updated January 2011, https://www.cdc.gov/std/treatment/2010/epididymitis.htm.

70. Centers for Disease Control and Prevention, "CDC Fact Sheet: Gonorrhea (Detailed)," February 13, 2017. May 19, 2016, https://www.cdc.gov/std/syphilis/stdfact-syphilis-detailed.htm

71. Ibid.

72. Ibid.

73. Ibid.

74. American Sexual Health Association, "Herpes: Fast Facts," Accessed June, 2017, www.ashasexualhealth.org/stdsstis/herpes/fast-facts-and-faqs; Centers for Disease Control and Prevention, "CDC Fact Sheet: Genital Herpes (Detailed)," February 2017, https://www.cdc.gov/std/herpes/stdfact-herpes.htm.

75. Ibid.

76. Centers for Disease Control and Prevention, "CDC Fact Sheet: Genital Herpes (Detailed)," February 2017, https://www.cdc.gov/std/herpes/stdfact-herpes.htm.

77. Ibid.

78. Centers for Disease Control and Prevention, "HPV Questions and Answers," November 2016, https://www.cdc.gov/hpv/parents/questions-answers.html.

79. Ibid.

80. Centers for Disease Control and Prevention, "Cervical Cancer," May 2017, http://www.cdc.gov/cancer/cervical.

81. American Cancer Society, "Cancer Facts ' Figures 2016," 2017, Available at http://www.cancer.org/acs/groups/content/@research/documents/document/acspc-047079.pdf.

82. Centers for Disease Control and Prevention, "Human Papillomavirus (HPV) and Oropharyngeal Cancer—Fact Sheet," January 2017, http://www.cdc.gov/std/hpv/stdfact-hpvandoropharyngealcancer.htm.

83. Centers for Disease Control and Prevention, "HPV Vaccine Information for Young Women," January 17, 2017, http://www.cdc.gov/std/hpv/STDFact-HPV-vaccine-young-women.htm; Centers for Disease Control and Prevention, "HPV Vaccine—Questions & Answers," November 2016, https://www.cdc.gov/hpv/parents/questions-answers.html.

84. Ibid.

85. Ibid.

86. Ibid.

87. Ibid.

88. Centers for Disease Control and Prevention, "Trichomoniasis: CDC Fact Sheet," March, 2017, www.cdc.gov/std/trichomonas/stdfact-trichomoniasis.htm.

89. Ibid.

Chapter 13

1. World Health Organization, *Global Status Report on Violence Prevention* (Geneva, Switzerland: World Health Organization, 2014), Available at www.undp.org/content/dam/undp/library/corporate/Reports/UNDP-GVA-violence-2014.pdf.

2. Centers for Disease Control and Prevention, "Ten Leading Causes of Death by Age Group, United States, 2014," Accessed March 2017, Available at https://www.cdc.gov/injury/wisqars/pdf/leading_causes_of_death_by_age_group_2014-a.pdf.

3. Federal Bureau of Investigation, "Crime in the United States, Preliminary Semiannual Uniform Crime Report for January–June 2016," 2016, https://www.fbi.gov/about-us/cjis/ucr/crime-in-the-u.s/2016/preliminary-semiannual-uniform-crime-report-januaryjune-2016/tables/table-3.

4. Ibid.

5. L. Langton and J. Truman, "Criminal Victimization—2015," Bureau of Justice Statistics, October 20, 2016., https://www.bjs.gov/index.cfm?ty=pbdetail & iid=5804.

6. Center for Public Integrity, "Sexual Assault on Campus: A Frustrating Search for Justice," Updated February 2013, www.publicintegrity.org/accountability/education/sexual-assault-campus.

7. American College Health Association, *American College Health Association—National College Health Assessment II: Reference Group Data Report, Fall 2016* (Baltimore, MD: American College Health Association, 2017).

8. Ibid.

9. Ibid.

10. World Health Organization Violence Prevention Alliance, "The Ecological Framework," Accessed June 2016, www.who.int/violenceprevention/approach/ecology/en/index.html; Centers for Disease Control and Prevention, National Center for Injury Prevention and Control, "Understanding School Violence: Fact Sheet—2015," Accessed June 2016, http://www.cdc.gov/violenceprevention/pdf/School_Violence_Fact_Sheet-a.pdf.

11. A. Martin et al., "Formal Controls, Neighborhood Disadvantage and Violent Crime in U.S. Cities: Examining (Un)intended Consequences," *Journal of Criminal Justice* 44 (2016): 58–65; American Psychological Association, "Violence and Socioeconomic Status," Accessed June 2014, www.apa.org/pi/ses/resources/publications/factsheet-violence.aspx.

12. C. Spencer et al., "Gender Differences in Risk Markers for Perpetration of Physical Partner Violence: Results from a Meta-analytic Review," *Journal of Family Violence* 31, no. 8 (2016): 981–84; E. Wright, "Less Social Support for Women in Disadvantaged Neighborhoods Means That They Are More Likely to Be the Victims of Intimate Partner Violence," *USApp—American Politics and Policy Blog*, May 12, 2016; World Health Organization Violence Prevention Alliance, "The Ecological Framework," Accessed June 2014, www.who.int/violenceprevention/approach/ecology/en/index.html.

13. C. Ferguson, "Does Media Violence Predict Societal Violence? It Depends on What You Look at and When?" *Journal of Communication* 65, no. 1 (2015): E1–E22; W. Gunter and K. Daley, "Causal or Spurious? Using Propensity Score Matching to Detangle the Relationship between Violent Video Games and Violent Behavior," *Computers in Human Behavior* 4, no. 28 (2012): 1348–55.

14. S. Calvert et al., "The American Psychological Association Task Force Assessment of Violent Video Games: Science in the Service of Public Interest," *American Psychologist* 72, no. 2 (2017): 126.

15. World Health Organization, *World Report on Violence and Health* (Geneva: World Health Organization, 2002).

16. Centers for Disease Control and Prevention, "Health, United States, 2015," April 2016, http://www.cdc.gov/nchs/data/hus/hus15.pdf.

17. Federal Bureau of Investigation, "Crime in the United States, 2016 Preliminary Semi-annual Uniform Crime Report," June 2016, Available at https://ucr.fbi.gov/crime-in-the-u.s/2016/preliminary-semiannual-uniform-crime-report-januaryjune-2016/tables/table-3.

18. Ibid.

19. Centers for Disease Control and Prevention, "Health, United States, 2015," April 2016, http://www.cdc.gov/nchs/data/hus/hus15.pdf

20. A. Lankford & S.Tomek, "Mass Killings in the United States from 2006-2013: Social Contagion or Random Clusters?" *Suicide and Life-Threatening Behavior*, 2017. doi: 10.1111/sltb.12366; A. Lankford. "Are America's Public Mass Shooters Unique? A Comparative Analysis of Offenders in the United States and Other Countries." *International Journal of Comparative and Applied Criminal Justice*, 40(2), 171–183

21. A. Anglemyer, et al. " The Accessibility of Firearms and Risk for Suicide and Homicide Victimization Among Household Members: A Systematic Review and Meta-analysis." *Annals of Internal Medicine*. 2014:160(2):101–110. DOI: 10.7326/M13-1301

I. C. Ingraham, "There Are Now More Guns Than People in the United States," *Washington Post*, October 5, 2015, https://www.washingtonpost.com/news/wonk/wp/2015/10/05/guns-in-the-united-states-one-for-every-man-woman-and-child-and-then-some; J. Davidson and H. Jones, "The Orlando Shooting Is a Haunting Reminder of Just How Many Guns Are in America," *Time*, June 14, 2016, http://time.com/4188456/orlando-shooting-mass-shootings-gun-control; National Conference of State Legislatures, "Guns on Campus: Overview," 2015, http://www.ncsl.org/research/education/guns-on-campus-overview.aspx.

22. Federal Bureau of Investigation, "Latest Hate Crime Statistics Released: Annual Report Sheds Light on Serious Issue," November 14, 2016, https://www.fbi.gov/news/stories/2015-hate-crime-statistics-released; Lynn Langton and Madeline Masucci, "Hate Crime Victimization, 2004–2015," U.S. Bureau of Justice Statistics, Hate Crime Series, National Crime Victimization Survey, June 29, 2017, NCJ 250653. https://www.bjs.gov/index.cfm?ty=pbdetail&iid=5967.

23. American Psychological Association, "Intimate Partner Violence—Facts and Resources," Accessed March 2017, http://www.apa.org/topics/violence/partner.aspx.

24. American Psychological Association, "Intimate Partner Violence—Facts and Resources," Accessed March 2017, http://www.apa.org/topics/violence/partner.aspx.

25. Ibid.

26. Centers for Disease Control and Prevention, "Intimate Partner Violence: Risk and Protective Factors." Accessed August 2017, https://www.cdc.gov/violenceprevention/intimatepartnerviolence/riskprotectivefactors.html.

27. L. Walker, *The Battered Woman* (New York, NY: Harper and Row, 1979).

28. L. Walker, *The Battered Woman Syndrome*, 3rd ed. (New York, NY: Springer, 2009).

29. Bureau of Justice Statistics, "Intimate Partner Violence, 1993–2011," February 2, 2016. https://www.bjs.gov/index.cfm?ty=pbdetail&iid=4801.

30. Child Welfare Information Gateway, Definitions of Child Abuse and Neglect (Washington, DC: U.S. Department of Health and Human Services, Children's Bureau, 2014), Available at www.childwelfare.gov/topics/systemwide/laws-policies/statutes/define; U. S. Department of Health and Human Services, Administration for Children and Families, "Definitions of Child Abuse and Neglect," February 2011, www.childwelfare.gov/systemwide/laws_policies/statutes/define.cfm.

31. M. Stoltenborgh et al., "The Current Prevalence of Child Sexual Abuse Worldwide: A Systematic Review and Meta-Analysis," *International Journal of Public Health* 58, no. 3 (2013): 469–83; Childhelp, National Child Abuse Statistics, "Child Abuse in America—2012," Accessed June 2014, www.childhelp.org/pages/statistics; U.S. Department of Health and Human Services, Children's Bureau, "Child Maltreatment–2015," January 2017, https://www.acf.hhs.gov/cb/resource/child-maltreatment-2015.

32. U.S. Department of Health and Human Services, Children's Bureau, "Child Maltreatment," 2017, https://www.acf.hhs.gov/cb/research-data-technology/statistics-research/child-maltreatment.

33. U.S. Department of Health and Human Services, Children's Bureau, "Child Maltreatment," 2017, https://www.acf.hhs.gov/cb/research-data-technology/statistics-research/

child-maltreatment; Childhelp, "Child Abuse in America—2012," Accessed June 2014, www.childhelp.org/pages/statistics.

34. Childhelp, "Child Abuse Statistics and Facts," Accessed July 2016, www.childhelp.org/child-abuse-statistics.

35. Centers for Disease Control and Prevention, "Understanding Elder Abuse, Fact Sheet 2016," Accessed March 2017, https://www.cdc.gov/violenceprevention/pdf/em-factsheet-a.pdf.

36. I. Quellet-Morin et al., "Intimate Partner Violence and New Onset Depression: A Longitudinal Study of Women's Childhood and Adult Histories of Abuse," *Depression and Anxiety* 32, no. 5 (2015): 316–24.

37. Federal Bureau of Investigation, "Preliminary Semiannual Uniform Crime Report. Data Declaration," 2015, https://www.fbi.gov/about-us/cjis/ucr/crime-in-the-u.s/2015/preliminary-semiannual-uniform-crime-report-januaryjune-2015/tables/table-3/table_3_january_to_june_2015_percent_change_for_consecutive_years.xls/@@template-layout-view?override-view=data-declaration.

38. White House Task Force to Protect Students from Sexual Assault, "Not Alone: First Report of White House Task Force to Protect Students from Sexual Assault," April 2014, www.whitehouse.gov/sites/default/files/docs/report_0.pdf.

39. Association of American Universities, "AAU Climate Survey on Sexual Assault and Sexual Misconduct," September 2015, https://www.aau.edu/key-issues/aau-climate-survey-sexual-assault-and-sexual-misconduct-2015; White House Task Force to Protect Students from Sexual Assault, "Not Alone: First Report of White House Task Force to Protect Students from Sexual Assault," April 2014, www.whitehouse.gov/sites/default/files/docs/report_0.pdf.

40. White House Task Force to Protect Students from Sexual Assault, "Not Alone: First Report of White House Task Force to Protect Students from Sexual Assault," April 2014, www.whitehouse.gov/sites/default/files/docs/report_0.pdf.

41. N. Anderson, "These Campuses Have the Most Reports of Rape," *Washington Post*, June 7, 2016, https://www.washingtonpost.com/news/grade-point/wp/2016/06/07/these-colleges-have-the-most-reports-of-rape.

42. California Legislative Information, "SB-967 Student Safety: Sexual Assault," 2013–2014, 2016.. https://leginfo.legislature.ca.gov/faces/billNavClient.xhtml?bill_id=201320140SB967.

43. B. Chappell, "California Enacts 'Yes Means Yes' Law, Defining Sexual Consent," September 29, 2014, www.npr.org/blogs/thetwo-way/2014/09/29/352482932/california-enacts-yes-means-yes-law-defining-sexual-consent.

44. A. Jackson, "State Contexts and the Criminalization of Marital Rape Across the United States," *Social Science Research* 51 (2015): 290–306.

45. Oregon State University, "Sexual Harassment and Sexual Violence," Accessed June 2016, http://eoa.oregonstate.edu/sexual-harassment-and-violence-policy.

46. Centers for Disease Control and Prevention, "Sexual Violence, Stalking, and Intimate Partner Violence Widespread in the US," NISVS 2010 Summary Report, Press Release, December 2011; NCVRW Resource Guide–2012, "Crime Victimization in the United States: Statistical Overviews," Accessed June 2014, www.ncjrs.gov/ovc_archives/ncvrw/2012/pdf/StatisticalOverviews.pdf.

47. D. Woodlock, "The Abuse of Technology in Domestic Violence and Stalking," *Violence against Women* 23, no. 5 (2017): 584–602.

48. P. Brady and L. Boufford, "Majoring in Stalking: Exploring Stalking Experiences between College Students and the General Public," *Crime Victims Institute—Series on Stalking* (2014), Available at http://dev.cjcenter.org/_files/cvi/Stalking%20Series3tInpdf.pdf.

49. U.S. Department of Justice, "Juvenile Justice Fact Sheet—Highlights of the 2012 National Youth Gang Survey," December 2014, www.ojjdp.gov/pubs/248025.pdf; Federal Bureau of Investigation, "2013 National Gang Threat Assessment—Emerging Trends," February 2015, www.fbi.gov/stats-services/publications/national-gang-report-2013.

50. Federal Bureau of Investigation, "National Gang Report, 2015," 2015, Available at https://www.fbi.gov/stats-services/publications/national-gang-report-2015.pdf; U.S. Department of Justice, "Juvenile Justice Fact Sheet—Highlights of the 2012 National Youth Gang Survey," December 2014, www.ojjdp.gov/pubs/248025.pdf; Federal Bureau of Investigation, "2013 National Gang Threat Assessment—Emerging Trends," February 2015, www.fbi.gov/stats-services/publications/national-gang-report-2013.

51. Violence Prevention Institute, "Why People Join Gangs and What You Can Do," Accessed June 2016, http://www.violencepreventioninstitute.com/youngpeople.html; Federal Bureau of Investigation, "What We Investigate: Cyber Crime," Accessed March 2017, https://www.fbi.gov/investigate/cyber.

52. U.S. Code of Federal Regulations, Title 28CFR0.85.

53. Centers for Disease Control and Prevention, Office of Public Health Preparedness and Response, "Overview," 2016, https://www.cdc.gov/phpr/about.htm.

54. Adapted from E. Allan and M. Madden, *Hazing in View: College Students at Risk* (Orono, ME: National Collaborative for Hazing Research and Prevention, 2008), Available at www.hazingstudy.org, Reprinted by permission of Elizabeth Allan; B.W. Chamberlin, "'Am I My Brother's Keeper?': Reforming Criminal Hazing Laws Based on Assumption of Care," *Emory Law Journal* 63, no. 4 (2014), http://law.emory.edu/elj/content/volume-63/issue-4/comments/reforming-criminal-hazing-laws.html.

55. Ibid.

56. National Highway Traffic Safety Administration, "Traffic Safety Facts, 2015 Data: Alcohol-Impaired Driving," December 2015, www.nrd.nhtsa.dot.gov/Pubs/812231.pdf.

57. National Highway Traffic Safety Administration. "Traffic Safety Facts: Crash Stats, March. 2017; Distraction.gov, "Facts and Statistics," Accessed March 2017, https://www.distraction.gov/stats-research-laws/facts-and-statistics.html.

58. T. Johnson, "Distraction and Teen Crashes: Even Worse Than We Thought," AAA Newsroom, March 25, 2015, http://newsroom.aaa.com/2015/03/distraction-teen-crashes-even-worse-thought.

59. National High Traffic Safety Administration. "Driver Electronic Device Uses in 2015." September, 2016. https://www.nhtsa.gov/sites/nhtsa.dot.gov/files/documents/driver_electronic_device_use_in_2015_0.pdf; National Traffic Law Center. "Investigation and prosecution of distracted driving cases ". (2017, May). (Report No. DOT HS 812 407). https://www.nhtsa.gov/sites/nhtsa.dot.gov/files/documents/812407-distracteddrivingreport.pdf https://www

.nhtsa.gov/sites/nhtsa.dot.gov/files/documents/812407-distracteddrivingreport.pdf

60. National Highway Traffic Safety Administration, "Distracted Driving Research: Teens and Young Drivers," Accessed March 2017, http://www.nsc.org/learn/NSC-Initiatives/Pages/distracted-driving-research-studies.aspx; Centers for Disease Control and Prevention. "Distracted Driving," March 7, 2016, https://www.cdc.gov/motorvehiclesafety/distracted_driving.

61. Insurance Institute for Highway Safety, "Distracted Driving," April 2017, http://www.iihs.org/iihs/topics/laws/cellphonelaws/maptextingbans.

62. National Highway Traffic Safety Administration, "Traffic Safety Facts, 2015 Data: Alcohol-Impaired Driving," December 2016, https://crashstats.nhtsa.dot.gov/Api/Public/ViewPublication/812350.

63. Ibid.

64. Ibid.

65. National Institute on Drug Abuse, "Drug Facts: Drugged Driving," Revised June 2016, www.drugabuse.gov/publications/drugfacts/drugged-driving.

66. Ibid.

67. S. Salomonsen-Sautel et al., "Trends in Fatal Motor Vehicle Crashes before and after Marijuana Commercialized in Colorado," *Drug and Alcohol Dependence* 140 (2014): 137–44.

68. National Institute on Drug Abuse, "Drug Facts: Drugged Driving," Revised June 2016, www.drugabuse.gov/publications/drugfacts/drugged-driving.

69. National Highway Traffic Safety Administration, "Traffic Safety Facts: 2014 Data," March 2016, www-nrd.nhtsa.dot.gov/Pubs/812246.pdf.

70. Insurance Institute for Highway Safety, "Vehicle Size and Weight," February 2014, www.iihs.org/iihs/topics/t/vehicle-size-and-weight/qanda.

71. Insurance Institute for Highway Safety, "Motorcycles Helmet Use," August 2017, http://www.iihs.org/iihs/topics/laws/helmetuse/mapmotorcyclehelmets; Insurance Institute for Highway Safety. Motorcycles and ATVs," November 2016, http://www.iihs.org/iihs/topics/t/motorcycles/fatalityfacts/motorcyclesTraf.

72. Ibid.

73. National Highway Traffic Safety Administration, "Aggressive Driving," www.nhtsa.gov/Aggressive.

74. National Highway Traffic Safety Administration, "Traffic Safety Facts: 2015 Data," May 2017.

75. National Highway Traffic Safety Administration, "Quick Facts—2015," May 2017, https://crashstats.nhtsa.dot.gov/Api/Public/ViewPublication/812348.

76. Insurance Institute for Highway Safety, "Pedestrians and Bicyclists," February 2016, http://www.iihs.org/iihs/topics/t/pedestrians-and-bicyclists/fatalityfacts/bicycles.

77. Centers for Disease Control and Prevention, "10 Leading Causes of Injury Deaths by Age Group Highlighting Unintentional Injury Deaths, United States, 2014," February 25, 2016, Available at www.cdc.gov/injury/wisqars/leadingcauses.html.

78. Centers for Disease Control and Prevention, "10 Leading Causes of Injury Deaths by Age Group Highlighting Unintentional Injury Deaths, United States, 2014," February 25, 2016, Available at www.cdc.gov/injury/wisqars/leadingcauses.html; Centers for Disease Control and Prevention, "Unintentional Drowning: Get the Facts," April 28, 2016, www.cdc.gov/HomeandRecreationalSafety/Water-Safety/waterinjuries-factsheet.html.

79. Centers for Disease Control and Prevention, "Unintentional Drowning: Get the Facts," April 28, 2016, www.cdc.gov/HomeandRecreationalSafety/Water-Safety/waterinjuries-factsheet.html.

80. Ibid.

81. U.S. Coast Guard, "Coast Guard News: U.S. Coast Guard Releases 2013 Recreational Boating Statistics Report," May 2014, http://coastguardnews.com/u-s-coast-guard-releases-2013-recreational-boating-statistics-report/2014/05/14/?utm_source=feedburner&utm_medium=feed&utm_campaign=Feed%3A+CoastGuardNews+(Coast+Guard+News).

82. Ibid.

83. Ibid.

84. U.S. Coast Guard, "Boating Safety Resource Center: Boating under the Influence Initiatives," April 2014, www.uscgboating.org/safety/boating_under_the_influence_initiatives.aspx.

85. American Boating Association, "Boating Safety—It Could Mean Your Life," 2013, www.americanboating.org/safety.asp.

86. H. Hoffman et al. "Declining Prevalence of Hearing Loss in U.S. Adults Aged 20–69 Years," *JAMA Otolaryngology–Head and Neck Surgery*, 143, no. 3 (2017): 274–85.

87. Ibid.

88. L. Clercq et al. "Music-Induced Hearing Loss in Children, Adolescents and Young Adults," *Otology and Neurotology*, 37, no. 9 (2016): 1208–16;.K. Hannah et al., "Evaluation of the Olivocochlear Efferent Reflex Strength in the Susceptibility to Temporary Hearing Deterioration after Music Exposure in Young Adults," *Noise Health* 16, no. 69 (2014): 108–15, doi:10.4103/1463-1741.132094.

89. National Institute on Deafness and Other Communication Disorders, "Noise-Induced Hearing Loss," February 7, 2017, https://www.nidcd.nih.gov/health/noise-induced-hearing-loss.

90. J.B. Mowry et al., "2015 Annual Report of the American Association of Poison Control Centers' National Poison Data System (NPDS): 33nd Annual Report," *Clinical Toxicology* 54, no. 10 (2016): 924-1109, Available at https://aapcc.s3.amazonaws.com/pdfs/annual_reports/2015_AAPCC_NPDS_Annual_Report_33rd_PDF.pdf.

91. American Association of Poison Control Centers, "Prevention," February 2015, www.aapcc.org/prevention.

92. Centers for Disease Control and Prevention, "10 Leading Causes of Injury Deaths by Age Group Highlighting Unintentional Injury Deaths, United States, 2014," February 25, 2016, Available at www.cdc.gov/injury/wisqars/leadingcauses.html.

93. Centers for Disease Control and Prevention, "Important Facts about Falls," January 20, 2016, www.cdc.gov/homeandrecreationalsafety/falls/adultfalls.html.

94. U.S. Fire Administration, "U.S. Fire Deaths, Fire Death Rates, and Risks of Dying in a Fire," Accessed March 2017, www.usfa.fema.gov/data/statistics/fire_death_rates.html.

95. U.S. Fire Administration, "Campus Fire Fatalities in Residential Buildings (2000–2015)," November 2015, https://www.usfa.fema.gov/downloads/pdf/publications/campus_fire_fatalities_report.pdf.

96. Ibid.

97. U.S. Bureau of Labor Statistics, "Table 3: Fatal Occupational Injury Counts and Rates for Selected Occupations—2015," November 2016, https://www.bls.gov/news.release/cfoi.nr0.htm.

98. National Institute of Neurological Disorders and Stroke, "Low Back Pain Fact Sheet," April 2014, www.ninds.nih.gov/disorders/backpain/detail_backpain.htm.

99. American College Health Association, *American College Health Association—National College Health Assessment II: Reference Group Executive Summary, Fall, 2016,* (Hanover, MD: American College Health Association, 2017), Available at: www.acha-ncha.org/reports_ACHA-NCHAII.html.

100. Mayo Clinic, "Carpal Tunnel Syndrome: Prevention," 2014, www.mayoclinic.org/diseases-conditions/carpal-tunnel-syndrome/basics/prevention/con-20030332.

Chapter 14

1. World Wildlife Fund, "Living Planet Report," Accessed June 2017, http://wwf.panda.org/about_our_earth/all_publications/lpr_2016.

2. U.N. Department of Economic and Social Affairs, "World Population Projected to Reach 9.8 Billion in 2050, and 11.2 Billion in 2100," June 21, 2017, https://www.un.org/development/desa/en/news/population/world-population-prospects-2017.html; Worldwatch Institute, "As Global Population Surpasses 7 Billion, Two Clear Strategies for a Sustainable Future," July 20, 2017, http://www.worldwatch.org/global-population-surpasses-7-billion-two-clear-strategies-sustainable-future.

3. U.N. Department of Economic and Social Affairs, "World Population Projected to Reach 9.8 Billion in 2050, and 11.2 Billion in 2100," June 21, 2017, https://www.un.org/development/desa/en/news/population/world-population-prospects-2017.html.

4. U.N. Environmental Programme, "Rate of Environmental Damage Increasing across the Planet but There Is Still Time to Reverse Worst Impacts If Governments Act Now, UNEP Assessment Says," May 19, 2016, www.unep.org/newscentre/Default.aspx?DocumentID=27074 & ArticleID=36180 & l=en.

5. Central Intelligence Agency, *The World Factbook: Country Comparison: Total Fertility Rate,* Accessed June 2016, https://www.cia.gov/library/publications/the-world-factbook/rankorder/2127rank.html.

6. U.N. Department of Economic and Social Affairs, "World Population Projected to Reach 9.8 Billion in 2050, and 11.2 Billion in 2100," June 21, 2017, https://www.un.org/development/desa/en/news/population/world-population-prospects-2017.html.

7. Ibid.

8. U.S. Census Bureau, "U.S. and World Population Clock," June 28, 2017, http://www.census.gov/popclock.

9. World Wildlife Fund, "Living Planet Report," Accessed June 2017, http://wwf.panda.org/about_our_earth/all_publications/lpr_2016; Global Footprint Network, "Key Findings of the National Footprint Accounts, 2016 Edition," June 8, 2016, http://www.footprintnetwork.org/en/index.php/GFN/page/footprint_data_and_results.

10. World Wildlife Fund, "Living Planet Report," Accessed June 2017, http://wwf.panda.org/about_our_earth/all_publications/lpr_2016.

11. United Nations, "UNEP Annual Report 2016," Accessed June 2017, http://www.unep.org/annualreport/2016/index.php?page=0 & lang=en.

12. G. Ceballos et al., "Accelerated Modern Human-induced Species Losses: Entering the Sixth Mass Extinction," *Science Advances* 1, no. 5 (2015): e1400253, doi:10.1126/sciadv.1400253.

13. The IUCN Red List of Threatened Species, "IUCN Red List Status: Mammals," July 2017, www

.iucnredlist.org/initiatives/mammals/analysis/red-list-status.

14. World Wildlife Fund, "Living Planet Report," Accessed June 2017, http://wwf.panda.org/about_our_earth/all_publications/lpr_2016.

15. The IUCN Red List of Threatened Species, "IUCN Red List Status: Amphibians," 2017.

16. United Nations, *Global Environment Outlook*," Accessed July, 2016, http://www.unep.org/geo.

17. United Nations, "UNEP Frontiers: 2016 Report: Emerging Issues of Environmental Concern," Accessed July 2017, http://www.unep.org/frontiers/sites/unep.org.frontiers/files/documents/unep_frontiers_2016.pdf.

18. Ibid.

19. C. Golden et al., "Fall in Fish Catch Threatens Human Health," *Nature* 534, no. 7607 (2016): 317–20; V. Christenson et al., "A Century of Fish Biomass Decline in the Ocean," *Marine Ecology Program Series* 512 (2014): 155–66, doi:10.3354/meps10946.

20. World Wildlife Fund, "Living Planet Report," Accessed June 2017, http://wwf.panda.org/about_our_earth/all_publications/lpr_2016; U.S. Department of Agriculture, "Overview: Agricultural Water Use," April 18, 2017, https://www.ers.usda.gov/topics/farm-practices-management/irrigation-water-use.aspx.

21. World Wildlife Fund, "Living Planet Report," 2016, Accessed June 2017, http://wwf.panda.org/about_our_earth/all_publications/lpr_2016; U.S. Department of Agriculture. "Overview: Agricultural Water Use," April 18, 2017. https://www.ers.usda.gov/topics/farm-practices-management/irrigation-water-use.aspx; U.S. Environmental Protection Agency, "Case Study Analysis of the Impacts of Water Acquisition for Hydraulic Fracturing on Local Water Availability," May 2015, Available at https://www.epa.gov/sites/production/files/2015-07/documents/hf_water_acquisition_report_final_6-3-15_508_km.pdf.

22. U.S. Energy Information Administration, "Independent Statistics and Analysis," July 2017, www.eia.gov.

23. J.P. Deaton , "Who Consumes the Most Fossil Fuels per Capita?," August 29, 2012, auto.howstuffworks.com/fuel-efficiency/fuel-consumption/consumes-most-fossil-fuel.htm.

24. U.S. Environmental Protection Agency, "Overview of Greenhouse Gases: Carbon Dioxide Emissions," April 2017, https://www3.epa.gov/climatechange/ghgemissions/gases/co2.html.

25. Ibid.

26. American Lung Association, "State of the Air—2017," Accessed July 2017, http://www.lung.org/assets/documents/healthy-air/state-of-the-air/state-of-the-air-2017.pdf.

27. American Lung Association, "State of the Air—2017," Accessed July 2017, http://www.lung.org/assets/documents/healthy-air/state-of-the-air/state-of-the-air-2017.pdf; American Lung Association, "Health Effects of Ozone and Particle Pollution," 2014, www.stateoftheair.org/2014/health-risks.

28. U.S. Environmental Protection Agency, "Acid Rain: Effects of Acid Rain—Surface Waters and Aquatic Animals," Updated December 2012, www.epa.gov/acidrain/effects/surface_water.html.

29. Ibid.

30. U.S. Environmental Protection Agency, "Effects of Acid Rain," July 2017. https://www.epa.gov/acidrain/effects-acid-rain

31. U.S. Environmental Protection Agency, "Overview of Greenhouse Gases: Emissions and Trends: Carbon Dioxide," Accessed July 2017; National

Aeronautics and Space Administration, "Ozone Hole Watch," July 2016, http://ozonewatch.gsfc.nasa.gov.

32. U.S. Environmental Protection Agency, "An Introduction to Indoor Air Quality," January 27, 2017, https://www.epa.gov/indoor-air-quality-iaq/introduction-indoor-air-quality.

33. Ibid.

34. U.S. Environmental Protection Agency, "Health Effects of Exposure to Secondhand Smoke," Updated November 2011, www.epa.gov/smokefree/healtheffects.html; American Cancer Society, "Secondhand Smoke," Revised February 2014. www.cancer.org/cancer/cancercauses/tobaccocancer/secondhand-smoke.

35. U.S. Environmental Protection Agency, "Indoor Air Quality," Updated July 11, 2017. https://www.epa.gov/indoor-air-quality-iaq

36. U.S. Environmental Protection Agency, "Health Risks of Radon," April, 2017, https://www.epa.gov/radon/health-risk-radon.

37. U.S. Environmental Protection Agency, "Ground Water and Drinking Water: Basic Information about Lead in Drinking Water," August 2017, https://www.epa.gov/ground-water-and-drinking-water/basic-information-about-lead-drinking-water.

38. Environmental Illness Resources, "Sick Building Syndrome (SBS)," September 1, 2017, http://www.ei-resource.org/illness-information/related-conditions/sick-building-syndrome.

39. T. Stafford, "A School Input That Matters: Indoor Air Quality and Academic Performance," University of New South Wales, Australian School of Business, School of Economics, 2012; Z. Bako-Biro et al., "Ventilation Rates in Schools and Pupil's Performance," *Building and Environment* 48, no. 1 (2012): 215–23.

40. U.S. Environmental Protection Agency, "IAQ Tools for Schools: Improved Academic Performance: Evidence from Scientific Literature," Updated January 2013, www.epa.gov/iaq/schools/student_performance/evidence.html.

41. U.S. Environmental Protection Agency, "Indoor Air Quality," Updated July 11, 2017. https://www.epa.gov/indoor-air-quality-iaq?

42. American Association for the Advancement of Science, "What We Know: The Reality, Risks, and Response to Climate Change," Accessed July 2017, Available at http://whatweknow.aaas.org/wp-content/uploads/2014/07/whatweknow_website.pdf; J. Cook et al., "Consensus on Consensus: A Synthesis of Consensus Estimates on Human-caused Global Warming," *Environmental Research Letters* 11, no. 4 (2016): 048002.

43. U.S. Global Research Program, "Understand Climate Change," Accessed July 2017, http://www.globalchange.gov/climate-change; American Association for the Advancement of Science, "What We Know: The Reality, Risks, and Response to Climate Change," Accessed July 2017, Available at http://whatweknow.aaas.org/wp-content/uploads/2014/07/whatweknow_website.pdf; J. Cook et al., "Consensus on Consensus: A Synthesis of Consensus Estimates on Human-caused Global Warming," *Environmental Research Letters* 11, no. 4 (2016): 048002.

44. A. Crimmins, and the U.S. Global Change Research Group, "The Impacts of Climate Change on Human Health in the United States: A Scientific Assessment," June 2016, https://health2016.globalchange.gov/downloads; National Aeronautics and Space Administration, "Climate Change: How Do We Know?," Accessed July 2016, http://climate.nasa.gov/evidence; U.S. Global Change Research Program, "The

Impacts of Climate Change on Human Health in the United States: A Scientific Assessment," April 2016, https://health2016.globalchange.gov.

45. U.S. Environmental Protection Agency, "Climate Change Facts: Answers to Common Questions," February 2016, https://www3.epa.gov/climatechange/basics/facts.html; National Academy of Sciences, "Attribution of Extreme Weather Events in the Context of Climate Change," 2016, https://nas-sites.org/americasclimatechoices/other-reports-on-climate-change/2016-2/attribution-of-extreme-weather-events-in-the-context-of-climate-change.

46. J. Olivier et al., "Trends in Global CO2 Emissions: 2016 Report," PBL Netherlands Environmental Assessment Agency, 2016, http://www.pbl.nl/sites/default/files/cms/publicaties/pbl-2016-trends-in-global-co2-emissions-2016-report.

47. National Aeronautics and Space Administration, "NASA, NOAA Data Show 2016 Warmest Year on Record Globally," January 18, 2017, https://www.nasa.gov/press-release/nasa-noaa-data-show-2016-warmest-year-on-record-globally; U.S. Environmental Protection Agency, "Climate Change Facts: Answers to Common Questions," 2016; J. Olivier et al., "Trends in Global CO2 Emissions: 2016 Report," PBL Netherlands Environmental Assessment Agency, 2016, http://www.pbl.nl/sites/default/files/cms/publicaties/pbl-2016-trends-in-global-co2-emissions-2016-report; National Aeronautics and Space Administration, "Global Climate Change: A Blanket around the Earth," Accessed July 2017, http://climate.nasa.gov/causes; National Oceanic and Atmospheric Administration, "Greenhouse Gases," Accessed July 2017, https://www.ncdc.noaa.gov/monitoring-references/faq/greenhouse-gases.php.

48. J. Cook et al., "Consensus on Consensus: A Synthesis of Consensus Estimates on Human-caused Global Warming," *Environmental Research Letters* 11, no. 4 (2016): 048002; National Aeronautics and Space Administration, "Global Climate Change: A Blanket around the Earth," Accessed July 2017, http://climate.nasa.gov/causes.

49. J. Cook et al., "Consensus on Consensus: A Synthesis of Consensus Estimates on Human-caused Global Warming," *Environmental Research Letters* 11, no. 4 (2016): 048002; National Aeronautics and Space Administration, "Global Climate Change: A Blanket around the Earth," Accessed July 2017, http://climate.nasa.gov/causes; J. Olivier et al., "Trends in Global CO2 Emissions: 2016 Report," PBL Netherlands Environmental Assessment Agency, 2016, http://www.pbl.nl/sites/default/files/cms/publicaties/pbl-2016-trends-in-global-co2-emissions-2016-report.

50 J. Cook et al., "Consensus on Consensus: A Synthesis of Consensus Estimates on Human-caused Global Warming," *Environmental Research Letters* 11, no. 4 (2016): 048002; National Aeronautics and Space Administration, "Global Climate Change: A Blanket around the Earth," Accessed July 2017, http://climate.nasa.gov/causes; J. Olivier et al., "Trends in Global CO2 Emissions: 2016 Report," PBL Netherlands Environmental Assessment Agency, 2016, http://www.pbl.nl/sites/default/files/cms/publicaties/pbl-2016-trends-in-global-co2-emissions-2016-report; U.S. Environmental Protection Agency, " Inventory of U.S. Greenhouse Gas Emissions and Sinks: 1990-2015," 2017, https://www.epa.gov/sites/production/files/2017-02/documents/2017_complete_report.pdf.

51. R. Scheen and D. Moss. "Deforestation and Its Extreme Effect on Global Warming." *Scientific American*. Accessed October, 2017. https://www.scientificamerican.com/article/deforestation-and-global-warming/; Environmental Protection Agency. "Sources of Greenhouse Gas Emissions." April, 2017. https://www.epa.gov/ghgemissions/sources-greenhouse-gas-emissions Ibid.

52. United Nations, "Sustainable Development Goals: 17 Goals to Transform our World," Accessed June 2017, http://www.un.org/sustainabledevelopment.

53. D. Vine, "Achieving the United States' Intended National Determined Contributions," Center for Climate and Energy Solutions, April 2016, http://www.c2es.org/docUploads/achieving-us-indc.pdf.

54. Ibid.

55. Environmental Defense Fund, "Cap and Trade—How Cap and Trade Works, Accessed July 2017, www.edf.org/climate/how-cap-and-trade-works.

56. Ibid.

57. Water Information Program, "Water Facts," Accessed July 2017, www.waterinfo.org/resources/water-facts.

58. Ibid.

59. Ibid.

60. Ibid.

61. Milken Institute Global Conference, "Solving the Global Water Challenge," May 3, 2016, http://www.milkeninstitute.org/events/conferences/global-conference/2016/panel-detail/6175; Water Information Program, "Water Facts," Accessed July 2017, www.waterinfo.org/resources/water-facts.

62. M. Kostich et al., "Concentrations of Prioritized Pharmaceuticals in Effluents from 50 Large Wastewater Treatment Plants in the U.S. and Implications for Risk Estimation," *Environmental Pollution* 184 (2014): 354–59.

63. J. Donn et al., "Pharmaceuticals Found in Drinking Water, Affecting Wildlife and Maybe Humans," *Associated Press*, Accessed July 2016, http://hosted.ap.org/specials/interactives/pharmawater_site/day1_01.html.

64. U.S. Environmental Protection Agency. "Drinking Water Contaminants: Standards and Regulations," May 2017, https://www.epa.gov/dwstandardsregulations; U.S. Geological Survey, "Contaminants Found in Ground Water," December 2016, https://water.usgs.gov/edu/earthgwquality.html; U.S. Environmental Protection Agency, "Assessment of the Potential Impacts of Hydraulic Fracturing for Oil and Gas on Drinking Water Resources" (External Review Draft), EPA/600/R-15/047, June 4, 2015, https://cfpub.epa.gov/si/si_public_record_report.cfm?dirEntryID=244651.

65. U.S. Environmental Protection Agency, "Drinking Water Contaminants- Standards and Regulations," May 2017, https://www.epa.gov/dwstandardsregulations; U.S. Geological Survey, "Contaminants Found in Ground Water," December 2016, https://water.usgs.gov/edu/earthgwquality.html; U.S. Environmental Protection Agency, "Assessment of the Potential Impacts of Hydraulic Fracturing for Oil and Gas on Drinking Water Resources" (External Review Draft), EPA/600/R-15/047, June 4, 2015, https://cfpub.epa.gov/si/si_public_record_report.cfm?dirEntryID=244651.

66. U.S. Environmental Protection Agency, "Advancing Sustainable Materials Management 2014. Fact Sheet: Assessing Trends in Material Generation, Recycling, Composting, Combustion with Energy Recovery and Landfilling in the United States," November 2016, https://www.epa.gov/sites/production/files/2016-11/documents/2014_smmfactsheet_508.pdf.

67. Ibid.

68. Ibid.

69. U. S. Environmental Protection Agency, "Basic Information about Electronics Stewardship." April 26, 2016, https://www.epa.gov/smm-electronics/basic-information-about-electronics-stewardship#01; National Cancer Institute, "Factsheet: Cell Phones and Cancer Risk," May 27, 2016, www.cancer.gov/cancertopics/factsheet/Risk/cellphones; American Cancer Society, "Cell Phones," Accessed June 2017, https://www.cancer.org/cancer/cancer-causes/radiation-exposure/cellular-phones.html.

70. U.S. Environmental Protection Agency, "Hazardous Waste," May 2016. www.epa.gov/osw/basic-hazard.htm; U.S. Environmental Protection Agency, "Household Hazardous Waste," April 2016, http://www.epa.gov/osw/conserve/materials/hhw.htm.

71. U.S. Environmental Protection Agency, "Superfund: Superfund National Accomplishments Summary, Fiscal Year 2016 May 2017, https://www.epa.gov/superfund/superfund-remedial-annual-accomplishments; U. S. Environmental Protection Agency , "Superfund National Priorities List (NPL) Sites by State," July 2017, https://www.epa.gov/superfund/superfund-national-priorities-list-npl.

72. U.S. Environmental Protection Agency, "Basic Information about Electronics Stewardship." April 26, 2016, https://www.epa.gov/smm-electronics/basic-information-about-electronics-stewardship#01; National Cancer Institute, "Factsheet: Cell Phones and Cancer Risk," May 27, 2016, www.cancer.gov/cancertopics/factsheet/Risk/cellphones; American Cancer Society, "Cell Phones," Accessed June 2017, https://www.cancer.org/cancer/cancer-causes/radiation-exposure/cellular-phones.html; National Cancer Institute, "Factsheet: Cell Phones and Cancer Risk," Accessed June 2014, www.cancer.gov; M.P. Little et al., "Mobile Phone Use and Glioma Risk: Comparison of Epidemiological Study Results with Incidence Trends in the United States," *British Medical Journal* 344 (2012): e1147, doi:10.1136/bmj.e1147; D. Aydin et al., "Mobile Phone Use and Brain Tumors in Children and Adolescents: A Multicenter Case-control study," *Journal of the National Cancer Institute* 103, no. 16 (2011): 1264–76, doi:10.1093/jnci/djr244.

73. U.S. Nuclear Regulatory Commission, "Radiation Basics," 2014, www.nrc.gov/about-nrc/radiation/health-effects/radiation-basics.html.

74. Ibid.

75. World Nuclear Association, "Fukushima Accident," April 2017, http://www.world-nuclear.org/information-library/safety-and-security/safety-of-plants/fukushima-accident.aspx.

76. International Atomic Energy Agency, "Climate Change and Nuclear Power 2016," September 2016, http://www-pub.iaea.org/MTCD/Publications/PDF/CCANP16web-86692468.pdf.

77. Thich Nhat Hanh, "The World We Have," *Lion's Roar: Buddhist Wisdom for Our Time*, April 6, 2017, https://www.lionsroar.com/the-world-we-have.

78. U.S. Environmental Protection Agency , "Basic Information about Electronics Stewardship." April 26, 2016, https://www.epa.gov/smm-electronics/basic-information-about-electronics-stewardship#01; National Cancer Institute, Factsheet, "Cell Phones and Cancer Risk," May 27, 2016, www.cancer.gov/cancertopics/factsheet/Risk/cellphones; American Cancer Society, "Cell Phones," Accessed June 2017, https://www.cancer.org/cancer/cancer-causes/radiation-exposure/cellular-phones.html.

Chapter 15

1. G.L. Petersen et al., "The Magnitude of Nocebo Effects in Pain: A Meta-Analysis," *Pain* 155, no. 8 (2014), 1426–34, doi:10.1016/j.pain.2014.04.016; L. Colloca and C. Grillon, "Understanding Placebo and Nocebo Responses for Pain Management," *Current Pain and Headache Reports* 18, no. 6 (2014): 419, doi:10.1007/s11916-014-0419-2.

2. A. Keitel et al., "Expectation Modulates the Effect of Deep Brain Stimulation on Motor and Cognitive Function in Tremor-dominant Parkinson's Disease," *PLOS ONE* 8, no. 12 (2013): e81878, doi:10.1371/journal.pone.0081878.

3. T. Bschor and L.L. Kilarski, "Are Antidepressants Effective? A Debate on Their Efficacy for the Treatment of Major Depression in Adults," *Expert Review of Neurotherapeutics* 16, no. 4 (2016): 367–74; J. Sarris et al., "St John's Wort (Hypericum Perforatum) versus Sertraline and Placebo in Major Depressive Disorder: Continuation Data from a 26-Week RCT," *Pharmacopsychiatry* 45, no. 7 (2012): 275–8, doi:10.1055/s-0032-1306348; R.A. Litten et al., "The Placebo Effect in Clinical Trials for Alcohol Dependence: An Exploratory Analysis of 51 Naltrexone and Acamprosate Studies," *Alcoholism, Clinical and Experimental Research* 37, no. 12 (2013): 2128–37, doi:10.1111/acer.12197; G.L. Petersen et al., "The Magnitude of Nocebo Effects in Pain: A Meta-Analysis," *Pain* 155, no. 8 (2014), 1426–34, doi:10.1016/j.pain.2014.04.016.

4. M.A. Hillen et al., " How Can Communication by Oncologists Enhance Patients' Trust? An Experimental Study," *Annals of Oncology* 25, no. 4 (2014): 896–901.

5. M. Paik et al., "Damage Caps and Defensive Medicine, Revisited," *Journal of Health Economics* 51 (2017): 84–97.

6. U.S. National Library of Medicine, "Patient's Rights," *Medline Plus* July 2017, https://medlineplus.gov/patientrights.html.

7. Centers for Disease Control and Prevention, "Therapeutic Drug Use," January 19, 2017, www.cdc.gov/nchs/fastats/drug-use-therapeutic.htm.

8. Ibid.

9. U.S. Department of Health and Human Services, "Facts about Generic Drugs," June 28, 2016, https://www.fda.gov/Drugs/ResourcesForYou/Consumers/BuyingUsingMedicineSafely/UnderstandingGenericDrugs/ucm167991.htm.

10. U.S. Food and Drug Administration, "The Possible Dangers of Buying Medicine over the Internet," May 2017, https://www.fda.gov/ForConsumers/ConsumerUpdates/ucm048396.htm.

11. National Center for Complementary and Integrative Health, "Complementary, Alternative, or Integrative Health: What's in a Name?," June 2016, https://nccih.nih.gov/health/integrative-health#types.

12. Ibid.

13. Ibid.

14. Ibid.

15. T.C. Clarke et al., "Trends in the Use of Complementary Health Approaches among Adults: United States, 2002–2012," *National Health Statistics Reports*, no. 79 (Hyattsville, MD: National Center for Health Statistics), February 2015, Available at www.cdc.gov/nchs/data/nhsr/nhsr079.pdf.

16. Ibid.

17. J.E. Stahl et al., "Relaxation Response and Resiliency Training and Its Effect on Healthcare Resource Utilization," *PLOS ONE* 10, no. 10 (2015): e0140212; M.D. Klatt et al., "A Healthcare Utilization Cost Comparison between Employees Receiving a Worksite Mindfulness or a Diet/Exercise Lifestyle Intervention to Matched Controls 5 Years post Intervention," *Complementary Therapies in Medicine* 27 (2016): 139–144.

18. J.E. Stahl et al., "Relaxation Response and Resiliency Training and Its Effect on Healthcare Resource Utilization," *PLOS ONE* 10, no. 10 (2015): e0140212.

19. National Center for Complementary and Integrative Health, "Traditional Chinese Medicine: In Depth," March 2017, https://nccih.nih.gov/health/whatiscam/chinesemed.htm.

20. National Center for Complementary and Integrative Health, "Traditional Chinese Medicine: In Depth," March 2017, https://nccih.nih.gov/health/whatiscam/chinesemed.htm; U.S. Food and Drug Administration, "Information for Consumers on Using Dietary Supplements," July 2016, https://www.fda.gov/Food/DietarySupplements/UsingDietarySupplements/default.htm.

21. National Center for Complementary and Integrative Health, "Ayurvedic Medicine: In Depth," April 2016, http://nccih.nih.gov/health/ayurveda/introduction.htm.

22. Ibid.

23. Ibid.

24. National Center for Complementary and Integrative Health, "Homeopathy," April 2016, http://nccih.nih.gov/health/homeopathy.

25. Ibid.

26. National Center for Complementary and Integrative Health, "Naturopathy," February 2016, https://nccih.nih.gov/health/naturopathy.

27. Ibid.

28. National Center for Complementary and Integrative Health, "Complementary, Alternative, or Integrative Health: What's in a Name?," June 2016, www.nccih.nih.gov/health/integrative-health.

29. American Chiropractic Association, "Facts about Chiropractic," Accessed May 2017, http://www.acatoday.org/News-Publications/News/Facts-About-Chiropractic.

30. National Center for Complementary and Integrative Health, "Spinal Manipulation," April 2016, https://nccih.nih.gov/health/spinalmanipulation; N. Paige et al., "Association of Spinal Manipulative Therapy with Clinical Benefit and Harm for Acute Low Back Pain: Systematic Review and Meta-analysis. *JAMA* 317, no. 14 (2017): 1451–60.doi:10.1001/jama.2017.308.

31. American Chiropractic Association, "Facts about Chiropractic," Accessed May 2017, http://www.acatoday.org/News-Publications/News/Facts-About-Chiropractic.

32. National Center for Complementary and Integrative Health, "Massage Therapy for Health Purposes," March 2017, https://nccih.nih.gov/health/massage/massageintroduction.htm.

33. Ibid.

34. Ibid.

35. Bureau of Labor Statistics, U.S. Department of Labor, "Massage Therapists," *Occupational Outlook Handbook*, 2016–2017 Edition, June 2017, http://www.bls.gov/ooh/healthcare/massage-therapists.htm.

36. National Center for Complementary and Integrative Health, "Acupuncture: In Depth," February 2017, https://nccih.nih.gov/health/acupuncture/introduction.

37. K. Linde et al., "Acupuncture for the Prevention of Tension-Type Headache," *Cochrane Database of Systematic Reviews* 48 (2016): CD007587.

38. C. Lowe et al., "Sham Acupuncture Is as Efficacious as True Acupuncture for the Treatment of IBS: A Randomized Placebo Controlled Trial," *Neurogastroenterology and Motility* 29, no. 7 (2017): e13040, doi:10.1111/nmo.13040.

39. R.L. Nahin et al., "Evidence-based Evaluation of Complementary Health Approaches for Pain Management in the United States," *Mayo Clinic Proceedings* 91, no. 9 (2016): 1292–1306.

40. National Center for Complementary and Integrative Health, "Acupuncture: In Depth," February 2017, https://nccih.nih.gov/health/acupuncture/introduction#hed2.

41. G.A. Kelley and K.S. Kelley, "Meditative Movement Therapies and Health-Related Quality-of-Life in Adults: A Systematic Review of Meta-Analyses," *PLoS ONE* 10, no. 6 (2015): e0129181, doi:10.1371/journal.pone.0129181.

42. S. Jain et al., "Clinical Studies of Biofield Therapies: Summary, Methodological Challenges, and Recommendations," *Global Advances in Health and Medicine* 4, suppl. (2015): 58–66; R. Hammerschlag et al., "Nontouch Biofield Therapy: A Systematic Review of Human Randomized Controlled Trials Reporting Use of Only Nonphysical Contact Treatment," *Journal of Alternative and Complementary Medicine* 20, no. 12 (2014): 881–92, doi:10.1089/acm.2014.0017.

43. M. Goretski and A. Zysk, "Using Mindfulness Techniques to Improve Student Wellbeing and Academic Performance for University Students: A Pilot Study." *Journal of Australian and New Zealand Student Services Association* 49, April (2017), http://isana.proceedings.com.au/docs/2014/paper_goretzki.pdf; D. Laneri et al., "Effects of Long-term Mindfulness Meditation on Brain's White Matter Microstructure and Its Aging," *Frontiers in Aging Neuroscience* 7 (2015); T. Ireland, "What Does Mindfulness Meditation Do to Your Brain?" *Scientific American*, June 12, 2014, https://blogs.scientificamerican.com/guest-blog/what-does-mindfulness-meditation-do-to-your-brain; H.H. Ching et al., "Effects of a Mindfulness Meditation Course on Learning and Cognitive Performance among University Students in Taiwan," *Evidence-Based Complementary and Alternative Medicine*, 2015 (2015): 254358; M.D. Mrazek et al., "Mindfulness Training Improves Working Memory Capacity and GRE Performance While Reducing Mind Wandering," *Psychological Science* 24, no. 5 (2013): 776–81; J.T. Ramsburg and R.J. Youmans, "Meditation in the Higher-education Classroom: Meditation Training Improves Student Knowledge Retention during Lectures," *Mindfulness* 5, no. 4 (2014): 431–41.

44. Ibid.

45. U.S. Food and Drug Administration, "'Natural' on Food Labeling," September 2016, www.fda.gov/Food/GuidanceRegulation/GuidanceDocumentsRegulatoryInformation/LabelingNutrition/ucm456090.htm.

46. U.S. Pharmacopoeial Convention, "USP-Verified Dietary Supplements," Accessed May 2017, http://www.uspverified.org/.

47. National Center for Complementary and Integrative Health, "Alerts and Advisories, 2017," Accessed May 2017, https://nccih.nih.gov/news/alerts.

48. National Center for Complementary and Integrative Health, "Using Dietary Supplements Wisely," June 2016, https://nccih.nih.gov/health/supplements/wiseuse.htm.

49. U.S. National Library of Medicine, "Managed Care," *MedlinePlus*, January 2016, https://www.nlm.nih.gov/medlineplus/managedcare.html.

50. U.S. Centers for Medicare and Medicaid Services, "National Health Expenditure Projections 2014–2024," July 2015, www.cms.gov/Research-Statistics-Data-and-Systems/Statistics-Trends-and-Reports/NationalHealthExpendData/Downloads/Proj2014.pdf.

51. National Committee to Preserve Social Security and Medicare, "Fast Facts about Medicare," February 2017, www.ncpssm.org/Medicare.

52. Centers for Medicare and Medicaid Services, "NHE Fact Sheet," March 21, 2017, https://www.cms.gov/research-statistics-data-and-systems/statistics-trends-and-reports/nationalhealthexpenddata/nhe-fact-sheet.html.

53. Henry J. Kaiser Family Foundation, "Medicaid in the United States," January 2017, http://files.kff.org/attachment/fact-sheet-medicaid-state-US.

54. U.S. Department of Health & Human Services, "2016 Poverty Guidelines," January 2016, https://aspe.hhs.gov/poverty-guidelines.

55. U.S. Department of Health & Human Services, "The Affordable Care Act Is Working," June 2015, http://www.hhs.gov/healthcare/facts-and-features/fact-sheets/aca-is-working/index.html.

56. Centers for Medicare and Medicaid Services, "Children's Health Insurance Program," July 2015, www.medicaid.gov/chip/chip-program-information.html.

57. National Conference of State Legislators, "Health Insurance: Premiums and Increases," January 2017, www.ncsl.org/issues-research/health/health-insurance-premiums.aspx.

58. National Center for Health Statistics, "Health Insurance Coverage: Estimates from the National Health Interview Survey, January–September 2016," February 2017, Available at https://www.cdc.gov/nchs/data/nhis/earlyrelease/insur201702.pdf.

59. Ibid.

60. Henry J. Kaiser Foundation, "State Health Facts: Totally Professionally Active Physicians," September 2016, http://kff.org/other/state-indicator/total-active-physicians/?currentTimeframe=0 & sortModel=%7B%22colId%22:%22Location%22,%22sort%22:%22asc%22%7D.

61. American Hospital Association, "Fast Facts on U.S. Hospitals," January 2017, www.aha.org/research/rc/stat-studies/fast-facts.shtml.

62. Centers for Medicare and Medicaid Services, "National Health Expenditure—Fact Sheet," March 2017.

63. Ibid.

64. U.S. Centers for Medicare and Medicaid Services, "The 80/20 Rule: How Insurers Spend Your Health Insurance Premiums," February 2013, https://www.cms.gov/CCIIO/Resources/Files/Downloads/mlr-report-02-15-2013.pdf.

65. L.S. Dafny, "Evaluating the Impact of Health Insurance Industry Consolidation: Learning from Experience," Commonwealth Fund, November 20, 2015, http://www.commonwealthfund.org/publications/issue-briefs/2015/nov/evaluating-insurance-industry-consolidation.

66. Ibid.

67. Central Intelligence Agency, "Country Comparison: Life Expectancy at Birth, 2016 Estimates," *The World Factbook*, April 2017, https://www.cia.gov/library/publications/the-world-factbook/rankorder/2102rank.html.

68. Ibid.

69. Central Intelligence Agency, "Country Comparison: Infant Mortality Rate, 2016 Estimates," *The World Factbook*, April 2017, https://www.cia.gov/library/publications/the-world-factbook/rankorder/2091rank.html.

70. U.S. Department of Health and Human Services, "The National Quality Strategy: Fact Sheet," January 2017, https://www.ahrq.gov/workingforquality/about/nqs-fact-sheets/fact-sheet.html.

Photo Credits

Chapter 1 1: Wavebreakmedia/Shutterstock; 2: Syda Productions/Shutterstock; 3: Michael Jung/Fotolia; 4: Grantly Lynch/UK Stock Images Ltd/Alamy Stock Photo; 4: Y Photo Studio/Shutterstock; 4: Webphotographeer/E+/Getty Images; 4: Stray_Cat/E+/Getty Images; 5: Brian A. Witkin/Shutterstock; 6: Shutterstock; 8: Tyler Olson/Shutterstock; 9: Tyler Olson/123RF; 10: Oliveromg/Shutterstock; 11: Maridav/123RF; 12: ML Harris/Iconica/Getty Images; 14: Manley099/E+/Getty Images; 15: Photographee.eu/Fotolia; 17: Jamie Grill/Blend Images/Brand X Pictures/Getty Images; 19: Fstop123/E+/Getty Images; 20: Shutterstock; 21: ESB Professional/Shutterstock

Chapter 2 25: Fat Camera/Getty Images; 27: Thinkstock/Stockbyte/Getty Images; 27: Terry Vine/Blend Images/Getty Images; 29: Stockbyte/Exactostock-1491/SuperStock; 30: Pascal Broze/Totem/AGE Fotostock; 31: WENN Ltd/Alamy Stock Photo; 32: Laszlo/Fotolia; 34: Chris Ammann/Baltimore Examiner/AP Images; 35: Espies/Shutterstock; 35: Neal & Molly Jansen/Superstock; 36: KN Studio/Shutterstock; 39: Johnaudrey/iStock/Getty Images; 40: Stock-Asso/Shutterstock; 42: Chris Rout/Alamy Stock Photo; 43: LTA WENN Photos/Newscom; 44: Simon Rawley/Alamy Stock Photo

Chapter 3 49: Lechatnoir/E+/Getty Images; 50: Wang Tom/123RF; 51: Pendygraft, John/St. Petersburg Times/PSG/Newscom; 51: Ariel Skelley/Blend Images/Getty Images; 51: Zwiebackesser/Shutterstock; 53: Oliver Furrer/Alamy Stock Photo; 54: Netris/iStock/Getty Images; 55: Nycshooter/iStock/Getty Images; 56: Elliott Kaufman/Corbis/Getty Images; 56: Radius Images/Getty Images; 58: Andrew S/Shutrrestock; 58: Masterchief Productions/Shutterstock; 58: Orhan Cam/Shutterstock; 58: JamieB/RooM the Agency/Alamy Stock Photo; 58: 06photo/Shutterstock; 58: Wong Sze Yuen/123RF; 58: Simone van den Berg/Shutterstock; 58: Radius Images/Corbis; 59: Rawpixel/iStock/Getty Images; 60: Hero Images/Getty Images; 61: Kate_sept2004/iStock/Getty Images; 62: Pressmaster/Shutterstock; 63: Cathy Yeulet/123RF; 64: Pressmaster/Shutterstock; 65: Parema//Getty Images; 66: Dorling Kindersley, Ltd.; 67: Uniquely India/Getty Images; 68: Susan Montgomery/Fotolia; 69: Solomiya Malovana/Shuttersstock

Chapter 4 71: FatCamera/Getty images; 72: Jetta Productions/Blend Images/Getty Images; 74: Air Images/Shutterstock; 76: Onoky/Eric Audras/Brand X Pictures/Getty Images; 77: Jim Purdum/Blend Images/Getty Images; 78: Mangostock/Fotolia; 79: BJI/Blue Jean Images/Getty Images; 80: Abfotolv/Fotolia; 81: Wavebreakmedia/Shutterstock; 83: Ryan McVay/Photodisc/Getty Images; 84: John Dowland/PhotoAlto Agency RF Collections/Getty Images; 86: Echo/Juice Images/Getty Images; 87: Hannibal Hanschke/Newscom; 87: Photo Image Press/Newscom; 90: David J. Green/Lifestyle themes/Alamy Stock Photo; 92: Tom Merton/OJO Images/Getty Images; 93: HuntstocK/Brand X Pictures/Getty Images; 94: Frederic Cirou/PhotoAlto/Alamy Stock Photo; 95: BananaStock/Getty Images; 96: Allison Michael Orenstein/Photodisc/Getty Images

Chapter 5 99: Hero Images/Getty Images; 101: Keith Brofsky/Photodisc/Getty Images; 102: Garo/Phanie/Science Source; 102: Debi Treloar/Jules Selmes/Dorling Kindersley, Ltd.; 105: Eric Audras/PhotoAlto Agency RF Collections/Getty Images; 106: Tomasz Trojanowski/Fotolia; 107: Phanie/Science Source; 107: Foto-begsteiger/Vario images GmbH & Co.KG/Alamy Stock Photo; 108: Saturn Stills/Science Source; 109: Pearson Education, Inc.; 112: Image Source/Photodisc/Getty Images; 113: David J. Green/Lifestyle Themes/Alamy Stock Photo; 116: Helder Almeida/Fotolia; 117: Yuri Arcurs/Hemera/Getty Images; 119: KidStock/Blend Images/Getty Images; 120: Moncherie/iStock/Getty Images; 123: Plush Studios/Blend Images/Getty Images; 124: 3bugsmom/iStock/Getty Images

Chapter 6 127: 1MoreCreative/Getty images; 129: ZUMA Press, Inc./Alamy Stock Photo; 130: Milenko Bokan/iStock/Getty Images; 130: Jupiterimages/Getty Images; 131: Adam Brown/UpperCut Images/Alamy Stock Photo; 133: Darren Green/Shutterstock; 134: Thomas M Perkins/Shutterstock; 136: Charles Tatlock, DDS, MPH; 136: Jannoon028/Shutterstock; 137: JamesBrey/E+/Getty Images; 138: RayArt Graphics/Alamy Stock Photo; 139: Svyatoslav Lypynskyy/123RF; 140: Gregor Buir/Shutterstock; 141: ZUMA Press Inc /Alamy Stock Photo; 142: Martyn Vickery/Alamy Stock Photo; 143: Alibi Productions/Alamy Stock Photo; 144: Janine Wiedel Photolibrary/Alamy Stock Photo; 145: Reuters/Alamy Stock Photo; 147: Manchan/Photographer's Choice RF/Getty Images; 148: Jupiterimages/Stockbyte/Getty Images

Chapter 7 151: Zoonar/Alexander Savchuk/Alamy Stock Photo; 154: Steve Gorton/Dorling Kindersley, Ltd.; 155: Willfried Gredler/Insadco Photography/Alamy Stock Photo; 157: Getty Images; 158: Martin M. Rotker/Science Source; 158: Martin M. Rotker/Science Source; 159: Dennis MacDonald/age fotostock/Alamy Stock Photo; 160: Joerg Lange/Vario Images/GmbH & Co.KG/Alamy Stock Photo; 161: Brent Hofacker/Fotolia; 162: Phanie/Super Stock; 165: Helen H. Richardson/Denver Post/Getty Images; 166: Oral Health America; 167: Pavlo Vakhrushev/Fotolia; 168: TPH special/AllOver images/Alamy Stock Photo; 169: American Cancer Society/Getty Images; 170: IS-200510/Image Source/Alamy Stock Photo; 171: Robert J. Beyers II/Shutterstock; 173: Comstock Images/Stockbyte/Getty Images

Chapter 8 177: Solis Images/Shutterstock; 178: Webphotographeer/iStock/Getty Images; 179: Spaxiax/Fotolia; 179: Chris Bence/Shutterstock; 179: Westmacott/Shutterstock; 179: Stargazer/Shutterstock; 179: Hurst Photo/Shutterstock; 180: George Muresan/Shutterstock; 181: Pearson Education, Inc.; 182: Mike Flippo/Shutterstock; 185: CSP_dmitrimaruta/AGE Fotostock; 186: Markus Mainka/123RF; 186: Antonov Roman/Shutterstock; 187: Ivaschenko Roman/Shutterstock; 187: Hal_P/Shutterstock; 187: V_blinov/Fotolia; 187: C Squared Studios/Photodisc/Getty Images; 188: Peter Zijlstra/Shutterstock; 188: Bluefern/Fotolia; 188: Martin Darley/Shutterstock; 189: PrzemysÅaw Ceynowa/123RF; 189: Vrozhko/123RF; 189: Thomas M Perkins/Shutterstock; 189: Stephen Mcsweeny/123RF; 190: Matka_Wariatka/iStock/Getty Images; 193: Voyagerix/Fotolis; 193: Pearson Education, Inc.; 195: Lopolo/Shutterstock; 196: Brian Hagiwara/Photolibrary/Getty Images; 197: ML Harris/Iconica/Getty Images; 199: MorePixels/iStock/Getty Images; 200: Vladimir Voronin/Fotolia

Chapter 9 203: David Buffington/Blend Images/Getty Images; 205: Big Cheese Photo LLC/Alamy Stock Photo; 206: ESB Professional/Shutterstock; 207: Timquo/Shutterstock; 207: Nitr/Shutterstock; 207: Mike Flippo/Shutterstock; 207: Davydenko Yuliia/Shutterstock; 208: Dennis MacDonald/Alamy Stock Photo; 211: David Madison/Photographer's Choice/Getty Images; 211: May/Science Source; 211: Phanie/Science Source; 211: Courtesy of COSMED USA, Inc; 211: Jamie Grill/Blend Images - JGI/Brand X Pictures/Getty Images; 211: Marcin Ciesielski/Sylwia Cisek/Alamy Stock Photo; 213: David C. Rehner/Shutterstock; 214: Luis Louro/Shutterstock; 215: Asia Images Group Pte Ltd/Alamy Stock Photo; 216: Byron Purvis/AdMedia/Newscom; 217: Howard Shooter/Dorling Kindersley, Ltd.; 218: Sakala/Shutterstock; 218: Custom Medical Stock Photo/Alamy Stock Photo; 220: Brand X Pictures/Stockbyte/Getty Images; 220: Gollykim/Getty Images; 221: Vladimirfloyd/Fotolia; 222: Barry Gregg/keepsake/Corbis; 223: Nico Blue/Vetta/Getty Images; 223: Photodisc/Getty Images

Chapter 10 225: Begalphoto/Shutterstock; 227: Pearson Education, Inc.; 227: Teo Lannie/PhotoAlto Agency RF Collections/Getty Images; 227: Photodisc/Getty Images; 227: Toxawww/iStock/Getty Images; 227: Graham Mitchell/Exactostock-1598/Superstock; 229: Georgijevic/Getty Images; 231: Rolf Adlercreutz/Alamy Stock Photo; 232: Bob Jacobson/Corbis/Getty images; 232: Walter Cruz/MCT/Newscom; 232: Cveltri/iStock/Getty Images; 232: PaulMaguire/iStock/Getty Images; 232: Kirstypargeter/iStock/Getty Images; 232: Enderbirer/iStock/Getty Images; 232: Gvictoria/Shutterstock; 232: Rod Ferris/Shutterstock; 232: DeymosHR/Shutterstock; 232: Ali Ender Birer/Shutterstock; 232: Stephen VanHorn/Alamy Stock Photo; 233: Dan Dalton/DigitalVision/Getty Images; 233: MIXA/Getty Images; 233: Daniel Grill/Alamy Stock Photo; 234: Pearson Education, Inc.; 234: Karl Weatherly/Photodisc/Getty Images; 235: Andrey Arkusha/Shutterstock; 236: Wavebreakmedia/Getty Images; 237: Pearson Education, Inc.; 237: Pearson Education, Inc.; 237: Blue Jean Images/Alamy Stock Photo; 238: Pearson Education, Inc.; 238: Pearson Education, Inc.; 238: Pearson Education, Inc.; 238: Pearson Education, Inc.; 238: Pearson Education, Inc.; 240: Nesharm/iStock/Getty Images; 241: Mark Cowan/UPI/Newscom; 242: Dmitry Morgan/Shutterstock; 242: Ludmila Smite/Fotolia; 244: Robert Babczynski/Shutterstock; 244: Chanchai Plongern/Shutterstock; 245: Dennis Welsh/UpperCut Images RF/AGE Fotostock; 246: Image Source/Stockbyte/Getty Images; 247: Shutterstock

Chapter 11 249: Sirtravelalot/Shutterstock; 252: Irina Iglina/123RF; 257: Radius Images/Alamy Stock Photo; 259: Jupiterimages/Stockbyte/Getty Images; 261: Levent Konuk/Shutterstock; 264: Stefano Giambra/123RF; 265: DawnPoland/E+/Getty Images; 266: Dnberty/iStock/Getty Images; 267: AfriPics/Alamy Stock Photo; 269: Tyler Olson/Shutterstock; 269: ZUMA Press Inc/Alamy Stock Photo; 271: James Stevenson/Science Source; 271: Dr P. Marazzi/Science Source; 271: Dr P. Marazzi/Science Source; 273: Dragon Images/Shutterstock; 274: Javier Larrea/Age Fotostock/Alamy Stock Photo; 276: Kamdyn R Switzer/Cal Sport Media/Newscom; 279: Paul Parker/Science Source; 279: BSIP SA/Alamy Stock Photo; 281: Dalaprod/Fotolia

Chapter 12 288: Photo Researchers/Science History Images/Alamy Stock Photo; 283: Eggeegg/Shutterstock; 284: Cathy Yeulet/123RF; 287: Paolese/Fotolia; 288: Dr. Gary Gaugler/Science Source; 288: Dr. Linda M. Stannard/University of Cape Town/Science Source; 288: Steve Gschmeissner/Science Source; 288: Eye of Science/Science Source; 288: Mediscan/Alamy Stock Photo; 289: Lezh/Getty Images; 291: Ricardo Funari/BrazilPhotos/Alamy Stock Photo; 291: Dan Wozniak/Southcreek Global/ZUMAPRESS/Alamy Stock Photo; 293: Lexx72/Fotolia; 294: Antagain/E+/Getty Images; 295: Nycshooter/E+/Getty Images; 296: Nyul/123RF; 297: Peter Bernik/Shutterstock; 299: Kevin Foy/Alamy Stock Photo; 300: Western Ophthalmic Hospital/Science Source; 301: Centers for Disease Control and Prevention (CDC); 302: SPL/Science Source; 303: Mediscan/Alamy Stock Photo; 304: Dr P. Marazzi/Science Source; 305: Eye of Science/Science Source

Chapter 13 307: Phovoir/Shutterstock; 308: Jochen Tack/Alamy Stock Photo; 309: Jochen Tack/imageBroker/Newscom; 310: Dean Millar/Getty Images; 311: Ryan Rodrick Beiler/Shutterstock; 311: Africa Studio/Shutterstock; 312: Janine Wiedel Photolibrary/Alamy Stock Photo; 314: Jason Malmont/The Sentinel/AP Images; 315: Bill Aron/PhotoEdit; 316: Iakov Filimonov/123RF; 317: Anthony Dunn/Alamy Stock Photo; 318: Tariq Zehawi/KRT/Newscom; 320: A. Ramey/PhotoEdit; 322: Adrin Shamsudin/Fotolia; 323: Paul Conklin/PhotoEdit; 324: Pearson Education, Inc.; 324: Pearson Education, Inc.; 324: Pearson Education, Inc.; 325: Erik Isakson/Getty Images; 327: Image Source/Alamy Stock Photo; 328: Science Photo Library/Getty images; 328: Science Photo Library/Getty images

Chapter 14 331: Majeczka/Shutterstock; 333: Brianindia/Alamy Stock Photo; 334: Anticiclo/Shutterstock; 335: Justin Sullivan/Getty Images; 336: Steve Froebe/iStock/Getty Images; 337: Moodboard/Alamy Stock Photo; 338: Dave King/Dorling Kindersley, Ltd.; 341: Qaphotos/Alamy Stock Photo; 343: Alterfalter/Shutterstock; 344: John Henley/Blend Images/

Text Credit

Chapter 1   2: Source: World Health Organization (WHO), "Constitution of the World Health Organization," Chronicles of the World Health Organization (Geneva: WHO, 1947), Available at www.who.int/governance/eb/constitution/en/index.html.; 3: Source: R. Dubos, So Human an Animal: How We Are Shaped by Surroundings and Events (New York: Scribner, 1968), 15.

Chapter 2   31: Source: K. Huffman and C. A. Sanderson, Real World Psychology (Hoboken, NJ: Wiley, 2014).; 33: Source: DanahZohar.com, "Learn the Qs," Accessed January 2014, http://dzohar.com/?page_id=622.; 34: "Source: Based on National Cancer Institute (NCI), "Spirituality in Cancer Care," November 2012, http://www.cancer.gov/cancertopics/pdq/supportivecare/spirituality/HealthProfessional/page1.; 39: "Source: Based on National Institute of Mental Health, "Anxiety Disorders," March 2016 https://www.nimh.nih.gov/health/topics/anxiety-disorders/index.shtml; 42: Source: American Psychiatric Association, Diagnostic and Statistical Manual of Mental Disorders, (DSM-5). 5th ed. (Washington, DC: American Psychiatric Association, 2013).; 44: Source: Based on American Foundation for Suicide Prevention, "Warning Signs of Suicide," Accessed February 2014, http://www.afsp.org/preventing-suicide/risk-factors-and-warning-signs.; 44: Source: Based on American Foundation for Suicide Prevention, "Warning Signs of Suicide," Accessed February 2014, http://www.afsp.org/preventing-suicide/risk-factors-and-warning-signs.

Chapter 3   50: Source: Data from American College Health Association (ACHA), American College Health Association–National College Health Assessment II (ACHA-NCHA II): Reference Group Data Report Spring, 2013 (Baltimore: American College Health Association, 2014.; 64: Source: Based on B. L. Seaward, Managing Stress: Principles and Strategies for Health and Well-Being. 7th ed. (New York: Barnes and Noble, 2012).

Chapter 4   80: Source: J. Wood, Interpersonal Communication: Everyday Encounters, 8th ed. (Boston, MA: Woodsworth Publishing, 2015).; 85: Source: The Gottman Institute, "Research FAQs," Accessed February 3, 2017, https://www.gottman.com/about/research/faq/.; 92: Source: F. Kelly, Sexuality Today, 11th ed. (New York: McGraw-Hill, 2014).

Chapter 5   114: Roe v. Wade, 410 U.S. 113 (1973).

Chapter 6   141: Source: Substance Abuse and Mental Health Services Administration, Results from the 2012 National Survey on Drug Use and Health: Summary of National Findings, NSDUH Series H-44, HHS Publication No. (SMA) 12-4713. Rockville, MD: Substance Abuse and Mental Health Services Administration, 2013.

Chapter 8   182: Sources: T. Huang et al., "Consumption of Whole Grains and Cereal Fiber and Total and Cause-Specific Mortality: Prospective Analysis of 367,442 Individuals," BMC Medicine 13, no. 1 (2015): 59; Scientific Report of the 2015 Dietary Guidelines Advisory Committee, "Advisory Report to the Secretary of Health and Human Services and the Secretary of Agriculture," 2015, Available at: http://health.gov/dietaryguidelines/2015-scientific-report.; 200: Source: Based on Centers for Disease Control and Prevention, CDC Estimates of Foodborne Illness in the United States, CDC 2011 Estimates: Findings, Updated January 8, 2014, from www.cdc.gov/foodborneburden/2011-foodborne-estimates.html; 201: Partnership for Food Safety Education, 2017, http://www.fightbac.org/free-resources/logos-and-graphics/

Chapter 9   214: Sources: Opinions on diet pros xand cons are based on U.S. News & World Report, "Best Diets Overall," 2017, http://health.usnews.com/best-diet/best-overall-diets?int=9c2508. Dietary reviews, particularly of fad diets, are available online from registered dieticians at the Academy of Nutrition and Dietetics, 2016; B. Johnson et al., "Comparisons of Weight Loss among Diet Programs in Overweight and Obese Adults: A Meta-analysis," Journal of the American Medical Association 312, no. 9 (2014): 923–33.; 219: Body Image Health, "The Model for Healthy Body Image and Weight," Accessed February 2016, http://bodyimagehealth.org/model-for-healthy-body-image.; 219: "10 Steps to Positive Body Image" from National Eating Disorders Association website, Accessed February 13, 2016. National Eating Disorders Association. Reprinted with permission. For more information, visit www.NationalEatingDisorders.org or call NEDA's helpline at 1-800-931-2237; 221: National Eating Disorders Association, "Anorexia Nervosa," Accessed February 2017, www.nationaleatingdisorders.org/anorexia-nervosa.

Chapter 10   234: Based on data from the American Heart Association

Chapter 11   254: Adapted from American Heart Association, "Warning Signs of Heart Attack, Stroke, and Cardiac Arrest," 2016, www.heart.org/HEARTORG/Conditions/911-Warnings-Signs-of-a-Heart-Attack_UCM_305346_SubHomePage.jsp.

Chapter 12   298-299: FDA, "Think Before You Ink: Are Tattoos Safe?" May 2017, https://www.fda.gov/ForConsumers/ConsumerUpdates/ucm048919.htm.; 302: CDC, "CDC Fact Sheet: Gonorrhea (Detailed)," May 19, 2016. http://www.cdc.gov/std/gonorrhea/stdfact-gonorrhea.htm.

Chapter 13   307: World Health Organization (WHO), Global Status Report on Violence Prevention (Geneva: World Health Organization, 2014), Available at www.undp.org/content/dam/undp/library/corporate/Reports/UNDP-GVA-violence-2014.pdf.; 307: Centers for Disease Control and Prevention, "Ten Leading Causes of Death by Age Group, United States, 2014," Accessed March 2017, Available at https://www.cdc.gov/injury/wisqars/pdf/leading_causes_of_death_by_age_group_2014-a.pdf; 315: SB-967, "Student Safety: Sexual Assault," 2013–2014, https://leginfo.legislature.ca.gov/faces/billNavClient.xhtml?bill_id=201320140SB967; 316: Oregon State University, Sexual Harassment and Sexual Violence, Accessed June 2016, http://eoa.oregonstate.edu/sexual-harassment-and-violence-policy; 317: U.S. Code of Federal Regulations, Title 28CFR0.85; 320: Adapted from E. Allan and M. Madden, Hazing in View: College Students at Risk (Orono, ME: National Collaborative for Hazing Research and Prevention, 2008), www.hazingstudy.org, Reprinted by permission of Elizabeth Allan. Emory Law Journal. "Am I My Brother's Keeper? Reforming Criminal Hazing Laws Based on Assumption of Care." 2014. http://www.law.emory.edu/fileadmin/journals/elj/63/63.4/Chamberlin.pdf; 323: National Highway Traffic Safety Administration, "Aggressive Driving," www.nhtsa.gov/Aggressive; 325: American Boating Association, "Boating Safety—It Could Mean Your Life," 2013, www.americanboating.org/safety.asp.; 327: American Association of Poison Control Centers, "Prevention," February 2015, www.aapcc.org/prevention; 329: Mayo Clinic, "Carpal Tunnel Syndrome: Prevention," 2014, www.mayoclinic.org/diseases-conditions/carpal-tunnel-syndrome/basics/prevention/con-20030332

Chapter 14   346: Thich Nhat Hanh, "The World We Have," Lion's Roar: Buddhist Wisdom for Our Time, April 6, 2017, https://www.lionsroar.com/the-world-we-have/

Chapter 15   352: NIH, U.S. National Library of Medicine-. "Patient's rights." Medline Plus. July, 2017. https://medlineplus.gov/patientrights.html.; 354: U.S. Food and Drug Administration, "The Possible Dangers of Buying Medicine over the Internet," May, 2017. https://www.fda.gov/ForConsumers/ConsumerUpdates/ucm048396.htm; 362: Used with permission of The United States Pharmacopeial Convention, 12601 Twinbrook Parkway, Rockville, MD 20851.; 365: MedlinePlus, "Managed Care," January 2016, https://www.nlm.nih.gov/medlineplus/managedcare.html.

Index

Index

Web Links for Health and Wellness

Chapter 1 Healthy Change

- **CDC Wonder.** A clearinghouse for information from the Centers for Disease Control and Prevention. http://wonder.cdc.gov

- **Mayo Clinic.** A reputable resource for information about health topics, diseases, and treatment options. www.mayoclinic.org

- **National Center for Health Statistics.** Information about health status in the United States, including key reports and national survey information. www.cdc.gov/nchs

- **healthfinder.gov.** A resource for consumer information about health. www.healthfinder.gov

- **World Health Organization.** A resource on global health; provides information on illness and disease statistics, trends, and outbreak alerts. www.who.int/en

Chapter 2 Psychological Health

- **American Foundation for Suicide Prevention.** Resources for suicide prevention; support for family and friends of those who have committed suicide. www.afsp.org

- **American Psychological Association Help Center.** Information on psychology at work, the mind-body connection, psychological responses to war, and other topics. www.apa.org/helpcenter

- **National Alliance on Mental Illness.** Support and advocacy for families and friends of people with severe mental illnesses. www.nami.org

- **National Institute of Mental Health (NIMH).** An overview of mental health information and research. www.nimh.nih.gov

- **Helpguide.** Resources for improving mental and emotional health, plus information on topics such as self-injury, sleep, depressive disorders, and anxiety disorders. www.helpguide.org

- **National Suicide Prevention Lifeline.** Help 24 hours a day for people in crisis via online chat, text, or phone. www.suicidepreventionlifeline.org or 1-800-273-8255.

Chapter 3 Stress

- **American College Health Association.** This site provides information and data from the National College Health Assessment survey. www.acha.org

- **Higher Education Research Institute.** This organization provides annual surveys of first-year and senior college students that cover academic, financial, and health-related issues. www.heri.ucla.edu

- **American College Counseling Association.** The website of the professional organization for college counselors offers useful links and articles. www.collegecounseling.org

Chapter 4 Relationships and Sexuality

- **American Association of Sexuality Educators, Counselors, and Therapists (AASECT).** Professional organization providing standards of practice for treating sexual issues and disorders. www.aasect.org

- **Go Ask Alice!** An interactive question-and-answer resource from the Columbia University Health Services. www.goaskalice.columbia.edu

- **Sexuality Information and Education Council of the United States (SIECUS).** Information, guidelines, and materials for advancement of healthy and proper sex education. www.siecus.org

- **The Human Rights Campaign.** Advocacy and resources about LGBT issues by the largest civil rights organization for lesbian, gay, bisexual, and transgender Americans. www.hrc.org

- **Advocates for Youth.** Current news, policy updates, research, and other resources about the sexual health of and choices particular to high school and college-aged students. www.advocatesforyouth.org

Chapter 5 Reproductive Choices

- **Guttmacher Institute.** This nonprofit organization is focused on sexual and reproductive health research, policy analysis, and public education. www.guttmacher.org

- **Association of Reproductive Health Professionals.** This independent organization, originally the educational arm of Planned Parenthood, provides education for health care professionals and the general public. It includes an interactive tool to help you choose a birth control method that will work for you. www.arhp.org

- **The American Pregnancy Association.** A wealth of resources to promote reproductive and pregnancy wellness. www.americanpregnancy.org

- **Planned Parenthood.** A range of up-to-date information on issues such as birth control, the decision of when and whether to have a child, STIs, and safer sex. www.plannedparenthood.org

Chapter 6 Addiction and Drug Abuse

- **National Council on Problem Gambling.** Information and help for people with gambling problems and their families. www.ncpgambling.org

- **National Institute on Drug Abuse (NIDA).** Information on the latest statistics and findings in drug research. www.drugabuse.gov

- **Substance Abuse and Mental Health Services Administration (SAMHSA).** An outstanding resource for information about national surveys, ongoing research, and national drug interventions. www.samhsa.gov

Chapter 7 Alcohol and Tobacco

- **Alcoholics Anonymous (AA).** General information about AA and the 12-step program. www.aa.org
- **College Drinking: Changing the Culture.** This resource center targets the student population as a whole, the college and its surrounding environment, and the individual at risk or alcohol-dependent drinker. www.collegedrinkingprevention.gov
- **American Lung Association.** Information on smoking trends, environmental smoke, and smoking cessation. www.lung.org
- **Action on Smoking and Health (ASH).** ASH takes legal actions and does other work to fight smoking and protect nonsmokers' rights. www.ash.org

Chapter 8 Nutrition

- **Academy of Nutrition and Dietetics.** Provides information on a range of dietary topics, including sports nutrition, healthful cooking, and nutritional eating. www.eatright.org
- **U.S. Food and Drug Administration (FDA).** The FDA provides information for consumers and professionals in the areas of food safety, supplements, and medical devices. www.fda.gov
- **Food and Nutrition Information Center.** This site offers a wide variety of information related to food and nutrition. www.nal.usda.gov/fnic
- **U.S. Department of Agriculture (USDA).** The USDA offers a full discussion of the USDA's Dietary Guidelines for Americans. www.usda.gov

Chapter 9 Weight Management and Body Image

- **ChooseMyPlate.gov.** USDA's ChooseMyPlate.gov offers extensive information about meal planning and physical activity for healthy living. www.choosemyplate.gov
- **The Rudd Center for Food Policy and Obesity.** The latest in obesity research, public policy, and ways to stop obesity at the community level. www.yaleruddcenter.org
- **National Eating Disorders Association.** Information for eating disorder sufferers and those wishing to help others with eating and body image issues. www.nationaleatingdisorders.org

Chapter 10 Fitness

- **ACSM Online.** The American College of Sports Medicine and all its resources. www.acsm.org
- **American Council on Exercise.** Information on exercise and disease prevention. www.acefitness.org

Chapter 11 CVD, Cancer, and Diabetes

- **American Heart Association.** Information, statistics, and resources regarding cardiovascular care, including an opportunity to test your risk for CVD. www.heart.org
- **American Cancer Society.** Information, statistics, and resources regarding cancer. www.cancer.org
- **American Diabetes Association.** Information and resources for those with diabetes. www.diabetes.org

Chapter 12 Infectious Conditions

- **American Sexual Health Association.** This site provides facts, support, resources, and referrals about sexually transmitted infections and diseases. www.ashastd.org
- **AVERT.** An international site with information on HIV/AIDS, global STI statistics, interactive quizzes, and graphics displaying current statistics for vulnerable populations. www.avert.org
- **San Francisco AIDS Foundation.** This community-based AIDS service organization focuses on ending the HIV/AIDS pandemic through education, patient services, advocacy, and global programs. www.sfaf.org

Chapter 13 Violence and Unintentional Injuries

- **National Center for Injury and Violence Prevention and Control.** Statistics and information on fatal and nonfatal injuries, both intentional and unintentional. www.cdc.gov/injury
- **National Center for Victims of Crime.** Resources for victims of crimes ranging from hate crimes to sexual assault. www.ncvc.org
- **National Sexual Violence Resource Center.** An excellent resource for victims of sexual violence. www.nsvrc.org
- **Men Can Stop Rape.** Practical suggestions and training for men interested in helping to protect women from sexual predators and assault. www.mencanstoprape.org
- **National Institute for Occupational Safety and Health (NIOSH).** Data and resources on a range of workplace safety issues. www.cdc.gov/workplace

Chapter 14 Environmental Health

- **Environmental Protection Agency (EPA).** The government agency responsible for overseeing environmental regulation and protection issues in the United States. www.epa.gov
- **National Center for Environmental Health (NCEH).** Information on a wide variety of environmental health issues; includes a series of helpful fact sheets. www.cdc.gov/nceh
- **National Environmental Health Association (NEHA).** Educational resources and opportunities for environmental health professionals. www.neha.org

Chapter 15 Consumerism and Complementary and Integrative Health Care Choices

- **Agency for Healthcare Research and Quality (AHRQ).** Links to sites that address health care concerns and provide information on making critical decisions about personal care. www.ahrq.gov
- **National Committee for Quality Assurance (NCQA).** Assessments and reports on managed care plans, including HMOs. www.ncqa.org
- **HealthCare.Gov.** Information regarding the Patient Protection and Affordable Care Act. www.healthcare.gov
- **National Center for Complementary and Integrative Health (NCCIH).** Information and research on complementary and integrative practices. www.nccih.nih.gov